Cancer and
Nutrition

Human Nutrition
A COMPREHENSIVE TREATISE

General Editors:
Roslyn B. Alfin-Slater, University of California, Los Angeles
David Kritchevsky, The Wistar Institute, Philadelphia

A Continuation Order Plan is available for this series. A continuation order will bring delivery of
each new volume immediately upon publication. Volumes are billed only upon actual shipment.
For further information please contact the publisher.

Cancer and Nutrition

Edited by

Roslyn B. Alfin-Slater
Schools of Public Health and Medicine
University of California, Los Angeles
Los Angeles, California

and

David Kritchevsky
The Wistar Institute
Philadelphia, Pennsylvania

PLENUM PRESS • NEW YORK AND LONDON

Library of Congress Cataloging-in-Publication Data

Cancer and nutrition / edited by Roslyn B. Alfin-Slater and David
  Kritchevsky.
       p.   cm. -- (Human nutrition ; v. 7)
    Includes bibliographical references.
    Includes index.
    ISBN 0-306-43425-3
    1. Cancer--Nutritional aspects.   I. Alfin-Slater, Roslyn, 1916-
  II. Kritchevsky, David, 1920-   . III. Series.
    [DNLM: 1. Diet--adverse effects. 2. Neoplasms--diet therapy.
  3. Neoplasms--etiology.   QU 145 H9183 1979 v. 7]
  QP141.A.H84 vol. 7
  [RC268.45]
  612'.3 s--dc20
  [616.99'4071]
  DNLM/DLC
  for Library of Congress   90-14318
                                                                     CIP

ISBN 0-306-43425-3

© 1991 Plenum Press, New York
A Division of Plenum Publishing Corporation
233 Spring Street, New York, N.Y. 10013

Printed in the United States of America

Contributors

Gabriele Angres • Institute of Toxicology and Chemotherapy, German Cancer Research Center, D-6900 Heidelberg, Federal Republic of Germany

Maren Beth • Institute of Toxicology and Chemotherapy, German Cancer Research Center, D-6900 Heidelberg, Federal Republic of Germany

Diane F. Birt • Eppley Institute for Research in Cancer and Allied Diseases, and Department of Biochemistry, University of Nebraska Medical Center, Omaha, Nebraska 68105

Edward Bresnick • Department of Pharmacology and Toxicology, Dartmouth Medical School, Hanover, New Hampshire 03756

Antonio C. L. Campos • Surgical Metabolism and Nutrition Laboratory, Department of Surgery, University Hospital, Syracuse, New York 13210

Kenneth K. Carroll • Department of Biochemistry, The University of Western Ontario Health Sciences Centre, London, Ontario, Canada N6A 5C1

Steven K. Clinton • The Dana-Farber Cancer Institute and Harvard Medical School, Boston, Massachusetts 02115

Graham A. Colditz • Channing Laboratory, Department of Medicine, Brigham and Women's Hospital and Harvard Medical School, and Department of Epidemiology, Harvard School of Public Health, Boston, Massachusetts 02115

Michael W. Conner • Department of Pathology, Boston University School of Medicine, Boston, Massachusetts 02118; *present address:* Merck, Sharp and Dohme, West Point, Pennsylvania, 19486

Ann T. Foltz • Departments of Biochemistry and Medicine, Emory University School of Medicine, Atlanta, Georgia 30322

John Higginson • Georgetown University Medical Center, Washington, D.C. 20007

David M. Klurfeld • The Wistar Institute of Anatomy and Biology, Philadelphia, Pennsylvania 19104

David Kritchevsky • The Wistar Institute of Anatomy and Biology, Philadelphia, Pennsylvania 19104

Donald B. McCormick • Departments of Biochemistry and Medicine, Emory University School of Medicine, Atlanta, Georgia 30322

Anthony John McMichael • Department of Community Medicine, University of Adelaide, South Australia 5000

Michael M. Meguid • Surgical Metabolism and Nutrition Laboratory, Department of Surgery, University Hospital, Syracuse, New York 13210

Alfred H. Merrill, Jr. • Departments of Biochemistry and Medicine, Emory University School of Medicine, Atlanta, Georgia 30322

Paul M. Newberne • Department of Pathology, Boston University School of Medicine, Boston, Massachusetts 02118

Adrianne E. Rogers • Department of Pathology, Boston University School of Medicine, Boston, Massachusetts 02118

Bruce Ruggeri • Department of Pathology, The Fox Chase Cancer Center, Philadelphia, Pennsylvania 19117

Michael J. Sheridan • Georgetown University Medical Center, Washington, D.C. 20007

Willard J. Visek • Division of Nutritional Sciences, Department of Internal Medicine, College of Medicine, University of Illinois, Urbana, Illinois 61801

Dan L. Waitzberg • Surgical Metabolism and Nutrition Laboratory, Department of Surgery, University Hospital, Syracuse, New York 13210

Walter C. Willett • Channing Laboratory, Department of Medicine, Brigham and Women's Hospital and Harvard Medical School, and Department of Epidemiology, Harvard School of Public Health, Boston, Massachusetts 02115

Preface

The role of nutrition in neoplasia has been of longstanding concern. The subject was addressed by investigators in the first decade of this century, but was dropped. Vigorous attention was paid to this area of oncology in the 1940s, primarily due to the efforts of Dr. A. Tannenbaum at the Michael Reese Hospital in Chicago and the group at the University of Wisconsin in Madison. However, interest waned again until the 1970s when the question of diet and cancer was addressed and it has since been at the forefront of cancer research.

The present volume (7) of *Human Nutrition: A Comprehensive Treatise* summarizes current knowledge in the area of nutrition and cancer. The first chapter is an overview written by John Higginson, whose contribution to understanding of cancer and nutrition spans several decades. The next essays cover epidemiology and physiology. The ensuing chapters address, in turn, those dietary factors relating to nutrition and cancer, namely, carbohydrates, protein, fat, cholesterol, calories, lipotropics, fiber, fruits and vegetables, vitamins, and alcohol. In a field moving as rapidly as this one is now, we can expect to miss a few late-breaking developments, but generally, the literature has been well covered through some time in 1988. Work relating to the effects of diet on oncogenes is in its very early development and has not been addressed as an entity per se. If this volume should help to review the field for some investigators and to stimulate research efforts in others, it has served its purpose.

David Kritchevsky
Roslyn B. Alfin-Slater

Contents

Chapter 2

Epidemiologic Approaches to the Study of Diet and Cancer

Graham A. Colditz and Walter C. Willett

Chapter 3

*A Comparison of the Changes in Carbohydrate, Fat, and Protein
Metabolism Occurring with Malignant and Benign Tumors and the
Impact of Nutritional Support*

Antonio C. L. Campos, Dan L. Waitzberg, and Michael M. Meguid

Chapter 4
Carbohydrate and Cancer
Kenneth K. Carroll

Chapter 5
Dietary Protein and Cancer
Willard J. Visek and Steven K. Clinton

Chapter 6
Fat and Cancer
David Kritchevsky and David M. Klurfeld

Chapter 7
Serum Cholesterol and Human Cancer
Anthony John McMichael

Chapter 8
Lipotropic Factors and Carcinogenesis
Paul M. Newberne and Adrianne E. Rogers

Chapter 9
The Effects of Caloric Restriction on Neoplasia and Age-Related Degenerative Processes
Bruce Ruggeri

Chapter 10

Dietary Fiber and Cancer

David Kritchevsky and David M. Klurfeld

Chapter 11

Chemoprevention by Nonnutrient Components of Vegetables and Fruits

Diane F. Birt and Edward Bresnick

Chapter 12

Vitamins and Cancer

Alfred H. Merrill, Jr., Ann T. Foltz, and Donald B. McCormick

Chapter 13

Interrelationships of Alcohol and Cancer

Adrianne E. Rogers and Michael W. Conner

Appendix

Effects of Dietary Constituents on Carcinogenesis in Different Tumor Models: An Overview from 1975 to 1988

Gabriele Angres and Maren Beth

Nutrition and Human Cancer

John Higginson and Michael J. Sheridan

1. Introduction

The role of diet in human carcinogenesis began to receive serious attention in the early twentieth century, following the demonstration that a number of dyes used as food colorants were carcinogenic in animals. The potential hazard of food additives and contaminants became of general concern by the mid-1930s and motivated much of the deliberations of the joint World Health Organization/Food and Agricultural Organization (WHO/FAO) Committee on food additives and pesticides in the postwar period (1958). This concern in the United States culminated in the 1958 passage of Public Law 85-929, known as the Delaney Amendment. Nonetheless, with the possible exception of aflatoxin, no animal carcinogen in food has been unequivocally demonstrated to produce cancer in humans following ingestion. Thus, despite their number, and after intensive examination, it has been concluded by the National Academy of Sciences (NAS) that food additives and contaminants do not account for a significant number of human cancers (1982). However, interpretation of data from animal studies on carcinogens in the diet remains of great importance for regulatory policies at both the national and international level.

The possibility that diet could *indirectly* modify cancer induction arose in the 1930s when it was observed that riboflavin deficiency enhanced liver cancer induction by *p*-dimethylaminoazobenzene. Later work by Tannenbaum and Silverstone on such macronutrients as fat, protein, carbohydrates, and caloric intake in rodent cancer delineated their important role in the genesis of many experimental cancers. Thus, excessive calories and fats enhanced, but undernutrition inhibited, carcinogenesis. For many years the view persisted that malnutrition, e.g., kwashiorkor (protein–calorie deficiency), was a major enhancing factor in human liver cancer (Higginson, 1956). Today it is believed that general undernutrition probably inhibits carcinogenesis in humans, a view consistent with animal studies (Tannenbaum and Silverstone, 1957; Ross and Bras, 1965, 1973; Ross *et al.*, 1970), but there are exceptions relating to specific micronutrients, such as iron deficiency and Plummer–Vinson syndrome.

John Higginson and Michael J. Sheridan • Georgetown University Medical Center, Washington, D.C. 20007.

Early dietary studies in America (Haenszel, 1961, Wynder *et al.*, 1963; Haenszel and Dawson, 1965; Wynder and Shigematsu, 1967), Europe (Stocks, 1970), and Africa (Higginson and Oettlé, 1960) were disappointing in identifying the role of specific dietary components in several cancers suspected to be dietary related. Although fiber, excessive calories, cereals, daily produce, and heated fats, among others, were all discussed generally, the results tended to be inconclusive. However, by the late 1960s, there was evidence in parts of Africa and Asia that a dietary mycotoxin (aflatoxin) contributed significantly to liver cancer morbidity (Linsell and Peers, 1977). Moreover, as the general effect of diet began to be accepted in cardiovascular disease, it was recognized that an indirect role for diet was biologically plausible with the multistage carcinogenesis theory. Reports attributed an increasing proportion of cancers in Western societies to diet, especially cancers of the gastrointestinal tract and such endocrine-dependent tumors as those of the breast, endometrium, ovary, and prostate (Wynder and Gori, 1977; Higginson and Muir, 1979; Doll and Peto, 1981). Such views were substantiated by a very large experimental base, although the impact of individual nutrients in humans was less clear. Accordingly, belief in the possibility of primary cancer prevention by dietary manipulation also expanded in scientific and lay circles, as indicated in the report *Diet, Nutrition, and Cancer* of the National Academy of Sciences (NAS, 1982) and a series of conferences on the subject (Lowenthal, 1983; Joossens *et al.*, 1985).

1.1. NAS Reports (1980 and 1982)

In view of its importance in influencing recent thinking on dietary carcinogenesis, the 1982 NAS report is worth considering. This report was written by a distinguished committee and provided the most complete compilation of the literature available on diet and cancer, as well as an introduction to current hypotheses of carcinogensis and their dietary implications. In commenting on the report, the National Academy strongly emphasized the role of diet in human cancer and made a number of definitive suggestions as to the benefits to be anticipated from specific changes in American eating habits. These relatively strong recommendations were to some extent inconsistent with the last paragraph of the 1982 report, which stated:

> The evidence reviewed by the committee suggests that cancers of most major sites are influenced by dietary patterns. However, the committee concluded that the data are not sufficient to quantitate the contribution of diet to the overall cancer risk or to determine the percent reduction in risk that might be achieved by dietary modifications. (Ch. 18, pp. 18–11)

This latter view did not significantly differ from that expressed in a 1980 report prepared by the Academy entitled *Toward Healthful Diets,* which concluded the data available were largely insufficient to make concrete recommendations on diet and cancer (NAS, 1980). *Toward Healthful Diets* was prepared by an equally distinguished panel with some differences in disciplinary backgrounds and experience. The differences and degree of emphasis between the two reports have caused considerable confusion among the public and controversy in the scientific community, which persists and reflects the scientific uncertainties still prevalent in the field.

The present reviewers, while convinced of the role of diet in human carcinogenesis, do not believe that the data published between the 1980 and the 1982 NAS reports were sufficient to justify differing scientific evaluations. Rather, the conclusions reflected different subjective judgments on how strongly the public should be advised. The 1980 report may have been unduly conservative as to the role of diet, whereas the 1982 report reflected a more positive viewpoint. Developments in scientific thinking on the importance of dietary carcinogenesis may also partly explain the difference in the two approaches (Higginson, 1982). This chapter will not attempt to review the extensive literature on diet and cancer, which is readily available in the 1982 NAS report. Rather it will attempt to briefly summarize the salient facts as seen by us and outline the conceptual issues involved. The enormous literature on experimental and domesticated animals will not be discussed except where pertinent.

1.2. Methodological Issues in Evaluating the Role of Diet in Human Cancer

The average diet contains a large number of chemicals with a wide and sometimes contradictory range of biological activities, as well as both macronutrients and micronutrients. Since carcinogenesis is a multistage process, dietary factors can be considered in two broad categories according to their potential mode of action: those that are initiators or complete carcinogens and those that indirectly modulate one or more stages of carcinogenesis. The latter group also includes dietary inhibitors as well as carcinogen activators.

In view of the numerous factors in diet and the potential complex interactions involved, there are obvious difficulties in demonstrating causal associations in epidemiological studies in humans with the same clarity as demonstrable with high exposures to individual carcinogens in the workplace. This is especially true where no component or factor can be pivotally related etiologically to a cancer. Many authors have emphasized the methodological difficulties of measuring intake of individual food components in diets consumed many years earlier (Lyon *et al.*, 1983) and the fact that the long latent period of most cancers makes causal association difficult (Zaridze *et al.*, 1985). Thus, to some extent, hypotheses and studies in humans are often dependent on ecological or laboratory data.

1.2.1. Laboratory Studies

The major recent experimental studies have been adequately referenced in the 1982 NAS report and in later conferences. In investigating chemical carcinogens, it is assumed with some reservations that animals predict qualitatively for humans, especially where there is evidence of common mechanisms. The situation is less satisfactory for diet since metabolic pathways may vary significantly both qualitatively and quantitatively from humans and between species and since multiple dietary factors and interactions may be involved. For example, rodent models of kwashiorkor or protein–calorie deficiency are unsatisfactory. While pigs or primates are preferable species, they are inconvenient for cancer studies. More important, experimental diets usually compare extreme or almost pharmacological variations in nutrient intake. These results may not be applicable to dietary effects in humans where dietary deficiencies and physiological variations usually occur within a modest range. Thus, the implications for humans of animal findings may be grossly exaggerated, especially in terms of modulation of carcinogenesis.

1.2.2. Dietary Assessment in Humans

A major limiting factor in all nutritional studies is the problem of dietary measurement. The human diet is a complex mass of nutrients and chemicals which are notoriously difficult to measure in observational studies (Lyon *et al.*, 1983; Zaridze *et al.*, 1985). Diet not only varies by season, but also from day to day and during the course of a week. Furthermore, perceived and actual dietary intake may differ significantly. Estimations of *per capita* intake are unlikely to be satisfactory for small-scale intergroup correlation studies where geographical dietary patterns may be so different as to make comparisons meaningless. Thus, there seems little point in drawing specific conclusions from comparisons of the diet of the South African Bantu and Western diets, as they do not permit evaluation of individual dietary components or very specific conclusions about food patterns. On the other hand, they may suggest inferences as to the overall impact of a dietary background, i.e., kwashiorkor and a low incidence of certain endocrine-dependent tumors in adults.

Further, all evidence indicates that most cancers suspected to be diet-related have a multifactorial origin. Thus, while a single factor may be examined in animals through dietary manipulation, this is rarely true in humans. Modification of one component in a diet usually is associated with a change in a second, so that an increase in calories from fat, for instance, reflects a reduced percentage of calories from other sources. This becomes important in determining dietary balance and the mechanism involved. As Zaridze *et al.* (1985) have pointed out, diet influences breast cancer risk primarily by altering the ages of menarche or menopause, both of which are risk factors in breast cancer.

1.3. Types of Epidemiological Studies Used in Nutritional Studies

The use of different epidemiological techniques has been reviewed recently by Zaridze *et al.* (1985), to whom reference should be made for more detailed discussion.

1.3.1. Correlation or Ecological Studies

In correlation studies the relationship between variables is examined at the population level. Due to the long induction period of cancer and the fact that average dietary patterns for a total population may contain enormous extremes, correlations between diet and cancer are especially difficult to evaluate (Zaridze *et al.*, 1985).

Correlation studies should be used only to generate hypotheses and not as bases for making definitive casual associations. Thomas *et al.* (1985) have reviewed the problems of multiple endpoints in ecological studies designed to generate hypotheses involving a simultaneous assessment of associations between many risk factors and disease outcomes. In such situations univariant hypothesis testing is not an appropriate basis for drawing inferences. Nonetheless, because large dietary variations often exist in countries at differing levels of development, comparisons between populations may be informative (Kolonel *et al.*, 1981a,b; Manousos *et al.*, 1983; Zaridze, 1983; Zaridze *et al.*, 1985) and should not be neglected, especially where dietary patterns are homogeneous, as in Africa and parts of Asia. In such situations case-control studies are unlikely to prove helpful. Inconsistent findings may prove valuable in refuting causal relationships or suggesting involvement of more complex mechanisms. Thus, while some reports support the role of fat in cancers of the breast, large bowel, and prostate (NAS, 1982), studies on Mormons (Enstrom, 1975a; Lyon and Sorenson, 1978), Seventh Day Adventists (Phillips and Snowden, 1983), vegetarian and nonvegetarian nuns (Kinlen, 1982), Scandinavians (IARC, 1977; Jensen *et al.*, 1982), and Japanese (Hirayama, 1985) are inconsistent and suggest that a simple causal association with fat alone is unlikely.

Studies in which individual dietary components are measured from representative samples of individuals, such as the Scandinavian studies of dietary fiber and rectal cancer (Reddy *et al.*, 1978; Jensen *et al.*, 1982), have considerable advantages over the general food disappearance data. Even in these studies significant individual variations occur and they can only provide relatively weak evidence for a causal relationship. Cross-sectional studies in which dietary characteristics are dependent on chemical endpoints, such as vitamin serum levels, also have deficiencies. Some of these problems are illustrated in the International Agency for Research on Cancer (IARC) esophageal cancer studies in Iran in trying to evaluate the relative role of nutrition and exogenous carcinogens (Day *et al.*, 1982).

A correlation between aflatoxin intake and liver cancer in Africa led to certain conclusions as to a causal relationship. Later studies on specific population samples in Taiwan showed that individuals who were hepatitis B carriers were much more susceptible to liver cancer (Beasley *et al.*, 1981). Thus, the earlier correlations were essentially meaningless as to dose responses, as these cancers almost certainly occurred only in a small segment of the population. Nevertheless, the results were regarded as sufficient to justify useful public health measures relating to the mycotoxin.

1.3.2. Case–Control Studies

Most early case–control studies on diet and cancer covered a range of foods and beverages and with a few exceptions proved disappointing. Their limitations are well known and include recent dietary modification due to the disease itself and inaccuracies in the quantification of dietary components based on recall. Where diets are relatively homogeneous, differences between controls and cancer cases may not be demonstrable. This is illustrated in the high-esophageal-cancer areas of China and Iran (Day *et al.*, 1982) where preneoplastic lesions are found in over 90% of the total population. Marked measurable differences in exposures are necessary to distinguish between cases and controls.

Zaridze *et al.* (1985) have also concluded that the inconsistent findings of many case–control studies result from dietary heterogenicity and the corresponding difficulty of relating a specific cancer to a pivotal causal factor. Case–control studies may be useful in migrant populations coming from low- to high-risk countries, such as Japanese migrants to the United States, where individuals can be classified according to their level of adoption of new dietary patterns.

1.3.3. Prospective Cohort Studies

The advantages of cohort studies in confirming strong causal associations are well recognized. The prospective approach has the advantage of examining a number of factors presumably before tumor initiation and of determining their relationship to later cancer development. The prospective approach is believed to be the most effective method to identify and evaluate biochemical markers related to diet. For example, analyses of blood, urine, feces, saliva, and hair may provide information as to the intake of certain micronutrients, such as minerals and vitamins.

If early dietary history turns out to be crucial, as believed, then prospective studies must be carried out over long periods to be meaningful. On the other hand, if the cohort is confined only to middle-aged individuals, then the impact of diet on early life, which may be fundamental, cannot be established. Attempts have been made to develop retrospective cohort studies based on previously collected material suitable for chemical analysis, such as vitamin levels in sera. These studies are also subject to limitations and often the most desirable variables are not available for study. The largest cohort follow-up studies are those of Framingham (Kannel, 1978) and of Hirayama in Japan (1981). Such studies have only begun to yield results after many years of follow-up and hindsight suggests many other variables that should have been studied. Zaridze *et al.* (1985) have suggested that ideally such studies should be set up in a number of widely separated areas simultaneously and include migrant populations that are adopting different dietary patterns. This would ensure that various racial and ethnic groups were represented and provide a variety of geographic, socioeconomic, and cultural information for consideration in determining the consistency of the findings.

Although the theoretical potential of such studies is widely accepted, they have so far been disappointing and far from adequately explored in view of the many logistic and technical problems involved and the wish to avoid expensive investigations on factors of doubtful biological significance.

1.3.4. Random Trials or Intervention Studies

The most scientifically rigorous approach is the randomized trial. This method is difficult to implement in the nutritional field since major dietary changes cannot easily be induced to order and ethical considerations require some potential benefit in human experiments. A random trial would theoretically be considered most suitable for the study of dietary factors that possibly could inhibit cancer induction, such as the addition of a particular vitamin or antioxidant to a dietary regimen. Zaridze *et al.* (1985) have suggested such trials when a particular nutrient of possible pivotal importance can be changed or modified. Such a study is limited by the low probability that a large population would follow a strictly prescribed diet. On the other hand, information may be obtainable from populations where certain dietary characteristics are adopted by individuals for religious or other reasons, for example, Seventh Day Adventist converts or migrants.

Random trials may be used to test theoretical cancer inhibitors, such as vitamin A or ascorbic acid. The result should be demonstrable within a relatively short period, theoretically, if the inhibitor affects late-stage carcinogenesis but not initiation. The only large-scale study of this type to date was carried out by the IARC in an area of China with a high incidence of esophageal cancers. After a year of dietary supplementation no decrease was observed in the prevalence of precancerous lesions of the esophagus in the test population as compared to controls (Muñoz *et al.*, 1985), but reevaluation has indicated a reduction in some dysplastic lesions.

In conclusion, the many uncertainties inherent in attempts to link individual dietary factors in humans with specific cancers explain the prevalence of conflicting opinions, since results tend to be inconsistent and causal associations weak, so that alternate explanations are possible.

2. Diet and Specific Cancers

In summarizing the relationship in humans between diet and cancer it is convenient to classify individual cancers according to their suspected relationship to nutritional factors. These include:

1. Cancers in which a defined carcinogenic agent in the diet is probable such as ethanol or aflatoxin.
2. Cancers possibly due to defined exogenous or endogenous agents related to diet, such as the formation of *N*-nitroso compounds from secondary amines and nitrite.
3. Cancers in which the role of diet is almost certainly indirect. This effect may be relatively specific, through the modification of defined carcinogen activating or deactivating enzymes in late-stage promotion by a specific dietary component, or be relatively nonspecific, as in the enhancing or inhibitory actions of calorie intake.

In this section, a number of human cancers are reviewed and current hypotheses regarding the potential role of dietary factors examined. In Section 3, the overall impact of specific dietary components is discussed in more depth.

2.1. Cancers of the Digestive System

2.1.1. Esophagus

The incidence of esophageal cancer is extremely variable, with high frequencies being found in the Middle East, in China, in Southern Africa, and in parts of South America and the Caribbean. In the same country there may be wide local differences. Certain occupations, such as barmen, military personnel, and salesmen, also show high frequencies. In Europe the incidence is relatively consistent, but in the United States there has been a slight fall of esophageal cancer among whites, but a fourfold increase in blacks over the last 50 years. Little is known of temporal traits in Africa and Asia.

2.1.1a. Ethanol-Related Esophageal Cancer. In North America and Europe case-control studies have confirmed a dose–response association between esophageal cancer and use of alcoholic beverages. The potential impact of other chemicals in such beverages has been examined, but Tuyns (1978) has shown that the correlation is predominantly with ethanol intake alone and not with type of beverage. It has been shown that the carcinogenic effect of cigarette smoking and alcoholic beverages is multiplicative in the esophagus. Since most drinkers in Tuyns's studies also indulged in cigarettes, the risk attributable to ethanol alone was somewhat difficult to measure, but substantial.

Laboratory studies on the possible carcinogenic role of ethanol in the esophagus have been negative. Some years ago ethanol was described as a promoter. Horie *et al.* (1965) have found that ethanol acts as a solvent facilitating the transport of polycyclic hydrocarbons through the esophageal mucosa. A definite toxic action has been demonstrated in the liver.

    2.1.1b. Non-Ethanol-Related Esophageal Cancer. No satisfactory explanation is available regarding the etiology of esophageal cancer in China, Southern Africa, and parts of Latin America. The extensive studies made by the IARC (Day *et al.*, 1982) in Iran uncovered more dietary deficiencies in the high-incidence area, including lower intakes of vitamins A, C, and riboflavin. However, more recent reports have suggested that dietary factors themselves are not likely to be as important as the chewing of certain opium products (Ghadirian *et al.*, 1985). In China no specific hypotheses have been formulated, but the possibilities include fungal contaminants, formation of N-nitroso compounds and dietary deficiency. High-incidence areas for esophageal cancer in both Iran and China show a high prevalence of preneoplastic lesions in over 90% of the population. Attempts to reverse these lesions in China by administration of various food and vitamin supplements have not been successful (Muñoz *et al.*, 1985). Hot drinks such as maté have been suggested as important in Latin America.

    In view of their importance in experimental esophageal cancer, the N-nitroso compounds, many of which are organ specific, have been the subject of great interest, but as yet there is no confirmatory evidence of their role in human esophageal cancer. No specific mycotoxins, although suspected, have been identified. Many authors have emphasized the potential role of multiple nutritional deficiencies in damaging the integrity of the esophageal mucosa, but this hypothesis, at least in Iran and Asia, is still unproven. A possible protective effect for vegetables in the poorer communities of the United States has been suggested (Ziegler *et al.*, 1981), but such results could equally be explained by the presence of inhibitors in the diet rather than as nutritional deficiency.

    In conclusion, whereas there is a general agreement that alcoholic beverages, especially in combination with cigarette smoking, are the major factors in Western countries, the causes of the high frequency of esophageal cancers as reported in parts of Africa, Asia, and Latin America have not been satisfactorily identified.

2.1.2. Cancer of the Oral Cavity, Larynx, and Oropharynx

    A number of studies have demonstrated a relationship between alcoholic beverages and these cancers in association with tobacco use in industrial countries (Tuyns, 1978; Austin, 1982; Mahboudi and Sayed, 1982). In India and other countries where betel use is prevalent, the enhancing role of dietary deficiencies remains speculative.

2.1.3. Stomach Cancer

    Dietary factors have long been accepted as playing a major role in stomach cancer, but the nature of the relationship remains to be established.

    2.1.3a. Laboratory Studies. Attempts have been made for many years to induce adenocarcinoma by the administration of carcinogens in the diet (Stewart, 1966). Early animal models using polycyclic aromatic hydrocarbons on rodents were unsatisfactory, and most induced cancers occurred in the forestomach. Recently, a more suitable model of gastric adenocarcinoma in experimental animals has been developed using N-nitroso compounds (Bartsch *et al.*, 1984). Studies on dietary deficiency have been unrewarding. The results of studies using heated fats and oils as related to fried foods have been essentially negative.

2.1.3b. Human Studies. The incidence of gastric adenocarcinoma and its subtypes has varied widely, both within and between countries. The most remarkable feature, however, has been the fall in incidence in many countries. This is most marked in the United States since the early 1930s, but is now occurring in other countries including Japan and is predominantly of the intestinal type. Any dietary hypothesis regarding gastric cancer must explain these geographic and temporal variations. Thus, migrant studies in North America suggest that the effects of diet must occur early in life, with lower frequencies being observed in second- and third-generation Japanese migrants.

The pathogenesis of gastric cancer is not fully understood, but in high-incidence areas chronic gastritis associated with hypochlorhydria and achlorhydria is frequent (Correa *et al.*, 1975; Broitman *et al.*, 1981). Dungal (1961) related gastric cancer in Iceland to smoked fish, and a high intake of smoked and salted foods and salt has been observed in other areas of high frequency (Geboers *et al.*, 1985b; Joossens, 1986). The NAS report recommended reduction of the use of such foodstuffs.

Early studies concentrated on polycyclic hydrocarbons (PAH) or compounds formed in cooking fats. Although there are some correlations, most case history studies examining cooking methods and diets have been essentially uninformative. Acheson and Doll (1964) and Wynder *et al.* (1963) found no association with dietary factors, whereas Meinsma (1964) and Higginson (1966) suggested some relationship with preserved meat and animal fats. Many studies, however, consistently show an inverse relationship with the use of fresh vegetables and dairy produce. Among Japanese migrants, Haenszel *et al.* (1972) concluded that pickled vegetables and dried or salted fish were important and that the more Europeanized the diet, the greater the reduction in gastric cancer. Hakama and Saxén (1967) reported a correlation between stomach cancer and cereals, but this has never been confirmed. No explanation can be offered for the sudden leveling off of gastric cancer decline that occurred in Norway after World War II, but a loss of a protective effect due to dairy products has been suggested.

N-nitroso compounds have been found in the human stomach, especially in individuals with chronic gastritis as well as in cancer patients (Correa *et al.*, 1975). An *in vivo* test for nitrosation has been developed by Bartsch and co-workers in humans (1984). It has been postulated that the inverse correlation of daily green vegetable and antioxidant intake with stomach cancer can be explained by the inhibition of this reaction. However, earlier reports of an association between nitrates in drinking water and gastric cancer have not been confirmed (Fraser, 1985). Thus, despite intense efforts to demonstrate a role for such *N*-nitroso compounds, the results remain inconclusive.

Others have ascribed the fall in gastric cancer to better refrigeration and increased use of antioxidants. The former could not be confirmed in a Kansas study (Higginson, 1966). Although low serum selenium concentrations have been associated with increased risk of cancer within countries (Shamberger *et al.*, 1976; Willett *et al.*, 1983; Salonen *et al.*, 1984, 1985), no correlations have been found between countries for gastric cancer with different serum levels of selenium. In view of the possible correlation between the fall in gastric cancer and increased use of antioxidants, such as butylated hydroxyanisole (BHA), efforts to reduce the latter possibly should be made with caution.

2.1.4. Colon and Rectal Cancer

Cancer of the large intestine is common in many developed countries, but is rare in Africa and Asia. In Japanese migrants to the United States, an increase occurs within the lifetime of the individual, suggesting that the impact of dietary effects is in late-stage carcinogenesis. Whereas in North America and parts of Europe slight temporal increases in colon and no increase in rectum cancers have been observed over the last three decades, there have been reports of an increase of both colon and rectal cancers in Japan (Kurihara et al., 1984). Although colon and rectal cancer tend to be considered together, there are differences, and a common simple etiology should not be assumed. The results of available case history studies have been inconclusive.

A number of models of large intestinal adenocarcinoma have been developed using a variety of chemicals, such as hydrazine, and while pathogenesis appears similar to the human disease, none of the tested compounds are likely to be directly relevant to humans. Such models are being used, however, to study the modulatory effects of various components of human diets such as bile salts (Reddy et al., 1977).

There is no evidence relating these cancers in humans to ingested carcinogens, with the possible exception of the association of beer and rectal cancer, which is not consistent (Tuyns, 1978). The NAS report emphasized the association between colon cancer and total dietary fat, but other studies, especially in Scandinavia, have failed to confirm this association (Jensen, 1985). Enstrom (1975b) emphasizes inconsistencies in incidence trends in the United States with per capita beef intake and points out that such a hypothesis cannot explain the lower frequencies of these cancers in Seventh Day Adventists or Mormons.

An inverse relationship between serum cholesterol levels and total and large-intestine cancer mortality and incidence has been reviewed by several authors who regard this finding as controversial (Lilienfeld, 1981; Feinleib, 1983, McMichael et al., 1984). The NAS report drew attention to the correlation between colon cancer mortality and that from coronary heart disease. This correlation, however, is questionable as coronary heart disease has fallen markedly over the last 15 years in the United States and Australia whereas no equivalent changes have occurred in the incidence of colon or rectal cancers.

Higginson and Oettlé commented on the inverse relation between colon cancer and roughage in the diet in Africa in 1960. The role of fiber has been extensively studied by Burkitt (1971), and a number of studies have indicated a definitive inverse relationship between total fiber intake and colorectal cancer. It is believed that pentose fraction (Cummings et al., 1978) is the effective component of the nonnutritive carbohydrates (see Section 3.5.2).

The NAS report (1982) stated that three dietary hypotheses are suggested by the epidemiological data: causal association with fat, a protective effect of dietary fiber, and, possibly, a protective effect of cruciferous vegetables. Unfortunately, these foodstuffs are interrelated and in-depth investigation of any individual compound is difficult. The present authors are less convinced of any simple causal association with fat. Marked changes have taken place in the U.S. diet over the last 30 years without any significant impact on colorectal cancer, and observations on the incidence of colon cancer in some population groups with varying fat intake remain inconsistent (Jensen et al., 1982; Jensen, 1985). There is also disagreement as to whether it is the type of fat or the total fat intake which is important.

2.2. Primary Liver Cancer

2.2.1. Laboratory Studies

There is extensive literature on the many experimental hepatocarcinogens that have been identified, of which only aflatoxin, a mycotoxin, appears pertinent to human dietary studies. In addition, a number of dietary factors, including protein and lipotrope deficiency, have been shown to modify hepatocarcinogenesis in rodents. Rodent studies have failed to demonstrate significant carcinogenic effects of ethanol on the liver, although a lesion corresponding to human "alcoholic" hepatitis can be produced in primates.

2.2.2. Human Studies

Primary cancer of the liver is rare in Europe and North America but is a common cancer in sub-Saharan Africa and parts of Southeast Asia. The original hypothesis that it was related directly to kwashiorkor (protein–calorie malnutrition) has now been discarded since the discovery of aflatoxin-contaminated foods in Africa and Asia. Although ecological studies have shown a correlation between aflatoxin ingestion and liver cancer, the hepatitis B virus carrier state appears to be an important cofactor, with the relative risk in carriers as compared to noncarriers in Taiwan being approximately 200-fold (Beasley *et al.*, 1981). If aflatoxin is the necessary initiator, this cancer represents a unique combination of a viral and a dietary factor. Theoretically, prevention could be possible either through reduction of aflatoxin in the diet or through preventing the hepatitis B carrier state through vaccination. Such a trial is now being undertaken in Gambia by the International Agency for Research on Cancer (IARC, 1985, p. 51). Attempts to associate liver cancer with aflatoxin in North America have been unconvincing.

The major factor in liver cancer in North America and Europe, from a pathogenic viewpoint, appears related to excessive alcohol ingestion. Although the NAS report regarded this association as equivocal, there are data suggesting a threshold effect so that cancer occurs only when the level of ingestion is sufficient to cause "alcoholic" hepatitis and consequent cirrhosis. The very high incidence of liver cancer in parts of Switzerland is believed to be related to alcohol, where at autopsy up to 18% of cirrhotic livers show hepatomas (Tuyns, 1978).

In summary, it appears that ingestion of foods contaminated with aflatoxin and the hepatitis B carrier state are important factors in the high-incidence areas of the world. Most hepatologists believe that excessive alcohol consumption is a major factor in liver cancer in Western countries and North America, and it is now becoming more important in developing Asian and African countries.

2.3. Pancreatic Cancer

In general, dietary studies of pancreatic cancer have been inconclusive. Pancreatic cancer tends to be most common in countries with a high standard of living and a Western type of diet, and thus the cancer has been ascribed to excess intake of fats and animal protein, among other foods. On the other hand, some workers have demonstrated a correlation with alcohol intake, including beer consumption. Others have related it predominantly to cigarette smoking. A report associating pancreatic cancer and coffee consumption has not been confirmed (Jensen, 1986).

Few authors have studied the relationship between per capita intake of foods and pancreatic cancers, but Lea (1967) found a strong correlation between intake of animal protein and pancreatic cancer. Ishii *et al.* (1968) reported an association of the disease with the consumption of high-meat diets in a case-control study in Japan study based primarily on the responses of relatives of deceased cases. In a large prospective cohort study, Hirayama (1981) reported a relative risk of 2.5 for daily meat intake and pancreatic cancer incidence in Japan.

2.4. Gallbladder Cancer

A high incidence of cancer of the gallbladder is found in Latin America and Southeast Asia, especially in females, and in North American Indians and Hispanics. Many primary cancers of the gallbladder are associated with gallstones and obesity so that a dietary role involving overnutrition is generally accepted as well as a possible racial component.

2.5. Breast Cancer

Breast cancer is frequent in many Western societies and comparatively rare in most of Africa and Asia. Diet has been considered a potential enhancing factor in breast cancer by many authors. However, sexual customs are involved and early pregnancy has a protective effect.

2.5.1. Laboratory Studies

The role of diet in experimental breast cancer in rodents was established early, especially the enhancing action of high-fat diets. High intakes of calories and certain carbohydrates may show similar enhancing activity, but also suggest some complexities as to the role of specific carbohydrates (Carroll, 1984).

2.5.2. Human Studies

The human data are largely dependent on ecological studies, and while studies on breast cancer mortality and fat intake suggest an association, correlations can also be shown with milk, total fat, beef calories, and protein—all components in Western diets— so that the influence of any individual component is difficult to evaluate. Improvements in living standards and diets in many countries have been associated with reduction in the age of menarche and an increase in that of the menopause, both factors that influence breast cancer (Miller *et al.*, 1978). Thus the proportion of breast cancer that can be attributed to diet remains uncertain. Greater weight and height are postulated to be associated with breast cancer among postmenopausal women but the extent to which this excess risk is due to overnutrition is far from clear (de Waard and Baanders-van Halewijn, 1974; de Waard, 1986). Experiments in animals support a relationship between excess caloric intake and cancer incidence, and breast cancer seems one of the most susceptible cancers to manipulations of this type. An increase in breast cancer is found in Japanese migrants to the United States. The rate change occurs over two to three generations, indicating that if dietary factors are important they impact in early life.

These issues have been reviewed by Willett and MacMahon (1984b), who concluded that a role for dietary fat in human breast cancer, while reasonable, was far from proven. It has been attractive to assume that a relationship between fat and carbohydrates is dependent on hormonal status, but this is uncertain. Although Hill *et al.* (1976) have demonstrated dietary-related endocrine changes in different ethnic groups, their significance in mammary cancer induction is unclear. Such hypotheses are dependent on observational studies which may be difficult to test for several reasons. First, the changes in the rate of breast cancer among some migrants occur slowly, suggesting that related risk factors are operative before age 20. Second, within certain populations such as that of the United States, there is considerably less variation in fat intake than in the intake of other nutrients. Third, dietary fat intake obtained from a variety of foods with variable fat content is difficult to estimate. Finally, a number of inconsistencies in the fat hypothesis have yet to be resolved.

2.6. Cancer of the Genitourinary System

2.6.1. Endometrial Cancer

Endometrial cancer has been associated with cancers of the breast, colon, and rectum. Thus far there have been no case history studies that directly compare the effects of diet and controls. If there is a dietary impact in endometrial cancer, it is believed to be indirect, possibly through the pituitary–hypophyseal axis. It should be pointed out that whereas endometrial cancer is a relatively common cancer in North America and Europe, the incidence in Africa and other countries, where the quality of diet and calorie intake may be reduced, is very low. For example, the incidence in the African Bantu is nearly one-thirtieth of that in Denmark or the United States.

2.6.2. Prostatic Cancer

There have been many attempts to associate incidence and mortality from prostatic cancer with diet (Howell, 1974; Rotkin, 1977; Hirayama, 1979; Schuman *et al.*, 1982). The NAS report (1982) was equivocal as to this relationship. Armstrong and Doll (1975) reported a nonsignificant correlation with total fat and oil intake. Reports from the United States have suggested that the highest mortality is in whites from countries with the greatest per capita intake of beef products, milk products, fats, and oils (Blair and Fraumeni, 1978). A correlation study based on dietary data from individual interviews in Hawaii indicated a significant association between prostatic cancer and animal fat (Kolonel *et al.*, 1981b).

The study of prostatic cancer is complicated by the high prevalence of "latent cancer" in the elderly. Thus, it is suggested that the role of diet, if any, is enhancing and not initiating. However, it is difficult to explain the very low incidence of latent cancer in Japan and China and a relatively high frequency in black Africans except on ethnic grounds. The geographic variation in prostate cancer between white and black Americans also is difficult to reconcile with any simple dietary hypothesis.

In conclusion, although the role of endocrine status and prostatic cancer has some biological plausibility, the role of environmental factors, including diet, remains unclear and probably cannot be elucidated by simple observational studies in humans in the absence of suitable hypotheses for testing.

2.6.3. Bladder Cancer

Most studies on the role of diet in bladder cancer relate to either coffee consumption or the use of nonnutritive sweeteners. In general, extensive studies have failed to confirm a causal relationship, and the NAS report (1982) concluded that the use of nonnutritive sweeteners was unlikely to be a significant risk factor.

2.6.4. Renal Cancer

There is little evidence that renal cancer is significantly related to diet.

3. Role of Specific Nutrients

3.1. Introduction

The following section discusses the role of specific nutrients in human carcinogenesis. Experimental studies have been largely reviewed elsewhere (NAS, 1982). The results of the major published human studies are presented in Tables I–III. We have tried to exclude studies whose results were incomplete, equivocal, or based on numbers too small for reliable estimates. These studies do not represent an exhaustive survey of the literature, but illustrate the difficulty of arriving at any definite dietary recommendations regarding food intake.

The weaknesses of such studies have been described in Section 1, and two points are especially important. First, attempts to quantitate macronutrients have many limitations and often depend on relatively crude calculations from food tables. Thus we have preferred to quote the authors' conclusions in this context without qualifications. Further, many authors have examined essentially the same epidemiological and dietary data sources, particularly in correlation studies, many of which have been used as the bases for public guidance. Thus the extent to which these can be regarded as separate studies is problematical.

3.2. Fats

Fats (lipids) have important biological functions, serving as structural components of membranes, as storage and transport forms of metabolic fuel, and as cell-surface components concerned with cell recognition, species specificity, and tissue immunity. Their role has been extensively studied and reviewed in relation to cancer (NAS, 1982; Graham, 1983a,b,c; Lowenthal, 1983; Willett and MacMahon, 1984b; Joossens *et al.*, 1985; Gori, 1986a). Nonetheless, there is still controversy as to the role of fat in individual human cancers and the extent to which it interacts with other factors.

3.2.1. Animal Studies

Laboratory studies have shown that dietary fats influence carcinogenesis. High-fat diets, especially polyunsaturated fats, increase tumor incidence at a number of sites (Carroll and Khor, 1970, 1971, 1975; Carroll, 1975, 1980; Broitman *et al.*, 1977;

Table 1. *Correlation Studies Relating Food Intake to Cancer Incidence and Mortality*

Author	Comments	Site	Association	Food source
Among countries				
Hakama and Saxén (1967)	Mortality (16 countries: Segi and Kurihara, 1964) Dietary factors (UN 1964)	Stomach (M&F)	Positive	Cereal used as flour
Lea (1967)	Morality (19–33 countries: Segi and Kurihara, 1964; WHO, 1959–1964) Dietary factors (FAO, 1965)	Colon/rectum (M&F) Ovary (F)	Positive	Fats, oils, animal protein
		Colon (M&F) Breast (F)	Inverse	Fish
		Prostate (M) Pancreas (M&F)	Positive	Fats, oils, animal protein, eggs, milk
		Uterus (F) Stomach (M&F)	Inverse	Fats and oils, sugar, animal protein, eggs
Drasar and Irving (1973)[a]	Incidence (37 countries: Doll, 1969) Dietary factors (FAO, 1969)	Colon (M&F)	Positive	Total fat, animal fat, animal protein, eggs
		Colon (M&F) Breast (F)	None	Fiber
		Breast (F)	Positive	Total protein, animal fat and protein, eggs
Berg and Howell (1974)	Incidence (58 registries: Doll et al., 1970) Mortality (41 countries: Segi et al., 1964) Dietary factors (FAO, 1971)	Colon/rectum (M&F)	Positive	Meat, especially beef
Bjelke (1974)	Mortality (27 countries: Segi et al., 1969) Dietary factors (FAO, 1969)	Colon (M&F)	Positive	Meat, animal protein, total fat
		Colon (M&F) Rectum (M&F) Breast (F)	Inverse	Cereals, nuts, seeds, pulses (beans, peas, etc.)
		Rectum (M&F)	Positive	Animal protein, total fat

(continued)

Table 1. (Continued)

Author	Comments	Site	Association	Food source
Howell (1974)	Mortality (41 countries: Segi et al., 1969)	Breast (F)	Positive	Meat, eggs, milk, fats & oils, animal protein, total fat
	Dietary factors (36 countries: FAO, 1971)	Stomach (M)	Positive	Starch
		Colon (M)	Positive / Inverse	Meats, eggs, sugar, milk / Rice
		Rectum (M)	Positive / Inverse	Meats, eggs, milk / Rice
		Lung (M)	Positive / Inverse	Meats / Pulses
		Prostate (M)	Positive / Inverse	Meat, fats and oils, milk, sugar / Pulses
Armstrong and Doll (1975)	Incidence (23 countries: Doll et al., 1966; Doll et al., 1970)	Colon/rectum (M&F)	Positive	Meat, total fat, animal protein (incidence and mortality)
	Mortality (32 countries: Segi et al., 1969; WHO, 1967–1969, 1970)	Colon (M&F)	Inverse	Cereal (mortality)
		Breast (F)	Positive	Total fat, animal protein, meat, sugar, eggs, fats and oils, milk (incidence and mortality)
	Dietary factors (FAO, 1959, 1960, 1971; UN, 1960, 1970)		Inverse	Cereals (incidence and mortality)
		Ovary (F)	Positive	Total fat, animal protein, fats and oils, milk (mortality)
		Uterus (F)	Positive	Total fat, meat, fats and oils, animal protein, eggs, milk (incidence)
		Testes (M)	Positive	Total fat, fats and oils (incidence)
		Stomach (F)	Inverse	Meat, total fat (incidence and mortality)
		Prostate (M)	Positive	Total fat, fats and oils, animal protein, milk (mortality)

Reference	Cancer site (sex)	Correlation	Dietary factor
	Kidney (M)	Inverse	Cereals (mortality)
	Kidney (M)	Positive	Sugar (incidence)
	Kidney (M&F)	Inverse	Pulses (mortality)
	Kidney (M&F)	Positive	Animal protein, milk, meat (incidence)
	Kidney (M)	Positive	Fats and oils, total fat (incidence and mortality)
	Kidney (F)	Positive	Total fat, total protein (incidence)
	Liver (M&F)	Positive	Potatoes (incidence)
	Liver (M&F)	Inverse	Sugar (incidence)
	Liver (F)	Inverse	Animal protein (incidence)
	Pancreas (M)	Positive	Animal protein (mortality)
Carroll (1975) Mortality (39 countries: Segi et al., (1969) Dietary factors (39 countries: FAO, 1971)	Breast (F)	Positive	Total dietary fat
	Breast (F)	None	Vegetable fat
Hems and Stuart (1975)[b] Mortality (10 countries: Various sources predominately pre-1961 [Single]; Segi and Kurihara, 1966 [Total]) Dietary factors (10 countries: UN, 1934–1965; FAO, 1960)	Breast (F) Prewar Single and married	Positive	Sugar
	Single and married	Inverse	Starch
	Postwar Single and married	Positive	Total calories, sugar
	Married	Positive	Fat
	Single	Inverse	Starch
Howell (1975) Mortality (37 countries: Segi et al., 1969) Dietary factors (37 countries: FAO, 1971)	Colon/rectum (M&F) Breast (F) Prostate (M)	Positive	Sugars, meats, eggs, milk, fats
	Colon/rectum (M&F) Breast (F) Prostate (M)	Inverse	Cereals, pulses
	Stomach (M&F)	Positive	Starch

(continued)

Table I. (Continued)

Author	Comments	Site	Association	Food source
Knox (1977)	Mortality (20 countries: WHO, 1973); Dietary factors (20 countries: OECD, 1970)	Colon (M&F)	Positive / Inverse	Meat (beef), eggs / Lard, pulses (beans, peas, etc.)
		Breast (F)	Positive / Inverse	Total fats, meat, animal protein, sugar, beer, eggs / Wheat, pulses, rice
Hems (1978)[c]	Mortality (41 countries: Segi, 1971, 1975; Segi et al., 1969, 1972, 1976; WHO, 1970); Dietary factors (FAO, 1970)	Breast (F)	Positive	Total fat, animal protein, animal calories, refined sugar
Gray et al. (1979)[d]	Incidence (8 countries: UICC, 1966, 1970); Mortality (12 countries: Segi et al., 1969; WHO, 1967–1970); Dietary factors (FAO, 1971)	Breast (F)	Positive	Animal protein, eggs, meat, sugar, total fat
Schrauzer (1976)	Mortality (17 countries: Segi et al., 1969); Dietary factors (OECD, 1970)	Colon (M&F)	Positive	Meat
		Rectum (M) / Rectum (F) / Lung (F)	Positive	Beer
		Prostate (M) / Bladder (M) / Ovary (F)	Positive	Fat
		Pancreas (M&F) / Breast (F) / Ovary (F) / Leukemia (M&F) / Bladder (F) / Skin (F)	Positive	Sugar

Reference	Cancer site	Correlation	Dietary factor
	Buccal cavity/pharynx (F)	Positive	Citrus
	Buccal cavity/pharynx (M)		
	Esophagus (M), Larynx (M)	Positive	Wine
	Thyroid (M), Liver (F)	Positive	Fruit
	Stomach (M&F), Liver (M)	Positive	Cereals
	Pancreas (F)	Inverse	Vegetables
	Lung (M)	Inverse	Fish
	Colon (M&F), Pancreas (M), Breast (F)		
	Ovary (F), Prostate (M), Bladder (F), Leukemia (M&F)	Inverse	Cereals
	Somach (M&F)	Inverse	Meat
	Liver (M&F)	Inverse	Sugar
Liu et al. (1979)[e] — Mortality (20 countries: WHO, 1967–1973), Dietary factors (20 countries: FAO, 1954–1965)	Colon (M&F)	Positive	Cholesterol
		None	Total fat, saturated and monounsaturated fat, fiber
Carroll (1980) — Mortality (48 countries: Segi et al., 1978), Incidence (Waterhouse et al., 1976), Dietary factors (FAO, 1971)	Colon (M&F)	Positive	Total fat (incidence and mortality)
	Rectum (M&F), Prostate (M), Ovary (F)	Positive	Total fat (mortality)
	Breast (F)	Positive	Total fat (incidence and mortality)
		None	Vegetable fat (mortality)

(continued)

Table I. (Continued)

Author	Comments	Site	Association	Food source
Between countries				
Gregor et al. (1969)*f*	Mortality (U.S. and Czecho-slovakia: Segi and Kurihara, 1966)	Uterus (F) Stomach (M&F) Liver (M&F)	None	Total fat (mortality)
	Dietary factors (Statistical Abstracts: U.S., 1964; Czechoslovakia, 1966)	Stomach (M) 1947–1948 1962–1963 Intestines (M) 1947–1948/ 1962–1963	Inverse None Positive	Animal protein (U.S. intake higher) Animal protein (U.S. intake higher)
Stocks (1970)	Mortality (England and Wales: Registrar General, 1949–1964)	Breast (F)	Positive	Liquid milk, cheese, butter, green vegetables
	Dietary factors (National Food Survey, 1957, 1964)		Inverse	Margarine
IARC (1977)*g*	Incidence [Denmark (1974) and Finland (1975): cancer registries]	Colon/rectum (M)	Positive None	High protein (low fiber) (Copenhagen) High protein (high fiber) (Kuopio)
	Dietary factors (food diaries and specimen analyses)			
Within countries				
Enstrom (1975b)	Incidence (U.S.: Dorn and Cutler, 1954; NCI, 1974) Mortality (U.S.: Buford, 1971; Cutler and Devesa, 1974; Mason and McKay, 1974)	Colorectal (M&F)	None	Beef and total fat
	Dietary factors (U.S.: Bureau of the Census, 1973)			

Reference	Source	Cancer site	Association	Dietary factor
Hirayama (1977)	Mortality (Japan: Vital Statistics, 1955–1975); Dietary factors (National Nutritional Survey, 1949–1973)	Stomach (M&F); Colon (M&F); Breast (F)	Inverse; Positive; Positive	Milk and eggs; Meat; Fat (especially pork)
Malhotra (1977)	Incidence (India: Cancer Registry, 1968–1973); Dietary factors (interviews)	Colon (M)	Inverse	Fermented milk products, cellulose, roughage, vegetable fiber
Blair and Fraumeni[h] (1978)	Mortality [U.S.: Mason and McKay (NIH), 1974]; Dietary factors (U.S.: Bureau of the Census, 1959, 1964; USDA, 1972)	Prostate (M)	Positive	Beef, milk products, fats, oil, pork, eggs
Enig et al. (1978)[i]	Mortality and incidence (U.S.: Devesa and Silverman, 1977); Dietary factors (Gordon et al., 1961; Bureau of the Census, 1972; Rizek et al., 1974)	Colon (M&F); Breast (F)	Positive; None; Positive; None; Inverse	Total fat, vegetable fat (especially *trans* fatty acids); Animal fat; Mortality: total fat, vegetable fat (especially *trans* fatty acids); Incidence: total fat, vegetable fat (especially *trans* fatty acids); Animal fat
Hirayama (1978)	Mortality and incidence (Japan: Vital Statistics, 1955–1975); Dietary factors (National Nutritional Survey, 1949–1973)	Breast (F)	Positive	Fat intake (especially pork)
Lyon and Sorenson (1978)	Incidence (U.S.: DHEW, 1974); Dietary factors (Utah Beef Council, 1972; dietary survey)	Colon (M&F) (white only: Mormons and non-Mormons)	None	Total protein, fat (meat), crude fiber
Bingham et al. (1979)	Mortality (U.K.: Registrar General, 1969–1973)	Colon (M&F)	None	Fat, animal protein (especially beef), total dietary fiber

(continued)

Table I. (Continued)

Author	Comments	Site	Association	Food source
	Dietary factors (National Food Survey, 1969–1973)		Inverse	Pentose fiber fraction, vegetables other than potatoes
Gaskill *et al.* (1979)[j]	Mortality (U.S.: NCHS, 1975) Dietary factors (USDA, 1970, 1974)	Breast (F)	Positive Inverse	Milk Eggs
Hems (1980)	Mortality (England and Wales: Case and Pearson, 1957; Case *et al.*, 1968; Registrar General, 1967–1974) Dietary factors (Greaves and Hollingsworth, 1966; National Food Survey Committee, 1952–1976)	Breast (F)	Positive	Fat and sugar (consumed 1 decade earlier) Animal protein (consumed 2 decades earlier)
Kolonel *et al.* (1981a)[k]	Incidence (U.S.: Hawaii Tumor Registry, 1973–1977) Dietary factors (interview)	Stomach (M&F) (M) (Caucasian F)	Positive Positive Inverse	Rice, pickled vegetables, carbohydrates Dry and salted fish Fresh fruit
Kolonel *et al.* (1981b)[k]	Incidence (U.S.: Hawaii Tumor Registry 1973–1977; Dept. of Health, 1975)	Lung (M&F) Larynx (M&F)	Positive	Cholesterol

Dietary factors (Household interview, USDA, 1972; Japan Dietary Association 1964; Philippine Food and Nutrition Research Center, 1968; Hawaii: Miller and Branthooven, 1957)	Breast (F) Corpus uteri (F)	Positive	Fat (total animal, saturated, unsaturated)
	Breast (F) Corpus uteri (F)	Inverse	Complex carbohydrates
	Prostate (M)	Positive	Fat (animal and saturated), protein (total and animal)
	Stomach (M&F)	Positive	Fish (fat and protein)

[a] Multiple regression analyses to control for socioeconomic variables; no separation of dietary factors was possible.

[b] Age-specific breast cancer rates between single and total (predominantly married) women in the 10 countries varied little by country, social class, urban–rural areas, or dietary factors.

[c] Partial correlation analysis indicated that breast cancer rates were positively correlated with total fat, animal protein, and animal calories, independently of other components of diet. These three components were correlated with one another so closely that it was not possible, with available data, to say whether any one was associated with breast cancer independently of the other.

[d] Correlation remained after controlling for height, weight, and age at menarche. No data were available for age at first birth or at menopause.

[e] Partial correlation coefficients between total fat, saturated and monounsaturated fats, and fiber and colon-cancer rates—controlling for cholesterol—were calculated and found to be no longer significant. On the other hand, the estimated partial correlation coefficient between cholesterol and colon cancer was still large (0.73–0.78) and highly significant ($p < 0.001$) when each of the other dietary factors was controlled. The two-way analyses of variance on mortality rates indicated a highly significant main effect for cholesterol but not for saturated fat or fiber, or for the interaction. Similar results were obtained when total fat or monounsaturated fat was considered. For polyunsaturated fat, the effect of cholesterol and the interaction were also significant.

[f] Intestine cancer mortality was higher for the United States (1.7×), but stomach cancer mortality was higher for Czechoslovakia (3×).

[g] Copenhagen had nearly 4.0× (M) and 3.0× (F) the incidence of colon and rectum caner, but Kuopio consumed greater protein (although less from meat).

[h] Mortality was higher in blacks than whites, in midwest and north-central regions, and in persons of Scandinavian descent.

[i] Significant positive correlation for vegetable fat could not always be explained by the effects of total unsaturated fatty acids, individual unsaturated fatty acids, or saturated fatty acids. Multiple partial correlation calculations showed a significant consistant role for *tran* fatty acids in the positive correlations for vegetable fats and additional multiple partial correlations using 10-year lag data increased their significance.

[j] Within the United States, age-adjusted breast cancer mortality was positively associated with consumption of milk, butter, and total milk fat, total calories, protein, fat, and beef, and negatively associated with egg demand. Only the associations with milk and egg demand, however, survived when the Southern states were eliminated from the analyses or when either age at first marriage or income was controlled. The associations with milk, and egg demand persisted despite multiple controls for other dietary and demographic variables, although the association with milk demand lost statistical significance in some second- and third-order partial correlations.

[k] Incidence rates in Hawaii, highest to lowest: Japanese immigrants, Japanese Hawaiian, Caucasian Hawaiian, Caucasian immigrants from U.S. mainland.

[l] Five ethnic groups in Hawaii: Japanese, Caucasian, Chinese, Filipino, Hawaiian.

Table II. Case–Control Studies Relating Food to Cancer Incidence and Mortality

Author	Comments	Site	Association	Food source
Pernu (1960)	Finland (7078 cases, 1773 controls	Colon (M)	Positive	Meat and animal fats
		(F)	None	
Wynder and Bross (1961)[a]	U.S. (150 cases, 150 controls)	Esophagus (M)	Inverse	Milk, butter, eggs, green and yellow vegetables
Meinsma (1964)	Netherlands [235 gastric cases, 262 "other cancer," and 223 "no cancer" controls (M); 105 gastric cases, 320 "other cancer," and 255 "no cancer" controls (F)]	Stomach (M&F)	Positive	Bacon
Higginson (1966)	U.S.: colon (340 cases, 1020 controls); stomach (93 cases, 279 controls)	Colon/rectum (M&F) Stomach (M&F)	None	Fried foods, meats, animal fats, dairy foods, fruits & vegetables
Wynder and Shigematsu (1967)	U.S. (794 cases, 409 controls)	Colon (M&F)	None	Smoked foods, charcoal foods, fats, green and yellow vegetables, fruit, cereals and potatoes
Wynder et al. (1969)[b]	Japan (151 cases, 307 controls)	Colon (M&F)	None	Salted and smoked meats, fried foods, butter, eggs, milk and fat, green and yellow vegetables, citrus fruit
Graham et al. (1972)	U.S. [160 matched pairs (M); 68 matched pairs (F)]	Stomach (M&F)	None	Fats and fried foods
		(M)	Inverse	Raw vegetables (especially coleslaw, lettuce, tomatoes)
		(M)	Positive	Potatoes
		(F)	Inverse	Beef
		(F)	Positive	Lamb
Haenszel et al. (1973)[c]	Hawaiian Japanese (179 cases, 357 controls)	Colon (M&F)	Positive	Meat (especially beef) and legumes (especially string beans)
Bjelke (1974)	Norway (228 stomach, 162 colon, 116 rectal cases, and 1394 controls)	Stomach (M&F)	Positive	Salted fish, cooked cereals, fruit soup
			Inverse	Vegetables and fruits high in vitamin C
		Colon/rectum (M&F)	Positive	Processed meats
			Inverse	Cereals, crude fiber

Reference	Study population	Cancer site	Association	Dietary factor
	U.S. (83 stomach, 259 colon, 114 rectal cases, and 1657 controls)	Colon (M&F)	Inverse	Coffee, carrots
		Stomach (M&F)	Positive	Cooked cereals, smoked fish, canned fruit
De Jong et al. (1974)[a]	Singapore Chinese (131 cases, 524 controls)	Colorectal (M&F)	Inverse	Vegetables
			Positive	Meats (especially among rectal patients)
			Inverse	Vegetables, crude fiber
			Inverse	Coffee (colon), fruits (rectal)
Modan et al. (1974)	Israel (151 cases, 151 colorectal cancer controls, 151 noncancer surgical controls, and 151 neighborhood controls)	Esophagus (M)	Inverse	Bread, potatoes, and bananas
		(M&F)	Positive	"Burning hot" beverages
		Stomach (M&F)	Positive	Noodles, cholent,[e] biscuits, chocolate, root beer
Modan et al. (1975)	Israel (194 matched pairs—neighborhood controls; 170 matched pairs—surgical controls)	Colon (M&F)	None	Fat, high-fat, animal, and vegetable protein
			Inverse	High-residue fiber foods
		Rectum (M&F)	None	High-residue fiber foods
Phillips (1975)	U.S. (Seventh Day Adventists: 41 colon cases, 123 controls; 77 breast cases, 221 controls)	Colon (M&F)	Positive	Meat (beef, lamb, fish), saturated fat, fried foods, and dairy products, except milk
			Positive	Fried potatoes
		Breast (F)	None	Coffee, meat, poultry, eggs, milk, seafood, and cheese
Armstrong et al. (1976)	England (139 cases, 139 controls)	Renal (M&F)	Positive	Eggs, margarine, cheese
Rotkin (1977)	U.S. (white and black: 111 cases, 111 controls)	Prostate (M)	None	Beef and meat, animal protein (beef, bacon, pork, lamb, and chicken)
Graham et al. (1978)	U.S. [256 colon cases, 783 controls (M); 330 rectal cases, 628 controls (M); 214 colon cases, 565 controls (F); 182 rectal cases, 416 controls (F)]	Colon/rectum (M&F)	Inverse	Cruciferous vegetables, raw vegetables
		Colon (M)	Positive	Fish
		Rectum (F)	None	Raw vegetables and cabbage
Miller et al. (1978)	Canada (pre- and postmenopausal women:	Breast (F)	Positive	Total fat

(continued)

Table II. (Continued)

Author	Comments	Site	Association	Food source
	100 cases, 300 neighborhood controls)			
Nomura et al. (1978)	U.S. (Japanese–Hawaiians: Spouses of women with breast cancer: 86 cases, 6774 controls)	Breast (F)	Positive Inverse	Meat (beef, veal, lamb, wieners), butter, margarine, and cheese Milk, green tea, nori, and other seaweeds
Dales et al. (1979)	U.S. (blacks: 99 cases, 189 hospital controls, 91 health checkup controls)	Colorectal (M&F)	Positive Inverse	High-saturated-fat–low-fiber foods High-fiber–low-fat foods
Martinez et al. (1979)[f]	Puerto Rico (461 cases, 461 neighborhood controls)	Colon (M&F)	Positive	Meat, total fats, cereals, total residue fiber
Cook-Mozaffari et al. (1979)[g]	Iran (344 esophageal cases, 688 village controls; 181 "other" cancer cases, 362 village controls)	Esophagus (M&F)	Inverse	Fresh fruit and vegetables
Mettlin and Graham (1979)	U.S. [377 cases, 645 controls (M); 112 cases, 256 controls (F)]	Bladder (M&F)	Inverse[h]	Vitamin A intake from foods (especially milk and carrots)
Mettlin et al. (1979)	U.S. (white males: 292 cases, 801 controls)	Lung (M)	Inverse[i] None None	Vitamin A from foods (especially milk and carrots) Fat, protein, vitamin C, carbohydrates Animal protein (especially beef), string beans, and starches
Haenszel et al. (1980)	Japan (588 cases, 1176 controls)	Colorectal (M&F)	Positive	Saturated fat, total fat, total protein, oleic acid
Jain et al. (1980)[j]	Canada (348 colon, 194 rectal cases; 542 neighborhood, 535 hospital controls)	Colon/rectum (M&F)	None	Crude fiber, linoleic acid
Mettlin et al. (1980)[k]	U.S. (white males: 147 cases, 264 controls)	Esophagus (M)	Inverse	Fresh fruit and vegetables
Lubin et al. (1981)[l]	Canada (577 cases, 826 disease-free controls)	Breast (F)	Positive	Beef and pork
Graham et al. (1981)	U.S. (white males: 374 cases, 381 controls)	Larynx (M)	Inverse[m] None	Vitamin A and vitamin C from foods Fats, meat, fiber, cruciferous vegetables

Reference	Population (cases/controls)	Site (sex)	Association	Dietary factor
Ziegler et al. (1981)[n]	U.S. (black males' next of kin: 120 cases; 250 controls)	Esophagus (M)	Positive	Processed and precooked meats and fish
			Inverse	Dairy products, eggs, fresh fruits and vegetables, fresh or frozen meat and fish consumption
Mettlin et al. (1981)	U.S. (white males: 122 cases, 235 controls)	Esophagus (M)	None[o]	Vitamin A from foods, mostly meat and fish consumption
			Inverse[p]	Vitamin C from foods, mostly fruit and vegetable consumption
Graham et al. (1982)	U.S. (white females: 2024 cases, 1463 controls)	Breast (F)	None	Foods containing vitamins A and C, cruciferous vegetables, animal fat
			Inverse	Foods containing vitamin A (women 55+ years)
Kinlen (1982)	U.K. (mortality: 1769 nuns eating no meat; 1044 nuns eating some meat)	Colon (F) Breast (F) Ovary (F)	None	Meat
Marshall et al. (1982)	U.S. (white males: 427 cases, 588 controls)	Oral cavity (M)	Inverse[p]	Vitamin A and vitamin C from foods
			None	Fats, fiber, cruciferous vegetables
Schuman et al. (1982)	U.S. (white males: 223 cases, 223 hospital, and 223 neighborhood controls)	Prostate (M)	Positive	Pork, smoked and salted ham, eggs, milk, ice cream
			Inverse	Chicken, fish, vegetables (especially carrots, cabbage, rutabagas, tomatoes), liver
Kolonel et al. (1983)	Hawaii (5 ethnic groups: 243 cases, 321 controls)	Prostate (M)	None[q]	Total fat, saturated fat, unsaturated fat (less than age 70)
			Positive[r] (n.s.)	Total fat, saturated fat, animal protein
	(Japanese: 137 cases, 152 hospital, and 152 neighborhood controls)	Breast (F)	Inverse[r] (n.s.)	Total fat, saturated fat (45–64 years)
			Positive[r] (n.s.)	Total fat, saturated fat (65+ years)
	(Caucasian: 131 cases, 143 hospital, and 144 neighborhood controls)	Breast (F)	Inverse[s]	Vitamin A from food (especially carotene) sources
	(5 ethnic groups: 267 cases, 444 controls)	Lung (M&F)	Positive	Meat, (especially lamb and beef) and high-meat–low-vegetable diet
Manousos et al. (1983)[t]	Greece (103 cases, 100 hospital controls)	Colorectal (M&F)	Inverse	Vegetables (especially beets, spinach, let-

(continued)

Table II. (Continued)

Author	Comments	Site	Association	Food source
Marshall *et al.* (1983)[a]	U.S. (white females: 513 cases, 490 hospital controls)	Cervix (F)	Positive	tuce, cabbage) and high-vegetable–low-meat diet
				Frequency of crucifous[a] vegetable consumption (especially cabbage, cole slaw, turnips, pickles), potatoes, fat[a] (especially bacon, pork)
			None	Protein, fiber, total calories, vitamin C from food sources
			Inverse	β-Carotene[a] from foods (especially carrots, tomatoes, broccoli), chicken, lamb
Miller *et al.* (1983)	Canada (348 colon cases, 194 rectal cases, 542 neighborhood, and 535 surgical controls)	Colon/rectum (M&F)	None	Dietary fiber
		Colon (F)	Inverse (weak)	Cruciferous vegetables
		Colon (M)	None	Cruciferous vegetables
		Colon (M&F)	Positive	Saturated fat

Rectum (F)	Positive	Saturated fat and pork
Rectum (M)	Positive	Eggs, beef, and veal

[a]The intake of milk and fresh vegetables was related to the consumption of alcohol and the author could not conclude from the data whether low intake of these foods had a direct bearing on the development of esophageal cancer or whether it was related only to the high intake of alcohol.

[b]Although no consistent differences were found, the colon cancer group tended to have a diet lower in rice and higher in fruits and milk, which probably reflected its higher socioeconomic status.

[c]Relative risks remained significant, even after adjustments for consumption of other foods within the same category and among different categories.

[d]When multivariate adjustment of the simultaneous effects of all variables was taken into account, only dialect group (Hokkien and Teochew) and beverage temperature continued to be significant. When bread, potatoes, and bananas were combined into a composite index in the regression, this index also continued to show a high significant inverse effect for males.

[e]An Eastern European Jewish dish composed of potatoes, dried beans, barley, beef, and fat cooked together on low heat for 24 hr.

[f]Cancer patients also had a higher frequency of other previous large bowel chronic diseases than controls.

[g]Increased risk was associated with low socioeconomic status and was significantly greater for esophageal tumors than for all other tumors combined. After multivariate adjustment, raw vegetables (especially cucumbers and tomatoes) and fresh fruit (especially oranges and lemons) remianed significantly negatively associated with esophageal cancer.

[h]Some significant risk reduction was found for the frequency of consumption of individual cruciferous vegetables, but the dose–response pattern observed was irregular.

[i]Adjusted for smoking status.

[j]Multivariate logistic regression indicated highest risk for saturated fat with evidence of a dose–response relationship. When these nutrients, which are highly correlated with saturated fat, were examined individually, most of the estiamtes were lower and less significant than for saturated fat. A history of bowel polyps for both sexes and regular use of laxatives by women were also significant risk factors.

[k]The effects of vegetables and fruit consumption remained significant after controlling for their possible association with smoking and drinking.

[l]This association remained after controlling for age at first birth, family history of breast cancer, previous benign biopsy, socioeconomic status, and ages at menarche and menopause.

[m]Adjusted for cigarette and alcohol consumption

[n]The least nourished third of the study population was at twice the risk of the most nourished third. None of these associations were markedly reduced by controlling for ethanol consumption, smoking, socioeconomic status, or other nutrition measures. Generally poor nutrition was the major dietary predicator of risk.

[o]A dose–response reduction in risk associated with increases in ingestion of vitamin A was observed, but this association disappeared when cigarette smoking and alcohol consumption were controlled.

[p]Adjusted for cigarette and alcohol consumption.

[q]Statistically adjusted for age, ethnicity, and socioeconomic status by multiple logistic regression analyses.

[r]Not significant (n.s.) after statistical adjustment for parity status, history of benign tumors, family history of breast cancer, use of exogenous estrogens, body height and weight, and special diets.

[s]Statistically adjusted for age, occupation, smoking history, cholesterol intake, ethnicity, and sex by multiple logistic regression analyses.

[t]No significant interactions were noted with respect to age, sex or anatomic localization (colon vs. rectum). A relative risk of 8.0 existed between the extreme diets (high meat-low vegetable vs. low meat-high vegetable).

[u]Cruciferous vegetables, fat consumption and β-carotene influenced risk in a statistically significant manner after controlling for number of marriages, age at first marriage, cigarette smoking, beer consumption and one another in a multiple logistic regression analysis.

Table III. Cohort Studies Relating Food Intake to Cancer Mortality

Author	Comments	Site	Association	Food source
Phillips and Snowden (1983)	Mortality (U.S. white Seventh Day Adventists: n = 21,295; follow-up = 21 years; age ≥35 years)	Colon (M&F)	Positive	Coffee
		Breast (F)	None	Meat and poultry
		Prostate (M)	None	Meat and poultry
Hirayama (1985)[a]	Mortality (Japan: n = 265,118; follow-up = 16 years; age ≥ 40 years)	Pancreas (M&F)	Positive	Daily meat consumption
		Lung[b] (F)		
		Breast[b] (F)		
		Colon[c] (M)	Inverse	Daily meat consumption (with daily green–yellow vegetable consumption)
		Colorectal[d] (M&F)	Inverse	Wheat and rice
		Stomach[b] (M&F)		
		Lung[b] (M&F)	Inverse	Green–yellow vegetable consumption
		Cervix[b] (F)		
		Prostate (M)		
		Stomach[b] (M&F)	Inverse	Soybean paste soup

[a]The highest cancer risk was observed in people who, on a daily basis, smoked, drank alcohol, consumed meat, and did not eat green–yellow vegetables. The lowest cancer risk was noted for those who, on a daily basis, neither smoked, nor drank alcohol, nor ate meat, but who ate green–yellow vegetables daily. Compared to the highest risk group, those who ate green–yellow vegetables daily showed considerably lower risk even when keeping other habits unchanged. Those men who were not daily consumers of green–yellow vegetables at the first survey (1965), but who increased their frequency of vegetable intake by the time of the second survey (1971), showed a decreased mortality from stomach cancer in the subsequent follow-up period compared to those who consumed green–yellow vegetables infrequently throughout the study period, yet their level of mortality remained higher than those who daily consumed vegetables at both the first and the second surveys.
[b]Adjusted for smoking and alcohol consumption.
[c]See also *Hirayama*, 1982.
[d]See also *Hirayama*, 1981.

Hopkins and Carroll, 1979; NAS, 1982; Kritchevsky *et al.*, 1984). Most studies on spontaneous and chemically induced mammary tumors suggest that the action is in the late (promotional) phase of carcinogenesis, but after the level of dietary fat reaches 20% the enhancing activity is less obvious. The nature of the enhancing effect has not been determined for mammary cancers. Experimental liver cancer induction by 2-acetyl-aminofluorene (AAF) is enhanced both by lipotrope-deficient diets and high-fat diets, illustrating the range of effects that may be produced by differing regimes of dietary fat. Promoting effects of high-fat diets have also been described for colon cancer in rodents. It has been suggested that high fat intake leads to increased bile acid and neutral steroid excretion in the feces, which may have a promoting effect on already initiated cells. Graham (1983c) also supports the view that high-fat diets may produce conditions in the gut possibly leading to the formation of powerful carcinogens, but such information was doubted by the NAS Committee (1982).

3.2.2. Human Studies

Some of the studies describing the association of fat intake and different cancers are presented in Tables I–III. Inconsistencies in certain studies can be seen which cannot easily be explained. While there is an association for a number of sites, the evidence is most persuasive for breast and large bowel cancer. On the other hand, the incidence of breast and colorectal cancer between Kuopio, Finland, and Copenhagen, Denmark, is the inverse of what would have been anticipated on dietary patterns (Jensen *et al.*, 1974, 1982; IARC, 1977). Other inconsistencies have been reported (Enstrom, 1980; Higginson, 1982; Kinlen, 1982).

The NAS report concluded that it was not possible to identify any specific fat components that were definitely related to carcinogenesis. In view of the potential magnitude of the effect of fat on mammary cancer and in view of the experimental results with different types of fat, it is somewhat surprising that the marked changes in the types of fats that have occurred in the U.S. population over the last three decades have had no apparent impact on mammary or colon cancer patterns. On the other hand, such data are consistent with the view that the essential impact is in childhood. As pointed out by many authors, dietary fat tends to correlate significantly with both protein and other potential modulating factors in affluent societies. Furthermore, since fats are a concentrated source of calories, the role of calories *per se* and their significance in relation to obesity need further exploration.

These inconsistencies are further reviewed by Willett and MacMahon (1984b), who conclude that while epidemiological studies of dietary intake among individual subjects provide contradictory support for the hypothesis that diet is related to colon cancer, there is sufficient data to suggest that a relationship may exist which should be further explored. In regard to breast cancer, they comment on the hypothesis that high levels of dietary fat may increase the rate of breast cancer through increased estrogen metabolism, referring to studies in which postmenopausal women switching from a low-fat vegetarian diet to a high-fat Western diet showed a decrease in luteinizing hormones, follicle-stimulating hormone, and prolactin. A relationship between dietary factors and hormonal levels in premenopausal women remains to be defined. Willett and MacMahon concluded that, while the hypothesis associating at least some types of dietary fat with breast cancer in humans was reasonable, it was not proven.

de Waard (1986) emphasizes that abundant availability of food leads to increased height and weight in many individuals and, in postadolescence, to obesity. The latter is most frequently related to endometrial cancer and cancer of the gallbladder. He states that the effect of large body size and mass cannot be disposed of lightly in such frequent cancers as those of the breast. He is of the opinion that 50% of the difference in breast cancer between Japan and the Netherlands can be explained statistically on the basis of weight and height alone. For the individual, the relationship between these factors is much greater than dietary fat, which may also influence breast cancer risk through its effect on body weight and height.

The European Organization for Cooperation on Cancer Prevention Studies/International Union of Nutritional Sciences (ECP/IUNS) (Geboers *et al.,* 1985a) concluded that the epidemiological and experimental evidence suggests that a high-fat diet is associated with an increased risk of several cancers, especially cancer of the breast, colon, and prostate, and recommended a reduction of fat to 30% of total calories. However, they and others (Pariza, 1984) also agree that the epidemiological and experimental evidence is not consistent enough to reach firm conclusions or to make recommendations about specific components. The data for prostatic cancer remain somewhat unconvincing (Higginson, 1982). Scandinavian data suggest that high intake of dietary fiber may be more important than intake of dietary fat, and the present authors believe that the interrelation between fiber and fat warrants further examination before this question can be satisfactorily answered. Whether dietary patterns must be instituted in early life to have an impact, at least on breast and prostatic cancers, also requires further investigation. Contrary to the view of the NAS report (1982), we are disturbed by the lack of effect that has been seen on breast, colon, and prostatic cancer patterns in the United States and Australia, despite the significant changes in the intake and types of fat that have occurred over at least three decades.

3.2.3. Conclusion

The overall data suggest that fat may be related to cancer induction, notably of the breast and the colon in humans. But there are many inconsistencies in the available evidence which make simple causal hypotheses unlikely, preventing specific advice regarding individual types of fat. On the other hand, it is difficult to argue categorically that reduction in fat calories from 40% to 30% would be without benefit for cancer as well as heart disease, although the data from Scandinavia suggest that other modifications in diet, notable increasing fiber, may be as effective. Until these complexities are further understood, it is difficult to recommend wholeheartedly that populations markedly modify their dietary fat habits on grounds of cancer causation alone.

3.3. Cholesterol

The data regarding the role of cholesterol in human cancer are inconsistent, and reports that low serum cholesterol is associated with a higher frequency of colon cancer have aroused interest. Many of the observational studies relating serum cholesterol to subsequent cancer come from long-term prospective cohort studies in which cardiovascular disease was the primary outcome of interest. While cancer mortality was usually well recorded, morbidity and confounding factors for cancer risk were often not measured.

Available studies indicate that dietary cholesterol is weakly to moderately linked to increased risk of cancers of the colon, breast, and, possibly, prostate and lung. However, the close correlation of cholesterol with other components of dietary fat, and with other nutrients, prevents a causal link from being inferred (Lilienfeld, 1981; Feinleib, 1983; McMichael *et al.*, 1984).

The NAS report (1982) concluded that the relationship between dietary cholesterol and cancer in humans was far from clear and that the inverse association between serum cholesterol levels and colon cancer mortality in males was inconsistent and inconclusive.

3.4. Protein

The importance of protein and the essential amino acids in the diet has been recognized for many years, and early studies examined their effects on experimental carcinogenesis in animals. Interest later concentrated on human liver cancer, since certain animal studies and the discovery of kwashiorkor suggested that protein deficiency played a role. More recently, however, most studies have given attention to the modulating effects of high-protein diets and foodstuffs.

3.4.1. Laboratory Studies

The earlier laboratory studies have been reviewed in the NAS report (1982). In brief, these studies showed that animals fed minimal amounts of protein tended to develop fewer tumors than the controls whether protein alone was considered or whether individual amino acids were used, notably cystine and lysine. The early studies of Tannenbaum (1942a,b, 1944, 1945a,b), Tannenbaum and Silverstone (1949, 1957), and Silverstone and Tannenbaum (1951) concluded that a low level of protein intake definitely reduced tumor responses but that when an adequate protein diet based on amino acid balance was fed, the expected incidence of tumors was approximately normal and was not further increased by excessive protein consumption. Further, the effect of protein was not confounded with total food or caloric intake nor related necessarily to change in body weight. These effects were observed in spontaneous tumors and in tumors induced by chemical carcinogens.

The relationship between protein and carcinogenesis is not straightforward. In general, a low-protein diet suppresses the carcinogenic process and subsequent growth and development of tumors, with an occasional exception. Thus low protein increases tumor yield in DMBA-treated animals. The NAS report (1982) could not determine whether general inhibition, at very high levels of protein, was due to reduced intake of food and total calories or to possibly toxic effects. Some authors have suggested changes in immune responses (Jose and Good, 1973). Although clearly demonstrated in severe protein deficiency in childhood, this hypothesis remains to be established. Earlier studies in Africa have been confusing owing to widespread stimulation of the immune system by parasites.

3.4.2. Human Studies

The data from human studies are confusing. Many conclusions are based on correlations and these are further confounded by the close association between high protein consumption and high-fat and -meat diets. Graham has pointed out that there is a fivefold range in protein ingested within the United States (1983c). Accordingly, he believes it is inappropriate to extrapolate from average per capita consumption to the comparatively few individuals who develop a specific cancer since few case history studies adequately cover the problem of early recall and protein intake over prolonged periods. Similar limitations apply to correlation with average fat consumption found in meats.

Tables I–III summarize part of the epidemiological literature and some of the inconsistencies and uncertainties reported. Thus, whereas a number of studies have found a correlation between protein and cancer of the breast, in some the correlation was stronger for fat, and thus at present it is inappropriate to draw definitive conclusions. Similar limitations are observed with colorectal cancer where a correlation was originally reported by Armstrong and Doll (1975), but again, the associations are stronger for fat and total protein. In the studies of Jensen (IARC, 1977; Jensen *et al.*, 1982) only fiber remained important when other variables were controlled. On the other hand, no such correlation was found in the United Kingdom by Bingham *et al.* (1979). Originally it was believed that the lower frequency of colorectal cancer in Mormons was due to a low intake of meat alone, but this was later shown not to be the case (Enstrom, 1975a, 1980).

The relationship to pancreatic cancer was described in Section 2.3.

3.4.3. Conclusion

In conclusion, the authors agree with the NAS report (1982) that while epidemiological studies have suggested possible associations, definite conclusions are difficult to establish in view of the high correlations between fat and protein, especially since many studies suggest that fat is the most active dietary component. The NAS report does not comment on the possible inhibitory benefits of a low-protein diet. However, as mentioned earlier, in countries where kwashiorkor (protein–calorie malnutrition) is prevalent, certain cancers prevalent in affluent societies tend to be rare. While animal studies suggest plausible biological explanations for attributing this effect to dietary deficiency, the relationship remains speculative. In the absence of definite proof, the authors believe that the present consensus of the scientific community is that protein intake has not been demonstrated to be significant in human carcinogenesis.

3.5. Carbohydrates (Including Fiber)

The human diet comprises two general classes of carbohydrate: monosaccharides, or simple sugars, and complex polysaccharides. The latter are subdivided into starch and nonstarch polysaccharides (NSP). NSP represent the cell walls of plant foods and may be considered the equivalent of dietary fiber (Cummings *et al.*, 1985).

The earlier literature on carbohydrates is reviewed in the NAS report (1982) and further evaluations were made by the American Association for Cancer Research (Lowenthal, 1983) and the joint European Organization for Cooperation in Cancer Prevention Studies/International Union of Nutritional Sciences (Joossens *et al.*, 1985). In contrast to fat and protein, little attention has been directed to the study of carbohydrates and the induction of cancer in humans. However, over the last two decades there has been growing interest in the inhibitory role of fiber or NSP.

3.5.1. Laboratory Studies

The experimental literature was fully reviewed in the 1982 NAS report and little can be added. Most laboratory studies suggest that a carbohydrate effect, when present, occurs in the later stages of carcinogenesis (promotion). To what extent this effect is specific, i.e., related to the type of carbohydrate, or nonspecific, i.e., related to caloric intake or obesity, is unclear and both possibilities may be involved. In the classical experiments of Tannenbaum (1942a,b, 1944, 1945a,b), the most striking and specific effect on carcinogenesis was through caloric restriction. However, the NAS concluded that most of the laboratory data were difficult to interpret because of generally poor experimental design and uncertainty as to the carbohydrate content of the foods used. Further, few studies were controlled for the caloric content of the experimental diets.

Some experimental animal studies suggest that the caloric effect may be most obvious in endocrine and endocrine-dependent tumors, but in view of the severe dietary manipulations involved and variations in species longevity, their relevance to humans is difficult to determine, in whom such variations are usually of a much lesser magnitude. Several authors (Bauer *et al.*, 1979; Hoehn and Carroll, 1979; Watanabe *et al.*, 1979; Glauert *et al.*, 1981; Kritchevsky, 1985) have shown that certain types of carbohydrate may promote experimental tumors in rats, and these findings need to be expanded.

Similar limitations affect the study of fiber on cancer induction in experimental animals. The inhibitory effect of fiber has been examined in terms of chemical carcinogens but, as pointed out by the NAS report (1982), such results are difficult to equate with epidemiological studies since most laboratory experiments have examined specific or individual components, whereas the latter have focused on fiber-containing foods. It is probably difficult to design an appropriate experiment since a strong carcinogen may mask the fiber effect. Further, it is necessary to consider fiber in relation to both direct intraluminal effects (i.e., bacterial flora) and more indirect systemic effects involving extraintestinal cancers.

3.5.2. Human Studies

The evaluation of the role of carbohydrates in modulating carcinogenesis in humans is complicated by a number of factors. The following confounding variables should be taken into consideration: (1) caloric intake, which is often related to carbohydrate intake, although other components of diet may be more important; (2) obesity, which is not necessarily related to excess carbohydrate ingestion; (3) the extent to which the enhancing activity of fat or protein in the diet may be dependent on the absolute or proportional amount in the diet; (4) recognition that in humans the impact of diet on cancer induction may be greatest in the preadolescent period, except possibly for colon or rectal cancer; (5) the fact that in Western industrial populations variations in dietary intake partly depend on cultural background and there may be considerable differences between social groups within the same country.

Further, in terms of fiber alone, the following are important: (1) type of carbohydrate, e.g., fiber, pentose or hextose sugar; there are now a number of informational studies on the physiological effects of different types of carbohydrates (Cummings, 1986); (2) interaction with caloric intake, including obesity or undernutrition; and (3) indirect effects, such as modifications of fecal flora. This large number of variables makes comparative studies both within and between countries difficult.

Some of the major epidemiological cancer studies are summarized in Tables I–III. Few of the studies are decisive in identifying a role for specific carbohydrate components. As stated in the NAS report (1982), correlation and case-control data are confusing and limited. While all reports confirm the role of obesity in cancers at certain sites, this cannot necessarily be attributed to carbohydrates. Willett and MacMahon (1984b) reviewed specific nutrients and only briefly mentioned caloric intake. They suggested the data were sufficient to accept an association between obesity and both endometrial and gallbladder cancers. They also concluded there was sufficient data to suggest an increase in breast cancer in postmenopausal women, but that height and other factors might also be related. In terms of cereals, early studies suggested that gastric cancer was associated with excessive cereal intake. However, in many parts of Africa where the diet is high in cereals, the incidence of both gastric cancer and colorectal cancer is low. In the extensive Japanese studies of Hirayama (1977, 1981, 1985), although the intake of rice was high and gastric cancer frequent, no positive correlation could be found with the amount of rice and wheat intake. In contrast, the higher the daily intake of rice and wheat, the lower the incidence of colorectal cancer. While this may reflect the quantity of fiber in the diet, other explanations are possible. The absence of a clear-cut consensus probably indicates that most scientists believe that the nutritive carbohydrates alone have no specific effect.

Nonstarch Carbohydrate. This subject has been extensively reviewed recently by Cummings (1985, 1986), who drew attention to the inconsistencies in the available data and has emphasized the importance of examining the chemistry of the fiber itself. In his report, Cummings points out that the hypothesis that dietary fiber prevents large-bowel cancer is largely due to Burkitt (1971), although its possible role had been identified earlier. While there are now over a dozen population studies showing a relation between large-bowel cancer mortality or incidence and fiber intake, Cummings has emphasized that there is still no general agreement as to the protective role. A recent experimental study in rats suggests an enhancing role for high fiber in colon cancer (Jacobs and Lupton, 1986).

The NAS report (1982) found "no conclusive evidence" to indicate that dietary fiber, as present in fruits, vegetables, and cereals, asserts a protective effect against colorectal cancer in humans. Both the NAS and Cummings now emphasize the need to study specific types of fiber components rather than total intake, a view supported by others (Jensen *et al.*, 1982; Bingham *et al.*, 1985). Preliminary studies emphasize the role of pentose NSPs (Bingham *et al.*, 1979). Cummings has emphasized several caveats in studying the physiological effects of dietary fiber in humans and making recommendations for increasing fiber intake. First, various fibers produce different effects at different sites and are known to differ in cholesterol-lowering and ion-binding properties. Second, fiber-containing foods often bind minerals and trace elements, such as iron, zinc, and calcium, leading to greater excretion. Finally, it is difficult to ascertain the relevance of physiological studies of the mode of fiber action in the gut in the absence of a proven mechanism for the cause of large-bowel cancer.

On the other hand, the Scandinavian data in particular strongly support the inverse relationship between fiber intake for breast and colorectal cancer and further suggest that fiber may counteract the effect of a high-fat diet at these two sites, even if the mechanism remains speculative (Jensen *et al.*, 1974, 1982). In view of its effect on other diseases of the large intestine, the present authors believe that an adequate dietary intake of fiber is advisable, as suggested by the ECP/IUNS group (Geboers *et al.*, 1985a).

4. Miscellaneous Dietary-Related Factors

4.1. Ingested Carcinogens

Aflatoxin is the only ingested carcinogenic contaminant for which reasonably strong evidence of an effect in humans is available. A toxic effect of bracken fern remains to be demonstrated. Although a number of man-made food additives or contaminants have been demonstrated to be animal carcinogens, studies in humans indicate no significant effects, and as yet no cancers have been attributed to such agents (NAS, 1982). This suggests that levels of exposure are so low as to be of no practical significance, especially if such exposures are considered in relation to the total burden of mutagens and naturally occurring carcinogenic initiators or enhancers found in the average diet (Ames, 1983). Nonetheless, prudence has dictated that obvious exposures to exogenous animal carcinogens should be controlled, and this is the basic policy in most industrial countries despite some controversy over the degree of control necessary for very small exposures. Reference should be made to the series of publications of the Joint FAO/WHO Expert Committee on Food Additives in this context.

4.2. N-Nitroso Compounds

There are, however, a class of compounds, notably the *N*-nitroso compounds, which are widely distributed in nature. These are potent carcinogens at many sites in many animal species (NAS, 1981). Nitrosamines are formed by the reaction of secondary or tertiary amines which are nitrosating agents. In foods, the agent is usually nitrous anhydride formed from nitrite in acidic solution.

Secondary and tertiary amines are found widely in nature, and nitrites, which occur frequently in plants, can be formed within the stomach from nitrates. There have been extensive studies of the formation of nitrosamines in foodstuffs and the amounts ingested by humans. Nonetheless, no specific cancer in humans has as yet been identified as resulting from exposure to exogenous nitrosamines (Preussmann and Eisenbrand, 1984).

There has been increasing interest in the significance of endogenous *N*-nitroso formation, especially in the human stomach, following its demonstration in experimental animals. Bartsch and co-workers (1984) have developed a noninvasive test for studying such a reaction, and a number of new compounds have been identified. Extensive collaborative studies are now being made in a number of countries of *in vivo* formation of *N*-nitroso compounds in human subjects (IARC, 1985, pp. 30–33).

A recent study of esophageal cancer in a high-incidence area of China indicates that the inhabitants had higher nitrate intakes than those living in a lower-incidence area and showed an increase in the formation of certain compounds (Xu, 1981). Similarly, Correa *et al.* (1983) have suggested that certain high-incidence areas of gastric cancer and chronic gastritis in Latin America are associated with *N*-nitroso compounds in the stomach. It is not clear, however, to what extent chronic gastritis with achlorhydria may contribute to the formation of these compounds or whether the compounds themselves are directly responsible for the precancerous lesions (Reed, 1985).

There have been a number of studies on nitrate ingestion and gastric cancer, but to date most studies have failed to demonstrate any definitive causal relationship. Thus, while the role of endogenous *N*-nitroso formation is attractive as a cause of some human cancers, notably of the stomach and esophagus, further confirmation is required. Nevertheless, recommendations have been made to reduce the amount of nitrite and nitrate in preserved foods as much as possible to avoid their ingestion.

4.3. Inhibitors and Other Biologically Active Compounds in Food

Since 1970, considerable effort has been directed to the examination of inhibitors and inactivators in foodstuffs and their potential role in human cancer. The general literature has been reviewed by Wattenberg (1979, 1985, 1986), and an excellent review of the many naturally occurring inhibitors and mutagens found in food has recently also been published by Ames (1983). More than 12 different classes of compounds present in foods

Table IV. Inhibitors of Carcinogenesis[a]

Category of inhibitor	Chemical class	Inhibitory compounds
Compounds preventing formation of carcinogens from precursor compounds	Reductive acids tocopherols Phenols	Ascorbic acid[b] α-Tocopherol,[b] γ-tocopherol, caffeic acid,[b] ferulic acid[b]
Blocking agents	Phenols	2(3)-Tert-butylhydroxyanisole,[c] butylated hydroxytoluene,[c] ellagic acid,[b] caffeic acid,[b] ferulic acid,[b] p-hydroxycinnamic acid[b]
	Indoles	Indole-3-acetonitrile,[b] indole-3-carbinol,[b] 3,3'-diindolymethane[b]
	Aromatic isothiocyanates	Benzyl isothiocyanate,[b] phenethyl isothiocyanate[b]
	Coumarins	Coumarin,[b] limettin[b]
	Flavones	Quercetin pentamethyl ether[d]
Suppressing agents	Diterpenes	Kahweol palmitate[b]
	Retinoids and carotinoids	Retinyl palmitate,[b] retinyl acetate,[b] β-carotene[b]
	Selenium salts	Sodium selenite,[b] selenium dioxide,[b] selenious acid[b]
	Protease inhibitors	Soybean protease inhibitors
	Cyanates and isothiocyanates	Benzyl isothiocyanate[b]
	Phenols	2(3)-Tert-butylhydroxyanisole[c]
	Plant sterols	β-Sitosterol[b]
	Methylated xanthines	Caffeine[b]
	Others	Fumeric acid[b]

[a]Reprinted with permission from: Wattenberg, 1985, p. 51.
[b]Naturally occurring compound present in food.
[c]Synthetic antioxidant used as a food additive.
[d]The closely related compounds tangeretin and nobilitin occur in citrus fruits.

have inhibiting capacity (see Table IV). They are divided into three major categories, although their mechanisms of action are poorly understood.

4.3.1. Compounds Inhibiting Formation of Carcinogens

This group of inhibitors includes, for example, the possible role of ascorbic acid in inhibiting the formation of *N*-nitroso compounds in the stomach. Willett and MacMahon (1984a) have found little empirical evidence that vitamin C protects against cancer in humans, although there are numerous theoretical reasons to explore such relationships further. It may well be that very high dose levels are necessary over prolonged periods, but the results of such studies are not available.

A number of other compounds in foods have been identified which inhibit the formation of carcinogens from precursor compounds, including electrophiles. Although long suspected as possibly important in gastric cancer, the role of antioxidants in human cancer remains to be confirmed (see Section 4.4).

4.3.2. Blocking Agents

Blocking agents prevent carcinogens from reaching or reacting with the critical target sites. They can be classified according to their mechanisms of action:

1. Inhibiting the activation of a carcinogen to its ultimate carcinogenic form
2. Inducing increases in enzyme systems which enhance carcinogen detoxification
3. Scavenging the reactive forms of carcinogens

Although theoretically attractive, there is no evidence that such agents have been important in human disease, but the hypothesis provides an approach to designing chemopreventive studies.

4.3.3. Suppressing Agents

A relatively small number of compounds have been identified which inhibit carcinogenesis when administered subsequent to a carcinogenic stimulus that would otherwise lead to cancer. One of the most intensely studied is vitamin A, which has been found to modify differentiation of epithelial tissues. Various analogs of vitamin A have also been synthesized and their inhibitory properties studied. Another group is made up of selenium salts, which in experimental systems appear to have considerable inhibiting effects.

Data on vitamin A have been reviewed by Willett and MacMahon (1984a) and by Graham (1983a,b,c). While case history and correlation studies suggest an inverse relationship between cancer and vitamin A, diets high in vitamin A and retinoids are also high in green and yellow vegetables. These diets contain many of the other inhibiting agents described by Wattenberg (1979, 1985, 1986), thus offering an alternative explanation for these suggestive findings and complicating the design of definitive preventive studies based on food intake. Graham argues that green and yellow vegetables may provide a more suitable approach to cancer inhibition as their use avoids determining the actual intake of vitamins A and C and allows for the testing of a number of hypotheses. A number of studies including that of Ziegler *et al.* (1981) on esophageal cancer in U.S. blacks, have shown lower cancer risks for larynx, lungs, esophagus, stomach, colon, rectum, and prostate with high levels of ingestion of these vegetables. Friedman *et al.* (1986) found no correlation between serum retinol and lung cancer.

In conclusion, Graham believes that it is premature to claim that large amounts of vitamin A or retinoids might inhibit cancer (Graham, 1983b,c).

4.4. Tocopherols and Other Antioxidants

There are good experimental reasons to postulate that agents such as selenium might influence cancer in humans. In addition to animal studies, it has been suggested that lower levels of selenium are found in cancer patients. Nonetheless, variations in serum selenium levels between countries are not consistent with cancer patterns. Thus, the serum selenium distributions of the Finnish and American populations differ so much that the lowest quintile of the U.S. population overlaps the highest quintile of the Finnish population (Huttunen, 1986). The association of increased cancer risk with such widely different intakes raises the question that serum selenium is a nonspecific marker of cancer risk. In other studies from Finland, it has been shown that serum selenium is correlated with a serum cholesterol index, blood hemoglobin, and indicators of general health (Willett *et al.,* 1983; Salonen *et al.,* 1984, 1985). These findings reinforce the views expressed by Willett and MacMahon (1984b) and the NAS report (1982) concerning the need for dose–response effects of selenium on the occurrence of cancer in humans.

4.5. Lipotropes

There have been extensive studies indicating that lipotrope deficiency (choline, methionine, folic acid, and vitamin B_{12}) may cause cancer of the liver in experimental animals. Although earlier experimental studies were flawed by possible dietary contamination with aflatoxin, there appears to be no doubt as to these findings. On the other hand, there is no evidence that lipotrope deficiency is of any significance in relation to human liver cancer, although such a possibility was hypothesized in the 1950s. It is very difficult to find a human diet that is markedly deficient in these micronutrients, although it is been suggested that relative deficiencies can occur in heavy drinkers.

4.6. Iron

Excessive iron intake has been related to cancer induction in experimental animals, especially of the liver, when administered in conjunction with hepatal carcinogens. However, there is little evidence that iron overload has a similar impact in humans, apart from certain specific conditions, such as idiopathic hemochromatosis. For example, southern blacks in Africa show enormous deposits of iron in the liver and other organs, but show no consistent evidence of any related increase of cancer at these sites. In contrast, cancers of the hypopharynx have been reported from Scandinavia and other countries, especially in women with iron and other deficiencies. The exact mechanisms, however, remain to be determined.

4.7. Effects of Cooking

In the 1940s and 1950s, there was considerable interest in carcinogens formed during cooking, especially in the effects of heat on oils and fats and, more recently, on proteins.

A number of studies have indicated the presence of animal carcinogens in such heated foods and several authors have emphasized the importance of mutagens formed from pyrolyzed amino acids (Matsumoto *et al.*, 1977, 1978; Nagao *et al.*, 1977a,b; Sugimura *et al.*, 1977). Nonetheless, case history studies to date, especially on the gastrointestinal tract, have failed to demonstrate any significant correlation between cooking methods and cancer. While guidelines have been offered regarding the potential role of bacon and many smoked foods, the possible formation of *N*-nitroso compounds offers another plausible hypothesis. It is unlikely that further studies in this area will add significantly to the present body of information.

4.8. Intestinal Flora

There has been considerable interest in the role of diet in modifying the bacterial flora within the intestinal tract and the possible formation of carcinogens by bacteria (Hill, 1985). While such bacterial modifications have been observed following different dietary patterns, it remains to be demonstrated that these are significantly related to intestinal cancer. Although carcinogens within the feces have been observed, their exact role remains uncertain. The subject is further complicated by the modifications such diets induce in terms of bile salts and other factors.

4.9. Age

Migrant and experimental studies indicate that diet, if important, has its action in early life. Thus migrants from Japan to North America show a relatively slow decrease in gastric cancer and increases in cancers of the prostate and breast. Such changes have been hypothesized to imply that dietary effects are associated with late-stage carcinogenesis, enhancing already initiated cells. However, no hypotheses have been put forward to explain why initiation in dietary-related tumors varies significantly between communities, and to what extent the effects may be dependent on changes in metabolism induced by childhood diet which may program enzymes for activating or deactivating carcinogens.

In contrast to the above sites, relatively rapid changes in incidence have been observed in cancer of the colon and rectum in migrants, suggesting that promoting factors in the diet may be involved. Experimental work does support a potential indirect role of diet operating through hormonal status and other factors and, presently, these seem the most plausible biological hypotheses. If, however, the age at which a dietary modification occurs is most important in the young, then dietary changes in adult life may not have significant impact. This may explain to some extent why no significant temporal changes have yet been observed in many dietary-related cancers which can be related to the major changes in the American and European dietary patterns that have occurred over the last four decades.

5. Conclusions and Recommendations

In evaluating the effects of diet, the total diet as well as particular components should be considered. Further, in considering macronutrients, the potential role of related micronutrients must be considered, as well as biologically active, naturally occurring chemicals and contaminants. Numerous guidelines have been promulgated, with varying degrees of emphasis, in recent years regarding diet and human cancer (Palmer, 1983) which have given rise to controversy (Pariza, 1984). However, more recent reports have tended to be less vigorous in making claims and more mindful of the inconsistencies in the data and the absence of simple relationships (Geboers *et al.*, 1985a; Gori, 1986b).

In fact, nearly all reports and guidelines include sufficient caveats to permit the informed reader to recognize the uncertainties involved, although often insufficiently emphasized. Whereas earlier reports stressed the role of fat, the ECP/IUNS group tended to be more emphatic about the potential role of vitamin A and carotene (Geboers *et al.*, 1985a; Gori, 1986b). They recommend a high and varied consumption of different types of vegetables and fruits, including green vegetables, legumes, and root vegetables, and lower fat sources of protein, such as fish and nonfat dairy products. A nutrient-rich diet is also recommended, including the reduction of processed foods high in fat, salt, and refined sugar which provide empty calories, although some might challenge the view that this represents meaningful physiological differences in terms of cancer.

The ECP/IUNS group did not believe that the current evidence for the role of vitamins and other dietary micronutrients in preventing human cancer justified any new dietary recommendations or reformulation of existing recommendations. The consensus statement on provisional dietary guidelines by this group reaffirmed the view that not more than 30% of total food energy should come from fat and that a widely varied diet was desirable, including foods that are rich in complex carbohydrates, although the Scandinavian data presented did not confirm this view. It was also suggested that maintaining appropriate body weight and a low-salt diet would be beneficial, as well as the use of fresh or minimally processed foods rather than cured, pickled, or traditionally smoked foods. Again, it is to be noted that, as in the case of other guideline reports, some of the above recommendations lack strong supportive data. Unfortunately, the ECP/IUNS group did not draw attention to the influence of age and the possibility that in later adult life such recommendations may have little impact.

The present authors believe that an optimum diet for cancer still remains to be defined in view of the many unresolved uncertainties. A balanced diet, with a moderate amount of undernutrition and adequate roughage beginning in early life, may have the strongest scientific base. However, diets may vary widely between individuals and between different ethnic groups living under a variety of conditions with similar cancer experiences. We concur with the final paragraph of the NAS (1982) report, which states:

> . . . the data are not sufficient to quantitate the contribution of diet to the overall cancer risk or to determine the percent reduction in risk that might be achieved by dietary modifications. (Ch. 18, pp. 18–11)

In conclusion, reaffirming our introductory remarks, we are of the view that strong recommendations tend to reflect the strength of personal convictions regarding the role of diet and cancer, rather than any real disagreement as to the data base for humans. It is disappointing to see how little real progress on human diet and cancer has been made since 1960, but perhaps not surprising considering the complexities of the relationship.

ACKNOWLEDGMENTS. We are indebted to Dana F. Flavin for collating some of the animal data and to Midge Young for her tireless preparations of the manuscript.

6. References

Acheson, E. D., and Doll, R., 1964, Dietary factors in carcinoma of the stomach: A study of 100 cases and 200 controls, *Gut* **5:**126–131.

Ames, B. N., 1983, Dietary carcinogens and anticarcinogens, oxygen radicals and degenerative diseases, *Science* **221:**1256–1264.

Armstrong, B., and Doll, R., 1975, Environmental factors and cancer incidence and mortality in different countries, with special reference to dietary practice, *Int. J. Cancer* **15:**617–631.

Armstrong, B., Garrod, A., and Doll, R., 1976, A retrospective study of renal cancer with special reference to coffee and animal protein consumption, *Br. J. Cancer* **33:**127–136.

Austin, D. F., 1982, Larynx, in: *Cancer Epidemiology and Prevention* (D. Schottenfeld and J. F. Fraumeni, Jr., eds.), Saunders, Philadelphia, pp. 554–563.

Bartsch, H., Ohshima, H., Muñoz, N., Crespi, M., Cassale, V., Ramazotti, V., Lambert, R., Minaire, Y., Forichon, J., and Walters, C. L., 1984, *In vivo* nitrosation, precancerous lesions and cancers of the gastro-intestinal tract: On-going studies and preliminary results, in: N-*Nitroso Compounds: Occurrence, Biological Effects and Relevance to Human Cancer,* IARC Scientific Publications No. 57 (I. K. O'Neill, R. C. von Borstel, J. E. Long, C. T. Miller, and H. Bartsch, eds.), International Agency for Research on Cancer, Lyon, pp. 955–962.

Bauer, H. G., Asp, N. G., Oste, R., Dahlqvist, A., and Fredlund, P. E., 1979, Effect of dietary fiber on the induction of colorectal tumors and fecal glucuronidase activity in the rat, *Cancer Res.* **39:**3752–3756.

Beasley, R. P., Lin, C. C., Hwan, L. Y., and Chien, C. S., 1981, Hepatocellular carcinoma and hepatitis B virus: A prospective study of 22,707 men in Taiwan, *Lancet* **2:**1129–1133.

Berg, J. W., and Howell, M. A., 1974, The geographic pathology of bowel cancer, *Cancer* **34:**805–814.

Bingham, S., Williams, D. R., Cole, T. J., and James, W. P., 1979, Dietary fibre and regional large-bowel cancer mortality in Britain, *Br. J. Cancer* **40:**456–463.

Bingham, S. A., Williams, D. R. R., and Cummings, J. H., 1985, Dietary fibre consumption in Britain; New estimates and their relation to large bowel cancer mortality, *Br. J. Cancer* **52:**399–402.

Bjelke, E., 1974, Epidemiologic studies of cancer of the stomach, colon and rectum with special emphasis on the role of diet, *Scand. J. Gastroenterol.* **31:**[Suppl.] 1–235.

Blair, A., and Fraumeni, J. F., Jr., 1978, Geographic patterns of prostate cancer in the United States, *J. Natl. Cancer Inst.* **61:**1379–1384.

Broitman, S. A., Vitale, J. J., Vavrousek-Jakuba, E., and Gottlieb, L. S., 1977, Polyunsaturated fat, cholesterol and large bowel tumorigenesis, *Cancer* **40:**2455–2463.

Broitman, S. A., Velez, H., and Vitale, J. J., 1981, A possible role of iron deficiency in gastric cancer in Colombia, *Adv. Exp. Med. Biol.* **135:**155–181.

Burkitt, D. P., 1971, Epidemiology of cancer of the colon and rectum, *Cancer* **28:**3–13.

Carroll, K. K., 1975, Experimental evidence of dietary factors and hormone-dependent cancers, *Cancer Res.* **35:**3374–3383.

Carroll, K. K., 1980, Lipids and carcinogenesis, *J. Environ. Pathol. Toxicol.* **3**(4):253–271.

Carroll, K. K., 1984, Influence of diet on mammary cancer, *Nutr. Cancer* **2:**232–236.

Carroll, K. K., and Khor, H. T., 1970, Effects of dietary fat and dose level of 7,12-dimethylbenz(α)anthracene on mammary tumor incidence in rats, *Cancer Res.* **30:**2260–2264.

Carroll, K. K., and Khor, H. T., 1971, Effects of level and type of dietary fat on incidence of mammary tumors induced in female Sprague–Dawley rats by 7,12-dimethylbenz(α)anthracene, *Lipids* **6:**415–420.

Carroll, K. K., and Khor, H. T., 1975, Dietary fat in relation to tumorigenesis, *Prog. Biochem. Pharmacol.* **10:**308–353.

Cook-Mozaffari, P. J., Azordegan, F., Day, N. E., Ressicaud, A., Sabai, D., and Aramesh, B., 1979, Oesophageal cancer studies in the Caspian Littoral of Iran: Results of a case–control study, *Br. J. Cancer* **39:**293–309.

Correa, P., Haenszel, W., Cuello, W., Tannenbaum, S., and Archer, M., 1975, A model for gastric cancer epidemiology, *Lancet* **2:**58–59.

Correa, P., Cuello, C., Fajardo, L. F., Haenszel, W., Bolanos, O., and de Raminez, B., 1983, Diet and gastric cancer: Nutrition survey in a high risk area, *J. Natl. Cancer Inst.* **70:**673–678.

Cummings, J. H., 1985, Cancer of the large bowel, in: *Dietary Fiber, Fiber-Depleted Foods and Disease* (H. S. Trowell, D. Burkitt, and K. W. Heaton, eds.), Academic Press, New York, pp. 161–189.

Cummings, J. H., 1986, Dietary carbohydrates and cancer, *Nutr. Cancer* **8**:10–14.

Cummings, J. H., Southgate, D. A. T., Branch, W., Houston, H., Jenkins, D. J., and James, W. P., 1978, Colonic response to dietary fibre from carrot, cabbage, apple, bran and guar gum, *Lancet* **1**:5–8.

Cummings, J. H., Englyst, H. N., and Wood, R., 1985, Determination of dietary fibre in cereals and cereal products. Collaborative Trials. Part I. Initial Trial, *J. Assoc. Off. Publ. Analysts* **23**:1–35.

Dales, L. G., Friedman, G. D., Ury, H. K., Grossman, S., and Williams, S. R., 1979, A case–control study of relationships of diet and other traits to colorectal cancer in American blacks, *Am. J. Epidemiol.* **109**:132–144.

Day, N. E., Muñoz, N., and Ghadirian, P., 1982, The epidemiology of oesophageal cancer: A review, in: *Epidemiology of Cancer of the Digestive Tract* (P. Correa and W. Haenszel, eds.), Martinus Nijhoff, The Hague, pp. 21–57.

De Jong, U. W., Breslow, N., Hong, J. G. E., Sridharan, M., and Shanmugaratnam, K., 1974, Aetiological factors in oesophageal cancer in Singapore Chinese, *Int. J. Cancer* **13**:291–303.

Delaney Amendment, Food Additives Amendment of 1958 to the Federal Food, Drug and Cosmetic Act, Public Law 85-929, Sept. 6, 1958.

de Waard, F., 1986, Dietary fat and mammary cancer, *Nutr. Cancer* **8**:5–8.

de Waard, F., and Baanders-van Halewijn, E. A., 1974, A prospective study in general practice on breast cancer risk in postmenopausal women, *Int. J. Cancer* **14**:153–160.

Doll, R., and Peto, R., 1981, The causes of cancer: Quantitative estimates of avoidable risks of cancer in the United States today, *J. Natl. Cancer Inst.* **66**:1192–1308.

Drasar, B. S., and Irving, D., 1973, Environmental factors and cancer of the colon and breast, *Br. J. Cancer* **27**:167–172.

Dungal, H., 1961, The special problem of cancer of the stomach in Iceland, *J.A.M.A.* **178**:789–798.

Enig, M. G., Munn, R. J., and Keeney, M., 1978, Dietary fat and cancer trends—A critique, *Fed. Proc.* **37**:2215–2220.

Enstrom, J. E., 1975a, Cancer mortality among Mormons, *Cancer* **36**:325–341.

Enstrom, J. E., 1975b, Colorectal cancer and consumption of beef and fat, *Br. J. Cancer* **32**:432–439.

Enstrom, J. E., 1980, Health and dietary practices and cancer mortality among California Mormons, in: *Cancer Incidence in Defined Populations,* Banbury Report 4 (J. Cairns, J. L. Lyon, and M. Skolnick, eds.), Cold Spring Harbor Laboratory, New York, pp. 69–92.

Feinleib, M., 1983, Review of the epidemiological evidence for a possible relatinship between hypo-cholesterolemia and cancer, *Cancer Res.* **43**[Suppl.]:2503s–2507s.

Fraser, P., 1985, Nitrates: Epidemiological evidence, in: *Interpretation of Negative Epidemiological Evidence for Carcinogenicity,* IARC Scientific Publication No. 65 (N. J. Wald and R. Doll, eds.), International Agency for Cancer Research, Lyon, pp. 183–194.

Friedman, G. D., Blaner, W. S., Goodman, D. S., Vogelman, J. H., Brind, J. L., Hoover, R., Fireman, B. H., and Orentreich, N., 1986, Serum retinol and retinol-binding protein levels do not predict subsequent lung cancer, *Am. J. Epidemiol.* **123**:781–899.

Gaskill, S. P., McGuire, W. L., Osborne, C. K., and Stern, M. P., 1979, Breast cancer mortality and diet in the United States, *Cancer Res.* **39**:3628–3637.

Geboers, J., Joossens, J. V., and Carroll, K. K., 1985a, Introductory remarks to the consensus statement on provisional dietary guidelines, in: *Diet and Human Carcinogenesis* (J. V. Joossens, M. J. Hill, and J. Geboers, eds.), Excerpta Medica, New York, pp. 337–342.

Geboers, J., Joossens, J. V., Kesteloot, H., 1985b, Epidemiology of stomach cancer, in: *Diet and Human Carcinogenesis* (J. V. Joossens, M. J. Hill, and J. Geboers, eds.), Excerpta Medica, New York, pp. 81–95.

Ghadirian, P., Stein, G., Gorodestzky, C., Roberfroid, M., Mahon, G. A. T., Bartsch, H., and Day, N. E., 1985, Oesophageal cancer studies in the Caspian Littoral of Iran: Some residual results, including opium use as a risk factor, *Int. J. Cancer* **35**:593–597.

Glauert, H. P., Bennink, M. R., and Sander, C. H., 1981, Enhancement of 1,2-dimethylhydrazine-induced colon carcinogenesis in mice by dietary agar, *Food Cosmet. Toxicol.* **19**:281–286.

Gori, G. B. (ed.), 1986a, A symposium: Proceedings of a Joint ECP–IUNS Workshop on Diet and Human Carcinogenesis (Aarhus, Denmark: June, 1985), *Nutr. Cancer* **8**:1–41.

Gori, G. B. (ed.), 1986b, Consensus statement on provisional dietary guidelines, *Nutr. Cancer* **8**:39–40.

Graham, S., 1983a, Results of case–control studies of diet and cancer in Buffalo, New York, *Cancer Res.* **43**:[Suppl.] 2409s–2413s.

Graham, S., 1983b, Toward a dietary prevention of cancer, *Epidemiol. Rev.* **5**:38–50.

Graham, S., 1983c, Diet and cancer: Epidemiologic aspects, in: *Reviews in Cancer Epidemiology,* Vol. 2 (A. M. Lilienfield, ed.), Elsevier, New York, pp. 1–45.

Graham, S., Schotz, W., and Martino, P., 1972, Alimentary factors in the epidemiology of gastric cancer, *Cancer* **30**:927–938.

Graham, S., Dayal, H., Swanson, M., Mittelman, A., and Wilkinson, G., 1978, Diet in the epidemiology of cancer of the colon and rectum, *J. Natl. Cancer Inst.* **61**:709–714.

Graham, S., Mettlin, C., Marshall, J., Priore, R., Rzepka, T., and Shedd, D., 1981, Dietary factors in the epidemiology of cancer of the larynx, *Am. J. Epidemiol.* **113**:675–680.

Graham, S., Marshall, J., Mettlin, C., Rzepka, T., Nemoto, T., and Byers, T., 1982, Diet in the epidemiology of breast cancer, *Am. J. Epidemiol.* **116**:68–75.

Gray, G. E., Pike, M. C., and Henderson, B. E., 1979, Breast-cancer incidence and mortality rates in different countries in relation to known risk factors and dietary practices, *Br. J. Cancer* **39**:1–7.

Gregor, O., Toman, R., and Prusova, F., 1969, Gastrointestinal cancer and nutrition, *Gut* **10**:1031–1034.

Haenszel, W., 1961, Cancer mortality among the foreign-born in the United States, *J. Natl. Cancer Inst.* **26**:37–132.

Haenszel, W., and Dawson, E. A., 1965, A note on mortality from cancer of the colon and rectum in the United States, *Cancer* **18**:265–272.

Haenszel, W., Kurihara, M., Segi, M., and Lee, R. K. C., 1972, Stomach cancer among Japanese in Hawaii, *J. Natl. Cancer Inst.* **49**:969–988.

Haenszel, W., Berg, J. W., Segi, M., Kurihara, M., and Locke, F. B., 1973, Large bowel cancer in Hawaiian Japanese, *J. Natl. Cancer Inst.* **51**:1765–1779.

Haenszel, W., Locke, F. B., and Segi, M., 1980, A case–control study of large bowel cancer in Japan, *J. Natl. Cancer Inst.* **64**:17–22.

Hakama, M., and Saxén, E. A., 1967, Cereal consumption and gastric cancer, *Int. J. Cancer* **2**:265–268.

Hems, G., 1978, The contribution of diet and child bearing to breast-cancer rates, *Br. J. Cancer* **37**:974–982.

Hems, G., 1980, Associations between breast-cancer mortality rates, child-bearing and diet in the United Kingdom, *Br. J. Cancer* **41**:429–437.

Hems, G., and Stuart, A., 1975, Breast cancer rates in populations of single women, *Br. J. Cancer* **31**:118–123.

Higginson, J., 1956, Primary carcinoma of the liver in Africa, *Br. J. Cancer* **10**:609–622.

Higginson, J., 1966, Etiological factors in gastro-intestinal cancer in man, *J. Natl. Cancer Inst.* **37**:527–545.

Higginson, J., 1982, Comments on the Diet, Nutrition and Cancer Report of the National Academy of Sciences 1982, in: *Diet, Nutrition and Cancer: A critique,* Council for Agricultural Science and Technology, Special Pub. No. 13, pp. 37–39.

Higginson, J., and Muir, C. S., 1979, Environmental carcinogenesis: Misconceptions and limitations to cancer control, *J. Natl. Cancer Inst.* **63**:1291–1298.

Higginson, J., and Oettlé, A. G., 1960, Cancer incidence in the Bantu and "Cape Colored" races of South Africa: Report of a cancer survey in the Transvaal (1953–55), *J. Natl. Cancer Inst.* **24**:589–671.

Hill, M. J., 1985, Mechanisms of colorectal carcinogenesis, in: *Diet and Human Carcinogenesis* (J. V. Joossens, M. J. Hill, and J. Geboers, eds.), Excerpta Medica, New York, pp. 149–163.

Hill, P., Wynder, E. L., Helman, P., Hickman, R., Rona, G., and Kuno, K., 1976, Plasma hormone levels in different ethnic populations of women, *Cancer Res.* **36**:2297–2301.

Hirayama, T., 1977, Changing patterns of cancer in Japan with special reference to the decrease in stomach cancer mortality, in: *Origins of Human Cancer, Book A: Incidence of Cancer in Humans* (H. H. Hiatt, J. D. Watson, and J. A. Winsten, eds.), Cold Spring Harbor Laboratory, New York, pp. 55–75.

Hirayama, T., 1978, Epidemiology of breast cancer with special reference to the role of diet, *Prev. Med.* **7**:173–195.

Hirayama, T., 1979, Epidemiology of prostate cancer with special reference to the role of diet, *Nat. Cancer Inst. Mono.* **53**:149–155.

Hirayama, T., 1981, A large-scale cohort study on the relationship between diet and selected cancers of the digestive organs, in: *Gastrointestinal Cancer, Endogenous Factors,* Banbury Report 7 (W. R. Bruce, P. Correa, M. Lipkin, S. R. Tannenbaum, and T. D. Wilkins, eds.), Cold Spring Harbor Laboratory, New York, pp. 409–429.

Hirayama, T., 1982, Epidemiology of human carcinogenesis: A review of food-related diseases, in: *Carcinogens and Mutagens in the Environment,* Volume 1 (H. F. Stich, ed.), CRC Press, Boca Raton, FL, pp. 13–30.

Hirayama, T., 1985, Diet and cancer: Feasibility and importance of prospective cohort study, in: *Diet and Human Carcinogenesis* (J. V. Joossens, M. J. Hill and J. Geboers, eds.), Excerpta Medica, New York, pp. 191–198.

Hoehn, S. K., and Carroll, K. K., 1979, Effects of dietary carbohydrate on the incidence of mammary tumors induced in rats by 7,12-dimethylbenz(α)anthracene, *Nutr. Cancer* **1**:27–30.

Hopkins, G. J., and Carroll, K. K., 1979, Relationship between amount and type of dietary fat in promotion of mammary carcinogenesis induced by 7,12-dimethylbenz(α)anthracene, *J. Natl. Cancer Inst.* **62**:1009–1012.

Horie, A., Kohchi, S., and Kuratsune, M., 1965, Carcinogenesis in the esophagus. II. Experimental production of esophageal cancer by administration of ethanolic solution of carcinogens, *Gann* **56**:429–441.

Howell, M. A., 1974, Factor analysis of international cancer mortality data and *per capita* food consumption, *Br. J. Cancer* **29**:328–336.

Howell, M. A., 1975, Diet as an etiological factor in the development of cancers of the colon and rectum, *J. Chronic Dis.* **28**:67–80.

Huttunen, J. K., 1986, Vitamins, trace elements and cancer, *Nutr. Cancer* **8**:19–22.

International Agency for Research on Cancer (IARC), Intestinal Microecology Group, 1977, Dietary fibre, transit-time, faecal bacteria, steroids and colon cancer in two Scandinavian populations, *Lancet* **2**:207–211.

International Agency for Research on Cancer (IARC), 1985, *Annual Report,* Lyon.

Ishii, K., Nakamura, K., Ozaki, H., Yamada, N., and Takeuchi, T., 1968, Epidemiological problems of pancreas cancer [In Japanese], *Jpn. J. Clin. Med.* **26**:1839–1842.

Jacobs, L. R., and Lupton, J. R., 1986, Relationship between colonic luminal pH, cell proliferation, and colon carcinogenesis in 1,2-dimethylhydrazine treated rats fed high fiber diets, *Cancer Res.* **46**:1727–1734.

Jain, M., Cook, G. M., Grace, F. G., Howe, M. G., and Miller, A. B., 1980, A case-control study of diet and colo-rectal cancer, *Int. J. Cancer* **26**:757–768.

Jensen, O. M., 1985, The role of diet in colorectal cancer, in: *Diet and Human Carcinogenesis* (J. V. Joossens, M. J. Hill, J. Geboers, eds.), Excerpta Medica, New York, pp. 137–147.

Jensen, O. M., 1986, Coffee and cancer, in: *Genetic Toxicology of the Diet,* Alan R. Liss, New York, pp. 287–297.

Jensen, O. M., Mosbech, J., Salaspuro, M., and Jhamäki, T., 1974, A comparative study of the diagnostic basis for cancer of the colon and cancer of the rectum in Denmark and Finland, *Int. J. Epidemiol.* **3**:183–186.

Jensen, O. M., MacLennan, R., and Wahrendorf, J., 1982, Diet, bowel function, fecal characteristics, and large bowel cancer in Denmark and Finland, *Nutr. Cancer* **4**:5–19.

Joossens, J. V., 1986, Salt and cancer, *Nutr. Cancer* **8**:29–32.

Joossens, J. V., Hill, M. J., and Geboers, J. (eds.), 1985, *Diet and Human Carcinogenesis,* Proceedings of the 3rd Annual Symposium of the European Organization for Cooperation in Cancer Prevention Studies (ECP), Aarhus, Denmark, June 19–21, Excerpta Medica, New York.

Jose, D. G., and Good, R. A., 1973, Quantitative effects of nutritional essential amino acid deficiency upon immune responses to tumors in mice, *J. Exp. Med.* **137**:1–9.

Kannel, W. B., 1978, Recent findings of the Framingham Study, *Resident Staff Physician* **24**:56–71.

Kinlen, L. J., 1982, Meat and fat consumption and cancer mortality: Study of strict religious orders in Britain, *Lancet* **1**:946–949.

Knox, E. G., 1977, Foods and diseases, *Br. J. Prev. Soc. Med.* **31**:71–80.

Kolonel, L. N., Nomura, A. M. Y., Hirohata, T., Hankin, J. H., and Hinds, M. W., 1981a, Association of diet and place of birth with stomach cancer incidence in Hawaii Japanese and Caucasians, *Am. J. Clin. Nutr.* **34**:2478–2485.

Kolonel, L. N., Hankin, J. H., Lee, J., Chu, S. Y., Nomura, A. M. Y., and Hinds, M. W., 1981b, Nutrient intakes in relation to cancer incidence in Hawaii, *Br. J. Cancer* **44**:332–339.

Kolonel, L. N., Nomura, A. M. Y., Hinds, M. W., Hirohata, T., Hankin, J. H., and Lee, J., 1983, Role of diet in cancer incidence in Hawaii, *Cancer Res.* **43**[Suppl.]:2397–2402.

Kritchevsky, D., 1985, Dietary fiber and cancer, *Nutr. Cancer* **6**:213–219.

Kritchevsky, D., Weber, M. M., and Klurfeld, D. M., 1984, Dietary fat versus caloric content in initiation and promotion of 7,12-dimethylbenz(α)anthracene induced mammary tumorigenesis in rats, *Cancer Res.* **44**:3174–3177.

Kurihara, M., Aoki, K., and Tominaga, S. (eds.), 1984, *Cancer Statistics in the World,* University of Nagoya Press, Nagoya.

Lea, A. J., 1967, Neoplasms and environmental factors, *Ann. R. Coll. Surg. Engl.* **41**:432–438.

Lilienfeld, A. M., 1981, The Humean fog: Cancer and cholesterol, *Am. J. Epidemiol.* **114**:1–4.

Linsell, C. A., and Peers, F. G., 1977, Aflaxtoxin and liver cell cancer, *Trans. R. Soc. Trop. Med. Hyg.* **71**:471–477.

Liu, K., Stamler, J., Moss, D., Garside, D., Persky, V., and Soltero, I., 1979, Dietary cholesterol, fat, and fibre, and colon cancer mortality: An analysis of international data, *Lancet* **2**:782–785.

Lowenthal, J. P., (ed.), 1983, Workshop conference on nutrition in cancer causation and prevention, *Cancer Res.* **43**[Suppl.]:2389s–2518s.

Lubin, J. H., Blot, W. J., Burns, P. E., Ziegler, R. G., Lees, A. W., and, Fraumeni, J. F., Jr., 1981, Dietary factors and breast cancer risk, *Int. J. Cancer* **28**:685–689.

Lyon, J. L., and Sorenson, A. W., 1978, Colon cancer in a low-risk population, *Am. J. Clin. Nutr.* **31**:S227–S230.

Lyon, J. L., Gardner, J. W., West, D. W., and Mahoney, A. M., 1983, Methodological issues in epidemiological studies of diet and cancer, *Cancer Res.* **43**[Suppl.]:2392s–2396s.

Mahboudi, E., and Sayed, G. M., 1982, Oval Cavity and Pharynx, in: *Cancer Epidemiology and Prevention* (D. Schottenfeld, and J. F. Fraumeni, Jr., eds.), Saunders, Philadelphia, pp. 583–595.

Malhotra, S. L., 1977, Dietary factors in a study of colon cancer from a cancer registry, with special reference to the role of saliva, milk and fermented milk products and vegetable fibre, *Med. Hypotheses* **3**:122–126.

Manousos, O., Day, N. E., Trichopoulos, D., Gerovassilis, F., Tzonou, A., and Polychronopoulou, A., 1983, Diet and colorectal cancer: A case–control study in Greece, *Int. J. Cancer* **32**:1–5.

Marshall, J., Graham, S., Mettlin, C., Shedd, D., and Swanson, M., 1982, Diet in the epidemiology of oral cancer, *Nutri. Cancer* **3**:145–149.

Marshall, J., Graham, S., Byers, T., Swanson, M., and Brasure, J., 1983, Diet and smoking in the epidemiology of cancer of the cervix, *J. Natl. Cancer Inst.* **70**:847–851.

Martinez, I., Torres, R., Frias, Z., Colon, J. R., and Fernandez, N., 1979, Factors associated with adenocarcinomas of the large bowel in Puerto Rico, in: *Advances in Medical Oncology, Research and Education,* Volume 3 (J. M. Birch, ed.), Pergamon Press, New York, pp. 45–52.

Matsumoto, T., Yoshida, D., Mizusaki, S., and Okamoto, H., 1977, Mutagenic activity of amino acid pyrolyzates in salmonella typhimurium TA 98, *Mutat. Res.* **48**:279–286.

Matsumoto, T., Yoshida, D., Mizusaki, S., and Okamoto, H., 1978, Mutagenicities of the pyrolyzates of peptides and proteins, *Mutat. Res.* **56**:281–288.

McMichael, A. J., Jensen, O. M., Parkin, D. M., and Zaridze, D. G., 1984, Dietary and endogenous cholesterol and human cancer, *Epidemiol. Rev.* **6**:192–216.

Meinsma, L., 1964, Nutrition and cancer, *Voeding* **25**:357–365.

Mettlin, C., and Graham, S., 1979, Dietary risk factors in human bladder cancer, *Am. J. Epidemiol.* **110**:255–263.

Mettlin, C., Graham, S., and Swanson, M., 1979, Vitamin A and lung cancer, *J. Natl. Cancer Inst.* **62**:1435–1438.

Mettlin, C., Graham, S., Priore, R., and Swanson, M., 1980, Diet and cancer of the esophagus [Abstr.], *Am. J. Epidemiol.* **112**:422–423.

Mettlin, C., Graham, S., Priore, R., Marshall, J., and Swanson, M., 1981, Diet and cancer of the esophagus, *Nutr. Cancer* **2**:143–147.

Miller, A. B., Kelly, A., Choi, N. W., Matthews, V., Morgan, R. W., Munan, L., Burch, J. D., Feather, J., Howe, G. R., and Jain, M., 1978, A study of diet and breast cancer, *Am. J. Epidemiol.* **107**:499–509.

Miller, A. B., Howe, G. R., Jain, M., Craib, K. J. P., and Harrison, L., 1983, Food items and food groups as risk factors in a case–control study of diet and colo-rectal cancer, *Int. J. Cancer* **32**:155–161.

Modan, B., Lubin, F., Barell, V., Greenberg, R. A., Modan, M., and Graham, S., 1974, The role of starches in the etiology of gastric cancer, *Cancer* **34**:2087–2092.

Modan, B., Barell, V., Lubin, F., Modan, M., Greenberg, R. A., and Graham, S., 1975, Low-fiber intake as an etiologic factor in cancer of the colon, *J. Natl. Cancer Inst.* **55**:15–18.

Muñoz, N., Wahrendorf, J., Lu, J. B., Crespi, M., Day, N. E., Thurnham, D. I., Zhang, C. Y., Zheng, H. J., Li, B., Li, W. Y., Lin, G. L., Lan, X. Z., Correa, P., Grassi, A., O'Conor, G. T., and Bosch, F. X., 1985, No effect of riboflavine, retinol, and zinc on precancerous lesions of the oesophagus: A randomized double-blind intervention study in a high-risk population of China, *Lancet* **2**:111–114.

Nagao, M., Honda, M., Seino, Y., Yahagi, T., Kawachi, T., and Sugimura, T., 1977a, Mutagenicities of protein pyrolysates, *Cancer Lett.* **2**:335–340.

Nagao, M., Yahagi, T., Kawachi, T., Seino, Y., Honda, M., Matsukura, N., Sugimura, T., Wakabayashi, K., Tsuji, K., and Kosuge, T., 1977b, Mutagens in foods, and especially pyrolysis products of protein, in: *Progress in Genetic Toxicology* (D. Scott, B. A. Bridges, and F. H. Sobels, eds.), Elsevier/North-Holland, New York, pp. 259–264.

National Academy of Sciences, 1980, *Toward Healthful Diets,* National Academy Press, Washington, DC.

National Academy of Sciences, 1981, *The Health Effects of Nitrate, Nitrite, and* N-*Nitroso Compounds,* Part 1 of a 2-Part Study by the Committee on Nitrite and Alternative Curing Agents in Food, National Academy Press, Washington, DC.

National Academy of Sciences, 1982, Committee on Diet, Nutrition, and Cancer, *Diet, Nutrition, and Cancer,* National Academy Press, Washington, DC.

Nomura, A., Henderson, B. E., and Lee, J., 1978, Breast cancer and diet among the Japanese in Hawaii, *Am. J. Clin. Nutr.* **31**:2020–2025.

Palmer, S., 1983, Diet, nutrition, and cancer: The future of dietary policy, *Cancer Res.* **43**[Suppl.]:2509s–2514s.

Pariza, M. W., 1984, A perspective on diet, nutrition, and cancer, *J.A.M.A.* **251**:1455–1458.

Pernu, J., 1960, An epidemiological study on cancer of the digestive organs and respiratory system: A study based on 7078 cases, *Ann. Med. Intern. Fenn.* **33**[Suppl.]:1–137.

Phillips, R. L., 1975, Role of life-style and dietary habits in risk of cancer among Seventh-Day Adventists, *Cancer Res.* **35**:3513–3522.

Phillips, R. L., and Snowden, D. A., 1983, Association of meat and coffee use with cancers of the large bowel, breast, and prostate among Seventh-Day Adventists: Preliminary results, *Cancer Res.* **43**[Suppl.]:2403s–2408s.

Preussmann, R., and Eisenbrand, G., 1984, Chemical carcinogens, in: *Am. Chem. Soc. Monograph No. 182,* Washington, DC, pp. 829–868.

Reddy, B. S., Watanabe, K., Weisburger, J. H., and Wynder, E. L., 1977, Promoting effect of bile acids in colon carcinogenesis in germfree and conventional F344 rats, *Cancer Res.* **37**:3238–3242.

Reddy, B. S., Hedges, A. R., Laakso, K., and Wynder, E. L., 1978, Metabolic epidemiology of large bowel cancer: Fecal bulk and constitutents of high-risk North American and low-risk Finnish populations, *Cancer* **42**:2831–2838.

Reed, P. I., 1985, The role of *N*-nitroso compounds in gastric cancer, in: *Diet and Human Carcinogenesis* (J. V. Joossens, M. J. Hill, and J. Geboers, eds.), Excerpta Medica, New York, pp. 97–107.

Ross, M. H., and Bras, G., 1965, Tumor incidence patterns and nutrition in the rat, *J. Nutr.* **87**:245–260.

Ross, M. H., and Bras, G., 1973, Influence of protein under- and overnutrition on spontaneous tumor prevalence in the rat, *J. Nutr.* **103**:944–963.

Ross, M. H., Bras, G., and Ragbeer, M. S., 1970, Influence of protein and caloric intake upon spontaneous tumor incidence of the anterior pituitary gland of the rat, *J. Nutr.* **100**:177–189.

Rotkin, I. D., 1977, Studies in the epidemiology of prostatic cancer: Expanded sampling, *Cancer Treat. Rep.* **61**:173–180.

Salonen, J. T., Alfthan, G., Huttunen, J. K., and Puska, P., 1984, Association between serum selenium and risk of cancer, *Am. J. Epidemiol.* **120**:342–349.

Salonen, J. T., Salonen, R., Lappeteläinen, R., Mäenpää, P. H., Alfthan, G., and Puska, P., 1985, Risk of cancer in relation to serum concentrations of selenium and vitamins A and E: Matched case-control analysis of prospective data, *Br. Med. J.* **290**:417–420.

Schrauzer, G. N., 1976, Cancer mortality correlation studies. II. Regional association of mortalities with the consumption of foods and other commodities, *Med. Hypotheses* **2**:39–49.

Schuman, L. M., Mandell, J. S., Radke, A., Seal, U., and Halberg, F., 1982, Some selected features of the epidemiology of prostatic cancer: Minneapolis–St. Paul, Minnesota case–control study, 1976–1979, in: *Trends in Cancer Incidence: Causes and Practical Implications* (K. Magnus, ed.), Hemisphere, New York, pp. 345–454.

Shamberger, R. J., Tytko, S. A., and Willis, C. E., 1976, Antioxidants and Cancer, VI, Selenium and age-adjusted human cancer mortality, *Arch. Environ. Health* **31**:231–235.

Silverstone, H., and Tannenbaum, A., 1951, Proportion of dietary protein and the formation of spontaneous hepatomas in the mouse, *Cancer Res.* **11**:442–446.

Stewart, H. L., 1966, Site variation of alimentary tract cancer in man and experimental animals as indicators of disease etiology, in: *Proceedings of the International Cancer Congress,* Tokyo, Vol. 9, 15–49.

Stocks, P., 1970, Breast cancer anomalies, *Br. J. Cancer* **24:**633–643.

Sugimura, T., Kawachi, T., Nagao, M., Yahagi, T., Seino, Y., Okamoto, T., Shudo, K., Kosuge, T., Tsuji, K., Wakabayashi, K., Iitaka, Y., and Itai, A., 1977, Mutagenic principle(s) in tryptophan and phenylalanine pyrolysis products, *Proc. Jpn. Acad.* **53**(1):58–61.

Tannenbaum, A., 1942a, The genesis and growth of tumors. II. Effects of caloric restriction per se, *Cancer Res.* **2:**460–467.

Tannenbaum, A., 1942b, The genesis and growth of tumors. III. Effects of a high-fat diet, *Cancer Res.* **2:**468–475.

Tannenbaum, A., 1944, The dependence of the genesis of induced skin tumors on the caloric intake during different stages of carcinogenesis, *Cancer Res.* **4:**673–677.

Tannenbaum, A., 1945a, The dependence of tumor formation on the degree of caloric restriction, *Cancer Res.* **5:**609–615.

Tannenbaum, A., 1945b, The dependence of tumor formation on the composition of the calorie-restricted diet as well as on the degree of restriction, *Cancer Res.* **5:**616–625.

Tannenbaum, A., and Silverstone, H., 1949, The genesis and growth of tumors. IV. Effects of varying the proportion of protein (casein) in the diet, *Cancer Res.* **9:**162–173.

Tannenbaum, A., and Silverstone, H., 1957, Nutrition and the genesis of tumours, in: *Cancer,* Volume 1 (R. W. Raven, ed.), Butterworth, London, pp. 306–334.

Thomas, D. C., Siemiatycki, J., DeWar, R., Robins, J., Goldberg, M., and Armstrong, B. G., 1985, The problem of multiple inference in studies designed to generate hypotheses, *Am. J. Epidemiol.* **122:**1080–1095.

Tuyns, A., 1978, *Alcool et Cancer,* International Agency for Research on Cancer, Lyon.

Watanabe, K., Reddy, B. S., Weisburger, J. H., and Kritchevsky, D., 1979, Effect of dietary alfalfa, pectin and wheat bran on azoxymethane or methylnitrosourea-induced colon carcinogenesis in F344 rats, *J. Natl. Cancer Inst.* **63:**141–145.

Wattenberg, L. W., 1979, Inhibitors of carcinogenesis, in: *Carcinogens: Identification and Mechanisms of Action* (A. C. Griffin and C. R. Shaw, eds.), Raven Press, New York, pp. 299–316.

Wattenberg, L. W., 1985, Inhibitors of carcinogenesis and their implications for cancer prevention in humans, in: *Diet and Human Carcinogenesis* (J. V. Joossens, M. J. Hill, and J. Geboers, eds.), Excerpta Medica, New York, p. 51.

Wattenberg, L. W., 1986, Micronutrients and other microconstituents, *Nutr. Cancer* **8:**22–24.

Willett, W. C., and MacMahon, B., 1984a, Diet and cancer, *N. Engl. J. Med.* **310:**633–638.

Willett, W. C., and MacMahon, B., 1984b, Diet and cancer, *N. Engl. J. Med.* **310:**697–703.

Willett, W. C., Polk, B. F., Morris, J. S., Stampfer, M. J., Pressel, S., Rosner, B., Taylor, J. O., Schneider, K., and Hames, C. G., 1983, Prediagnostic serum selenium and risk of cancer, *Lancet* **2:**130–134.

World Health Organization, 1958, Procedures for the testing of intentional food additives to establish their safety for use. Second report of the joint FAO/WHO Expert Committee on Food Additives, *WHO Tech. Rep. Ser.* **144:**1–19.

Wynder, E. L., and Bross, I. J., 1961, A study of etiological factors in cancer of the esophagus, *Cancer* **14:**389–413.

Wynder, E. L., and Gori, G. B., 1977, Contribution of the environment to cancer incidence: An epidemiologic exercise, *J. Natl. Cancer Inst.* **58:**825–832.

Wynder, E. L., and Shigematsu, T., 1967, Environmental factors of cancer of the colon and rectum, *Cancer* **20:**1520–1561.

Wynder, E. L., Kmet, J., Dungal, N., and Segi, M., 1963, An epidemiological investigation of gastric cancer, *Cancer* **16:**1461–1496.

Wynder, E. L., Kajitani, T., Ishekawa, S., Dodo, H., and Takano, A., 1969, Environmental factors of cancer of the colon and rectum, II. Japanese epidemiological data, *Cancer* **23:**1210–1220.

Xu, G., 1981, Gastric cancer in China: A review, *J. Roy Soc. Med.* **74:**210–211.

Zaridze, D. G., 1983, Environmental etiology of large-bowel cancer, *J. Natl. Cancer Inst.* **70:**389–400.

Zaridze, D. G., Muir, C. S., and McMichael, A. J., 1985, Diet and cancer: Value of different types of epidemiological studies, in: *Diet and Human Carcinogenesis* (J. V. Joossens, M. J. Hill, and J. Geboers, eds.), Excerpta Medica, New York, pp. 221–233.

Ziegler, R. G., Morris, L. E., Blot, W. J., Pottern, L. M., Hoover, R., and Fraumeni, Jr., J. F., 1981, Esophageal cancer among black men in Washington, D. C. II. Role of nutrition, *J. Natl. Cancer Inst.* **67**:1199–1206.

2

Epidemiologic Approaches to the Study of Diet and Cancer

Graham A. Colditz and Walter C. Willett

1. Introduction

Laboratory workers have known for decades that tumor incidence in animals can be modified by nutritional manipulation (Tannenbaum, 1942). However, the potential importance of diet in the cause and prevention of cancer in human beings has received major attention only recently. This interest has, to a great extent, been stimulated by the large international differences in cancer incidence rates (Armstrong and Doll, 1975; Schrauzer *et al.*, 1977).

Many laboratory methods have been developed to determine the effects of environmental substances, including diet, on carcinogenesis (IARC Working Group, 1980). Among these are microbial mutagenicity tests (such as the Ames test), which have been widely used to study components of human diets. Although these tests are unquestionably helpful in directing human research and elucidating mechanisms of action, they cannot by themselves provide information that is directly relevant to human beings. For example, there are many substances, such as asbestos, that influence the risk of cancer but are not mutagenic. They may act by affecting the permeability of host tissues to carcinogens, by altering hormone balances that modify tumor growth, or by changing the immune response of the host. These higher-level functions are not replicated in bacterial testing systems, thus resulting in false-positive and false-negative results.

Experimental exposure of laboratory animals to substances that may influence cancer incidence is more likely to simulate the effect of a chemical or food substance on the incidence of cancer in human beings. However, higher doses that do not reflect human experience are generally used, and species differ in the way their enzymatic systems activate or deactivate potentially carcinogenic substances. Factors such as these preclude direct extrapolation of findings from animal experiments to human beings.

Graham A. Colditz and Walter C. Willett • Channing Laboratory, Department of Medicine, Brigham and Women's Hospital and Harvard Medical School, and Department of Epidemiology, Harvard School of Public Health, Boston, Massachusetts 02115.

The establishment of an association between a dietary component and risk of human cancer and the quantification of the magnitude of this risk thus require evidence from human beings. The study of nutritional determinants of cancer risk in human populations is a relatively new area of investigation and few associations can be considered established at this time. Therefore, instead of reviewing the largely conflicting data for many specific relationships, we will focus this chapter on the principles and methodologic issues of studies relating diet to cancer. Specifically, we will discuss study designs that are being employed, the methods by which diet is assessed, and the principles of the analysis, reporting, and interpretation of such data. These principles will be supplemented with examples when possible, primarily using data relating intake of green and yellow vegetables (sometimes assumed to represent β-carotene intake) to risk of lung cancer. Of all the diet and cancer associations being addressed, this association is the only one for which there exists a substantial body of consistent supporting epidemiologic evidence at this time.

2. Study Designs

2.1. Randomized Controlled Trials

In a scientific investigation of an hypothesized association between a dietary (or any other) exposure and cancer, an investigator would test the hypothesis with empirical data. In defining exposure to a dietary factor, we must consider many details, such as the dose or duration of exposure and other variables that may alter or modify the effect of the dietary factor in a given subject.

Ideally, the investigator creates an experimental group and a control group, the two groups being identical in all aspects except for the experimental treatment, which is clearly defined and the same for all subjects in the experimental group. Operationally, assignment to experimental and control groups is best done on a random basis to avoid any bias in selecting healthier subjects for one group or another. Using this design, any differences between the two groups can be ascribed to the experimental exposure. Optimally a randomized trial is conducted as a double-blind experiment. Neither the investigator nor the subjects in the trial know which treatment group a subject is allocated to. This is particularly important for the assessment of outcomes that require judgment in the application of criteria (e.g., the presence or absence of colon polyps) in contrast to, say, mortality.

Several randomized trials addressing hypotheses that relate diet and cancer are being conducted at present (Greenwald *et al.*, 1986). Among these is the Physicians' Health Study in which some 22,000 U.S. male physicians have been randomized to either 30 mg β-carotene or placebo, on alternate days. These subjects are being followed to observe the impact of this exposure on total mortality and on cancer incidence rates (Hennekens *et al.*, 1985).

This trial is typical of the experimental studies that are practical in the study of diet and cancer. That is, minor components of the diet, such as trace elements or vitamins which may prevent cancer, can feasibly be administered to human subjects in the form of a pill. There are many dietary factors that may be related to cancer, but for which the investigator cannot feasibly randomize the study subjects to experimental or control groups. For example, it would be unethical to randomize nondrinking men to alcohol or abstinence to study the impact on subsequent mortality or the incidence of heart disease or cancer. Similarly, it would be extremely difficult to randomize men who drink alcohol to cessation or continuance, since compliance would almost certainly be poor. Many other components of diet are similarly limited as to the likely degree of compliance that could be achieved in a long-term experimental study.

Even if feasible, randomized trials of dietary factors and cancer may be inconclusive because of the length of time between changing a dietary factor and a change in the incidence of cancer. This time interval is uncertain but may be many years; thus trials must be of long duration to eliminate the possibility that the lack of an observed difference between treatment groups is not merely due to an insufficient length of follow-up.

In these situations we are largely dependent on observational epidemiologic studies that accurately measure dietary exposures and disease outcomes. In such studies the investigator observes differences in cancer risks among subjects with contrasting levels of dietary factors; it is thus possible to describe and quantify associations between diet and cancer. Despite inherent methodologic difficulties, such studies are often the only possible means to study the relationships between diet and human cancer. Furthermore, experiments among human beings are justifiable only after considerable nonexperimental data have been collected to ensure both that a benefit is reasonably probable and that an adverse outcome is unlikely.

2.2. Observational Studies

2.2.1. International Correlation Studies

International studies have compared the rates of cancer between countries and described large differences for many malignancies. For example, age-adjusted rates of breast and colon cancer in many parts of the world are less than one-fifth those in the United States. The lowest incidence rates of colon cancer per 100,000 males are recorded for Dakar (0.6), Poona, India (3.1), and Bombay, India (3.5). In contrast, the highest rates are from the United States, where Connecticut has recorded a rate of 32.3, and New York State 31.4 (Boyle *et al.*, 1985). Moreover, strong nutritional correlates exist for specific cancers. In these studies (sometimes called ecological studies) the country, or other geographic area, is the unit of measure rather than the individual. Comparing *per capita* total fat intake and national breast cancer mortality rates among women, Armstrong and Doll (1975) described a correlation of 0.89. Comparing per capita fat intake and mortality from colon cancer, these authors observed a correlation of 0.85 for men and 0.81 for women.

Many factors other than dietary differences distinguish countries with a high incidence from those with a low incidence and can thus provide an alternate explanation for differences in cancer rates. Countries that are more industrialized will not only have diets with a higher proportion of total calories from fat, but will also have shifted from an agrarian to an industrialized, sedentary society with lower total energy needs. Thus exposure to many aspect of life in an industrialized society will vary inversely with exercise and directly with fat intake. For example, international data have been analyzed to show that differences in body size can explain a large portion of the variation in national rates of breast cancer (Gray *et al.*, 1979). This is consistent with the hypothesis that energy restriction sufficiently severe to reduce stature reduces risk of human breast cancer. The substantial gain in stature by Japanese migrants to the United States provides clear evidence that caloric restriction has occurred in Japan (Insull *et al.,* 1968). Thus the interrelationships of total calorie intake, physical activity, dietary fat, and other factors make interpretation of international studies quite difficult. Nevertheless, such correlation studies provide a rich source for hypotheses relating diet to cancer incidence.

2.2.2. Cohort Studies

The term "cohort" was originally a Roman military term: a cohort was a tenth of a legion. Typically, the members of a cohort would be recruited from young men of a single age in a single place. The cohort would undergo attrition, never being replenished, and would be disbanded when the term of enlistment was up.

Since the occurrence of illness is manifest in populations of individuals, we may define a particular set of individuals and observe them for the onset of disease. A cohort, like its Roman counterpart, has no replacements during its lifetime. It may be defined by all its members experiencing a membership-defining event. For example, in the Nurses' Health Study, the cohort is made up of those women who responded to the mailing of a questionnaire (121,700 women) in 1976 (Barton *et al.,* 1980). The return of the questionnaire defines entry to the cohort and the beginning of follow-up for each participant. Such a cohort is finite, as indicated by the count 121,700. The cohort is followed through time and observed for the occurrence of new cases of disease in subjects previously free from disease (incident cases).

During or at the end of follow-up, the disease frequency within a cohort may be measured as either a cumulative incidence rate (a measure of risk that is the number of incident cases divided by the population that gave rise to the cases) or incidence-density rate (the number of incident cases divided by the person-time of follow-up). The usual measures of effect due to an exposure (e.g., a dietary factor) are the rate difference (sometimes called attributable risk) and rate ratio (sometimes called relative risk). The latter measure is the rate of disease in the exposed subjects (e.g., these with high intake of dietary factor) divided by the rate of disease in the unexposed (e.g., those with low intake of a dietary factor).

For illustration, among the cohort of 121,700 women in the Nurses' Health Study we identified a group of participants free from cancer in 1976 and followed them through June 1980 to measure the cumulative incidence of breast cancer (Willett *et al.,* 1985a). This outcome was defined as histologically confirmed cases of breast cancer. In one analysis, the primary exposure of interest was relative weight (Quetelet's Index = weight/height^2). We calculated cumulative incidence rates of breast cancer for women by level of Quetelet's Index. These cumulative incidence rates were used to calculate relative risk of breast cancer, using the group with lowest relative weight as the comparison group. Among 13,730 premenopausal women in the highest quintile of Quetelet's Index, there were 58 cases of breast cancer (cumulative incidence = 422.4 per 100,000), compared to 79 cases among the 15,637 women in the lowest quintile (cumulative incidence = 505.2 per 100,000). This gave a relative risk (without adjustment for age) of 0.84 for those in the highest quintile of relative weight compared to those in the lowest quintile.

Another example of a cohort study comes from Norway, where Bjelke (1975) fol-

Table I. Strengths and Limitations of Cohort Studies of Diet and Cancer

Strengths
1. In principle, provides a complete description of experience subsequent to exposure, including rates of progression and natural history.
2. Allows study of multiple potential effects of a given dietary exposure, thereby obtaining information on potential benefits as well as risks.
3. Allows for the calculation of rates of disease in subjects with different levels of intake of a food or nutrient.
4. Avoids the possibility that the presence of disease alters the measurement of diet or other exposures.
5. Allows study of multiple potential causes of disease.

Limitations
1. Large numbers of subjects are required to study rare diseases.
2. Potentially long duration for follow-up.
3. Current practice, suage, or exposure to study factors may change over the duration of the follow-up.
4. Relatively expensive to conduct.
5. Maintaining follow-up is expensive.
6. Control of extraneous variables may be incomplete.

lowed 11,038 men, 45 years old or more, for whom an index of dietary vitamin A was computed based on self-administered questionnaires. During 5 years of follow-up, 53 cases of lung cancer were recorded. An inverse association was observed between the dietary vitamin A index and lung cancer incidence. After controlling for cigarette smoking, the relative risk of those with a high vitamin A index compared to a low index was 0.38 ($p < 0.01$).

The use of a cohort approach has many advantages when studying diet and cancer (see Table I). One particular strength is the fact that this allows the study of multiple effects of a given dietary exposure. For example, both the beneficial effects of alcohol on the risk of gallstone formation (Scragg *et al.*, 1984) and coronary heart disease (Hennekens, 1983) and the potential deleterious effects of alcohol on cancer can be weighed against each other in a cohort study. In addition, the absolute rates of disease can be measured according to the level of a food or nutrient intake.

An alternative approach to the analysis of data from a cohort is to use a nested case–control study. Here cases are compared to a sample of the noncases in the cohort. This approach is most often employed when biological specimens have been collected from all cohort members, but for practical reasons it is not feasible to analyze all the specimens. Using this approach, Willett and colleagues utilized a nested case–control analysis in their study of serum selenium and cancer (Willett *et al.*, 1983b). Bloods had been collected and stored from participants in the Hypertension Detection and Follow-up Program at entry to the study in 1973. It was deemed most efficient to identify the subjects who had developed cancer during a 5-year follow-up period and then select controls for these cases from within the cohort. One the 111 cases and controls (two were selected for each case) were identified, their blood specimens could be retrieved from storage and analyzed for serum selenium concentration. Thus, with prospectively collected specimens on hand, a case–control sampling scheme (see below) was used to efficiently study the association of serum selenium and risk of cancer.

Several groups have used nested case–control analyses to study the association between β-carotene levels and risk of lung cancer in prospectively collected blood samples. Menkes and Comstock (1984) analyzed sera collected prospectively from 88 lung cancer cases and 176 controls matched by age, sex, month of serum donation, and smoking history. Cases had significantly lower levels of β-carotene at baseline (25.5 μg/dl) than the controls (28.7 μg/dl), and a statistically significant trend for increasing risk of lung cancer with decreasing β-carotene levels was observed. Using sera collected prospectively from 6800 Hawaiian men, Nomura *et al.* (1985) also observed significantly lower mean β-carotene concentration in baseline bloods from 74 lung cancer cases (20.0 μg/dl) as compared with 302 controls (29.0 μg/dl). After categorizing current cigarette smokers into three groups and β-carotene into tertiles, the age-adjusted relative risk for heavy smokers in the lowest β-carotene subgroups was 4.9 times that of heavy smokers in the highest β-carotene subgroup. Similarly, among a cohort of 4224 men, Stahelin *et al.* (1984) observed a mean β-carotene concentration of 14.8 μg/dl among 35 individuals who later developed lung cancer compared to 23.7 μg/dl among 102 control subjects.

These examples led us to consider the principles underlying case–control studies.

2.3. Case–Control Studies

Although cohort studies are conceptually desirable because it is clear that exposure level (e.g., intake of a dietary factor) precedes disease, they are usually expensive and of long duration. For practical reasons, case–control studies are often employed as an alternate mode of investigation. In a case–control study, persons with a disease are compared with a sample of "control" subjects without disease with respect to a possible risk factor (e.g., level of a dietary factor). Such data may be used to evaluate the hypothesis that the risk factor is a cause of the disease. In such a sampling design, individuals are selected on the presence of absence of disease. When employing this design, exposures are based on measurements of previously collected specimen (as in a nested case–control study) or it is presumed that information measured at present (sometimes based on recall by subjects) reflects that preceding the disease.

Conceptually, the cases selected for such a study arise from a defined population that may be either clearly defined, as in a cohort, or not specifically enumerated, as in a county population. The population represents those at risk of developing the disease under study; thus by definition, all previous (prevalent) cases are not in the population. Each time someone in the population develops the disease, this subject joins the case series, and the remainder of the population remain at risk of developing the disease. As a case arises from the population, one or more controls should also be sampled to estimate the prevalence of the exposures among those remaining free of disease. In this setting a person sampled as a control at one time is at risk of later developing the disease and may subsequently become a case. Thus for each case, a control or set of control subjects is selected. The controls may be chosen as any sample of individuals who provide valid information about those at risk for the disease. For practical reasons it is not always possible to select a random sample from the population at risk. Convenience may dictate the choice of controls; these have sometimes included neighbors, hospitalized patients with other disease, or persons with randomly selected telephone numbers. It is most essential to choose controls so that their probability of selection is unrelated to the exposure being studied.

As an example of a case–control study, MacLennan *et al.* (1977) identified all cases of lung cancer diagnosed during an 18-month period from 1972 in three Singapore

*Table II. Strengths and Limitations of Case–Control Studies
in the Study of Diet and Cancer*

Strengths
  1. Well suited to the study of rare diseases.
  2. Relatively quick to mount and conduct.
  3. Relatively inexpensive.
  4. Requires comparatively few subjects.
  5. No risk to subjects.
  6. Allows study of multiple potential causes of a disease.
Limitations
  1. Relies on recall for information on past dietary exposures.
  2. Validation of dietary information is usually impossible.
  3. Disease status may modify recall of past diet and alter many biochemical
     parameters.
  4. Control of extraneous variables may be incomplete.
  5. Selection of an appropriate comparison group may be difficult.
  6. Rates of disease in exposed and unexposed individuals usually cannot be
     determined.

hospitals. Controls were identified from other hospital patients who did not have smoking-related diseases. A total of 233 cases and 300 controls were interviewed regarding frequency of consumption of dark-green leafy vegetables and food preparation habits. In this study an increased risk of lung cancer was related to low consumption of dark-green leafy vegetables.

Among the most important of the limitations is the comparability of information between the cases and controls (see Table II). In contrast with a randomized, double-blind controlled trial, where subjects are randomized to an exposure and followed over time to observe the development of an outcome state, or a cohort, where data are collected from healthy subjects who subsequently go on to develop disease, these case–control studies collect data from subjects who (in most situations) know their own disease status, and the person collecting the data will often also know the disease status. This may, of course, influence the accuracy of the data collected, either through differential recall by cases and controls, or by an interviewer being more persistent in questioning cases than controls. Ultimately, the investigator must appeal to either subjective or semiquantitative arguments to the effect that the information from cases and controls is equivalent in quality. There are several ways to reduce this bias; one such approach is to collect data from patients who, though referred to a center for diagnosis, have not yet been diagnosed. Information may thus be collected from all subjects under similar circumstances, and the diagnostic process may classify subjects as either cases or controls.

Another limitation of the case–control study is its implication for analysis. One can only compare the prevalence of an exposure among the cases with that among the controls. Using case–control analysis, it is thus not possible to measure incidence rates. Data for cases and controls are shown in Table III to illustrate the measure of association that is used in these analyses. As implied from the previous discussion of case and control selection, the total number of cases ($a + c$) and of controls ($b + d$) is determined by the investigator. Since this is often done without any knowledge of the actual total number in

Table III. Association of Risk Factor and Disease
in Case–Control Sample[a]

Risk factor classification	Cases	Controls
High intake	*a*	*b*
Low intake	*c*	*d*
Total	*a + c*	*b + d*

[a]Relative risk = *ad/bc*; *a ÷ c/b ÷ d = ad/bc.*

the population, it is impossible to use any ratio of cases to controls to reflect the risk of disease for a level of exposure. The ratio $a/(a+b)$, for example, does not estimate the risk of disease for those with a high dietary intake; as can be seen, this ratio depends in part on the number of controls selected for each case. Instead, this study design provides information on the likelihood of exposure, given case–control status. Thus, from the total number of cases $(a+c)$, the relationship of a to c provides an estimate of how all cases are divided into those with high (a) or low (c) intake. Likewise, the ratio of b to d estimates the distribution of intake among those at risk of becoming cases (the controls). The ratio a/c to b/d estimates the relative risk of disease (ad/bc). This relative risk approximates the rate ratio calculated from follow-up studies and is sometimes referred to as an odds ratio.

Most nutrient intakes can be measured with sufficient accuracy (see Section 3) so that an important effect will not be missed (given a sufficient sample size). However, systematic bias (e.g., differential recall due to the diagnosis of cancer) remains a potential problem in case–control studies. Although bias may not actually be a problem in any particular study, it is extremely difficult to rule out that a 5–10% systematic error due to recall has not occurred. Since differences of 5–10% in means between cases and controls translate into potentially important relative risks (Miller *et al.*, 1978), some uncertainty will necessarily attend most traditional case–control studies. Our concern regarding this issue has been heightened by the consistent finding that responses to questions about remote dietary intake are biased by recent intake (Rohan and Potter, 1984; Jensen *et al.*, 1984), which can well have been altered by cancer or its treatment in the typical case–control setting. We believe this argues strongly for large cohort studies to complement case–control investigations (which do serve an important exploratory and developmental role). Since recent intake influences recall of diet in the remote past, case–control studies are particularly limited in their ability to address important issues of latency, i.e., the time from an exposure to the development of a cancer. In contrast, using a cohort study with periodically updated dietary exposure information will allow for analyses of specific subgroups who have consumed known levels of nutrients at defined intervals prior to the development of disease.

3. Measuring Dietary Exposure

3.1. Interview, Questionnaire, and Diary

In any study relating dietary exposure to cancer incidence, it is imperative that the long-term exposure status be accurately measured. An assessment of dietary intake that could accurately measure long-term exposure was, until recently, thought to be impossible for large-scale studies. However, a number of useful methods for assessing long-term dietary intake have recently been developed and refined (Block, 1982). These methods include the use of food diaries in which subjects record all the foods they eat on a meal-by-meal basis (Heady, 1961), interviews about previous dietary intake (Burke, 1947), short-term recall (Beaton *et al.,* 1979), and questionnaires relating to the usual frequency of consumption of a selected list of foods (Stefanik and Trulson, 1962). Food diaries require subjects to keep a record of all that they eat, by either weighing, measuring, or estimating. Though this method gives a reasonably accurate estimate of actual intake, it nevertheless requires a high degree of cooperation on the part of subjects and is usually impractical for large-scale epidemiologic studies. The diet history interview is more appealing since it is an attempt to ascertain long-term usual intake patterns. However, it requires an extensive interview by a trained nutritionist, again limiting its usefulness in epidemiologic studies. Short-term recall is more feasible: although dietary intake may be estimated with reasonable accuracy, the day-to-day variation in individual dietary intake will usually make recall of a single day unrepresentative of usual intake.

Although each method has advantages in particular applications, the food frequency method is the most practical for large studies. The aim of the food frequency questionnaire is to characterize food intake over an extended period, even though this may sacrifice some information on details of an individual's food consumption. A food frequency questionnaire consists of two basic parts: a list of foods and a set of frequency response options to indicate how often each food is consumed during a specified time period. Questions relate to usual intake over an extended period of time, such as a year. This contrasts with the periods of a few days or weeks which were used in more traditional methods. The longer time interval is likely to be more appropriate for studies of diet and cancer since an assessment of longer-term average intake is required. Data obtained from a food frequency questionnaire may be used directly to examine the association between frequency of using a specific food and risk of cancer. Alternatively, nutrient scores may be calculated by multiplying the frequency of consumption for a food by the nutrient content of specified portions and then summing the contribution of each food to intake of a nutrient. This food frequency approach is sometimes used to categorize subjects in one of several levels of relative intake, such as quintiles, rather than to obtain an absolute quantification of intake.

In a typical application of a food frequency questionnaire, Bjelke calculated a vitamin A index by multiplying the frequency of consumption of various dietary items by a weight estimated from Norwegian food tables to represent average vitamin A or vitamin A equivalents in a standard quantity of the edible portion. Food (and their respective weights) included in the calculation of the index were potatoes (0.0115), salted, fresh, or frozen fish (0.010), salted meat or ham (0.0075), eggs (0.050), fruit soup (0.010), cabbage (0.0063), rutabaga (0.030), carrots (0.44), cauliflower (0.0025), lettuce (0.0107), tomatoes (0.040), peas (0.010), beans (0.010), rhubarb (0.008), berry juice (0.001), fruit juice (0.001), garden berries (0.0059), wild berries (0.0015), canned fruits (0.0051), oranges (0.0045), apples (0.0045), grapes (0.002), bananas (0.027), and milk (0.820) (Kvale *et al.,* 1983). The total vitamin A index (the sum of the products of food frequency multiplied by food weight) was used in the previously cited prospective study (Bjelke, 1975).

Byers *et al.* (1985) have clearly demonstrated that a high proportion of the between-person variance in nutrient intake can be explained by a relatively small number of foods. Rohan and Potter (1984) found nutrient intakes measured by a food frequency questionnaire reproducible over a 3-year period, and Byers *et al.* (1983) have found that a vitamin A index is reproducible over 24 years. Furthermore, results obtained with these questionnaires correlate with intakes determined by more detailed dietary methods (Heady, 1961; Stefanik and Trulson, 1962; Balogh *et al.*, 1968; Willett *et al.*, 1985b). We have also shown significant correlations between biochemical indexes of nutrient intake (plasma carotenoids and α-tocopherol) and rankings derived from a food frequency questionnaire (Willett *et al.*, 1983a).

Sacks *et al.* (1982) have shown that a food frequency questionnaire can reasonably measure change in diet. Among 22 adults who consumed a typical, nonvegetarian diet, intakes of protein, fat, carbohydrate, and total calories were all significantly correlated with intakes measured by a 7-day diet record ($r = 0.50$–0.67). Subjects were switched to a primarily lactovegetarian diet and a second food frequency questionnaire was completed at that time. Individual changes in plasma cholesterol were correlated with changes in dietary cholesterol ($r = 0.49$), animal fat ($r = 0.41$), and vegetable fat and linoleic acid ($r = 0.65$) as measured by the food frequency questionnaires.

The precision of dietary questionnaires or interviews varies widely among nutrients, being dependent on the consistency of the concentration of a nutrient in a given food. For some nutrients these methods may be useless. For example, cholesterol intake can be reasonably assessed since it is largely derived from a fairly small number of foods with relatively constant concentrations of cholesterol. Selenium, on the other hand, varies greatly in concentration within foods, depending largely on the soils on which the foods were grown. Since people are, in general, unaware of the sources of their foods, intakes or selenium and some other trace elements may not be amenable to meaningful estimation from food frequency questionnaires or interviews.

One limitation of the food frequency approach is that, in general, it provides rankings of relative intake rather than a quantification of absolute intake. This therefore limits the usefulness of this instrument for estimating dose–response relationships between diet and the disease expressed in terms of grams of nutrient per day. However, this situation may be rectified by the use of more detailed methods of diet recording to quantify the intake that corresponds to each of the categories of relative intake as estimated by the food frequency approach. A record of all foods eaten on a meal-by-meal basis may be obtained from a sample of the study population to determine the absolute intakes that correspond to the quintiles of intake for each nutrient. We used this approach, collecting detailed diet records from 197 women for four 1-week periods over a 12-month interval to quantify intakes and rankings on a food frequency questionnaire (Willett *et al.*, 1985b).

3.2. Biochemical Indicators of Nutrient Intake

For some nutrients, biological specimens may provide the only feasible means of assessing past dietary intake. This appears to be the case for selenium, for reasons noted earlier. For example, Morris *et al.* (1983) demonstrated that toenail clippings from different toes represent an integrated intake of selenium over an extended period. Similarly, serum levels of carotene and vitamin E are sensitive to dietary intake and can therefore be used to study the relationship between intakes of these nutrients and cancer (Willett *et al.*,

1983a). Since disease status often alters dietary intake, as well as the digestion and metabolism of many nutrients, the collection of blood specimens for biochemical assessments of diet is most appropriate in the setting of a cohort study.

4. Measuring Correlates of Dietary Exposure

Dietary factors are likely to be associated with other possible determinants of cancer, including other dietary variables. For example, alcohol intake is associated with smoking. Smoking could distort the association between alcohol intake and lung cancer since smoking is associated with the exposure and the outcome. Smoking is thus said to confound the association between alcohol and lung cancer. Such a confounding variable may partly account for the apparent association in a study, or it may mask a true underlying association. If information on the potentially confounding variable is available, one can adjust for the effect of the confounder in the analysis (Kleinbaum *et al.*, 1982; Schlesselman, 1982; Cochran, 1983). For example, in a cohort study of Japanese men in Hawaii, Pollack *et al.* (1984) analyzed data on alcohol intake and lung cancer incidence, controlling for smoking status and age in a multivariate model. This analysis showed that the risk of lung cancer for those who consumed alcohol was double that of nondrinkers.

As another example of confounding, we consider data from a hypothetical case–control study of lung cancer patients and control patients with nonrespiratory, nonneoplastic disease. We observed an association between the number of cigarettes smoked and dietary vitamin A intake; heavier smokers consumed less dietary vitamin A (Table IV). Cigarette smoking, a risk factor for lung cancer, is thus also associated with vitamin A intake and therefore confounds the association between vitamin A and lung cancer.

Table IV. Hypothetical Data Demonstrating Confounding of the Association between Vitamin A Intake and Lung Cancer Risk

	One pack of cigarettes or less/day		More than one pack of cigarettes/day	
	Lung cancer	Control	Lung cancer	Control
Vitamin A $\leq$ 74	7	75	90	100
Vitamin A $\geq$ 125	3	75	10	20
RR	2.33		1.8	

$$\text{Crude relative risk} = \frac{97 \times 95}{13 \times 175} = 4.0$$

$$\text{Adjusted relative risk} = \frac{\Sigma a_i d_i/t_i}{\Sigma b_i c_i/t_i} \quad \text{where } a_i,b_i,c_i,d_i = \text{cell frequencies for stratum i, and } t_i \text{ is the stratum total}$$

$$= \frac{(7 \times 75)/160 + (90 \times 20)/220}{(3 \times 75)/160 + (10 \times 100)/220}$$

$$= \frac{11.46}{5.95}$$

$$= 1.9$$

Among control patients, those who smoked more than a pack of cigarettes per day were five times more likely to have low dietary vitamin A intake compared to those smoking one pack of cigarettes per day or less $(100 \times 75) \div (75 \times 20)$. For those smoking one pack of cigarettes per day or less the relative risk of lung cancer was 2.33 for those with low vitamin A intake compared to high intake. For those smoking more than a pack per day this relative risk was 1.8. As seen in Table IV, if smoking is not taken into account in the analysis, the crude relative risk of lung cancer is 4.0 for low intake of vitamin A compared to high intake. However, after controlling for the confounding due to smoking, the relative risk is 1.9, less than half the crude estimate. This illustrates that lack of control for the effect of smoking would grossly overestimate the impact of dietary vitamin A on the risk of lung cancer.

5. Analysis and Reporting

In contrast with a randomized trial where all factors other than the exposure under investigation are equally distributed in each group, observational epidemiologic studies often have many factors varying from subject to subject in addition to the exposure that is of prime interest to the investigator. Methods to control for the influence of the age distribution of cases and noncases are presented in detail elsewhere (Kleinbaum *et al.*, 1982; Schlesselman, 1982). Since age is an important determinant of cancer risk and is also associated with dietary intake, all analyses are usually presented as age-adjusted. When a rate ratio or rate difference is reported as the measure of association between diet and cancer, a measure of the statistical stability of this estimate should also be reported. This is typically presented as the 95% confidence interval.

5.1. Nutrient–Disease Relationships

Relationships between nutritional factors and cancer may be examined in terms of absolute intake or in relation to total caloric intake. The analytical approach will depend on both the nature of the biological relationship and public health considerations. A major concern in the analysis of epidemiologic data on diet and cancer is the between-person variation in total caloric intake. Among free-living individuals neither height nor weight accounts for a major portion of this variation in total caloric intake (Gordon *et al.*, 1984; Thompson and Billewicz, 1961). Thus physical activity, metabolic efficiency, and net energy balance remain to account for this variation. Although measurement of physical activity and metabolic efficiency is at best crude, long-term net energy balance is accurately assessed through measures of obesity or change in weight.

Intakes of most nutrients in free-living populations tend to be positively correlated with caloric intake (Jain *et al.*, 1980). These positive correlations result from the contribution of macronutrients to caloric intake. In addition, more active and larger individuals generally eat more of everything, resulting in correlations between nutrients without caloric value and total energy intake. Thus for the interpretation of individual nutrients, total caloric intake is particularly important.

Long-term total caloric intake is largely beyond an individual's direct control (Hegstead, 1985) unless accompanied by major changes in weight or physical activity.

Thus, changes in absolute nutrient intake must be accomplished by altering the composition of the diet rather than the total food intake. For this reason, dietary recommendations are often made in reference to total caloric intake. From a public health standpoint, analysis of nutrient intake in relation to total caloric intake is more relevant than analyses based on crude nutrient intake.

When total caloric intake is associated with disease, analysis and interpretation of individual nutrients is complex (Willett and Stampfer, 1986). Specific nutrients will be associated with disease simply because of their correlation with caloric intake (Lyons *et al.*, 1983). For example, in almost every study of diet and coronary heart disease, individuals who subsequently develop disease have lower total caloric intakes, on average, than individuals who remain free from disease (Thompson and Billewicz, 1961; Garcia-Palmieri *et al.*, 1980; Gordon *et al.*, 1981; McGee *et al.*, 1984a; Kromhout and Coulander, 1984). As a result, individual nutrient intakes also tend to be lower among cases. Difference in body size is an unlikely explanation of this lower caloric intake, and variation in metabolic efficiency is impossible to eliminate as an explanation. However, decreased physical activity is associated with an increased risk of coronary heart disease (Thompson and Billewicz, 1961; Paffenbarger *et al.*, 1978). Thus an appropriate interpretation of the inverse association between total caloric intake and risk of coronary heart disease is not that one should increase food intake, but rather that an increase in physical activity may reduce the risk of disease.

Variation in caloric intake between individuals is largely secondary to nonnutritional factors, such as physical activity, metabolic efficiency, and body size. If the association between a nutrient and cancer is simply the result of a difference in caloric intake, then this association is unlikely to be of direct etiologic importance. Thus, in the analysis of nutrient–cancer relationships it is important to remove the effect of caloric intake, that is, to demonstrate that the effect of the nutrient is independent of caloric intake.

Controlling for Caloric Intake

The traditional approach used to control for total caloric intake is to divide nutrient values by caloric intake (i.e., to compute "nutrient densities"). This approach, though simple, is particularly limited when addressing diet–cancer relationships and does not necessarily remove or control for the effect of total caloric intake (Willett and Stampfer, 1986). When total caloric intake is associated with disease, dividing nutrient values by this caloric intake creates a variable that will be associated with disease in the opposite direction from total caloric intake.

A simple way to avoid this problem is to include caloric intake and absolute nutrient intake as terms in a multivariate model, with disease outcome as the dependent variable. However, high colinearity between nutritional factors (e.g., fat and total calories) often complicates their simultaneous inclusion in multivariate models (McGee *et al.*, 1984b). To overcome this problem Willett and Stampfer (1986) have suggested the use of "calorie-adjusted" nutrient intakes, calculated as the residuals from the regression model, with total calorie intake as the independent variable and absolute nutrient intake as the dependent variable. If the usual assumptions for regression are met, these calorie-adjusted nutrient intakes will be uncorrelated with caloric intake.

5.2. Foods

Although analysis of diet and cancer relationships has typically focused on specific nutrients, there are several limitations to such an analysis. A focus on nutrients may mask a net adverse effect of a food. Ames (1983) has emphasized that a food may contain substances potentially protective against cancer, as well as materials that is potentially carcinogenic. The balance of these influences can best be determined by directly examining the association between a food and the disease outcome of interest.

Furthermore, foods need to be examined carefully for possible associations with cancers, since evidence continues to accumulate that certain vegetables and fruits contain antimutagens that are not represented by nutrient scores typically computed. For example, a consistent body of evidence from cohort and case–control studies supports a protective effect against lung cancer of some factor, possibly β-carotene, in fruits and vegetables (MacLennan *et al.*, 1977; Kvale *et al.*, 1983; Mettlin *et al.*, 1979; Hirayama, 1979; Shekelle *et al.*, 1981). A more detailed examination of which specific foods are protective might provide further clues as to the protective factor as well as a practical basis for dietary recommendations even while awaiting the identification of the active agent.

Another major reason for analyzing and reporting results for individual foods arises from the possibility of replicating nutrient effects within the same study. When different foods contain a common nutrient, the finding of similar associations between these foods and cancer incidence may strengthen the hypothesis than the nutrient is related to cancer. For example, when investigating the effect of alcohol on risk of coronary heart disease, the finding of a protective effect for each type of beverage supports the hypothesis that alcohol itself is responsible rather than some other factors (Yano *et al.*, 1977; Hennekens *et al.*, 1979).

Analyses of relationships between specific foods and cancer risk also offer the potential to express results in terms of change in risk per unit change in food intake. Such reporting has clear meaning to the public and lends itself to a more relevant set of recommendations for dietary change. Because of the complexity of diet, recommendations should be based on individual foods that have been studied for their association with cancer. For example, Kvale *et al.* (1983) reported results for diet and squamous and small cell lung cancer. Comparing consumption of four glasses of milk per day to less than one glass per day, they observed a relative risk of 0.32.

6. Interpretation of Diet–Cancer Relationship

Any diet–cancer relationship from an epidemiologic study must be carefully considered before a causal relationship is concluded. An association may be noncausal and may arise due to chance. Though *p* values offer an arbitrary cutoff level for chance, statistical significance does not ensure that an association is causal or biologically important.

Bias within a study may explain an observed association. In case–control studies of diet and cancer, a systematic error due to recall of diet may yield a biased result that is still highly statistically significant. This is particularly important since recent diet influences recall of past diet, and for many cancers patients have modified their diet by the time they are included in a case–control study. Such bias cannot be controlled in the analysis of data. In contrast, confounding may be controlled in the analysis of a study, as we discussed in the preceding section.

In assessing a causal association, several criteria are often considered. The consistency of the data with results from other investigations adds strength to a causal interpretation, as does the presence of a dose–response effect. The existence of a similar effect in animal models adds further credence to a causal interpretation. Although the existence of a biological mechanism may be useful, lack of an obvious mechanism should not be viewed as evidence against a causal effect, since the etiology of most cancers is so poorly understood.

7. Conclusion

Evidence from international studies, laboratory and animal data, and observational studies among human beings suggests that dietary factors have important causative and protective roles in carcinogenesis. To identify and quantify the effects of specific dietary determinants of cancer, a variety of epidemiologic approaches is required. Underlying each of these is the need for reliable and valid measures of exposure and outcome and careful analyses that control for the influences of the many covariates of diet that also modify cancer risk.

8. References

Ames, B. N., 1983, Dietary carcinogens and anticarcinogens, *Science* **221:**1256–1264.

Amstrong, B., and Doll, R., 1975, Environmental factors and cancer incidence and mortality in different countries with special reference to dietary practices, *Int. J. Cancer* **15:**617–631.

Balogh, M., Medalie, J. H., Smith, H., and Groen, J. J., 1968, The development of a dietary questionnaire for an ischemic heart disease study, *Isr. J. Med. Sci.* **4:**195–203.

Barton, J., Bain, C., Hennekens, C. H., Rosner, B., Belanger, C., Roth, A., and Speizer, F. E., 1980, Characteristics of respondents and non-respondents to a mailed questionnaire, *Am. J. Public Health* **70:**823–825.

Beaton, G. H., Milner, J., and Corey, P., 1979, Sources of variance in 24-hour dietary recall data: Implications for nutrition study design and interpretation, *Am. J. Clin. Nutr.* **32:**2546–2559.

Bjelke, E., 1975, Dietary vitamin A and human lung cancer, *Int. J. Cancer* **15:**461–565.

Block, G., 1982, A review of validations of dietary assessment methods, *Am. J. Epidemiol.* **115:**492–505.

Boyle, P., Zaridze, D. G., and Smans, M., 1985, Descriptive epidemiology of colorectal cancer, *Int. J. Cancer* **36:**9–18.

Burke, B. S., 1947, The dietary history as a tool in research, *J. Am. Diet. Assoc.* **23:**1041–1046.

Byers, T. E., Rosenthal, R. J., Marshall, J. R., Thomas, F., Rzepka, K., Cummings, M., and Graham, S., 1983, Dietary history from the distant past: A methodologic study, *Nutr. Cancer* **5:**69–77.

Byers, T., Marshall, J., Fiedler, R., Zielenzny, M., and Graham, S., 1985, Assessing nutrient intake with an abbreviated dietary interview, *Am. J. Epidemiol.* **122:**41–50.

Cochran, W. G., 1983, *Planning and Analysis of Observational Studies,* Wiley, New York.

Garcia-Palmieri, M. R., Sorlie, P., and Tillotson, J., 1980, Relationship of dietary intake to subsequent coronary heart disease incidence: The Puerto Rican Heart Health Program, *Am. J. Clin. Nutr.* **33:**1818–1827.

Gordon, T., Kagan, A., and Garcia-Palmieri, M. R., 1981, Diet and its relationship to coronary heart disease and death in three populations, *Circulation* **63:**500–515.

Gordon, T., Fisher, M., and Rifkind, B., 1984, Some difficulties inherent in the interpretation of dietary data from free-living populations, *Am. J. Clin. Nutr.* **39**:152–6.

Gray, G. E., Pike, M. C., and Henderson, B. E., 1979, Breast cancer incidence and mortality rates in different countries in relation to known risk factors and dietary practices, *Br. J. Cancer* **39**(1):1–7.

Greenwald, P., Sondik, E., and Lynch, B. S., 1986, Diet and chemoprevention in NCI's research strategy to achieve national cancer control objectives, *Ann. Prev. Public Health* **7**:267–291.

Heady, J. A., 1961, Diets of bank clerks: Development of a method of classifying the diets of individuals for use in the epideiologic studies, *J. R. Stat. Soc. (A)* **124**:366–361.

Hegstead, D. M., 1985, Dietary standards: Dietary planning and nutrition education, *Clin. Nutr.* **4**:159–163.

Hennekens, C. H., 1983, Alcohol, *in: Prevention of Coronary Heart Disease. Practical Management of the Risk Factor,* (N. M. Kaplan and J. Stamler, eds.), Saunders, Philadelphia, pp. 130–138.

Hennekens, C. H., Willett, W. C., and Rosner, B., 1979, Effects of beer, wine and liquor in coronary deaths, *JAMA* **242**:1973–1974.

Hennekens, C. H., Eberlein, K. A., and the Physicians' Health Study Research Group, 1985, A randomized trial of aspirin and beta-carotene among U.S. physicians, *Prev. Med.* **14**:165–168.

Hirayama, T., 1979, Diet and cancer, *Nutr. Cancer* **1**:67–81.

IARC Working Group, 1980, An evaluation of chemicals and industrial processes associated with cancer in humans based on human and animal data: IARC Monographs Volumes 1 to 20, *Cancer Res.* **40**:1–12.

Insull, W., Oiso, T., and Tsuchiya, K., 1968, Diet and nutritional status of Japanese, *Am. J. Clin. Nutr.* **21**:753–777.

Jain, M., Cook, G. M., Davis, F. G., Grace, M. G., Howe, O. R., and Miller, A. B., 1980, A case–control study of diet and colo-rectal cancer, *Int. J. Cancer* **26**:757–768.

Jensen, D. M., Wahrendorf, J., Rosenquist, A., and Geser, A., 1984, The reliability of questionnaire derived historical dietary information and temporal stability of food habits in individuals, *Am. J. Epidemiol.* **120**:281–290.

Kleinbaum, D. G., Kupper, L. L., and Morgensten, H., 1982, *Epidemiologic Research, Principles and Quantitative Methods,* Lifetime Learning Publications, Belmont, CA.

Kromhout, D., and Coulander, C. L., 1984, Diet, prevalance, and 10 year mortality from coronary heart disease in 871 middle-aged men: The Zutphen Study, *Am. J. Epidemiol.* **118**:733–741.

Kvale, G., Bjelke, E., and Gart, J. J., 1983, Dietary habits and lung cancer risk, *Int. J. Cancer* **31**:397–405.

Lyons, J. L., Gardner, J. W., West, D. W., and Mahoney, A. M., 1983, Methodologic tissues in epidemiologic studies of diet and cancer, *Cancer Res.* **43**:2392S-2396S.

MacLennan, R., DaCosta, J., Day, N. E., Law, C. H., Ng, Y. K., and Shanmugaratnan, K., 1977, Risk factors for lung cancer in Singapore Chinese, a population with high female incidence rates, *Int. J. Cancer* **20**:854–860.

McGee, D. L., Reed, D. M., and Yano, K., 1984a, Ten-year incidence of coronary heart disease in the Honolulu Heart Study Program: Relationship nutrient intake, *Am. J. Epidemiol.* **119**:667–676.

McGee, D., Reed, D., and Yano, K., 1984b, The results of logistic analyses when the variables are highly correlated: An empirical example using diet on CHD incidence, *J. Chron. Dis.* **37**:713–719.

Menkes, M., and Comstock, G. W., 1984, Vitamin A and E and lung cancer (Abstr.), *Am. J. Epidemiol.* **120**:491.

Mettlin, C. S., Graham, S., and Swanson, M., 1979, Vitamin A and lung cancer, *J. Natl. Cancer Inst.* **62**(6):1435–1438.

Miller, A., 1980, A case–control study of diet and colorectal cancer, *Int. J. Cancer* **26**:757–768.

Miller, A. B., Kelly, A., Choi, N. W., Matthews, V., Morgan, R. V., Munan, L., Burch, J. D., Feather, J., Howe, G. R., and Jain, M., 1978, A study of diet and breast cancer, *Am. J. Epidemiol.* **107**:499–509.

Morris, J. S., Stampfer, M. J., and Willett, W. C., 1983, Dietary selenium in humans. Toenails as an indicator, *Biol. Trace Element Res.* **5**:529–537.

Nomura, A. M. Y., Stammermann, G. N., Heilbrun, L. K., Salkeld, R. M., and Vuilleumier, J. P., 1985, Serum vitamin levels and the risk of cancer of specific sites in men, of Japanese ancestry in Hawaii, *Cancer Res.* **45**:2369–2372.

Paffenbarger, R. S., Wing, A. L., and Hyde, R. T., 1978, Physical activity as an index of heart attack risk in college alumni, *Am. J. Epidemiol.* **161**:175.

Pollack, E. S., Nomura, A. M. Y., Heilbrun, L., Stemmerman, G. N., and Green, S. B., 1984, Prospective study of alcohol consumption and cancer, *N. Engl. J. Med.* **310**:617–621.

Rohan, J. E., and Potter, J. D., 1984, Retrospective assessment of dietary intake, *Am. J. Epidemiol.* **120:**876–887.

Sacks, F. M., Willett, W. C., Handysides, G., Mavas, G., and Bowden, N., 1982, Use of a self-administered food frequency questionnaire for dietary assessment in a short-term clinical trial, (Abstr.), *Circulation* **66:**(Suppl. II):315.

Schlesselman, J. J., 1982, *Case–Control Studies: Design, Conduct, Analysis,* Oxford University Press, New York.

Schrauzer, G. N., White, D. A., and Schenider, C. J., 1977, Cancer mortality correlation studies. III. Statistical associations with dietary selenium intakes, *Bioinorgan. Chem.* **7:**23–31.

Scragg, R., McMichael, A. J., and Baghurst, P. A., 1984, Diet, alcohol and relative weight in gallstone disease: A case–control study, *Br. Med. J.* **288:**1113–1119.

Shekelle, R. B., Lepper, M., Liu, S., Malizac, C., Raynor, W. J., and Rossof, A. H., 1981, Dietary vitamin A and risk of cancer in the Western Electric Study, *Lancet* **2:**1185–1190.

Stahelin, H. B., Rosel, F., Buess, E., and Brubacker, G., 1984, Cancer, vitamins, and plasma lipids, Prospective Basil Study, *J. Natl. Cancer Inst.* **73:**1463–1468.

Stefanik, P. A., and Trulson, M. C., 1962, Determining the frequency of intakes of foods in large groups studies, *Am. J. Clin. Nutr.* **11:**335–343.

Tannenbaum, A., 1942, The genesis and growth of tumors. III. Effects of high fat diet, *Cancer Res.* **2:**468–475.

Thompson, A. M., and Billewicz, W. Z., 1961, Height, weight and food intake in men, *Br. J. Nutr.* **15:**241–252.

Willett, W. C., and Stampfer, M. J., 1986, Total energy intake: Implications of epidemiologic analyses, *Am. J. Epidemiol.* **124:**17–27.

Willett, W. C., Stampfer, M. J., Underwood, B. A., Taylor, J. O., and Hennekens, C. H., 1983a, Vitamins A, E, and carotene: Effects of supplementation on their plasma levels, *Am. J. Clin. Nutr.* **38:**559–566.

Willett, W. C., Polk, B. F., Morris, J. S., Stampfer, M. J., Pressel, S., Schenider, K., and Hames, C. G., 1983b, Prediagnostic serum selenium and risk of cancer, *Lancet* **2:**130–134.

Willett, W. C., Browne, M. L., Bain, C., Lipnick, R. J., Stampfer, M. J., Rosner, B., Colditz, G. A., Hennekens, C. H., and Speizer, F. E., 1985a, Relative weight and risk of breast cancer among premenopausal women, *Am. J. Epidemiol.* **122:**731–740.

Willett, W. C., Sampson, L., Stampfer, M. J., Rosner, B., Bain, C., Witschi, J., Hennekens, C. H., and Speizer, F. E., 1985b, Reproducibility and validity of a semiquantitative food frequency questionnaire, *Am. J. Epidemiol.* **122:**51–55.

Yano, K., Rhoads, G. G., and Kagan, A., 1977, Coffee, alcohol and risk of coronary heart disease among Japanese men living in Hawaii, *N. Engl. J. Med.* **297:**405–409.

3

A Comparison of the Changes in Carbohydrate, Fat, and Protein Metabolism Occurring with Malignant and Benign Tumors and the Impact of Nutritional Support

Antonio C. L. Campos, Dan L. Waitzberg, and Michael M. Meguid

1. Introduction

Cachexia is a common feature of advanced malignancy. In many patients, anorexia or alterations in gastrointestinal function seem to contribute to the observed weight loss. However, weight loss occurs in some patients even without an obvious cause, which is widely believed to be due to increased energy expenditure associated with the presence of a neoplasm. Although this concept has not been confirmed in a number of studies (Knox *et al.*, 1983; Hansell *et al.*, 1986), Lundholm *et al.* (1981a) suggested that anorexia is the primary event, based on data showing that food intake in cancer-bearing patients relative to matched controls is diminished. Data from animal experiments and pair-fed studies indicate that malignant tumor-or host-secreted factors may play a major role in weight loss by interfering with the normal carbohydrate, fat, and protein metabolism (Burt *et al.*, 1983a; Devereux *et al.*, 1985; Brennan, 1977; Heber *et al.*, 1982; Norton *et al.*, 1981; Pain *et al.*, 1984; Warren *et al.*, 1987). The changes in host metabolism induced by malignant tumors are in contrast with the effects of benign tumors. Although benign tumors demonstrate similar significant growth, they appear to cause little systemic disturbance unless endocrinologically active or anatomically strategically sited.

Human studies of the influence of a cancer on carbohydrate, fat, and protein metabo-

Antonio C. L. Campos, Dan L. Waitzberg, and Michael M. Meguid • Surgical Metabolism and Nutrition Laboratory, Department of Surgery, University Hospital, Syracuse, New York 13210.

lism are few because of the obvious difficulties in carrying out such studies. Also, the relevance of animal models using transplantable tumors may be questionable, primarily because the average tumor burden in such models may reach as much as 30–40% of body weight (Mider *et al.*, 1948), while human tumors are considered clinically large when still less than 1% of body weight (Costa, 1977). Reports regarding the metabolic effects of benign tumors are scarce, possibly because of a dearth of suitable experimental models and because of the lack of scientific interest in humans with benign tumor, in whom there is no visible disturbance in metabolic homeostasis and, thus, the lack of impetus for their study.

We attempt here to compare the changes in carbohydrate, fat, and protein metabolism and their effect on energy expenditure and protein–energy metabolism as associated with malignant and benign tumors, and to analyze the influence of nutritional support, as provided on a daily basis in clinical practice, on these metabolic features in the light of current knowledge. What is the relevance of the knowledge concerning carbohydrate, fat, and amino acid metabolism? In part, this lies in the clinical practice of providing cancer-bearing patients with nutritional support (Meguid and Dudrick, 1986). Nutritional support, either parenteral or enteral, usually consists of a mixture of glucose, fat, and amino acids together with a limited number of trace elements and all the vitamins. Nutritional support is given to patients who cannot eat or who are unable to eat sufficiently. It is given in amounts equal to or greater than the energy expenditure (usually 35–45 kcal/kg per day and 0.2–0.3 g N/kg per day) of a particular patient with a particular diagnosis—cancer-bearing state in this discussion—on the assumption that nutritional support has therapeutic benefit (Meguid *et al.*, 1990a,b).

Cancer patients are at high risk of developing malnutrition because the presence of a malignant disease is often associated with reduced oral intake (Meguid *et al.*, 1986) from anorexia and with altered metabolism. Also, cancer treatment, i.e., extensive resective surgery, chemotherapy, and radiation therapy, may produce additional nutritional wasting in already nutritionally compromised patients. A clear association between preoperative malnutrition and poor surgical outcome exists (Campos and Meguid, 1990), and the purpose of nutritional support is to effectively reduce the observed excess morbidity: thus, the preoccupation with the provision of nutritional support and, hence, the interest that nutritional support evokes in the cancer-bearing patient on carbohydrate, fat, and protein metabolism.

2. Changes in Carbohydrate Metabolism Associated with Malignant and Benign Tumors

Warburg (1956) observed that the high anaerobic glycolysis characteristic of malignant tumors was not totally suppressed in the presence of oxygen, implying that the cancer tissue has a diminished Pasteur effect. According to Warburg, the high anaerobic glycolysis of malignant growth is caused by a defect in respiration secondary to an irreversible injury in the respiration mechanism due to the malignant growth, resulting in an adapting fermentative metabolism which allows growing in an uncontrolled fashion. However, many nonmalignant tissues, such as embryonic tissue, also have high anaerobic glycolysis rates.

Table I. Glucose Metabolism in Cancer Patients and Normal Subjects[a]

	Total glucose turnover[b] (TGT)	Cori cycle[b] (CC)	TGT–CC
Normal, overnight fast	200	36	164
Normal, 7-day fast	144	36	108
Cancer, stable weight	187	33	154
Cancer, progressive weight loss	268	115	153
Cancer, progressive weight loss with increased basal metabolic rate	370	212	158

[a]Reproduced from Holroyde *et al.*, 1981, with permission.
[b]gm/1.73 m² per 24 hr.

Isotope tracer techniques have shed light on the rates of glucose flux in cancer patients. Although no differences were observed in rates of glucose production and oxidation, glucose recycling was increased (Reichard *et al.*, 1964). A comparison between glucose metabolism in normal volunteers and in cancer patients with and without progressive weight loss is summarized in Table I (Holroyde *et al.*, 1975). Patients with progressive weight loss have increased rates of total glucose turnover and Cori cycle activity (the conversion of glucose to lactic acid by glycolysis and its hepatic reconversion to glucose), differing from the pattern seen in normal individuals without cancer. This increased glucose turnover may explain 50% or more of the elevated energy expenditure seen in some cancer patients and would be responsible for 0.5–1.0 kg weight loss per month (Eden *et al.*, 1984). The increased cycling of glucose carbons may explain the high glucose turnover. It is caused by elevated gluconeogenesis from lactate, glycerol, and amino acids (alanine), corresponding to interorgan cycling of glucose carbons. The increased plasma glucose turnover may represent the summation of tumor glucose uptake, increased uptake by immune cells, and altered substrate preference by some tissues, especially the liver.

Using isotope tracer studies, Weinhouse (1951) showed that tumors could oxidize glucose to CO_2 at rates comparable to those of normal tissues. However, in contrast to normal cells, supplying tumor cells with glucose inhibits endogenous respiration, turning the available glucose into the preferential nutrient for cancer cells (Guillino *et al.*, 1967).

The cellular differentiation of the tumor may also play a role in the carbohydrate metabolism disturbances seen in cancer patients. Experimental studies with the Morris hepatoma indicated that respiration decreases with loss of cellular differentiation. In contrast, there is a low rate of or no glycolysis in the well-differentiated hepatomas (Weber *et al.*, 1961; Elwood *et al.*, 1963). These metabolic alterations could be ascribed to differences in specific isoenzyme activities. Weinhouse studied the switch in pyruvate kinase patterns as the cause for competition for adenosine diphosphate between respiration and glycolysis (1972). In slow-growing, highly differentiated hepatomas, type II pyruvate kinase is increased but it is absent in fast-growing, poorly differentiated hepatomas. However, type I pyruvate kinase is much increased in poorly differentiated hepatomas, and that could explain their high glycolytic activity, as shown in Fig. 1.

Additional evidence for altered glucose metabolism in cancer patients is based on

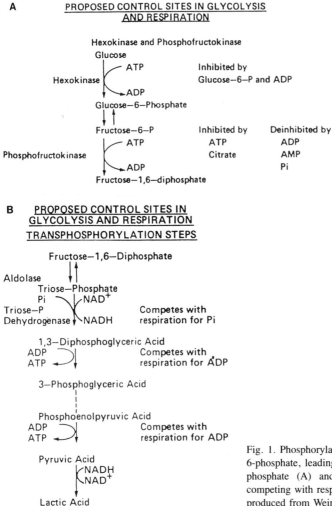

A   PROPOSED CONTROL SITES IN GLYCOLYSIS
                     AND RESPIRATION

Fig. 1. Phosphorylation sites of glucose and fructose 6-phosphate, leading to formation of fructose 1,6-diphosphate (A) and transphosphorylating enzymes competing with respiration for ADP and P_i (B). (Reproduced from Weinhouse, 1972, with permission.)

glucose tolerance studies (Jasani *et al.*, 1978; Schein *et al.*, 1979). Cancer patients are known to have high blood glucose concentrations and delayed blood clearances after glucose loads, due partly to tissue resistance to insulin. These alterations occur in the presence of normal fasting blood glucose concentrations. Some factors that impair glucose tolerance include starvation, bed rest, sepsis, and malnutrition; since these are often found in cancer patients as well, it is difficult to incriminate cancer as the primary agent responsible for the glucose intolerance found in these patients (Marks and Bishop, 1959).

In addition to the carbohydrate metabolic disturbances already described, hypoglycemia is sometimes observed. While hypoglycemia could result from excessive consumption of glucose by large bulky mesenchymal tumors (Unger, 1966), it is not usually found in cancer because of compensatory and counterregulatory hormones that result in glycogenolysis and glyconeogenesis.

In a study of the metabolic changes accompanying growth of a methylcholanthrene (MCA)-induced tumor in rats, blood glucose levels were significantly lower in tumor-bearing rats as compared to controls (Kurzer *et al.*, 1988). However, blood glucose levels in tumor-bearing rats did not differ from those of their pair-fed controls, suggesting that decreased food intake rather than the tumor was responsible for the relative hypoglycemia observed in the tumor-bearing animals. We also investigated the metabolic changes associated with growth of a carrageenan-induced benign tumor (Kawashima *et al.*, 1989). Rats given carrageenan subcutaneously were compared to controls receiving normal saline for 21 days. Blood glucose levels in the benign tumor rats did not differ significantly from those observed in controls (data not presented), suggesting that the benign tumor model does not interfere with normal glucose levels. In contrast, in another experimental model of nonmalignant rapid cell proliferation, i.e., liver regeneration, major changes occurred in the intermediary carbohydrate metabolism after 70% hepatectomy in the rabbit (Irie *et al.*, 1983). Significant increases were found in the concentrations of pyruvate, lactate, glucose-6-phosphate, and fructose-6-phosphate. A glucose tolerance test was abnormal in the rabbits during the maximum cellular replication period, during the first 48 hr after hepatectomy, suggesting a preferentially anaerobic metabolism during the period of rapid liver growth.

Another contributory factor to the elevated glucose turnover in cancer appears to be increased production of lactate secondary to tumor growth (Holroyde *et al.*, 1977). The association of lactic acidosis with malignancy has been described in leukemia (Block, 1974), bronchogenic carcinoma, and hepatocarcinoma (Spechler *et al.*, 1978). The etiology of this lactic acidosis in cancer is unknown, but may result from increased lactic acid production unattended by adequate lactate clearance. Holroyde *et al.* have studied lactate metabolism in metastatic colorectal cancer (1979). As shown in Fig. 2, the patients with cancer presented a moderately increased rate of lactate oxidation and twofold increases in monoxidative lactate disposal. The authors suggest that conversion of lactate to glucose

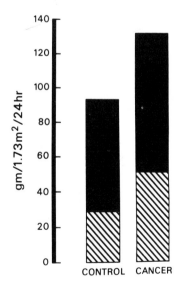

Fig. 2. Rates of lactate metabolism in 13 control subjects and 20 cancer patients. The height of the bars represents rates of lactate production. The solid portion of each bar is the rate of lactate oxidation and the hatched portion represents nonoxidative disposal. (Reproduced from Holroyde *et al.*, 1981, with permission.)

may account for the greater difference observed in monoxidative disposal in cancer patients. However, the observed lactate production correlated poorly with tumor burden.

There is also increased glucose transport in malignant cells as compared to normal cells, which appears to favor the development of poorly vascularized and oxygen-deficient tumors in their ability to use glucose (Weber, 1973).

3. Impact of Nutritional Support on Carbohydrate Metabolism in Tumor-Bearing Hosts

Table II summarizes the effects of total parenteral nutrition (TPN) on carbohydrate metabolism in tumor-bearing patients (Brennan, 1981). Gluconeogenesis can be suppressed by administration of substrate in the form of TPN (Waterhouse *et al.*, 1979), although there is no uniform consensus as to the optimal glucose infusion rate for cancer patients. Glucose infusion rates of up to 7 mg/kg per min in postoperative patients was associated with increased glucose oxidation and CO_2 production derived from glucose (Wolfe *et al.*, 1980). TPN also induces a moderate lactic acidemia and an increased lactate turnover in cancer patients (Holroyde *et al.*, 1977). The increase in plasma lactate may be due to increased lactate production by the tumor or it may be due to insulin resistance, thus influencing the intermediary metabolism of other tissues.

The fate of the infused glucose from TPN is poorly understood. The glucose turnover rate increases (Holroyde *et al.*, 1977; Burt *et al.*, 1982); depending on the isotope tracer used, it may be increased as much as 415%. After the administration of glucose, there is an increase in the glucose oxidation rate, showing that the caloric substrate is used for energy. However, complete oxidation may account for only half or less of body glucose turnover (Holroyde *et al.*, 1977).

Eden *et al.* (1984) evaluated the effects of enteral nutrition on carbohydrate metabo-

Table II. Carbohydrate Metabolism in Cancer Patients before and after Total Parenteral Nutrition[a]

	Pre-TPN tumor-bearing vs. pre-TPN non-tumor-bearing	Tumor-bearing during TPN vs. pre-TPN tumor-bearing
Glucose	No change	Significant increase
Lactate	Significant increase	Significant increase
Serum insulin	No change	Significant increase
Plasma glucagon	No change	No change
Glucose tolerance	Significant decrease	(Unknown)
Whole-body glucose turnover	Significant increase	Significant increase
Endogenous glucose production		No change
Glucose oxidation rate	No change	Significant increase
Gluconeogenesis from alanine	Significant increase	Significant decrease
Gluconeogenesis from lactate	Significant increase	Significant decrease

[a]Adapted from Brennan, 1981.

lism of cancer patients. After 14 days of continuous enteral nutrition, simultaneous measurements of energy expenditure and glucose cycling in cancer patients showed that the whole-body flux of glucose for oxygen uptake increased twofold in the cancer patients and remained unaltered in the control patients, indicating that glucose was channeled into nonoxidative pathways and was stored as glycogen and lipids.

4. Changes in Fat Metabolism Associated with Malignant and Benign Tumors

Tumor cells exhibit very active metabolism of fatty acids, which are required as oxidative substrates for replacement of membrane lipid components and for the manufacture of new cell membranes needed for growth and cell dividing. The fatty acids present in the tumor seem to be derived in large part from the host, although fatty acid synthesis from glucose also occurs (Medes *et al.*, 1953, 1957). Studies with Ehrlich ascites tumor suggest that glucose exerts a stimulatory effect on fatty acid synthesis either by providing NADPH through the pentose phosphate pathway (Kimura *et al.*, 1964) or by being converted to triose acceptors for incorporation of the newly formed fatty acids into lipid esters (Spector and Steinberg, 1966). The pathway for *de novo* fatty acid biosynthesis is operative in experimental cancer (Kimura *et al.*, 1964).

Tumor cells are able to desaturate and elongate fatty acids (Sabine *et al.*, 1968).Regulation of fatty acids biosynthesis is different in tumor-bearing animals when compared to controls; hepatic fatty acid biosynthesis, normally depressed in animals on a high-fat diet, is not inhibited in hepatoma-bearing rats (Sabine *et al.*, 1966). Fasting reduced acetate incorporation in control rat livers but not in those with hepatoma (Sabine *et al.*, 1967). When fasted rats were refed with a high-carbohydrate diet, hepatoma-bearing rats failed to increase acetate incorporation. The disturbed dietary regulation of fatty acid biosynthesis in tumor-bearing animals is not from fundamental differences in responsiveness of the fatty acid synthetic enzymes, but seems related to inability of the inhibitors to regulate the synthesis of the enzyme system (Sabine *et al.*, 1968; Sabine and Chaikoff, 1967). This aberrant metabolic control also compromises dietary regulation of cholesterol synthesis (Watson, 1972).

Studies of the fractional rate of lipid incorporation into tumor cells tended to show that most of the glucose incorporated into lipids was in glycerol backbones of lipid esters rather than in fatty acids (Miras *et al.*, 1967). These data suggest that, although many tumors derive a large fraction of their fatty acids from the host, in at least a few experimental tumor models the *de novo* hepatic fatty acid biosynthesis is equal to or greater than that observed in controls (Henderson and PePage, 1959).

The host responds to the presence of a tumor by increasing plasma glycerol turnover (Lundholm *et al.*, 1982) and by increasing lipolysis in peripheral tissues (Bennegard *et al.*, 1982). Although hyperlipidemia is not always associated with the presence of cancer in humans, increased free fatty acid turnover does occur. The loss of fat is attributed to excessive free fatty acid mobilization from the adipose tissue (Mays, 1969), only partly suppressed by high rates of glucose infusion (Edmonson, 1966).

In lipid kinetic studies of patients with cachexia associated with cancer, it was recently shown that free fatty acids and glycerol plasma concentrations and turnover rates were higher than reported values for healthy normals (Legaspi et al., 1987). Complete hydrolysis of triglycerides was observed, as was the absence of any extensive reesterification of free fatty acids in adipose tissue. The authors concluded that fat is efficiently mobilized and utilized as a fuel source in hypermetabolic cancer patients in the postabsorptive state. Another study observed similar findings in weight-losing patients with gastrointestinal cancer when compared to normals or cancer patients without weight loss (Shan and Wolfe, 1987). It is possible that the extent of carcass lipid depletion is related to tumor type, as suggested experimentally (Hollander et al., 1986).

It was also observed that some human tumors are associated with type IV hyperlipidemia (Dilman et al., 1981) and that very-low-density-lipoprotein hyperlipidemia is found in leukemia and lymphomas (Spiegel et al., 1982), indicating the existence of a defect in lipoprotein lipase function in cancer patients. Moreover, the reduced activity of lipoprotein lipase was strongly correlated with weight loss (Vlassara et al., 1986). It is important to note that the decrease in lipoprotein lipase in cancer associated with normal or increased insulin levels that, together with reduced food intake and weight loss, characterize a maladaptative host response that is completely different from the response expected in starvation (Vlassara et al., 1986).

The metabolism of free fatty acid in tumors involves uptake, oxidation, and sterification. Experimentally it was shown that tumor uptake of fatty acids is not dependent on metabolic energy, in contrast to what happens in nonmalignant cells (Spector et al., 1965; Wright and Green, 1971). The entry of fatty acids into Enrlich tumor cells is regulated by the molar ratio of fatty acids to albumin (directly) (Spector et al., 1965), pH (indirectly) (Spector, 1969), and fatty acid chain size (directly) (Spector and Steinberg, 1967a). With respect to the chain size, short-chain and medium-chain fatty acids are taken up very poorly; this might represent a future approach to specific nutritional support for the host, with depletion of tumor nutrition.

Fatty acid oxidation in cancer cells also occurs in the mitochondria and is mediated by the tricarboxylic acid cycle (Brown et al., 1956). Another possible metabolic pathway of fatty acids after uptake is incorporation into phospholipids, glycerides, and cholesterol esters. Certain of the esterified fatty acids in tumor cells, particularly those in lecithin, have a high turnover rate (Spector and Steinberg, 1967b). It appears that fatty acid metabolic pathways are, in general, the same in tumors as in nonmalignant tissues. However, this conclusion should be interpreted cautiously, because almost all data about fatty acid metabolism in cancer come from the Ehrlich ascites carcinoma. It is unknown whether other types of tumors will maintain the same metabolic activity, and thus, further research using other tumor models is needed to support the current data base.

Another important feature of fat metabolism in the presence of malignancy is the demonstration of lipolytic factors in the serum of tumor-bearing animals. It was observed that surgical removal of experimental tumors in rats was accompanied by the normalization of serum free fatty acid levels known to be increased in cancer (Frederick and Begg, 1954). This observation and others (Kralovic et al., 1977) suggest the existence of a fat-mobilizing substance produced by the tumor, which, when injected into normal mice, produces an immediate massive fat mobilization that is not suppressed by feeding (Kamada et al., 1980). Recent work has focused on the macrophage-produced monokine cachectin/tumor necrosis factor (TNF) as the cause of host weight loss and hyperlipidemia, biological effects similar to those frequently seen in cancer cachexia (Beutler and Cerami, 1986, 1987). Cachectin/TNF produces hyperlipidemia by reducing lipopro-

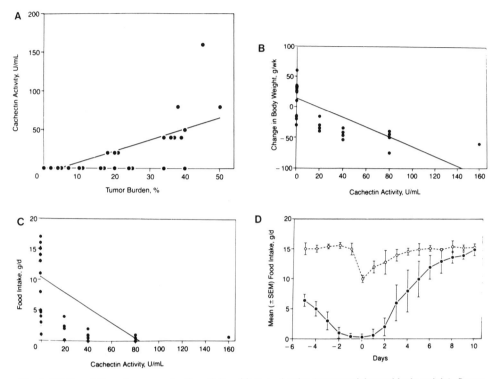

Fig. 3. (A) Correlation of serum cachectin activity with tumor burden (tumor weight/total body weight). Serum cachectin activity increased directly with tumor burden ($r = 0.72$; $p < 0.001$). (B) Correlation of serum cachectin activity with tumor-bearing rat change in body weight. Serum cachectin activity levels correlate inversely with tumor-bearing rat change in body weight ($r = -0.75$; $p < 0.001$). (C) Correlation of serum cachectin activity with tumor-bearing rat food intake. Serum cachectin activity correlated inversely with tumor-bearing rat food intake ($r = -0.66$; $p < 0.001$). (D) Food intake of tumor-bearing (closed circles) and non-tumor-bearing (open circles) rats before and after tumor resection or sham operation. Food intake of cachectic tumor-bearing rats progressively declined as non-tumor-bearing rats consumed 15 g/day ($p < 0.05$). Tumor was resected or sham operation was performed on day 0. (Reproduced from Stovroff *et al.*, 1989, with permission.)

tein lipase activity, thereby inhibiting the clearance of lipids from plasma (Kawakami *et al.*, 1982); it also impedes accumulation of fat within adipose cells. With the help of a new sensitive bioassay (Stovroff *et al.*, 1989), it was possible to detect circulating cachectin activity in the serum of sarcoma-bearing rats; these increased cachectin levels correlated with progressive weight loss and extension of disease. After tumor resection, food intake and body weight increased and serum cachectin activity became undetectable (Fig. 3). Further, serum triglyceride levels, which were higher in cachectic tumor-bearing rats than in pair-fed nontumor controls, decreased after tumor resection (Stovroff *et al.*, 1989).

There are few reports regarding the effects of benign tumors on fat metabolism. In a model of rapid nonmalignant cell proliferation, i.e., liver regeneration in dogs, we investigated the effects of the infusion of TPN with or without lipids (Campos *et al.*, 1984). In the group not receiving lipids parenterally, we observed a decrease in linoleic acid and an increase in palmitoleic, stearic, and oleic acids in hepatic tissue. By contrast, in the group receiving lipids, a significant increase in hepatic linoleic, oleic, and steraric acids was found. These results suggest that a relative essential fatty acid (linoleic acid) deficiency may occur in the fast-growing phase of a benign tissue. This concept is supported by the finding that the parenteral infusion of lipids is able to prevent the tissue linoleic acid deficiency. Whether these changes occur in rapid malignant cell proliferation needs investigating, considering the important role played by lipids in the composition of lipoproteins and new cell membranes.

5. Impact of Nutritional Support on Fat Metabolism in Tumor-Bearing Hosts

Nutritional support is able to restore body fat in depleted animal models (Popp *et al.*, 1984). In patients who received TPN for 6 weeks, a mean increase in body weight was observed, equally distributed between total body fat and total body water (Cohn *et al.*, 1982). During intravenous nutritional support, plasma free fatty acid levels appear to decrease in cancer patients receiving glucose-based intravenous nutrition (Waterhouse and Kemperman, 1971). The fractions that exhibited the most prominent decrease were low-density and high-density lipoproteins (Tashiro *et al.*, 1986). In contrast, the infusion of a 10% long-chain triglyceride fatty emulsion caused a marked increase in low-density lipoproteins together with increases in phospholipids and cholesterol, especially free cholesterol (Waterhouse and Kemperman, 1971).

As previously stated, some tumors consume relatively large quantities of glucose or gluconeogenic precursors during active growth. Theoretically, caloric provision by non-gluconeogenic precursors such as lipids would provide no utilizable energy substrate increase for the tumor. Experimentally it was shown that the infusion of adequate caloric substrate (as fat plus amino acids) produced no significant increase in tumor growth as compared to chow-fed controls, and slower tumor growth as compared to diets with equal caloric amounts of carbohydrate and protein (Buzby *et al.*, 1980). Unfortunately, these promising results have not been convincingly duplicated (Hak *et al.*, 1984; Mahaffey *et al.*, 1985; Bevilacqua *et al.*, 1984), suggesting that they may be specific to the experimental model used instead of being a general metabolic response.

Because ketone bodies can preserve lean body mass during periods of weight loss and yet be poor metabolic substrates for tumors (Rofe *et al.*, 1986), the administration of medium-chain triglycerides as efficient ketosis inducers was investigated in tumor-bearing mice (Tisdale and Brennan, 1988). When compared to normal controls receiving a high-carbohydrate, low-fat diet, animals fed medium-chain triglycerides showed a reduced weight loss and a marked reduction in tumor size. In contrast, neither weight loss nor tumor size differed significantly from controls in animals fed long-chain triglyceride diet. These differences were attributed to the increases of ketone body concentration rather than just replacement of the carbohydrate diet by fat.

6. Changes in Energy Metabolism Associated with Malignant and Benign Tumors

The maintenance of cell and organ function requires energy. Adequate knowledge of the metabolism and utilization of fuel sources and of the regulation of whole-body energy

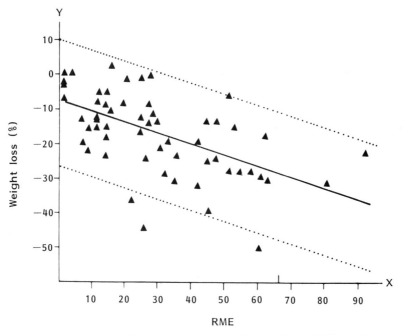

Fig. 4. Percentage of weight loss as a function of resting metabolic expenditure (RME) in 65 patients with advanced cancer. $Y = 0.193$, $X = -8.33$. Regression test, $F = 12.96$, $p < 0.005$. (Reproduced from Bozzetti *et al.*, 1980, with permission.)

expenditure is important for understanding nutritional derangements in cancer patients, and therefore for planning nutritional support in such patients.

Cancer-induced malnutrition is a clinical condition due to a complex interrelationship between anorexia, altered physical activity, modifications in the protein–energy metabolism, activation of the immune system (including cell proliferation), tumor metabolism, and, eventually, paraneoplastic changes. While it is generally accepted that anorexia is a major contributor to the weight loss commonly observed in cancer patients (Morrison, 1976), there is no uniform acceptance that increased energy expenditure is a major factor responsible for the weight loss in cancer. Reports in the literature are conflicting; while some authors reported increased resting energy expenditure, others found resting energy expenditure normal or even low. Resting energy metabolism represents the combustion of fuel sources needed to provide energy for the processes maintaining function and integrity of cells and organs, and for the processes involved in keeping the body alive (Young, 1977).

The considerable variations in resting metabolic expenditure among and within the various reported studies (Warnold *et al.*, 1978; Arbeit *et al.*, 1984; Bozzetti *et al.*, 1980; Burke *et al.*, 1980) may represent differences in methodologic and biological variables as well as possible metabolic effects of different cancers and severity and stage of disease. One of the first studies of resting metabolic expenditure found it increased in 20–60% of patients with advanced cancer. There was a significant correlation between resting metabolic expenditure and tissue wasting, evaluated as weight loss and decreased serum transferrin (Bozzetti *et al.*, 1980). These results are shown in Fig. 4.

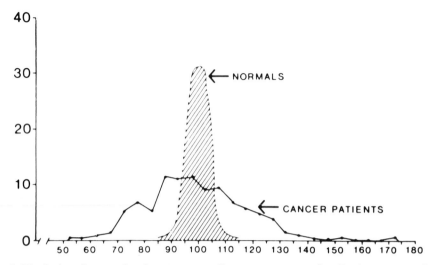

Fig. 5. Distribution of measured resting energy expenditure as a percentage of predicted energy expenditure in "normals" and in 200 cancer patients. (Reproduced from Knox *et al.*, 1983, with permission.)

Other studies, however, failed to support this conclusion; it was observed that increased resting energy expenditure was not a consistent finding in cancer patients (Hansell *et al.*, 1986; Young, 1977; Burke *et al.*, 1980). It seems that the adaptation of cancer patients to starvation is abnormal. In one study, the difference in energy expenditure between malnourished cancer patients and noncancer patients was 148 kcal/24 hr. This amount would represent wasting of about 0.5 kg of body fat/month or 1.1 kg of muscle mass/month (Lundholm, 1984). Over a longer period of time this could explain at least part of the weight loss seen in patients with progressive malignant disease.

One study examined energy expenditure in weight-losing and non-weight-losing cancer patients and compared the results to a similar population without malignancy. Oxygen uptake and resting energy expenditure, expressed per kilogram of body weight, were elevated in weight-losing cancer patients compared to their non-tumor-bearing controls (Lindmark *et al.*, 1984). In another study evaluating 200 hospitalized cancer patients, most patients were outside the range of energy expenditure predicted by the Harris–Benedict equation. Hypometabolism was found in 33%, normometabolism in 41%, and hypermetabolism in 26% of the patients (Fig. 5). It is interesting to note that hypermetabolic patients had a significantly longer duration of disease than did normometabolic patients.

In a similar study of 173 malnourished patients with gastrointestinal cancer, distribution according to energy expenditure was similar to the previous study (Demsey and Mullen, 1985). However, the primary tumor site influenced the basal metabolic expenditure. Patients with pancreatic and hepatobiliary tumors were more frequently hypometabolic, while patients with gastric cancer were more frequently hypermetabolic. When resting energy expenditure was compared in patients with diffuse as opposed to localized disease, patients with extensive metastatic disease had an increase in energy expenditure.

In a recent controlled study, resting energy expenditure and body composition were

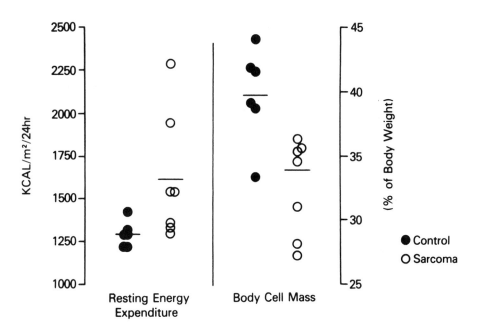

Fig. 6. Plot of resting energy expenditure (REE) and body cell mass (BCM) data for control subjects and sarcoma patients. Note that REE/m^2 per 24 hr is higher in sarcoma patients than in controls ($p < 0.05$), and that BCM as percent of body weight is lower in sarcoma patients ($p < 0.05$). m^2, Meters squared (BSA); (———), mean. (Reproduced from Peacock *et al.*, 1987, with permission.)

examined in noncachectic patients with sarcomas, a metabolically active tumor type (Peacock *et al.*, 1987). As shown in Fig. 6, an inverse relationship between resting energy expenditure and body cell mass was observed, in contrast to what occurs in normal subjects. When resting energy expenditure was corrected for body cell mass, it was higher in sarcoma patients before anorexia and cachexia were apparent. The increased resting metabolic expenditure, despite weight loss and undernutrition, indicates that the adaptive mechanisms that usually follow semistarvation are impaired in patients with uncontrolled cancer growth.

Several possibilities have been proposed to explain this adaptive homeostatic impairment found in cancer patients. Since tumor tissue is only a very small fraction of total body tissue (Costa, 1977) (except for the huge sarcomas), it is unlikely that the tumor burden is responsible for the increased oxygen consumption. Utilization of lactate for hepatic glucose synthesis could be responsible for the increased energy expenditure in the tumor-bearing patient (Gold, 1974). However, increased Cori cycle activity does not appear to account for a significant fraction of daily energy expenditure (Young, 1977). As shown in Fig. 7, the increased activity of some futile cycles (glucose-6-phosphate, fructose-6-phosphate, and phosphoenolpyruvate) has been proposed as an explanation for the energy waste. Another possibility may be a high substrate consumption by the tumor cell. However, most tumors have a lower metabolic rate than their tissues of origin (Guillino, 1976), although some exceptions occur; some huge sarcomas may consume up to 700 kcal/day.

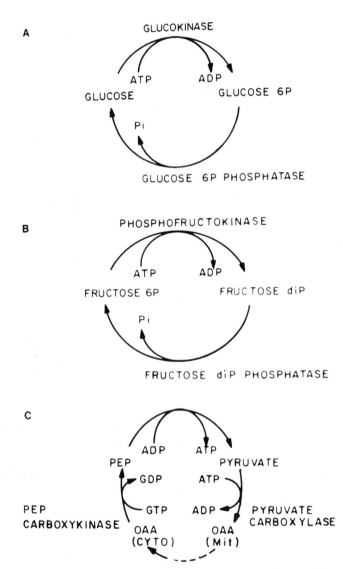

Fig. 7. Three futile cycles in carbohydrate metabolism: the glucose 6-phosphate (glucose 6F), fructose 6-phosphate (glucose 6P), and phosphoenolpyruvate (PEP) cycles. The variable activity of these cycles, which do not involve a net change in the levels of reactants (e.g., glucose, fructose 6-phosphate, or phosphoenolpyruvate), will result in changes in rates of ATP generation, relative to rates of ATP hydrolysis. OAA, Oxaloacetic acid; CYTO, cytoplasmic; Mit, mitochondrial. (Reproduced from Young, 1977, with permission.)

Previously we showed a significant decrease in DNA, RNA, total protein (Meguid *et al.*, 1987), and amino acid (Landel *et al.*, 1987) content of skeletal muscle in 21-day tumor-bearing rats. As this may adversely affect the contractile proteins and thus muscle function, we studied the effects of tumor on muscle performance and associated energy utilization within the three fiber types of skeletal muscle. MCA tumor was implanted into

Fischer rats. Twenty days later the gastrocnemius–soleus muscle group was stimulated with an *in situ* preparation. Muscles ($n = 6$) were stimulated for 10 min at 7.5, 15, and 30 tetani/min and for 5 min at 60 tetani/min. A control group of non-tumor-bearing rats was similarly stimulated. ATP content of white and red gastrocnemius and soleus was measured. No significant differences in force output and ATP content were observed. Data indicate that despite observed changes in DNA, RNA, total protein, and amino acid content in tumor-bearing rats at 21 days, no changes in muscle performance or muscle energy status were observed (Whitlock and Meguid, 1988).

It is possible that several organs or tissues could be involved in explaining the elevated energy expenditure found in some cancer patients. The sympaticoadrenergic system may have elevated activity, because high levels of circulating catecholamines have been found (Russell *et al.*, 1984), leading to hyperfunction of the heart and activation of brown adipose tissue thermogenesis (Brooks *et al.*, 1981). The liver is normally a high-energy-consuming organ and increased enzyme activity has been reported in tumor host livers, suggesting an elevated metabolic rate (Greengard and Cayanis, 1983). However, these findings have not been confirmed by other investigators (Lundholm *et al.*, 1983). Finally, the alterations of energy metabolism in tumor-bearing host could be related to changes in the intracellular intermediary metabolism of amino acids, carbohydrate, and lipids.

7. Changes in Protein Metabolism Associated with Malignant and Benign Tumors

The weight loss that accompanies progressive malignant disease is associated with a reduction of not only body fat stores, but also body protein mass. The most clinically obvious manifestation of cachexia of malignancy is the extensive skeletal muscle wasting. Other body proteins are also depleted (Stein *et al.*, 1981), which may simply result from decreased intake (DeWys, 1977) or antineoplastic therapy (Lawrence, 1977), although there is increasing evidence of a more direct tumor effect on host protein metabolism (Lundholm *et al.*, 1981a; Brennan, 1977; Jeevanandam *et al.*, 1984; Meguid *et al.*, 1987). Thus, protein turnover is disturbed in the cancer-bearing host, and there is a net loss of nitrogen from nonmalignant tissues as protein degradation exceeds synthesis.

Some tumor effects on host protein metabolism which are not readily measurable in humans have been studied in animal models. In 1948 it was demonstrated that the nitrogen content of a large rodent tumor (Walker carcinoma 256) exceeds the amount of nitrogen stored by its host during the period of tumor growth (Mider *et al.*, 1948). Therefore, part of the nitrogen contained in such a tumor must have been derived from the host's organs and tissues (Sherman *et al.*, 1950). From this observation, the concept that the malignant tissue acts as a "nitrogen trap" was derived. More recently, stable isotope techniques provide a new metabolic approach to investigate protein turnover in the cancer-bearing state. Using labeled amino acids, tumor-bearing animals have been shown to have higher liver fractional synthetic rates, higher muscle catabolic rates, higher whole-body protein turnover rates, and lowered skeletal muscle fractional synthetic rates than do normal controls (Norton *et al.*, 1981; Sherman *et al.*, 1950; Goodgame *et al.*, 1979; Stein *et al.*, 1976; Buzby *et al.*, 1980; Kawamura *et al.*, 1981). Even before decreases in food intake

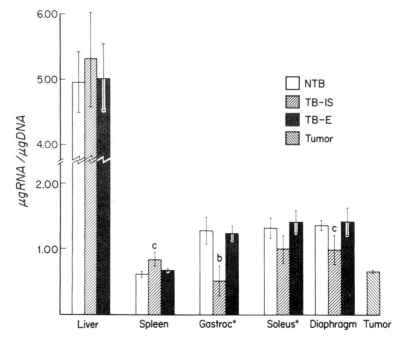

Fig. 8. Ratio of RNA to DNA in the liver, spleen, gastrocnemius, soleus, and diaphragm of non-tumor-bearing controls (NTB, $n = 8$), tumor-bearing rats whose tumor was left *in situ* (TB-IS, $n = 6$), and tumor-bearing rats after tumor was excised (TB-E, $n = 8$). Tumor ratio is also shown. TB-IS vs. NTB and TB-E. $b = p < 0.01$; $c = p < 0.05$. (Reproduced from Meguid *et al.,* 1987, with permission.)

can be measured, changes in body weight and nitrogen balance occurred, suggesting that these metabolic effects were primarily induced by the biological activity of the tumor.

As the tumor grows, it competes with the host for nutrients. Tumor cells have a higher and more efficient capacity for concentrating amino acids than do normal cells (Christensen, 1961) and also have the ability to draw directly from host tissue proteins (Sherman *et al.,* 1950). Thus, the tumor changes the patterns of protein synthesis in the host tissues (Landel *et al.,* 1987). Some enzymes and proteins for tumor use are synthesized by the host while production of similar substances for host use is suppressed (Goodlad, 1964).

We have shown (Meguid *et al.,* 1987; Landel *et al.,* 1987) that removal of tumor stopped the processes just outlined, with restoration to normal of the abnormal profiles of plasma amino acids found during the tumor-bearing state (Fig. 8). We subsequently investigated whether these changes were due only to malnutrition or to more complex alterations in protein metabolism, using pair-fed control (non-tumor-bearing) and malnourished control rats (Kurzer *et al.,* 1988). Plasma levels of each of the three branched-chain amino acids (BCAA) were found to be significantly lower in tumor-bearing rats than in both control and pair-fed rats, as were arginine, serine, and citrulline. In contrast, tumor-bearing rats exhibited higher levels of lysine, glycine, and proline. The finding of reduced levels of BCAA in both tumor-bearing and pair-fed rats (much more marked in the former) implies either increased tissue uptake or decreased tissue output or, more likely, a combination of the two. The primary site of BCAA catabolism is in skeletal muscle. The amino groups are converted to alanine, the primary gluconeogenic precursor of the liver.

The results of these animal experiments are confirmed by some reports of protein metabolism measurements in cancer-bearing patients. The rate of incorporation of labeled leucine into muscle protein is decreased and the fractional degradation rate of proteins is found to be increased in cancer patients (Lundholm *et al.*, 1976). Labeled leucine is incorporated more into hepatic proteins of cancer patients than controls, indicating increased synthesis of hepatic proteins (Lundholm *et al.*, 1978). The turnover of muscle protein is found to be controlled by alterations of protein synthesis rather than by increased breakdown (Rennie *et al.*, 1983). Whole-body protein turnover is found to be increased in patients with colorectal carcinoma (Carmichael *et al.*, 1980), non-small-cell lung cancer (Heber *et al.*, 1982), and even in children with leukemia (Kien and Camitta, 1983), implying that disordered protein metabolism may participate in the altered energy expenditure observed in cancer patients.

When compared to malnourished patients with benign disease or fasted normal controls, cancer patients are found to have markedly elevated rates of whole-body protein turnover and synthesis (Jeevanandam *et al.*, 1984). Nitrogen balance studies, a time-honored way to assess protein status, can be misleading in tumor-bearing subjects, be-

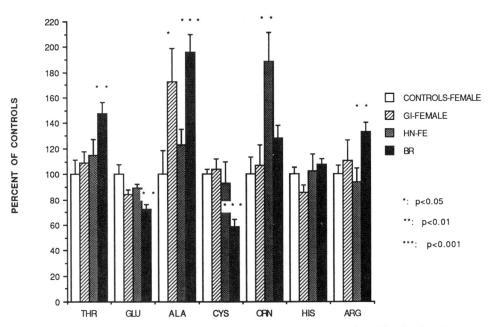

Fig. 9. Changes in plasma amino acids in females with breast, gastrointestinal, and head and neck cancer expressed as a percent of controls. (Reproduced from Kubota *et al.*, 1990.)

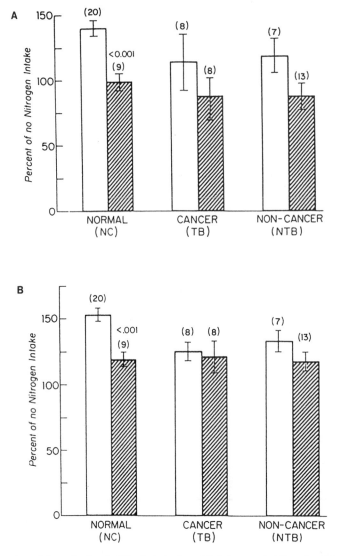

Fig. 10. Changes in protein synthesis rate (A), whole-body protein turnover rate (B), and protein breakdown rate (C) during oral and intravenous feeding. The results are normalized to no nitrogen intake as 100%. (Reproduced from Jeevanandam *et al.*, 1987, with permission.)

cause nitrogen retention in tumor growth may outweigh the negative nitrogen balance occurring in the rest of the host from lean tissue catabolism (Lowry and Brennan, 1986).

Most plasma amino acid levels in cancer-bearing patients with minimal weight loss were similar to those in controls. The venous concentrations of leucine, isoleucine, and valine are in the normal range in malnourished cancer patients (Norton *et al.*, 1985). It appears that increased protein breakdown, the major mechanisms for increased BCAA levels in early starvation, declines with prolonged starvation, a metabolic adaptation that does not occur in cancer.

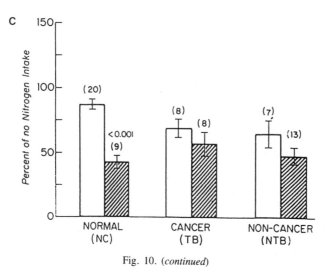

Fig. 10. (*continued*)

Although plasma amino acids represent less than 1% of the body's total free amino acid pool, they are sensitive to and reflect the host metabolic changes that accompany a variety of disease states (Kubota *et al.*, 1990). We have shown that total plasma amino acids in breast cancer patients are significantly higher than in female controls. There is also a strong correlation between seven plasma amino acid levels (glutamine, threonine, histidine, cysteine, alanine, arginine, and ornitine) and the organ site of three kinds of malignant tumors, as shown in Fig. 9. These changes in plasma amino acid profiles reflect the net result of host production and tumor utilization.

In a carrageenan-induced benign tumor model, we have noted that serum albumin decreases significantly as the benign tumor grows, as compared to controls (Kawashima *et al.*, 1989). It is likely that rapidly growing benign tumors also have avidity for amino acids to support their growth.

8. Impact of Nutritional Support on Protein Metabolism of Tumor-Bearing Hosts

As previously stated, in times of reduced nutrient supply from cancer anorexia, the tumor has an inherent biological advantage and acts to direct substrate toward itself (Sherman *et al.*, 1950). This could explain why total starvation has little, if any, effect on the DNA synthesis, the protein synthesis, or the growth of a tumor (Goodgame *et al.*, 1974; Reilly *et al.*, 1977), although feeding tumor-bearing rats a protein-free diet leads to significantly smaller tumors than in their normal chow-fed controls (Waitzberg *et al.*, 1989). In a similar study, protein-depleted rats have a longer survival when compared to controls receiving a regular diet (Gerry *et al.*, 1982).

Although these findings suggest caution concerning the indiscriminate use of nutritional support in cancer patients, especially those who still have significant tumor burdens, it has been observed that cancer patients improved their protein-synthesizing capacity after 14 days of TPN, as reflected by an increased RNA content in muscle tissue

Table III. The Effect of 10 Days of TPN on Whole-Body Protein Kinetics
of Weight-Losing Cancer Patients[a]

	Condition		Starved normals[b] (n = 5)
	Benign (n = 9)	Malignant (n = 5)	
% Weight loss[c]	15 ± 2	18 ± 2	8 ± 1
N balance (mg/kg per day)	−91 to +76	−84 to +52	−99 to +110
Protein turnover (g/kg per day)	↑ 1%	↑ 15%**	↑ 24%*
Protein synthesis (g/kg per day)	↓ 33%*	↓ 21%*	↓ 1%
Protein breakdown (g/kg per day)	↓ 59%**	↓ 49%**	↓ 54%*

[a]Adapted from Jeevanandam *et al.*, 1985.
[b]Adapted from Rose *et al.*, 1983.
[c]Change from basal (pre-TPN).
*$p < 0.05$, **$p < 0.005$, study 1 (pre-TPN) vs. study 2 (during TPN), paired *t*-test.

(Lundholm *et al.*, 1981b) and an increased leucine incorporation into muscle proteins *in vitro*. Also, in weight-losing cancer patients the provision of enteral nutrition resulted in an improved tyrosine balance across the leg, suggesting a net protein synthesis (Bennegard *et al.*, 1983). While the peripheral tissues remained in net negative nitrogen balance, a whole-body positive nitrogen balance was achieved (Lundholm *et al.*, 1982).

As shown in Fig. 10, protein kinetics are increased by oral feeding and by TPN in depleted patients. However, while oral feedings have a greater effect on total protein synthesis, TPN is associated with a greater decrease in total protein breakdown rates (Jeevanandam *et al.*, 1987). Nutritional support may preferentially enhance protein synthesis in the visceral compartment in patients with chronic weight loss, with or without cancer. In a controlled trial in patients with esophageal squamous cell carcinoma, it was shown that nutritional repletion increased turnover of whole-body proteins, stimulated protein synthesis, decreased muscle breakdown, and improved nitrogen balance and body weight (Burt *et al.*, 1983b, 1984). Using body composition techniques, cancer patients improved their lean body mass (Shizgal, 1985), increased muscle glycogen (Sandstedt *et al.*, 1985), and retained potassium (Bozzetti *et al.*, 1987), as summarized in Table III. These data suggest that nutritional support in cancer patients can lead to an increase in lean body mass, but only to a limited extent and requiring prolonged TPN administration.

Because there are similarities between the metabolic response to injury and to active tumor growth, BCAA have been used to modify the metabolic response of the tumor-bearing host (Brennan, 1981). Continuous oral administration of BCAA to tumor-bearing rats significantly increased survival time by 32% and reduced tumor size by 33% after 3 weeks of growth (Schaur *et al.*, 1980). When 50% BCAA-enriched amino acid TPN solutions were administered to malnourished advanced-cancer patients, there was improvement in whole-body leucine flux, oxidation, leucine balance, and fractional synthetic rates of albumin (Tayek *et al.*, 1986). In other experiments using tyrosine as the amino acid tracer, it was shown that tumor-bearing rats receiving BCAA-enriched amino acid solutions had decreased tyrosine oxidation; the net tyrosine balance was improved. These data suggest that BCAA-enriched TPN solutions increase amino acid utilization for net protein synthesis preferentially by reducing amino acid oxidation without stimulating tumor growth (Crosby *et al.*, 1988).

We prospectively evaluated 60 depleted postoperative cancer patients who received either a standard TPN or BCAA-enriched TPN solution with either a high or a low leucine content (Campos and Meguid, 1990). A sustained increase in plasma BCAA levels was observed with the high-leucine BCAA–TPN solution, together with a positive nitrogen balance not achieved with the standard TPN solution. However, the low-leucine BCAA–TPN solution failed to sustain a positive nitrogen balance, providing results similar to those obtained with standard TPN. These data suggest that the ability of BCAA to promote nitrogen retention is dependent on the leucine content of the solution, although BCAA–TPN promotes better nitrogen retention than does standard TPN at similar leucine contents. We also investigated leucine kinetics in normal volunteers by the continuous infusion of ^{13}C-leucine. We demonstrated that when leucine intake increased, leucine flux increased due to higher rates of leucine oxidation; the rate of whole-body protein breakdown decreased relative to the rate of whole-body protein synthesis. These results confirm that leucine content is an important controlling mechanism in protein turnover and that the effects of leucine infusion are more consistently related to decreasing protein breakdown than to increasing protein synthesis.

Exercise is another approach for improving host muscle uptake of nutrients. Muscles of tumor-bearing rats submitted to exercise maintain their mass, whereas nonexercising muscles lose muscle mass (Norton *et al.*, 1979). As anorexia and host weight loss are the main components of cachexia, the use of insulin as an anabolic hormone has also been investigated. In tumor-bearing rats, exogenous insulin improved food intake and host body composition, inhibited host protein waste, shifted nutrient flow from tumor to host, and improved survival when given for short periods during the development of cachexia (Moley *et al.*, 1985a,b; Peacock and Norton, 1988).

Attempts have also been made to starve the tumor selectively, through a biochemically rational chemotherapy with depleting enzymes and antimetabolites for specific amino acids. The most used antimetabolites are those of L-glutamine, with the drug azaserine, 6-diazo-5-oxo-L-norleucine (DON). Although DON is not primarily an antagonist to protein synthesis, it works as an antagonist to glutamine in its role of *de novo* purine synthesis. Exogenous L-asparaginase has been used to obtain asparagine deprivation in lymphoid malignancies, being highly effective in some leukemias (Sallan *et al.*, 1983).

The effectiveness of amino acid deprivation in cancer was also investigated in association with chemotherapy and radiotherapy; results of the therapies were improved by the administration of TPN without methionine and cysteine (Goseki *et al.*, 1982). The infusion of arginine-enriched amino acid solution was reported to suppress both the early stages of tumor growth and the appearance of metastases in tumor-bearing rats (Tachibana *et al.*, 1985). These beneficial effects were attributed to the immune stimulatory effect of the solution. Finally, the eventual stimulation of tumor growth by TPN in human malignancy was also assessed. In operatively obtained tumor specimens, no increases in fractional protein synthetic rates were found in the intravenously fed patients (Mullen *et al.*, 1980), clearly suggesting that TPN does not stimulate tumor growth.

ACKNOWLEDGMENT. Work presented in this paper was supported in part by Grant AM36275 from the National Institute of Arthritis, Diabetes, Digestive and Kidney Disease, NIH.

9. References

Arbeit, J. M., Lees, D. E., Corsey, R., and Brennan, M. F., 1984, Resting energy expenditure in controls and cancer patients with localized and diffuse disease, *Ann. Surg.* **199**:292–298.

Bennegard, K., Eden, E., Ekman, L., Scherstein, T., and Lundholm, K., 1982, Metabolic balance across the leg in weight-losing cancer patients compared to depleted patients without cancer, *Cancer Res.* **42**:4293–4299.

Bennegard, K., Eden, E., Ekman, L., Scherstein, T., and Lundholm, K., 1983, Metabolic response of whole body and peripheral tissues to enteral nutrition in weight-losing cancer and non-cancer patients, *Gastroenterology* **85**:92–99.

Beutler, B., and Cerami, A., 1986, Cachectin and tumor necrosis factor as two sides of the same biological coin, *Nature* **326**:584–588.

Beutler, B., and Cerami, A., 1987, Cachectin: More than a tumor necrosis factor, *New. Engl. J. Med.* **316**:379–385.

Bevilacqua, R. G., Gomes, M. C. C., Bevilacqua, L. R., Margarido, N. F., Waitzberg, D. L., and Lima, G. L., 1984, Efeitos da utilizacao da dieta hiper lipidica sobre o desenvolvimento tumoral. Estudo experimental com o carcinossarcoma de Walker 256, *Rev. Paul. Med.* **102**:249–255.

Block, J. B., 1974, Lactic acidosis in malignancy and observations on its possible pathogenesis, *Ann. NY Acad. Sci.* **230**:94–102.

Bozzetti, F., Pangnomi, A. M., and DelVecchio, M., 1980, Excessive caloric expenditure as a cause of malnutrition in patients with cancer, *Surg. Gynecol. Obstet.* **150**:229–234.

Bozzetti, F., Ammatuna, M., Migliavacca, S., Banalumi, M. G., Facchetti, G., Pupar, A., and Terno, G., 1987, Total parenteral nutrition prevents further nutritional deterioration in patients with cancer cachexia, *Ann. Surg.* **205**:138–143.

Brennan, M. F., 1977, Uncomplicated starvation versus cancer cachexia, *Cancer Res.* **37**:2359.

Brennan, M. F., 1981, Total parenteral nutrition in the cancer patient, *N. Engl. J. Med.* **305**:375–382.

Brooks, S. L., Neville, A. M., Rothwell, N. J., Stock, M. J., and Wilson, S., 1981, Sympathetic activation of brown-adipose tissue thermogenesis in cachexia, *Biosci. Rep.* **1**:509–517.

Brown, G. W., Jr., Katz, J., and Chaikoff, I. L., 1956, The oxidative metabolic pattern of mouse hepatoma C 954 as studied with C^{14}-labeled acetate, propionate, octanoate and glucose, *Cancer Res.* **16**:509–519.

Burke, M., Bryson, E. I., and Kark, A. E., 1980, Dietary intakes, resting metabolic rates, and body composition in benign and malignant gastrointestinal disease, *Br. Med. J.* **280**:211–215.

Burt, M. E., Gorschboth, C., and Brennan, M. F., 1982, A controlled, prospective randomized trial evaluating the metabolic effects of enteral and parenteral nutrition in the cancer patient, *Cancer* **49**:1092–1102.

Burt, M. E., Aoki, T. T., Borschboth, C. M., and Brennan, M. F., 1983a, Peripheral tissue metabolism in cancer-bearing man, *Ann. Surg.* **198**:685–691.

Burt, M. E., Stein, T. P., and Brennan, M. F., 1983b, A controlled randomized trial evaluating the effects of enteral and parenteral nutrition on protein metabolism in cancer-bearing man, *J. Surg. Res.* **34**:303–314.

Burt, M. E., Stein, T. P., Schwade, J. G., and Brennan, M. F., 1984, Whole body protein metabolism in cancer bearing patients: Effect of total parenteral nutrition and associated serum insulin response, *Cancer* **53**:1246–1252.

Buzby, G. P., Mullen, J. L., Stein, T. P., Miller, E. F., Hobbs, C. L., and Rosato, E. F., 1980, Host tumor interaction and nutrient supply, *Cancer* **45**:2940–2948.

Campos, A. C. L., and Meguid, M. M., 1990, Mechanism of improved nitrogen-sparing of branched chain amino acid TPN solutions enriched with different leucine concentration in malnourished postoperative cancer patients, *Am. J. Surg.* (submitted).

Campos, A. C. L., Vic, P., Crastes de Paulet, P., Astre, C., Liu, Y. Y., Saint-Aubert, B., Crastes de Paulet, A., and Joyeux, H., 1984, Beneficial effect of lipid infusion during liver regeneration after 65% hepatectomy in the dog, in: *Advances in Hepatic Encephalopathy and Urea Cycle Diagnosis* (G. Kleinberger, P. Ferenci, P. Riederer, and H. Thaler, eds.) Karger, Basel, pp. 720–724.

Campos, A. C. L., Chen, M., and Meguid, M. M., 1990, Comparisons of body composition derived from anthropomorphic and bioelectrical impedance methods, *J. Am. Coll. Nutr.* **8**:484–489.

Carmichael, M. J., Clague, M. B., Keir, M. J., Johnston, I. D. A., 1980, Whole body protein turnover, synthesis and breakdown in patients with colorectal carcinoma, *Br. J. Surg.* **67**:736–739.

Christensen, H. N., 1961, Free amino acids and peptides in tissues, in: *Mammalian Protein Metabolism,* Volume 1 (H. N. Munro and J. B. Allison, eds.), Academic Press, New York, pp. 105–124.

Cohn, S. H., Vartsky, D., Vaswani, A. N., Sawitsky, A., Rai, K., Gartenhaus, W., Yasumura, S., and Ellis, K. J., 1982, Changes in body composition of cancer patients following combined nutritional support, *Nutr. Cancer* **4:**107–119.

Costa, G., 1977, Cachexia, the matabolic component of neoplastic diseases, *Cancer Res.* **37:**2327–2335.

Crosby, L. E., Bistrian, B. R., Ling, P., Istfan, N. W., Blackburn, B. L., and Hoffman, S. B., 1988, Effects of branched chain amino acid-enriched total parenteral nutrition on amino acid utilization in rats bearing yoshida sarcoma, *Cancer Res.* **48:**2698–2702.

Demsey, D. T., and Mullen, J. L., 1985, Macronutrient requirements in the malnourished cancer patient, *Cancer* **197:**152–162.

Devereux, D. F., Redgrave, T. G., Loda, M., Clowes, G. H. A., Jr., and Deckers, P. J., 1985, Tumor-associated metabolism in the rat is a unique physiologic entity, *J. Surg. Res.* **38:**149–153.

DeWys, W. D., 1977, Anorexia in cancer patients, *Cancer Res.* **37:**2354–2358.

Dilman, V. M., Berstein, L. M., Ostroumova, M. N., Tsyrlina, Y. V., and Goluber, A. G., 1981, Peculiarities of hyperlipidemia in tumor patients, *Br. J. Cancer* **43:**637–643.

Eden, E., Edstrom, S., Bennegard, K., Scherstein, T., and Lundholm, K., 1984, Glucose flux in relation to energy expenditure in malnourished patients with and without cancer during periods of fasting and feeding, *Cancer Res.* **44:**1718–1724.

Edmonson, J. H., 1966, Fatty acid mobilization and glucose metabolism in patients with cancer, *Cancer* **19:**277–280.

Elwood, J. C., Lin, Y. C., Cristofalo, V. J., Weinhouse, S., and Morris, H. P., 1963, Glucose utilization in homogenates of the Morris hepatoma 5123 and related tumors, *Cancer Res.* **23:**906–913.

Frederick, G. L., and Begg, R. W., 1954, Development of lipidemia during tumor growth in rat, *Proc. Am. Assoc. Cancer Res.* **1:**14–18.

Gerry, K. L., Witt, B. H., Track, N. S., McDonnell, M., Makowka, L., and Falk, R. E., 1982, The effect of protein depletion upon tumor growth and host survival, *J. Surg. Res.* **33:**332–336.

Gold, J., 1974, Cancer cachexia and gluconeogenesis, *Ann. NY Acad. Sci.* **230:**103–110.

Goodgame, J. T., Lowry, S. F., Reilly, J. J., Jones, D. C., and Brennan, M. F., 1974, Nutritional manipulations and tumor growth. I. The effects of starvation, *Am. J. Clin. Nutr.* **32:**2277–2284.

Goodgame, J. T., Lowry, S. F., and Brennan, M. F., 1979, Nutritional manipulations and tumor growth II. The effects of intravenous feeding, *Am. J. Clin. Nutr.* **32:**2285–2292.

Goodlad, G. A., 1964, Protein metabolism and tumor growth, in: *Mammalian Protein Metabolism,* Volume 2, (H. N. Munro and J. B. Allison, eds.), Academic Press, New York, pp. 415–444.

Goseki, N., Onodera, T., Mori, S., and Menjo, M., 1982, Nippon Gan Chiryo, *Gakkai Shi* **17(7):**1980–1916.

Greengard, O., and Cayanis, E., 1983, Hormonal and dietary regulation of hepatic enzymes in tumor-bearing rats, *Cancer Res.* **43:**1575–1580.

Guillino, P. M., 1976, *In vivo* utilization of oxygen and glucose by neoplastic tissue, *Adv. Exp. Med. Biol.* **75:**521–536.

Guillino, P. M., Grantham, F. M., Courtney, A. M., and Losonczy, I., 1967, Relationship between oxygen and glucose consumption by transplanted tumors *in vivo, Cancer Res.* **27:**1041–1052.

Hak, L. J., Haasch, R. H., Hammer, V. B., Mathes, T., Sandler, R. S., and Heizer, W. D., 1984, Comparison of intravenous glucose and fat calories on host and tumor growth, *J. Parent. Ent. Nutri.* **8:**657–659.

Hansell, D. T., Davies, J. W., and Burns, J. H., 1986, The relationship between resting energy expenditure and weight loss in benign and malignant disease, *Ann. Surg.* **203:**240–245.

Heber, D., Chlebowski, R. T., Ishibashi, D. E., Harrold, J. N., and Block, J. B., 1982, Abnormalities in glucose and protein metabolism in noncachetic lung cancer patients, *Cancer Res.* **42:**4815–4819.

Henderson, J. F., and PePage, G. A., 1959, The nutrition of tumors: A review, *Cancer Res.* **19:**887–902.

Hollander, D. M., Ebert, E. C., Roberts, A. I., and Devereux, D. F., 1986, Effects of tumor type and burden on carcass lipid depletion in mice, *Surgery* **100:**292–297.

Holroyde, C. P., Gabuzda, T. G., Putnam, R. C., Paul, P., and Reichard, G. A., 1975, Altered glucose metabolism in metastatic carcinoma, *Cancer Res.* **35:**3710–3714.

Holroyde, C. P., Myers, R. N., Smink, R. D., Putnam, R. C., Paul, P., and Reichard, G. A., 1977, Metabolic response to total parenteral nutrition in cancer patients, *Cancer Res.* **37:**3109–3114.

Holroyde, C. P., Axelrod, R. S., Skutches, C. L., Haff, A. C., Paul, D., and Reichard, G. A., 1979, Lactate metabolism in metastatic colorectal cancer, *Cancer Res.* **39:**4900–4904.

Holroyde, C. P., and Reichard, G. A., 1981, Carbohydrate metabolism in cancer cachexia, *Cancer Treat. Rep.* **65**(suppl.)**:**55–59.

Irie, R., Kono, Y., Aoyama, H., Nakatani, T., Yasuda, K., Ozawa, K., and Tobe, T., 1983, Impaired glucose tolerance related to changes in the energy metabolism of the remnant liver after major hepatic resection, *J. Lab. Clin. Med.* **101:**692–698.

Jasani, B., Donaldson, L. J., Ratcliffe, J. G., and Sohki, G. S., 1978, Mechanism of impaired glucose tolerance in patients with neoplasia, *Br. J. Cancer* **38:**287–292.

Jeevanandam, M., Lowry, S. F., Horowitz, G. D., and Brennan, M. F., 1984, Cancer cachexia and protein metabolism, *Lancet* **1:**1423–1426.

Jeevanandam, M., Horowitz, G. D., Lowry, S. F., Legaspi, A., and Brennan, M. F., 1985, Cancer cachexia: Effect of total parenteral nutrition on whole body protein kinetics in man, *J. Parent. Ent. Nutr.* **9:**108 (abstr.).

Jeevanandam, M., Lowry, S. F., and Brennan, M. F., 1987, Effect of the route of nutrient administration on whole body protein kinetics in man, *Metabolism* **36:**968–973.

Kamada, S., Hay, E. F., and Mead, J. S., 1980, A lipid mobilizing factor in serum of tumor-bearing mice, *Lipid* **15:**168–174.

Kawakami, M., Pekala, P. H., Lane, M. D., and Cerami, A., 1982, Lipoprotein lipase suppression in 3T3-L1 cells by an endotoxin-induced mediator from exudate cells, *Proc. Natl. Acad. Sci. USA* **79:**912–916.

Kawamura, I., Moldawer, L. L., Bistrian, B. R., and Blackburn, G. L., 1981, Altered protein turnover in rats with progressive tumor growth, *Surg. Forum* **32:**441–444.

Kawashima, Y., Campos, A. C. L., Meguid, M. M., Kurzer, M., and Oler, A., 1989, Ability of a benign tumor to decrease spontaneous food intake and body weight in rats, *Cancer* **63:**693–699.

Kien, C. L., and Camitta, B. M., 1983, Increased whole-body protein turnover in sick children with newly diagnosed leukemia or lymphoma, *Cancer Res.* **43:**5586–5592.

Kimura, Y., Niwa, T., Wada, E., and Komeiji, T., 1964, Incorporation of labeled glucose carbon into different fractions of Ehrlich ascites tumor cells with special references to lipogenesis from glucose, *Jpn. J. Exp. Med.* **34:**267–269.

Knox, L. S., Crosby, L. O., Feurer, I. D., Buzby, G. P., Miller, C. L., and Mullen, J. L., 1983, Energy expenditure in malnourished cancer patients, *Ann. Surg.* **197:**152–162.

Kralovic, R. C., Repp, E. A., and Cenedella, R. J., 1977, Studies on the mechanism of carcass fat depletion in experimental cancer. *Eur. J. Cancer* **18:**1071–1079.

Kubota, A., Meguid, M. M., and Hitch, D. C., 1990, Free amino acids profiles correlate diagnostically with organ site or origin of three kinds of malignant tumor, *Cancer* (submitted).

Kurzer, M., Janiszewski, J., and Meguid, M. M., 1988, Amino acid profiles in tumor bearing and non-tumor bearing malnourished rats, *Cancer* **62:**1492–1496.

Landel, A. M., Lo, C.-C., Meguid, M. M., and Rivera, D., 1987, Effect of methylcholanthrene-induced sarcoma and its removal on rat plasma and intracellular free amino acid content, *Surg. Res. Commun.* **1:**273–287.

Lawrence, S. J., 1977, Nutritional consequences of surgical resection of the gastrointestinal tract for cancer, *Cancer Res.* **37:**2379–2386.

Legaspi, A., Jeevanandam, M., Starnes, H. F., and Brennan, M. F., 1987, Whole body lipid and energy metabolism in the cancer patient, *Metabolism* **36:**958–963.

Lindmark, L., Bennegård, K., Eden, E., Ekman, L., Schersten, T., Svaninger, G., and Lundholm, K., 1984, Resting energy expenditure in malnourished patients with and without cancer, *Gastroenterology* **87:**402–408.

Lowry, S. F., and Brennan, M. F., 1986, Intravenous feeding of the cancer patient, in: *Parenteral Nutrition,* Volume 2 (J. L. Rombeau and M. D. Caldwell, eds.), Saunders, Philadelphia, pp. 445–470.

Lundholm, K., 1984, Energy and substrate metabolism in the cancer-bearing host, in: *Nutrition in Cancer and Trauma Sepsis* (F. Bozzetti and I. Dionigi, eds.), Proceedings of the 6th Congress of the European Society of Parenteral and Enteral Nutrition (ESPEN), Milan, Oct. 1–3.

Lundholm, K., Bylund, A. C., Holm, J., and Schersten, T., 1976, Skeletal muscle metabolism in patients with malignant tumor, *Eur. J. Cancer* **12:**465–473.

Lundholm, K., Edstrom, S., Ekman, L., Karlberg, I., Bylund, A. C., and Schersten, T., 1978, A comparative study of the influence of malignant tumors on host metabolism in mice and man: Evaluation of an experimental model, *Cancer* **42**:453–461.

Lundholm, K., Karlberg, I., Ekman, L., Edstrom, S., and Schersten, T., 1981a, Evaluation of anorexia as the cause of altered protein synthesis in skeletal muscles from non-growing mice with sarcoma, *Cancer Res.* **41**:1989–1996.

Lundholm, K., Edstrom, S., Ekman, L., Karlberg, I., and Schersten, T., 1981b, Metabolism in peripheral tissues in cancer patients, *Cancer Treat. Rep.* **65**(S):79–83.

Lundholm, K., Edstrom, S., Karlberg, I., Ekman, L., and Scherstein, T., 1982, Glucose turnover, gluconeo-genesis from glycerol and estimation of net glucose cycling in cancer patients, *Cancer* **50**:1142–1150.

Lundholm, K., Edstrom, S., Ekman, L., Karlberg, I., Bylund-Fellenius, A. C., and Schersten, T., 1983, Activities of key enzymes in relation to glucose flux in tumor host livers, *Int. J. Biochem.* **15**:65–72.

Mahaffey, S. M., Copeland, E. M., and Citrin, E. M., 1985, Host and tumor compositional changes due to qualitative nutritional manipulation in TPN fed mice, *J. Parent. Ent. Nutr.* **9**:112.

Marks, P. A., and Bishop, J. S., 1959, Studies on carbohydrate metabolism in patients with neoplastic disease II. Response to insulin administration, *J. Clin. Invest.* **38**:668–672.

May, E. T., 1969, Serum lipids in human cancer, *J. Surg. Res.* **9**:273–277.

Medes, G., Thomas, A. J., and Weinhouse, S., 1953, Metabolism of neoplastic tissues. IV. A study of lipid synthesis in neoplastic tissue slices in vitro, *Cancer Res.* **13**:27–29.

Medes, G., Paden, G., and Weinhouse, S., 1957, Metabolism of neoplastic tissues. XI. Absorption and oxidation of dietary fatty acids by implanted tumors, *Cancer Res.* **17**:127–133.

Meguid, M. M., and Dudrick, S. (eds.), 1986, Introduction to nutrition and cancer, in: *Surgical Clinics of North America,* Volume 66, Nos. 5 and 6, Saunders, Philadelphia.

Meguid, M. M., Mughal, M. M., Debonis, D., Meguid, V., and Terz, J., 1986, Influence of nutritional status on the resumption of adequate food intake in patients recovering from colo-rectal cancer operation, *Surg. Clin. North Am.* **66**:1167–1176.

Meguid, M. M., Landel, A. M., Lo, C.-C., and Rivera, D., 1987, Effect of tumor and tumor removal on DNA, RNA, protein tissue content and survival of methylcholanthrene sarcoma-bearing rat, *Surg. Res. Commun.* **1**:261–271.

Meguid, M. M., Campos, A. C., and Hammond, W. G., 1990a, Nutrition support in surgical practice: Current knowledge and research needs: Part I, *Am. J. Surg.* **159**:345–358.

Meguid, M. M., Campos, A. C., and Hammond, W. G., 1990b, Nutrition support in surgical practice: Current knowledge and research needs: Part II, *Am. J. Surg.* **159**:427–443.

Mider, G. B., Tesluk, H., and Morton, J. J., 1948. Effects of Walker carcinoma 256 on food intake, body weight and nitrogen metabolism of growing rats, *Acta Union inter contre cancer* **6**:409–420.

Miras, C. J., Legakis, N. J., and Lewis, G. M., 1967, Conversion of glucose to lipids by normal and leukemic lymphocytes, *Cancer Res.* **27**:2153–2158.

Moley, J. F., Morrison, S. D., and Norton, J. A., 1985a, Insulin reversal of cancer cachexia in rats, *Cancer Res.* **45**:4925–4931.

Moley, J. F., Peacock, J. E., Morrison, S. D., and Norton, J. A., 1985b, Insulin reversal of cancer-induced protein loss, *Surg. Forum* **36**:416–419.

Morrison, S. D., 1976, Theoretical Review. Control of food intake in cancer cachexia. A challenge and a tool, *Physiol. Behav.* **17**:705–714.

Mullen, J. L., Buzby, G. P., Gertner, M. H., Stein, T. P., Hargrove, W. C., Oram-Smith, J., and Rosato, E. F., 1980, Protein synthesis of dynamics in human gastrointestinal malignancies, *Surgery* **87**:331–338.

Norton, J. A., Lowry, S. F., and Brennan, M. F., 1979, Effect of work induced hypertrophy on skeletal muscle of tumor and nontumor-bearing rats, *J. Appl. Physiol.* **46**:654–657.

Norton, J. A., Shamberger, R., Stein, T. P., Milne, G. W. A., and Brennan, M. F., 1981, The influence of tumour-bearing on protein metabolism in the rat, *J. Surg. Res.* **30**:456–462.

Norton, J. A., Gorschboth, C. M., Wesley, R. A., Burt, M. E., and Brennan, M. F., 1985, Fasting plasma amino acid levels in cancer patients, *Cancer* **56**:1181–1186.

Pain, V. M., Randall, D. P., and Garlick, P. J., 1984, Protein synthesis in liver and skeletal muscle of mice bearing an ascites tumor, *Cancer Res.* **44**:1054–1057.

Peacock, J. L., and Norton, J. A., 1988, Impact of insulin on survival of cachexia tumor-bearing rats, *J. Parent. Ent. Nutr.* **12**:260–264.

Peacock, J. L., Inculet, R. I., Corsey, R., Ford, D. B., Rumble, W. F., Lawson, D., and Norton, J. A., 1987,

Resting energy expenditure and body cell mass alterations in noncachetic patients with sarcomas, *Surgery* **102**:465–472.

Popp, M. B., Kirkemo, A. K., Morrison, S. D., and Brennan, M. F., 1984, Tumor and host carcass changes during total parenteral nutrition in an anorectic rat-tumor system, *Ann. Surg.* **199**:205–210.

Reichard, G. A., Jr., Moury, N. F., Jr., Hochella, N. J., Putnam, R. C., and Weinhouse, S., 1964, Metabolism of neoplastic tissue. XVII. Blood glucose replacement rates in human cancer patients, *Cancer Res.* **24**:71–76.

Reilly, J. J., Goodgame, J. T., Jones, D. C., and Brennan, M. F., 1977, DNA synthesis in rat sarcoma and liver; the effects of starvation, *J. Surg. Res.* **22**:281–286.

Rennie, M. J., Edwards, R. H. T., Emery, P. W., Halliday, D., Lundholm, K., and Millward, D. J., 1983, Depressed protein synthesis is the dominant characteristic of muscle wasting and cachexia, *Clin. Physiol.* **3**:387–398.

Rofe, A. M., Bais, R., and Conyers, R. A. J., 1986, Ketone-body metabolism in tumor-bearing rats, *Biochem. J.* **233**:485.

Rose, D., Horowitz, G. D., Jeevanandam, M., Brennan, M. F., Shires, G. T., and Lowry, S. F., 1983, Whole-body protein kinetics during acute starvation and intravenous refeeding in normal man, *Fed. Proc.* **42**:1070 (abstr.).

Russell, D. McR., Shike, M., Marliss, E. B., Detsky, A. S., Shepherd, F. A., Feld, R., Evans, W. K., and Jeejeebhoy, K. N., 1984, Effects of total parenteral nutrition and chemotherapy on the metabolic derangements in small cell lung cancer, *Cancer Res.* **44**:1706–1711.

Sabine, J. R., and Chaikoff, I. L., 1967, Control of fatty acid synthesis in homogenate preparations of mouse hepatoma BW 7756, *Aust. J. Exp. Biol. Med. Sci.* **4**:541–548.

Sabine, J. R., Abraham, S. and Chaikoff, I. L., 1966, Lack of feedback control fatty acid synthesis in a transplantable hepatoma, *Biochim. Biophys. Acta* **11**:407–409.

Sabine, J. R., Abraham, S., and Chaikoff, I. L., 1967, Control of lipid metabolism in hepatomas. Insensitivity of the rate of fatty acid and cholesterol synthesis by mouse hepatoma BW 7756 to fasting and to feedback control, *Cancer Res.* **27**:793–799.

Sabine, J. R., Abraham, S., and Morris, H. P., 1968, Defective dietary control fatty acid metabolism in four transplantable rat hepatomas; numbers 51230, 7793, 7795 and 7800, *Cancer Res.* **28**:45–61.

Sallan, S. E., Hitchcock-Bryan, S., Gelber, R., Cassady, J. R., Frei, E., 3d, and Nathan, D. G., 1983, Influence of intensive asparaginase in the treatment of childhood non T cell acute lymphoblastic leukemia, *Cancer Res.* **43**:5601–5607.

Sandstedt, C., Lennmarken, C., Symreng, T., Vinnars, E., and Larsson, J., 1985, The effect of preoperative total parenteral nutrition on energy rich phosphates, electrolytes and free amino acids in skeletal muscle of malnourished patients with gastric carcinoma, *Br. J. Surg.* **72**:920–924.

Schaur, R. J., Semmelrock, H. J., Schreibmayer, W., Tillian, H. M., and Schwastein, E., 1980, Tumor host relations, *J. Cancer Res. Clin. Oncol.* **97**:285–293.

Schein, P. S., Kasner, D., Haller, D., Blecher, M., and Hamosh, M., 1979, Cachexia of malignancy; potential role of insulin in nutritional management, *Cancer* **43**:2070–2076.

Shan, L. H. F., and Wolfe, R. R., 1987, Fatty acid and glycerol kinetics in septic patients and in patients with gastrointestinal cancer. The response to glucose infusion and parenteral feeding, *Ann. Surg.* **205**:368–376.

Sherman, C. D., Jr., Morton, J. J., and Mider, G. B., 1950, Potential sources of tumor nitrogen, *Cancer Res.* **10**:374–378.

Shizgal, H. M., 1985, Body composition of patients with malnutrition and cancer. Summary of methods of assessment, *Cancer* **55**:250–253.

Spechler, S. J., Esposito, A. L., Koff, R. S., and Hong, W. K., 1978, Lactic acidosis in oat cell carcinoma with extensive hepatic metastases, *Arch. Intern. Med.* **138**:1663–1664.

Spector, A. A., 1969, Influence of pH on the medium on free fatty acid utilization by isolated mammalian cells, *J. Lipid Res.* **10**:270–215.

Spector, A. A., and Steinberg, D., 1966, Relationship between fatty acid and glucose utilization in Ehrlich ascites tumor cells, *J. Lipid Res.* **7**:657–663.

Spector, A. A., and Steinberg, D., 1967a, The effect of fatty acid structure on utilization of Ehrlich ascites tumor cells, *Cancer Res.* **27**:1587–1594.

Spector, A. A., and Steinberg, D., 1967b, Turnover and utilization of esterified fatty acids in Ehrlich ascites tumor cells, *J. Biol. Chem.* **242**:3057–3062.

Spector, A. A., Steinberg, D., and Tanaka, A., 1965, Uptake of free fatty acids by Ehrlich ascites tumor cells, *J. Biol. Chem.* **240:**1032–1041.

Spiegel, R. J., Schaefer, E. J., Magrath, I. T., and Edwards, B. K., 1982, Plasma lipid alterations in leukemia and lymphoma, *Am. J. Med.* **72:**775–782.

Stein, T. P., Oram-Smith, J. C., Leskiw, M. J., Wallace, H. W., and Miller, E. F., 1976, Tumor caused changes in host protein synthesis under dietary situations, *Cancer Res.* **36:**2926–2940.

Stein, T. P., Buzby, G. P., Rosato, E. F., and Mullen, J. L., 1981, Effect of parenteral nutrition on protein synthesis in adult cancer patients, *Am. J. Clin. Nutr.* **34:**1484–1488.

Stovroff, M. C., Fraker, D. L., and Norton, J. A., 1989, Cachectin activity in the serum of cachetic, tumor-bearing rats, *Arch. Surg.* **124:**94–99.

Tachibana, K., Mukai, K., Hiraoka, I., Moriguchi, S., Takama, S., and Kishino, Y., 1985, Evolution of the effect of arginine enriched amino acid solution on tumor growth, *J. Parent. Ent. Nutr.* **9:**428–434.

Tashiro, T., Mashima, Y., Yamamori, H., and Okui, K., 1986, Alteration of lipoprotein profile during total parenteral nutrition with Intralipid 10%, *J. Parent. Ent. Nutr.* **10:**622–626.

Tayek, J. A., Bistrian, B. R., Ling, P., Istfan, N. W., Blackburn, B. L., and Hoffman, S. B., 1986, Effects of branched chain amino acid-enriched total parenteral nutrition on amino acid utilization in rats bear yoshida sarcoma, *Cancer Res.* **48:**2698–2702.

Tisdale, M. J., and Brennan, R. A., 1988, A comparison of long-chain triglycerides and medium-chain triglycerides on weight loss and tumor size in a cachexia model, *Br. J. Cancer* **58:**580–583.

Unger, R. H., 1966, The riddle of tumor hypoglycemia, *Am. J. Med.* **40:**325–330.

Vlassara, H., Spiegel, R. J., Doval, D. S., and Cerami, A., 1986, Reduced plasma lipoprotein lipase activity in patients with malignancy-associated weight loss, *Horm. Metabol. Res.* **18:**698–703.

Waitzberg, D. L., Goncalves, E. L., and Faintuch, J., 1989, Effect of diets with different protein levels on the growth of Walker 256 carcinosarcoma in rats, *Brazilian J. Med. Biol. Res.* **22:**447–455.

Warburg, O., 1956, On the origin of cancer cells, *Science* **123:**309–314.

Warnold, I., Lundholm, K., and Scherstein, T., 1978, Energy balance and body composition in cancer patients, *Cancer Res.* **38:**1801–1807.

Warren, R. S., Jeevanandam, M., and Brennan, M. F., 1987, Comparison of hepatic protein synthesis *in vivo* versus *in vitro* in the tumor-bearing rat, *J. Surg. Res.* **42:**43–50.

Waterhouse, C., and Kemperman, J. H., 1971, Carbohydrate metabolism in subjects with cancer, *Cancer Res.* **31:**1273–1278.

Waterhouse, C., Jeanpetre, N., and Keilson, J., 1979, Gluconeogenesis from alanine in patients with progressive malignant disease, *Cancer Res.* **39:**1968–1972.

Watson, J. A., 1972, Regulation of lipid metabolism in *in vitro* cultured minimal deviation hepatoma 7288C, *Lipids* **7:**146–155.

Weber, M. J., 1973, Hexose transport in normal and in Rous sarcoma virus-transformed cells, *J. Biol. Chem.* **248:**2978, 2983.

Weber, S., Banerjee, G., and Morris, H. P., 1961, Comparative biochemistry of hepatomas. I. Carbohydrate enzymes in Morris hepatoma 5123, *Cancer Res.* **21:**933–937.

Weinhouse, S., 1951, Studies on the fate of isotopically labeled metabolites in the oxidative metabolism of tumors, *Cancer Res.* **11:**585–591.

Weinhouse, S., 1972, Glycolysis, respiration, and anomalous gene expression in experimental hepatomas, *Cancer Res.* **32:**2007–2016.

Whitlock, D., and Meguid, M. M., 1988, Muscle performance and ATP status in 21 day MCA-tumor bearing rats, *Clin. Res.* **36:**774A.

Wolfe, R. R., O'Donnell, T. F., Stone, M. D., Richmand, D. A., and Burke, J. F., 1980, Investigation of factors determining the optimal glucose infusion rate in total parenteral nutrition, *Metabolism* **29:**892–900.

Wright, J. D., and Green, C., 1971, The role of the plasma membrane in fatty acid uptake by rat liver parenchymal cells, *Biochem. J.* **123:**837–844.

Young, V. R., 1977, Energy metabolism and requirements in the cancer patient, *Cancer Res.* **37:**2336–2347.

4

Carbohydrate and Cancer

Kenneth K. Carroll

1. Introduction

As noted by the Committee on Diet, Nutrition, and Cancer (1982), dietary intake of carbohydrate in relation to cancer has received much less attention than intake of fat and protein, the two other macronutrients of the diet.

The carbohydrate in foods consists mainly of sugars, starches, and indigestible polysaccharides. Sugars and starches will be considered in this chapter, and the indigestible polysaccharides will be discussed under dietary fiber.

2. Epidemiologic Evidence

One of the difficulties in relating specific dietary components to chronic diseases such as cancer is the interdependence of different dietary variables. As illustrated in Table I, dietary fat, protein, and calories each show strong positive correlations with one another. Dietary carbohydrate shows weak positive correlations with calories and with protein and a weak negative correlation with dietary fat.

Analysis of epidemiologic data on cancer incidence and mortality has shown strong positive correlations between cancer at certain sites, such as breast and colon, and the amount of dietary fat available for consumption (Armstrong and Doll, 1975; Carroll and Khor, 1975). In view of the correlations between dietary variables just referred to, it is not surprising that these types of cancer show strong positive correlations with calories and protein as well (Carroll and Khor, 1975). Conversely, when there is a positive correlation with dietary fat, a negative correlation with dietary carbohydrate can be expected (Fig. 1).

The different components that make up the major macronutrients in food can vary independently of one another and hence do not necessarily show the same type of correla-

Kenneth K. Carroll • Department of Biochemistry, The University of Western Ontario Health Sciences Centre, London, Ontario, Canada N6A 5C1.

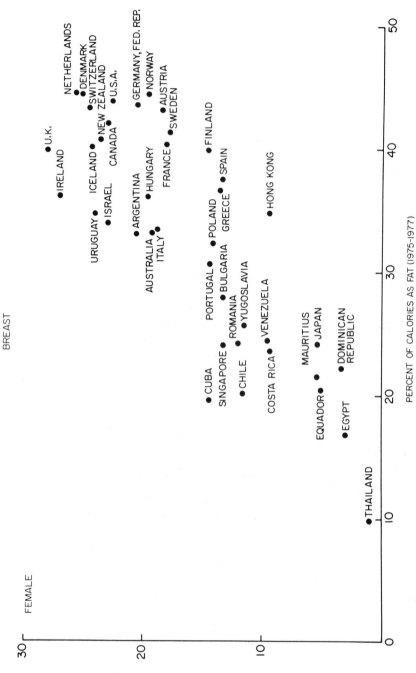

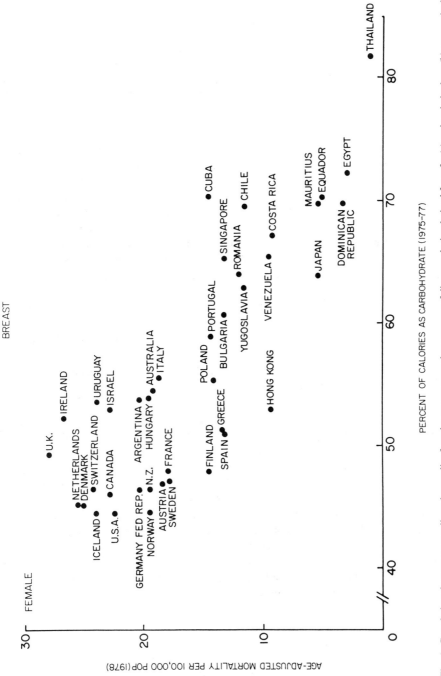

Fig. 1. Correlations between age-adjusted mortality from breast cancer and percentage of dietary calories derived from fat (a) and carbohydrate (b), respectively. (Reproduced from Carroll, 1986b.)

Table I. Correlations between Different Dietary
Ingredients[a]

	Calories	Protein	Fat
Protein	+0.943		
Fat	+0.844	+0.792	
Carbohydrate	+0.256	+0.248	−0.263

[a]Data from Carroll and Khor (1975).

tion as the macronutrient as a whole. As an example, breast cancer incidence and mortality show positive correlations with dietary sugars but are negatively correlated with complex carbohydrate (Hems and Stuart, 1975; Carroll, 1977; Hems, 1978; Committee on Diet, Nutrition, and Cancer, 1982). Seely and Horrobin (1983) reported that the positive correlation between dietary sugar and breast cancer was stronger for women in the older age groups. They suggested insulin as a possible connecting link between sugar consumption and breast cancer. In a recent case–control study in Belgium, Tuyns *et al.* (1987) observed a positive correlation between dietary mono- and disaccharides and colorectal cancer. Polysaccharides showed a negative correlation with colon cancer but not with rectal cancer.

A positive correlation between mortality from stomach cancer and *per capita* intake of cereal used as flour was reported by Hakama and Saxén (1967). In a case–control study of gastric cancer, Modan *et al.* (1974) found that starchy foods were eaten more frequently by cases than controls. Risch *et al.* (1985) likewise found an association between gastric cancer and consumption of carbohydrate. However, in many parts of Africa and Asia, the incidence of gastric cancer is low although the diet is high in cereals (Higginson, 1986).

Correlations observed in analyzing epidemiologic data do not necessarily imply cause and effect but provide leads for further data-gathering and experimental studies. The higher incidence of certain types of cancer associated with high-fat diets could be due to specific effects of dietary fat but could also be related to the reduced intake of carbohydrate associated with such diets.

It is also possible that the observed correlations are influenced by caloric intake. High-fat diets normally have a higher caloric density than low-fat diets and thus tend to be associated with increased caloric intake, which by itself may affect carcinogenesis (Carroll, 1986a; Reddy, 1986; Kritchevsky, 1986). In a case–control study of large-bowel cancer, Bristol *et al.* (1985) observed that cases consumed significantly more energy than controls, with the excess being mainly accounted for by fiber-depleted sugar and fat–sugar combinations. Thus, sugar as well as fat may influence cancer indirectly by encouraging increased caloric intake (Cummings, 1986).

3. Experimental Evidence

In their survey of the literature, the Committee on Diet, Nutrition, and Cancer (1982) found relatively few studies on the relationship between dietary carbohydrates and cancer.

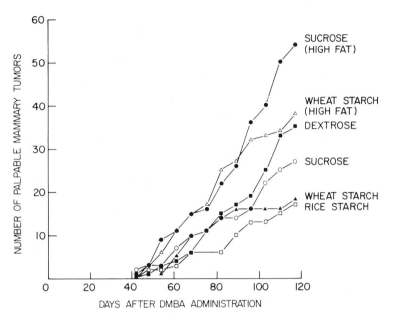

Fig. 2. Effects of dietary sugars and starches on yield of mammary tumors induced by DMBA in groups of 20 female, Sprague-Dawley rats. (Based on data of Hoehn and Carroll, 1979.)

In general, the results tend to show little or no effect of dietary carbohydrate and are sometimes difficult to interpret because of poor experimental design and uncertainty about the actual carbohydrate content of foods used in the test diets.

In our studies on mammary tumors induced by 7,12-dimethylbenz(α)anthracene (DMBA), rats fed diets containing sugar developed more tumors than those fed starch-containing diets, and this difference was observed at both high and low levels of fat intake (Hoehn and Carroll, 1979) (Fig. 2). In subsequent studies on this tumor model, Klurfeld *et al.* (1984) reported that mammary tumor incidence was similar in rats fed sucrose and cornstarch but lower in rats fed lactose. Gridley *et al.* (1983) compared the effects of diets high in sucrose or dextrin on development of spontaneous mammary tumors in C3H/HeJ mice and found a significantly higher incidence in sucrose-fed mice, beginning at 90 weeks of age.

In studies on hepatocarcinogenesis induced by diethyl nitrosamine in rats, Hei and Sudilovsky (1985) observed that rats fed a diet containing 65% sucrose had twice as many γ-glutamyltranspeptidase-positive foci as those fed a diet containing 65% glucose. Sucrose-fed rats also had heavier livers than those fed glucose. Sato *et al.* (1984) studied the effect of dietary carbohydrate on 3'-methylaminoazobenzene-induced liver carcinogenesis in rats fed liquid or powder diets. They made the surprising observation that tumorigenesis was enhanced by reducing the sugar intake while maintaining the intake of other nutrients at the same level.

Thus, although effects of dietary carbohydrate have been studied much less intensively than those of other macronutrients, the evidence indicates that carcinogenesis can be significantly affected in animals by the amount and type of carbohydrate in the diet.

4. References

Armstrong, B. A., and Doll, R., 1975, Environmental factors and cancer incidence and mortality in different countries, with special reference to dietary practices, *Int. J. Cancer* **15:**617–631.

Bristol, J. B., Emmett, P. M., Heaton, K. W., and Williamson, B. C. N., 1985, Sugar, fat and the risk of colorectal cancer, *Br. Med. J.* **291:**1467–1470.

Carroll, K. K., 1977, Dietary factors in hormone-dependent cancers, in: *Current Concepts in Nutrition, Volume 6 Nutrition and Cancer* (M. Winick, ed.), Wiley, New York, pp. 25–40.

Carroll, K. K., 1986a, Dietary fat and cancer: Specific action or caloric effect? *J. Nutr.* **116:**1130–1132.

Carroll, K. K., 1986b, Experimental studies on dietary fat and cancer in relation to epidemiological data, in: *Progress in Clinical Biological Research, Volume 222, Dietary Fat and Cancer* (C. Ip, D. F. Birt, A. E. Rogers, and C. Mettlin, eds.), Alan R. Liss, New York, pp. 231–248.

Carroll, K. K., and Khor, H. T., 1975, Dietary fat in relation to tumorigenesis, *Prog. Biochem. Pharmacol.* **10:**308–353.

Committee on Diet, Nutrition, and Cancer, Assembly of Life Sciences, National Research Council, 1982, *Diet, Nutrition, and Cancer,* National Academy Press, Washington, D.C.

Cummings, J. H., 1986, Dietary carbohydrates and cancer, *Nutr. Cancer* **8:**10–14.

Gridley, D. S., Kettering, J. D., Slater, J. M., and Nutter, R. L., 1983, Modification of spontaneous mammary tumors in mice fed different sources of protein, fat and carbohydrate, *Cancer Lett.* **19:**133–146.

Hakama, M., and Saxén, E. A., 1967, Cereal consumption and gastric cancer, *Int. J. Cancer* **2:**265–268.

Hei, T. K., and Sudilovksy, O., 1985, Effects of a high-sucrose diet on the development of enzyme-altered foci in chemical hepatocarcinogenesis in rats, *Cancer Res.* **45:**2700–2705.

Hems, G., 1978, The contributions of diet and childbearing to breast-cancer rates, *Br. J. Cancer* **37:**974–982.

Hems, G., and Stuart, A., 1975, Breast cancer rates in populations of single women, *Br. J. Cancer* **31:**118–123.

Higginson, J., 1986, Cancer, carbohydrates, and fiber, *Nutr. Cancer* **8:**14–17.

Hoehn, S. K., and Carroll, K. K., 1979, Effects of dietary carbohydrate on the incidence of mammary tumors induced in rats by 7,12-dimethylbenz(α)anthracene, *Nutr. Cancer* **1**(3):27–30.

Klurfeld, D. M., Weber, M. M., and Kritchevsky, D., 1984, Comparison of dietary carbohydrates for promotion of DMBA-induced mammary carcinogenesis in rats, *Carcinogenesis (Lond.)* **5:**423–425.

Kritchevscky, D., 1986, Fat, calories and fiber, in: *Progress in Clinical Biological Research, Vol. 222, Dietary Fat and Cancer* (C. Ip, D. F. Birt, A. E. Rogers, and C. Mettlin, eds.), Alan R. Liss, New York, pp. 495–515.

Modan, B., Lubin, F., Barell, V., Greenberg, R. A., Modan, M., and Graham, S., 1974, The role of starches in the etiology of gastric cancer, *Cancer* **34:**2087–2092.

Reddy, B. S., 1986, Dietary fat and cancer: Specific action or caloric effect, *J. Nutr.* **116:**1132–1135.

Risch, H. A., Jain, M., Choi, N. W., Fodor, G., Pfeiffer, C. J., Howe, G. R., Harrison, L. W., Craib, K. J. P., and Miller, A. B., 1985, Dietary factors and the incidence of cancer of the stomach, *Am. J. Epidemiol.* **122:**947–959.

Sato, A., Nakajima, T., Koyama, Y., Shirai, T., and Ito, N., 1984, Dietary carbohydrate level as a modifying factor on 3'-methyl-4-dimethylaminoazobenzene liver carcinogenesis in rats, *Gann* **75:**665–671.

Seely, S., and Horrobin, D. F., 1983, Diet and breast cancer: The possible connection with sugar consumption, *Med. Hypotheses* **11:**319–327.

Tuyns, A. J., Haelterman, M., and Kaaks, R., 1987, Colorectal cancer and the intake of nutrients: Oligosaccharides are a risk factor, fats are not. A case–control study in Belgium, *Nutr. Cancer* **10:**181–196.

5

Dietary Protein and Cancer

Willard J. Visek and Stephen K. Clinton

1. Introduction

The average life expectancy for Americans has increased by almost 25 years since 1900. Eighty-five years ago infectious diseases were the leading cause of death. In the growing population of industrial workers of that time, accidents were also a major cause of morbidity and shortened lifespan. The significant gains in life expectancy have been largely due to improved preventive measures facilitated by advances in sanitation, nutrition, and industrial health. Prolongation of survival has produced a population of aged people with high rates of cardiovascular disease and cancer. Together, these diseases currently account for approximately 70% of deaths in the United States. Consequently, a major fraction of our health care expenditures and allocations of funds for biomedical research has been directed to the treatment of these diseases. Despite these efforts, overall age-adjusted mortality from cancer has remained remarkably constant, although there have been dramatic reductions in mortality from some of the rarer forms of neoplasia, like Hodgkin's disease, childhood leukemia, and testicular cancer. The slow progress in the therapy of major cancers, as perceived by the public and lawmakers, has stimulated a resurgence of interest in cancer causation and prevention.

Most malignancies have a multifactorial etiology in which both environmental and genetic factors contribute to cancer risk. In the early years of experimental oncology, Moreschi (1909) and Rous (1914) observed that the diet was an environmental factor which could modify tumor growth in laboratory animals. During subsequent decades, new information about the nutritional requirements of laboratory animals and the development of animal models for a number of human malignancies laid the groundwork for exploring the relationship of nutrition to carcinogenesis. Over the past 30 years, improved methods of nutritional and metabolic epidemiology have expanded our knowledge of associations between the incidence of certain human cancers and specific dietary components. Books,

Willard J. Visek • Division of Nutritional Sciences, Department of Internal Medicine, College of Medicine, University of Illinois, Urbana, Illinois 61801.   *Steven K. Clinton* • The Dana-Farber Cancer Institute and Harvard Medical School, Boston, Massachusetts 02115.

reports of symposia, and reviews have become more common and funding agencies have increased allocations of resources for studying the role of the diet in cancer causation and prevention.

Protein requirements of humans and other animals have been one of the most studied topics in nutrition. Although epidemiologic studies indicate that dietary protein is associated with cancer of various organs, other nutrients, such as vitamin A, selenium, lipids, and energy intake have been more extensively investigated (NAS, 1982). Since protein-rich foods and the diets that contain them tend to be low in fiber and rich in other nutritional factors, like fat and calories, human epidemiologic studies have failed to delineate the unique effects of protein. The use of experimental models for human cancers has allowed examination of the effects of specific nutrients alone or in combination with other variables. Animal models have been used in attempts to quantitate the effects of dietary protein concentration and quality on tumor incidence and to explore the underlying mechanisms whereby protein influences carcinogenesis.

2. Methodology

Epidemiologic studies have provided a basis for developing hypotheses pertaining to the role of diet in carcinogenesis. These studies show large differences in the incidence of specific cancers between countries (Carroll and Khor, 1975; Armstrong and Doll, 1975; Doll and Peto, 1981). Studies of migrant populations show that these differences cannot be totally explained by genetic predisposition (Staszewski and Haenszel, 1965). For instance, the progeny of Japanese migrants to the United States experience a higher incidence of breast cancer in succeeding generations as they acquire American cultural and eating habits (Buell, 1973). Subpopulations within countries likewise emphasize the importance of dietary and cultural habits. This is well demonstrated by the Seventh Day Adventists, who practice vegetarianism extensively and, compared to national averages in the United States, show a lower incidence of cancer at a number of organ sites (Phillips, 1975).

Investigations of nutrient–cancer relationships in humans require accurate estimates of food composition and intake. For many nations the nutrient content of foods is not known, reliable records of consumption are not available, and correlations are based on food availability in the marketplace rather than on actual nutrient intake. The development of reliable questionnaires and interviewing methods for estimating nutrient intake is an active area of investigation. USDA publications (Watt and Merrill, 1975) provide estimates of protein and other nutrient content for most foods of the United States. New, more reliable indices of nutritional status based on the analysis of blood, urine, or tissue biopsies are needed.

Reports of retrospective and prospective studies relating nutrition to cancer have become more frequent in the scientific literature. Retrospective studies compare nutrient intake in individuals with cancer to control subjects without cancer. Unfortunately, the lag time between cancer initiation and clinical manifestation may be 10–30 years and current dietary habits which may also be influenced by the present illness or therapy may have little relationship to dietary habits at the critical time in cancer development. Prospective studies follow a selected population over time, with monitoring of nutrient intakes and subsequent cancer development. Few such studies have been conducted because they require long observation periods and large numbers of participants. Furthermore, the variation in individual protein intakes within relatively homogeneous populations like that of the United States may be insufficient to cause detectable differences in tumor incidence. The ideal nutritional study would be a randomized trial involving volunteers assigned to specific diets with careful monitoring of compliance and subsequent cancer incidence. Interventional studies of this type provide quantitative information directly applicable to humans, without the uncertainties of extrapolations from laboratory animals. Unfortunately, such trials require large numbers of participants, are costly, and need to be of long duration because the time between dietary change and tumor development may be years or decades. In actual practice, compliance with the experimental protocols over long periods is likely to vary and the control population may also change its dietary habits, thereby introducing uncertainties of interpretation. With those constraints and requirements, such trials need to be justified by extensive correlational data in humans, supported by a large body of experimental data from animals.

Guidelines have been established for making sound inferences about causal relationships based on associations observed in epidemiologic data. To support a causal relationship between diet and cancer, the following criteria should be satisfied: a graded response with intake; independence from other variables; appropriate temporal relationships; consistency of data from multiple studies; and concurrence with known biological characteristics of the malignancy (Woteke *et al.*, 1987; Hill, 1965). In addition, supporting data from carefully controlled laboratory studies strengthen the likelihood of causality.

Animal studies can be designed to rigorously examine the effects of nutrients and their interactions. Despite these opportunities, numerous animal studies have failed to yield definitive data because they employed inappropriate dietary and nutritional protocols. A common shortcoming has been the failure to record feed (energy) intake. Since caloric intake significantly influences experimental tumor incidence (Tannenbaum, 1959; Albanes, 1987), recording food consumption and body weight should be considered an important aspect of the protocol. This is especially true in experiments where protein is a variable because both protein quantity and quality influence calorie intake and growth.

Occasionally, commercial, open-formula, cereal-based laboratory chows have served as control or "normal" protein diets for comparison against semipurified diets with different concentrations of protein. Although commercial laboratory chows contain the stated minimal content of nutrients, they vary in the source of natural ingredients as a function of market availability. Consequently, they also vary in the content of man-made contaminants and natural substances which may influence carcinogenesis. Experimental diets should be formulated so that the influence of single variables can be determined. The nutrient requirements of most laboratory animals have been well characterized (National Research Council, 1978) and assistance in diet preparation and formulation can be found in other publications (Newberne *et al.*, 1978; AIN, 1977, 1980).

In summary, the logistics and cost of definitive prospective intervention studies are likely to limit future testing of diet and cancer hypotheses in humans. Thus, diet recommendations will be based on a consensus derived from descriptive epidemic data, supported by limited studies in humans and information from carefully d experiments in laboratory animals. Such recommendations will require careful

tion of the effects of dietary changes on cancer risk, with cognizance that they can alter physiological and developmental processes and the susceptibility to other diseases.

3. Breast Cancer

Approximately 1 of every 11 American women will develop breast cancer. Currently, over 120,000 new cases are diagnosed each year and 38,000 deaths occur annually due to this disease (Silverberg and Lubera, 1987). Breast cancer remains the leading cause of cancer deaths in American women, although lung cancer may soon assume this dubious distinction. The principal risk factors include a positive family history, previous benign breast disease, nulliparity or later age of first pregnancy, and late menopause (Kelsey, 1979). Some reduction in risk is associated with pregnancy at an early age or pre-menopausal ovariectomy (Kelsey, 1979).

The relationship of diet to breast cancer incidence has been examined in numerous epidemiologic studies and in laboratory animals. Protein has attracted much less research interest than dietary fat, even though epidemiologic studies have found similar correlations between protein intake and breast cancer incidence (NAS, 1982). Armstrong and Doll (1975) observed that the incidence of breast cancer in different nations was highly correlated with marketplace availability of total protein, especially animal protein, and total fat. The incidence rates for breast cancer, colon cancer, and prostate cancer, highly correlated with each other, are most common in Western, industrially developed nations, where diets are rich in fat, animal products, and total calories but low in fiber. An exception is Japan, where intakes of total calories, fat, and animal protein are lower than in other highly developed nations and the incidence of cancers of breast, colon, and prostate is also lower (Armstrong and Doll, 1975; Carroll and Khor, 1975).

Hems (1978) reported that breast cancer incidence and mortality rates were highly correlated with dietary factors in 41 countries in 1970–1971. Partial correlation analysis indicated that breast cancer rates were positively correlated with total fat, animal protein, and calories from animal products. However, these three dietary components were so closely correlated with each other that it was impossible to discern if the association with any one was independent. Subsequent studies by Hems (1980) in England and Wales showed a stronger association of breast cancer mortality with fat than with protein. Gray et al. (1979) analyzed rates of incidence and mortality from breast cancer in different countries and found both correlated with height, weight, and earlier menarche. However, they also found correlations with total fat and per capita animal protein consumption even controlling for the three anthropometric variables. The authors suggested that the diet ...ed directly in addition to its promotion of more rapid growth and develop-

...ned age-adjusted breast cancer mortality in relation to other foods by state within the United States. They milk products, total calories, fat, protein, beef, and this was not statistically significant after control for tor of age at first pregnancy. Subsequently, Kolonel et cancer risk within the Caucasian, Japanese, Chinese, ...lations of Hawaii. They found a direct correlation between breast cancer risk and the intake of saturated fat, unsaturated fat, total animal fat, and animal protein. The nutrient intakes were based on food consumption interviews. Two case–control studies have revealed an association between breast cancer and dietary fat but not with protein (Miller *et al.*, 1978; Phillips, 1975). However, a third study showed an association with the consumption of beef and pork (Lubin *et al.*, 1981). The majority of epidemiologic evidence suggests an association of protein with breast cancer, but a unique role of protein, independent of total caloric intake, dietary fat, or animal products, has not been established.

Extensive studies in laboratory rodents support the roles of increased dietary fat or caloric intake as promoters of mammary carcinogenesis (NAS, 1982). The incidence of virally transmitted or chemically induced breast cancer is reduced by restriction of caloric intake (NAS, 1982; Albanes, 1987). 7,12-Dimethylbenz(α)anthracene (DMBA)-induced breast cancer risk is also reduced in rats with lower *ad libitum* food intake (Clinton *et al.*, 1984, 1986). Diets high in fat have been found to increase the incidence of chemically induced, spontaneous, and radiation-induced breast cancer and the growth of transplantable mammary carcinomas (Clinton and Visek, 1986; Cohen, 1986). Fewer laboratory studies examining the relationship of dietary protein to mammary carcinogenesis have been conducted and the results have been less consistent than for fat or caloric intake. Several investigators reported no effect on breast cancer from increasing dietary protein (Tannenbaum and Silverstone, 1949; Ross and Bras, 1973), whereas some have reported enhancement (Shay *et al.*, 1964; Hawrylewicz *et al.*, 1982; Hawrylewicz, 1986) and others, inhibition (Clinton *et al.*, 1979b, 1986a).

Our laboratory examined the effects of dietary protein on DMBA-induced mammary carcinogenesis in rats (Clinton *et al.*, 1979b). We found that increasing dietary protein from 7.5% to 15% or 45%, for the period from weaning until carcinogen administration 4 weeks later (initiation phase), was associated with lower tumor incidence (Table I). In contrast, varying protein intake following DMBA administration had no significant effect on final tumor yield (promotion phase). We have postulated that the mechanism underlying the influence of protein on the initiation phase of DMBA-induced tumorigenesis is related to carcinogen metabolism. Our studies showing elevated activity of hepatic xenobiotic metabolizing enzymes (Fig. 1) with increased protein intake (Clinton *et al.*, 1979b, 1980) support the hypothesis that dietary protein modifies the carcinogenic re-

Table I. Initiation and Promotion of 7,12-Dimethylbenz(a)anthracene-Induced Mammary Carcinogenesis in Rats Fed Different Concentrations of Dietary Protein[a]

Dietary protein (% of kcal)	Initiation			Promotion		
	Incidence (%)	Latency (days)	Tumors per rat	Incidence (%)	Latency (days)	Tumors per rat
7.5	85	84 ± 7	2.2 ± 0.4	55	125 ± 7	1.4 ± 0.1
15.0	52	119 ± 7	1.4 ± 0.2	55	133 ± 14	1.4 ± 0.1
45.0	30	126 ± 7	1.1 ± 0.1	40	119 ± 14	1.1 ± 0.1

[a]Weanling female Sprague–Dawley rats were utilized in each study and DMBA was administered after 4 weeks of feeding. For the initiation-phase study, diets varied in protein only for the 4 weeks prior to DMBA administration. Diets varying in protein were fed only following carcinogen administration in the promotion-phase study. (Data from Clinton *et al.*, 1979a.)

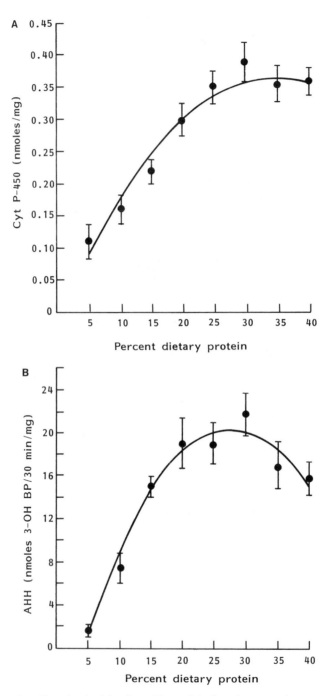

Fig. 1. Dietary protein and hepatic mixed-function oxidase activity (cytochrome c-reductase, cytochrome P-450, aryl hydrocarbon hydroxylase) in weanling rats fed casein-based diets varying in protein from 5 to 40% by weight for 2 weeks. (Clinton *et al.*, 1980; reprinted by permission of *Journal of Dairy Science*, Vol. 67, No. 3, p. 493.)

sponse by enhancing DMBA conversion to noncarcinogenic, more readily excretable metabolites. This agrees with other studies where pretreatment with inducers of hepatic xenobiotic metabolizing enzymes prior to DMBA administration reduced the number of tumors (Wattenberg, 1975). Human studies also show that the metabolism and clearance of various pharmacological agents are enhanced when protein intakes are raised (Kappas *et al.*, 1976). The effects of dietary protein on DMBA metabolism have been examined by Singletary and Milner (1984, 1987a,b). They observed that hepatic S-9 preparations from rats fed higher amounts of protein produced fewer DNA-binding metabolites of DMBA *in vitro* (1984). In the subsequent study, rat mammary cells isolated from rats fed 15% protein showed 20% greater DNA binding of DMBA metabolites than cells from rats fed 7.5% protein (1987a). However, hepatocytes isolated from rats fed 15% protein displayed increased formation of extracellular water-soluble DMBA metabolites and decreased release of DNA-binding metabolites (Singletary and Milner, 1987a). Although the details of DMBA absorption, metabolism, conjugation, distribution to various tissues, and their interaction with changes in diet have not yet been defined, we believe that low-protein diets decrease the production of detoxified products of DMBA, thereby increasing the quantity of potentially carcinogenic metabolites that can act on mammary tissue. It appears that the production of detoxified metabolites of DMBA by the liver of rats fed higher-protein diets greatly exceeds formation of active DNA-binding carcinogens in mammary tissue.

Our studies (Clinton *et al.*, 1979b), showing no effect of protein on the promotion phase of DMBA-induced mammary cancer in rats, agree with others (Tannenbaum and Silverstone, 1949; Ross and Bras, 1973) showing no effect of protein on spontaneous breast tumorigenesis in mice and rats, respectively. In contrast, Shay *et al.* (1964) reported increased 3-methylcholanthrene-induced breast cancer as rats were fed greater concentrations of protein. Significant differences were reported, but the interpretation is open to question because the higher-protein experimental diets were based on purified ingredients whereas the control diet, containing 20% protein, was standard laboratory chow.

Hawrylewicz *et al.* (1982), using a two-generation experimental model, reported more DMBA-induced mammary tumors in rats fed increasing amounts of casein. The experimental diets were fed throughout the initiation and promotion phases to offspring of dams fed the same diets during mating, gestation, and lactation (Hawrylewicz *et al.*, 1982). Since certain hormones are critical in rodent breast carcinogenesis (Welsch, 1986), modulation of their action by varying dietary protein was subsequently examined (Huang *et al.*, 1982). Compared to rats fed 19.5% or 31% casein, rats fed 8% casein, weaned from dams also fed 8% casein, showed reduced growth, delayed vaginal opening, and diminished proestrus surges of prolactin, estradiol, and progesterone at 3 weeks after vaginal opening. Wholemount preparations of mammary glands from the low-protein-fed rats also showed reduced ductal development (Hawrylewicz, 1986). Hawrylewicz (1986) proposed that female rats, obtained from dams fed the same low-protein diets throughout gestation and following birth, developed fewer breast tumors because of delayed sexual maturation, with altered hormonal and morphological characteristics of their mammary glands. At the same age, the body weights of rats fed 8% protein were under 200 g compared to more than 260 g for rats fed 19 or 31% casein. These studies show important effects of protein on mammary carcinogenesis in a multigeneration model. Additional studies of the mechanisms whereby protein acts *in utero* and during early development to modify future risk of mammary carcinogenesis are needed.

Studies in our laboratory (Clinton *et al.*, 1985) with female rats fed 8, 16, or 32% of calories as casein beginning at weaning also show reduced initial growth, delayed vaginal opening, and delayed first estrus if the rats were fed low-protein diets. However, we observed no differences in serum prolactin, serum estrogen, or the secretion of prolactin following pituitary stimulation with perphenazine after 20 weeks of feeding. The final body weights for rats fed the three diets were similar and did not show the persistent differences seen in multigeneration studies (Hawrylewicz, 1986).

We have recently completed studies evaluating the interactions of protein, fat, and caloric intake on DMBA-induced breast cancer (Clinton *et al.*, 1984, 1986a, 1988b). Again, the higher-protein diets fed during the initiation phase reduced breast cancer incidence with no effects on promotion. We observed no significant interactions of dietary protein, fat, and calories, although each exerted independent effects. Dietary fat consistently increased mammary carcinogenesis during both the initiation and promotion phases. Statistical analysis of *ad libitum* feed intakes revealed that each additional kcal ingested (average consumption, 44 kcal/day) increased the odds of an adenocarcinoma or tumor of any type being present at necropsy by 10 and 20%, respectively. Few studies have attempted to evaluate the effects of protein source on mammary cancer, although epidemiologic studies suggest stronger correlations with animal proteins. Carroll (1975) found no difference in DMBA-induced breast cancer in rats fed protein supplied by isolated soybean protein or casein.

Formulating a unifying hypothesis about the effects of dietary protein on mammary cancer is not possible at this time. Limited published data with experimental mammary carcinogenesis show inconsistent results. Studies to date have employed a variety of experimental models and protocols, with inappropriate dietary controls in some instances. Human epidemiologic data are suggestive, but show no clear relationship of dietary protein which is independent of dietary fat or total calories. Overall, human and laboratory studies suggest that dietary fat and caloric intake are much more important than protein intake.

4. Colon Cancer

Colon and rectal cancers account for over 138,000 new cases annually, accounting for approximately 16% of all diagnosed cancers in the United States (Silverberg and Lubera, 1987). Fortunately, many are diagnosed when surgical resection is possible, so that annual mortality is reduced to 60,000 (Silverberg and Lubera, 1987). Nevertheless, colon cancer ranks second as the most common fatal cancer in Americans. As with most cancers, it is more common in older individuals. Two-thirds of colon cancers are diagnosed in patients after the age of 50. Persons with familial polyposis or ulcerative colitis experience increased risk of colon cancer at a younger age, and prophylactic colon resections are frequently recommended (Lennard-Jones *et al.*, 1977). Adenomatous polyps and villous adenomas are considered precursor lesions, resulting in intensive efforts directed at their identification and removal before malignant change (Muto *et al.*, 1975). More precise nondietary risk factors have not been reported.

Diets high in fat or low in fiber have been most extensively evaluated in epidemiologic and laboratory studies for their role in colon cancer etiology (Jensen, 1986). Several epidemiologic studies also show correlations between protein intake and colon cancer incidence. However, most investigations suggest equally strong correlations with fat, low dietary fiber, dairy products, and meat. Dairy products and meat both supply abundant protein, fat, and total calories. When Gregor *et al.* (1969) studied the variation in colon cancer incidence in 28 countries, they observed correlations between mortality from colon cancer and higher intakes of animal protein, total protein, and total lipid. Subsequently, Gregor *et al.* (1971) reported data that suggest the decreasing rate for stomach cancer and the increasing rate for colon cancer within these same countries were correlated with increasing animal protein intake. Studies by Berg and Howell (1974) and Howell (1975) showed that international mortality rates for colon cancer were most highly correlated with food consumption patterns in which meat, especially beef, was an important dietary constituent. Armstrong and Doll (1975) also found the correlations to be higher with meat than with total protein or animal protein. Knox (1977) found the relationship between cancer of the large intestine to be strongest for eggs, beef, and pork.

Other studies have failed to detect a relationship between colon cancer and protein intake. Enstrom (1975), using time-trend data, did not find an association between beef consumption or protein and fat intake with colorectal cancer in Americans. Enstrom's studies were based on secular, socioeconomic, and urban rural gradients and on geographic differences in beef and fat consumption within the United States compared to corresponding data on colorectal cancer incidence and mortality rates. In contrast with other studies, Hirayama's (1981) large cohort study in Japan showed a correlation between a higher daily intake of meat and a reduced risk of colorectal cancer. Bingham *et al.* (1971) calculated the average intakes of various foods, nutrients, and fiber in different regions of Great Britain and related them to the geographic pattern of death from colon and rectal cancers between 1969 and 1973. They found no significant association with total protein or animal protein intake. Phillips and Snowdon (1985) reported a survey of 21,295 Seventh Day Adventists (SDA) in California. SDA lifestyles include refraining from smoking and alcoholic beverages, and an adherence by about 50% to a lactoovovegetarian diet. The age-adjusted mortality from colon cancers was lower than the national average. Contrary to earlier work by Phillips (1975), Phillips and Snowden (1985) suggested that large-bowel cancer in the SDA group was not related to meat intake.

Several case–control studies evaluated the frequency of consumption of different foods in an attempt to find relationships with colon cancer. Haenszel *et al.* (1973) found that bowel cancer patients of Japanese ancestry living in Hawaii ate meat, especially beef, more frequently than controls. When extended to colon cancer patients in Japan, the significant associations with beef consumption were not seen (Haenszel *et al.*, 1980). The investigators attributed this difference to the high homogeneity in protein consumption patterns in Japan. Failure to reproduce the findings in Hawaii (Haenszel *et al.*, 1973) was also reported for similar studies in Norway and Minnesota (Bjelke, 1978) and for the continental United States (Graham *et al.*, 1978). A case–control study from Canada involving 348 cases of colon cancer, 194 cases of rectal cancer, and matched controls examined the relationship of dietary patterns to cancer incidence (Jain *et al.*, 1980). Higher intakes of dietary protein were associated with increased risk of both cancers, although the association was stronger with saturated fat.

Table II. Incidence and Total Number of DMH-Induced Tumors
in the Small and Large Intestine and the Inner Ear of Rats
Fed Different Levels of Protein[a]

	Percent of rats with tumors			Average number of tumors/rat	
Diet (n)	Small intestine	Large intestine	Inner ear	Small intestine	Large intestine
7.5% Protein (32)	31	84	47	0.37	1.03
15.0% Protein (31)	65	87	58	0.74	1.68
22.5% Protein (33)	52	91	78	0.78	1.67

[a]Male rats were given DMH via intraperitoneal injection at 15 mg/kg body weight each week for 24 weeks. Rats were necropsied between 28 and 32 weeks after the initiation of the experiment. (Data from Topping and Visek, 1976.)

Few laboratory studies have examined the relationship of dietary protein to colon carcinogenesis. Topping and Visek (1976) studied 1,2-dimethylhydrazine (DMH)-induced carcinogenesis in male rats *ad libitum*-fed purified diets containing 7.5, 15.0, or 22.5% casein. The total number of tumors per rat was greater with 15.0 or 22.5% protein (Table II). In addition, DMH-induced tumors of the inner ear developed earlier and with a higher incidence as the percentage of protein in the diet was increased. We have investigated changes in DMH metabolism (Fig. 2) as one possible mechanism whereby protein may influence DMH-induced colon carcinogenesis. Kari *et al.* (1983) found that the percentage of DMH metabolized to mutagenic end-products in protein-deficient mice was lowered, apparently because higher quantities of the volatile metabolite azomethane were expired. Examination of the data implicated decreased conversion of the subsequent metabolite, azoxymethane, to its metabolic product, methylazoxymethanol. Methylazoxymethanol is converted to the ultimate carcinogen, and inhibition of its formation allowed a buildup of axoxymethane with consequently greater expiration of its volatile precursor, azomethane (Table III). The evidence was compatible with greater amounts of the ultimate carcinogen formed metabolically by rats fed the higher-protein diets.

The possibility that dietary protein stimulates colon carcinogenesis via alterations in fecal lipids or associated factors, such as bile acids, was suggested by recent findings. Hevia *et al.* (1984) and Anderson *et al.* (1985) found that concentrations of crude lipids doubled in feces of both sexes of mice when protein content of their diet was raised from 10% to 40% while the dietary concentration of corn oil was unchanged. Epidemiologic data show an association between dietary lipids, fecal lipids, fecal bile acid excretion, and colon cancer in humans (Reddy, 1983, 1986). Similar evidence has been published for rodents (Reddy, 1983, 1986). The evidence from mice suggests that protein intake may influence the colon milieu by changing the lipid composition of the intestinal contents. Intracolonic lipids may directly influence mucosal cells or change the action of carcinogenic or promoting agents which generally are lipophilic and present in the intestinal lumen.

It is generally believed that tissue polyamine levels are related to cell proliferation and carcinogenesis (Tabor and Tabor, 1976). Ornithine decarboxylase (ODC) catalyzes the

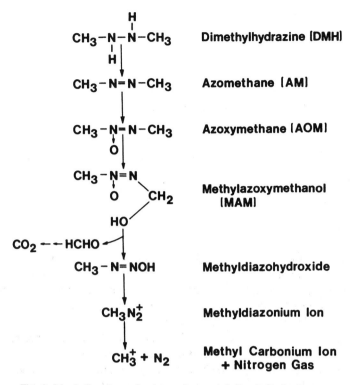

Fig. 2. Metabolic scheme for the carcinogen 1,2-dimethylhydrazine.

rate-limiting enzymatic step in polyamine biosynthesis. Activity of this enzyme rises before cell division and is correlated with elevated levels of tissue polyamines (Russell and Snyder, 1968). Classic tumor-promoting agents stimulate ODC activity in various tissues (O'Brian *et al.*, 1975). Siegler and Kazarinoff (1983, 1984) postulated that dietary protein exerts some of its effects on colon carcinogenesis via changes in polyamine biosynthesis. However, they observed that basal levels of ODC did not change after feeding of diets containing 5 or 20% casein. Furthermore, induction of colonic ODC by sodium deoxycholate was more pronounced with the low-protein diet. Preliminary studies

Table III. Distribution of [^{14}C]-DMH Metabolites of Mice Fed Different Concentrations of Dietary Protein[a]

Protein (%)	Expired AM[b]	Expired $^{14}CO_2$	Other expired metabolites	Urine, feces cage rinse	Carcass	Total
2.5	60.8	2.9	6.6	2.6	26.1	99.0
10.0	39.4	6.6	6.8	3.4	43.4	99.6
40.0	45.0	9.1	3.4	1.9	38.0	97.4

[a]Data represent cumulative percentage of the administered dose after 7 hr.
[b]Azoxymethane.

Table IV. The Effects of Intrarectally Administered Ammonium Acetate
on the Frequency, Morphology, and Histopathology of MNNG-Induced Colon Cancer in Rats[a]

| | Number of rats | Adenocarcinomas | | Morphology[b] | | | |
| | | | | Polypoid | | Sessile | |
		Percent[c]	Number	Percent[c]	Number	Percent[c]	Number
Control	54	46	28[d]	16[d]	9[e]	33	19
Ammonia	53	63	52	44	28	38	24

[a]Data from Clinton et al., 1988a.
[b]Benign lesions and carcinomas.
[c]Percentage of rats with at least one lesion.
[d]Significantly different at $p < 0.003$.
[e]Significantly different at $p < 0.001$.

in our laboratory show a 50% increase in ODC activity in the colon mucosa of rats after consuming diets containing 32% vs. 8% protein for 9–11 weeks (Lin and Visek, 1988).

There is evidence suggesting that ammonia produced by the bacterial flora and other cells in proportion to dietary protein intake promotes experimental colon cancer. Urea is the main nitrogen detoxication product in mammals. About 25% of the urea formed daily enters the alimentary tract with the secretions and is hydrolyzed by bacterial ureases to CO_2 and ammonia. Ammonia in the gastrointestinal tract is either absorbed and reincorporated into urea by the liver, utilized by colonic bacteria for protein synthesis, or retained within the intestinal contents. Ammonia has several effects on cells which suggest that it may influence colon carcinogenesis. It reduces colonic epithelial cell lifespan, alters DNA synthesis, disrupts intermediary metabolism, increases mucosal cell turnover rates, and reaches highest concentrations in those segments of the large intestine where colon cancer incidence is highest (Visek, 1972, 1978). We have examined the effects of ammonium acetate on N-methyl-N'-nitro-N-nitrosoguanidine (MNNG)-induced colon carcinogenesis in rats (Clinton et al., 1988a) (Table IV). Male Sprague–Dawley rats given MNNG intrarectally were subsequently given intrarectal ammonium acetate solutions (24.8 mg NH_3/0.3 ml per rat) or distilled water, 3 times weekly for 52 weeks (Clinton et al., 1988a). Ammonium acetate shortened the latency period for the appearance of fecal blood, increased the frequency of adenocarcinomas, and increased the percentage of rats with polypoid lesions. The earlier appearance of fecal blood correlated with the presence of polypoid lesions, which showed a greater propensity to bleed than sessile, plaquelike carcinomas. Although the possible influence of acetate was not evaluated, this study supports the hypothesis that ammonia acts directly on the colon mucosa to promote colon carcinogenesis. Production of the RAS oncogene protein (p21), detected immunohistochemically, was higher in MNNG-induced adenocarcinomas, the normal mucosa, or benign lesions, but ammonium acetate produced no detectable enhancement (Clinton et al., 1987). Earlier, Topping and Visek (1976) had included urea in the diet of rats given DMH in an attempt to incease colon ammonia concentration. However, no differences in intraluminal ammonia concentrations or cancer incidence were observed. Our preliminary studies show, however, that the intrarectal instillation of ammonia increases the mean ODC activity of the colon mucosa approximately threefold, but the response is highly variable.

Epidemiologic studies often show that meat consumption is more strongly associated with colon cancer than total protein, but few laboratory studies have examined the effects of protein source on colon carcinogenesis. When our laboratory compared DMH-induced tumorigenesis in rats fed diets containing protein from different sources, charcoal-broiled beef was included as one of the dietary treatment variables to determine whether polycyclic aromatic hydrocarbons (Lijinsky and Shubik, 1964) or other factors produced during the cooking of beef would modify the carcinogenic response (Clinton *et al.*, 1979a). The raw or charcoal-broiled beef was lyophilized and incorporated into purified diets with a final concentration of 20% protein and 20% beef fat. No evidence was obtained that source of protein (raw beef, charcoal-broiled beef, or isolated soybean protein) influenced the incidence of DMH-induced small intestinal or colon tumors. This study and the results of Topping and Visek (1976) indicate that the concentration of protein rather than its source has a greater influence on experimental colon carcinogenesis.

In summary, a number of epidemiologic studies suggest correlations between colon cancer incidence and diets high in protein, especially animal protein. However, since human diets rich in animal products generally are also high in fat and other nutrients, it has been impossible to determine effects of protein *per se*. Laboratory studies suggest that increasing protein enhances colon carcinogenesis. The specific mechanisms whereby protein acts are not known. Some studies show that raising protein intake alters carcinogen metabolism, stimulates intestinal ODC activity, and increases the presence of promoting agents, such as ammonia or lipids, within the colon lumen. Laboratory studies indicate that protein source does not influence experimental colon carcinogenesis even though epidemiologic studies in humans suggest that animal proteins are more highly correlated with human colon cancer incidence than vegetable proteins.

5. Pancreatic Cancer

The incidence of pancreatic cancer in the United States has tripled during the last 50 years, and it ranks as the fifth most frequently diagnosed cancer in the United States (Silverberg and Lubera, 1987). The disease causes high mortality, with less than 2% of the patients surviving 5 years following diagnosis. No specific etiology has been identified, although cigarette smoking, chronic pancreatitis, or diabetes may be contributing factors (MacMahon, 1982).

Several international epidemiologic studies suggest a correlation between pancreatic cancer incidence and diets rich in fat and protein (Armstrong and Doll, 1975; Lea, 1967; Ishii *et al.*, 1968; Hirayama, 1977; Wynder, 1975; Wynder *et al.*, 1973; Meyer, 1977; Zaldivan *et al.*, 1981). However, the role of diet in pancreatic cancer has been less extensively evaluated than for cancers of the breast and colon. This difference stems in part from the greater difficulty in diagnosing pancreatic cancer and confirming its actual incidence, especially in underdeveloped nations. Countries with Western culture and diet generally employ more reliable diagnostic techniques and reporting of cases. An early study by Lea (1967) and the more comprehensive study by Armstrong and Doll (1975) showed a strong correlation between mortality from pancreatic cancer in different countries and animal protein intake. Epidemiologic studies in Japan by Ishii *et al.* (1968), which employed questionnaires answered by relatives of the deceased from pancreatic cancer, agree with these findings and showed an association in Japanese men with high intakes of meat. Hirayama (1977) also reported that the relative risk of pancreatic cancer was increased 2.5-fold among daily meat consumers in a large cohort of subjects in Japan.

Two recently developed animal models have been used to investigate the role of diet in pancreatic carcinogenesis. Single injections of N-nitrosobis[2-oxopryl]amine (BOP) induce high yields of ductal pancreatic carcinomas in Syrian golden hamsters (Birt *et al.*, 1981). Multiple injections of azaserine or its inclusion in the diet produce acinar cell pancreatic carcinomas in rats (Longnecker *et al.*, 1981). Several studies suggest that both dietary protein and fat influence pancreatic cancer in these models. Roebuck *et al.* (1981, 1985) found that diets containing larger amounts of unsaturated fat increased the incidence of azaserine-induced pancreatic premalignant foci or tumors. Birt *et al.* (1981) showed that a greater total concentration of dietary fat enhanced BOP-induced pancreatic tumors in both male and female Syrian golden hamsters. Roebuck *et al.* (1981) examined the effects of 11, 20, and 50% casein on azaserine-induced pancreatic carcinogenesis and found decreased incidence in rats fed higher-protein diets. Underlying this observation may have been the reduced food intake and body weight seen with high-protein feeding. Pour *et al.* (1983) observed that a protein-free diet prior to or following BOP administration inhibited tumor incidence. Further studies showed that females fed 9% casein developed fewer BOP-induced cancers than those fed 18 or 36% casein. However, Pour and Birt (1983) observed no differences in the number of lesions in males. Birt *et al.* (1983) also suggested a significant interaction between dietary fat and protein on BOP-induced tumor incidence and multiplicity. Enhanced carcinogenesis by a diet containing 42% of calories as corn oil occurred only in hamsters fed the high-protein diet. Conversely, the stimulatory effects of high-protein diets were seen only with diets also high in fat. These results suggest positive effects of both dietary protein and fat and possible interactions which warrant further investigation.

Several recent studies have investigated the stimulating effect of raw soy protein isolate on pancreatic carcinogenesis (Roebuck *et al.*, 1987). Non-heat-treated soy protein isolate stimulated carcinogen-induced pancreatic carcinogenesis and caused hypertrophy and hyperplasia in non-carcinogen-treated rats. These effects have been attributed to soybean trypsin inhibitor activity and associated elevation of cholecystokinin secretion by raw soybean protein.

6. Liver Cancer

Hepatocellular carcinoma accounts for only 2% of all cancers in the United States (Silverberg and Lubera, 1987). However, the frequency is much higher in other areas of the world, such as Africa and Southeast Asia, where liver cancer may account for 5–8% of all deaths. The possible roles of cirrhosis, parasitism (schistosomiasis), hemochromatosis, and hepatitis B infection have been investigated. Specific hepatocarcinogens that have been investigated include alcohol, safrol, pyrrolizidine alkaloids, cycasin, aflatoxins, and certain steroid hormones used in pharmacological preparations (Anthony, 1977). Human epidemiologic studies have not revealed strong associations between protein intake and liver cancer, although areas where protein–calorie malnutrition is common show higher rates. Several animal models have shown effects of dietary protein on hepatic tumor development. Studies with the azo dye dimethylaminoazobenzene suggested that low-protein diets (8%) reduced the growth rate of rats, but also caused more liver tumors (Silverstone, 1948). In contrast, male and female mice of two strains fed 9% casein developed fewer spontaneous benign hepatomas than those fed 18% casein (Silverstone and Tannenbaum, 1951). These results were obtained in mice fed isocalorically or maintained at equivalent body weights. The 9% casein diet supplemented with 9% gelatin caused no change, but small amounts of added methionine, the first limiting amino acid in casein, raised tumor incidence to that seen with 18% casein (Silverstone and Tannenbaum, 1951).

Madhavan and Gopalan (1965) initially reported markedly enhanced aflatoxin-induced liver toxicity in rats fed diets low in protein. In contrast, their long-term studies with lower dosages of aflatoxin B_1 showed that 36% of the rats fed 20% casein developed hepatomas compared to 0% in those fed 5% casein (Madhavan and Gopalan, 1968). Wells *et al.* (1976) obtained similar results with male rats fed 8, 22, or 30% casein, showing aflatoxin B_1-induced hepatomas in 0/16, 6/9, and 8/10, respectively. Temcharoen *et al.* (1978) found no differences in hepatocarcinogenicity of a mixture of aflatoxin-B_1 and G_1 in rats fed either 5% or 20% protein for 33 weeks. However, the incidence of cystic lesions, cirrhosis, hyperplastic nodules, and cholangiofibroses was higher in the 5% casein-fed animals, suggesting that higher protein intakes protect against these toxic manifestations of aflatoxin. In general, these studies suggest that low-protein diets inhibit aflatoxin-induced liver carcinogenesis but enhance aflatoxin toxicity.

Campbell and associates (1983a,b) have conducted extensive studies to determine the mechanisms whereby aflatoxin-induced tumorigenesis is modified by dietary protein. They found that 5% dietary protein decreases hepatic aflatoxin–DNA adduct formation and that 30% dietary casein enhances covalent binding to DNA (Preston *et al.*, 1976). These studies suggested that the reduced carcinogenicity seen with low-protein diets is partially due to reduced covalent binding of aflatoxin-B_1 to critical genomic macromolecules. However, subsequent studies indicated that the effects of dietary protein on the promotion phase of aflatoxin-induced liver carcinogenesis were very important. When the effects of variations in protein intake before, during, or following aflatoxin-B_1 dosing were examined (Appleton and Campbell, 1983a,b), rats fed 5% casein during dosing developed more severe hepatomegaly, bile duct proliferation, and cholangiofibrosis, and more γ-glutamyltransferase (GGT)-positive foci compared to rats fed 20% casein. Conversely, rats fed 5% protein during the promotion phase showed a large decrease in the number of preneoplastic GGT-positive foci compared to those fed 20%. It was postulated that the effect of protein deprivation on the promotion of preneoplastic liver lesions may be more important than its effect on initiation.

7. Other Cancers

Cancer of the prostate is the second most common carcinoma in American males, accounting for an estimated 96,000 new cases in 1987 (Silverberg and Lubera, 1987). Epidemiologic and clinical studies have examined heredity (Woolf, 1960), social class (Ernster *et al.*, 1978; Graham *et al.*, 1960; Richardson, 1965), marital status (King *et al.*, 1963), viral infections (Sandford *et al.*, 1977), venereal disease (Krain, 1974; Steel *et al.*, 1971), sexual maturation (Rotkin, 1977), benign prostatic hypertrophy (Greenwald *et al.*,

1974), and endocrine changes (Hill *et al.*, 1979, 1981, 1982) for their relation to prostate cancer risk, but the etiology of this disease remains obscure. The wide variation between nations and the changes in incidence with migration from low- to high-risk countries suggest involvement of environmental variables (Haenszel and Kurihara, 1968; Staszewski and Haenszel, 1965). There is a 40-fold difference between the Japanese, who show a low incidence, and black Americans, the population group with the highest rate in the world (Doll, 1978; Hutchinson, 1976). The incidence in black Africans appears to be significantly lower (Higginson and Oettle, 1960). Armstrong and Doll (1975) analyzed international statistics and reported a correlation between prostate cancer mortality and meat intake, especially beef, and with total protein and fat. Kolonel *et al.* (1981) also noted that the incidence of prostate cancer correlated with differences in total protein and with animal protein intake between regions in Hawaii. A subsequent study (Kolonel *et al.*, 1983) confirmed these findings. The calculated correlation coefficients for positive associations with prostate cancer were 0.90, 0.87, 0.78, and 0.83 for animal fat, saturated fat, total protein, and animal protein, respectively. Hirayama (1977) found a relationship between the increase in prostate cancer in Japan since 1950 and the increase in consumption of animal protein and lipids during the same period. A case–control study of prostate cancer in blacks and whites in Southern California showed that total fat intake increased risk, but no consistent relationship with protein was noted (Ross *et al.*, 1987). We have not found studies of dietary protein–prostate cancer relationships with experimental models in the published literature.

The incidence of endometrial cancer tends to be high in countries where cancers of the breast, colon, and prostate are most frequent. Similarly, endometrial cancer incidence is correlated with high intakes of total fat, total protein, and animal products (Armstrong and Doll, 1975; Kolonel *et al.*, 1981). No epidemiologic or experimental studies specifically addressing the role of protein in endometrial cancer appear to have been reported.

Armstrong and Doll (1975) initially noted a correlation between the incidence of renal cancer and animal protein intake in humans. This finding was not confirmed in a subsequent case–control study (Armstrong *et al.*, 1976). McLean and Magee (1970) reported that protein deficiency at the time of dimethylnitrosamine (DMN) administration reduced the acute toxicity but increased the number of renal tumors in rats. Further studies (Swann and McLean, 1971) showed that DMN metabolism was reduced by 50% in liver slices from rats fed the protein-free diet for 7 days. The reduction in liver metabolizing capacity probably left more unmetabolized DMN in the circulation with greater distribution to other body tissues. This was suggested by threefold higher methylation of guanine by DMN in the kidney nucleic acids and a higher tumor incidence. Unfortunately, the studies of DMN-induced kidney cancer were done without recording feed intake and a semipurified protein-free diet fed to the experimental group was compared against commercial laboratory pellets as the dietary control.

Cancer of the lung remains the most frequent malignancy in the United States (Silverberg and Lubera, 1987), and its clear association with cigarette smoking makes it the single most important preventable cause of cancer mortality. Few studies have examined the effects of protein nutrition on lung cancer. Walters and Roe (1964) treated newborn BALB/C mice with DMBA, which causes pulmonary adenomas and adenocarcinomas under these conditions. Pregnant females were fed diets containing casein, wheat flour, and wheat germ meal at 31 or 22% protein equivalent. Newborn pups were treated with DMBA and maintained on the diets of their dams after weaning. Although all mice in both groups developed tumors, the 31%-protein-fed animals developed 50% more lesions than those fed 22% protein.

Experimentally induced skin cancer models have been extensively used to investigate mechanisms of initiation and promotion. Few investigators have evaluated the role of dietary protein. Studies by Tannenbaum and Silverstone (1949) showed no effect of casein-based diets on benzopyrene-induced skin tumors when protein was varied between 9 and 45%.

Ross and Bras (1970, 1973) evaluated spontaneous tumor incidence in long-term studies with rats under *ad libitum* or restricted feeding with different protein–calorie ratios. The direction and magnitude of the influence of these changes differed with the mode of feeding and depended on the tissue of origin, the tumor type, and malignancy of the tumor. Generally higher calorie and protein intakes and faster attainment of mature weight were associated with higher tumor incidence.

8. Amino Acids

The nutritional adequacy of protein is based on its content and balance of specific amino acids. It has been postulated that rapidly growing tumors could be adversely influenced by deficiencies of indispensable amino acids or imbalances of dietary amino acids which impair tissue synthesis. The details of a number of these studies have been reviewed (NAS, 1982; Jose, 1979). A large fraction of studies employing diets deficient in an indispensable amino acid show an inhibition of tumorigenesis. However, such diets generally reduce feed intake and depress growth, making it impossible to assess the specific effects of the amino acid supply. Several clinical case reports have also been reported; Demopoulos (1966) and Lorincz and Kuttner (1965) observed that diets low in phenylalanine and tyrosine, usually given to children with phenylketonuria, seemed to benefit patients with malignant melanoma, Hodgkin's disease, or carcinoma of the uterus. The systematic evaluation of specific amino-acid-deficient diets in treating human malignancies has not been reported.

The effects of excess intake of certain amino acids on tumorigenesis have also been examined. Defining the relationship of excess dietary tryptophan to an increase in urinary bladder carcinogenesis has been a problem in experimental oncology since the original studies by Dunning *et al.* (1950). Feeding excess tryptophan to dogs (Radmoski *et al.*, 1971) or rats (Miyakowa *et al.*, 1973) produced hyperplasia of the urinary bladder epithelium. The incidence of bladder cancer induced by N-2-fluorenylacetamide (AAF) or N-[4-(5-nitro-2-furyl)-2- thiazolyl] (FANFT) formamide increased with the added tryptophan (Dunning *et al.*, 1950; Cohen *et al.*, 1979). However, all studies have not shown this response (Sakata *et al.*, 1984; Birt *et al.*, 1987), and it appears that other modifying factors, such as vitamin B_6, may play a role.

The inhibition of rodent mammary carcinogenesis by excess arginine has also been an area of active investigation. L-Arginine added at a 5% final dietary concentration was fed to rats given DMBA. Lower breast tumor incidence and total number of tumors was subsequently observed (Takeda *et al.*, 1975). Burns and Milner (1984) made similar observations for N-methyl-N-nitrosourea-induced breast cancer in rats. The mechanism of inhibition is unknown and deserves further study since the addition of arginine to the diet was not associated with significant toxicity.

Recent studies related to arginine metabolism are also of interest relative to carcinogenesis. It is well established that excess ammonia or a relative deficiency of arginine will elevate the production of orotic acid, a pyrimidine synthesized by the liver (Visek, 1978). Arginine counteracts ammonia intoxication and the associated elevation of orotic acid formation. Recently, orotic acid feeding (Laurier *et al.*, 1984; Rao *et al.*, 1985; Elliott *et al.*, 1987) and arginine-free diets (Rao *et al.*, 1984) have been shown to promote 1,2-dimethylhydrazine-induced liver tumors. The conditions necessary for ammonia or orotic acid to modify tumor incidence and its relationship to dietary arginine remain to be defined.

9. Summary

Present information precludes the formulation of a unifying hypothesis concerning the role of dietary protein in cancer. Numerous epidemiologic studies in human populations show strong correlations between protein intake and the incidence of cancer at a number of organ sites. Since human diets high in protein are also rich in total calories and total fat, it has been difficult to delineate the specific role of protein. In laboratory animals, the effects of dietary protein on cancer are diverse. They depend on the animal model, tissue of origin, the carcinogenic agent, and dietary protocols. Frequently, diets that support suboptimal growth due to quantity or quality of protein inhibit tumorigenesis. This may be secondary to decreased calorie intake, which often accompanies inadequate intakes of total protein or imbalances in essential amino acids. The more extensive epidemiologic and experimental literature about dietary fat and caloric intake suggests that these dietary factors may have more consistent and quantitatively more important roles in carcinogenesis at several organ sites.

10. References

Albanes, D., 1987, Total calories, body weight, and tumor incidence in mice, *Cancer Res.* **47**:1987–1992.

American Institute of Nutrition, 1977, Report of the AIN *Ad Hoc* Committee on Standards for Nutritional Studies, *J. Nutr.* **107**:1340–1348.

American Institute of Nutrition, 1980, Second Report of the *Ad Hoc* Committee on Standards for Nutritional Studies, *J. Nutr.* **110**:1726.

Anderson, P. A., Alster, J. M., Clinton, S. K., Imrey, P. B., Mangian, H. J., Truex, C. R., and Visek, W. J., 1985, Plasma amino acids and excretion of protein end products by mice fed 10% or 40% soybean protein diets with or without dietary benzo(a)pyrene or 1,2-dimethylhydrazine, *J. Nutr.* **115**:1515.

Anthony, P. D., 1977, Cancer of the liver: Pathogenesis and recent aetiological factors, *Trans. R. Soc. Trop. Med. Hyg.* **71**:466–470.

Appleton, B. S., and Campbell, T. C., 1983a, Effect of high and low dietary protein on the dosing periods of aflatoxin B₁-induced hepatic preneoplastic lesion development in the rat, *Cancer Res.* **43**:2150–2154.

Appleton, B. S., and Campbell, T. C., 1983b, Dietary protein intervention during the postdosing phase of aflatoxin B₁-induced hepatic preneoplastic lesion development, *J. Natl. Cancer Inst.* **70**:547–549.

Armstrong, B., and Doll, R., 1975, Environmental factors and cancer incidence and mortality in different countries with special reference to dietary practices, *Int. J. Cancer* **15**:617–631.

Armstrong, B., Garrod, A., and Doll, R., 1976, A retrospective study of renal cancer with special reference to coffee and animal protein consumption, *Br. J. Cancer* **33**:127–136.

Berg, J. W., and Howell, M. A., 1974, The geographic pathology of bowel cancer, *Cancer* **34**:805–814.

Bingham, S., Williams, D. R. R., Cole, T. J., and James, W. P. T., 1979, Dietary fibre and regional large-bowel cancer mortality in Britain. *Br. J. Cancer* **40**:456–463.

Birt, D., Salmasi, S., and Pour, P., 1981, Enhancement of experimental pancreatic cancer in Syrian golden hamsters by dietary fat, *J. Natl. Cancer Inst.* **67**:1327–1332.

Birt, D., Stepan, K., and Pour, P., 1983, Interaction of dietary fat and protein on pancreatic carcinogenesis in Syrian golden hamsters, *J. Natl. Cancer Inst.* **71**:355–360.

Birt, D., Julius, A., Hagesawa, R., St. John, M., and Cohen, S., 1987, Effect of L-tryptophan excess and vitamin B_6 deficiency on rat urinary bladder cancer promotion, *Cancer Res.* **47**:1244–1250.

Bjelke, E., 1978, Dietary factors and the epidemiology of cancer of the stomach and large bowel. *Aktuel. Ernaehrungsmed. Klin. Prax. Suppl.* **2**:10–17.

Buell, P., 1973, Changing incidence of breast cancer in Japanese–American women, *J. Natl. Cancer Inst.* **51**:1479–1483.

Burns, R. A., and Milner, J. A., 1984, Effect of arginine on the carcinogenicity of 7,12-dimethyl-benz(a)anthracene and N-methyl-N-nitrosourea, *Carcinogenesis* **5**:1539–1542.

Carroll, K. K., 1975, Experimental evidence of dietary factors and hormone-dependent cancers, *Cancer Res.* **35**:3374–3383, 1975.

Carroll, K. K., and Khor, K. T., 1975, Dietary fat in relation to tumorigenesis, *Prog. Biochem. Pharm.* **10**:308–353.

Clinton, S. K., and Visek, W. J., 1986, The macronutrients in experimental carcinogenesis of the breast, colon, and pancreas, in: *Dietary Fat and Cancer,* Volume 222 (A. Rogers, D. Birt, and C. Ip, eds.), Prog. Clin. Biol. Res., Alan R. Liss, New York, pp. 377–401.

Clinton, S. K., Destree, R. J., Anderson, D. B., Truex, C. R., Imrey, P. B., and Visek, W. J., 1979a, 1,2-Dimethylhydrazine-induced intestinal cancer in rats fed beef or soybean protein, *Nutr. Rep. Int.* **20**:335.

Clinton, S. K., Truex, C. R., and Visek, W. J., 1979b, Dietary protein, aryl hydrocarbon hydroxylase and chemical carcinogenesis in rats, *J. Nutr.* **109**:55–62.

Clinton, S. K., Truex, C. R., Imrey, P. B., and Visek, W. J., 1980, Dietary protein and mixed function oxidase activity, in: *Microsomes, Drug Oxidations, and Carcinogenesis* (M. J. Coon, ed.), Academic Press, New York, pp. 1129–1132.

Clinton, S. K., Imrey, P. B., Alster, J. M., Simon, J., Truex, C. R., and Visek, W. J., 1984, The combined effects of dietary protein and fat on 7,12-dimethylbenz(a)anthracene-induced breast cancer in rats, *J. Nutr.* **114**:1213–1223.

Clinton, S. K., Li, S., and Visek, W. J., 1985, The combined effects of dietary protein and fat on prolactin in female rats, *J. Nutr.* **115**:311–318.

Clinton, S. K., Alster, J. M., Imrey, P. B., Nandkumar, S., Truex, C. R., and Visek, W. J., 1986, Effects of dietary protein, fat and energy intake during an initiation phase study of 7,12-dimethylbenz(a)anthracene-induced breast cancer in rats, *J. Nutr.* **116**:2290–2302.

Clinton, S. K., Dieterich, M., Bostwick, D. G., Olson, L. M., Montag, A. G., Michelassi, F., and Visek, W. J., 1987, The effects of ammonia on N-methyl-N'-nitrosoguanidine (MNNG)-induced colon carcinogenesis and RAS oncogene (p21) expression, *Fed. Proc.* **46**:585 (Abstr. 1567).

Clinton, S. K., Bostwick, D. G., Olson, L. M., Mangian, H. J., and Visek, W. J., 1988a, Ammonia and cholic acid as promoters of N-methyl-N'-nitrosoquanidine (MNNG)-induced colon carcinogenesis in rats, *Cancer Res.* **48**:3035–3039.

Clinton, S. K., Imrey, P. B., Alster, J. M., Simon, J., and Visek, W. J., 1988b, The combined effects of dietary protein and fat intake during the promotion phase of 7,12-dimethylbenz(a)anthracene-induced breast cancer in rats, *J. Nutr.* **118**:1577–1585.

Cohen, L. A., 1986, Dietary fat and mammary cancer, in: *Diet, Nutrition, and Cancer: A Critical Evaluation* (B. S. Reddy, L. A. Cohen, eds.), CRC Press, Boca Raton, FL, Chapter 6.

Cohen, S. M., Arai, M., Jacobs, J. B., and Friedell, G. H., 1979, Promoting effect of saccharin and DL-tryptophane in urinary bladder carcinogenesis, *Cancer Res.* **39**:1207–1217.

Demopoulos, H. B., 1966, Effects of reducing the phenylalanine–tyrosine intake of patients with advanced malignant melanoma, *Cancer* **19**:657–664.

Doll, R., 1978, Geographic variation in cancer incidence: A clue to causation, *World J. Surg.* **2**:595–602.

Doll, R., and Peto, R., 1981, *The Causes of Cancer,* Oxford University Press, New York.

Dunning, W. F. Curtis, M. R., and Mann, M. E., 1950, The effect of added dietary tryptophan on the occurrence of 2-acetylaminofluorene-induced liver and bladder cancer, *Cancer Res.* **10**:454–459.

Elliott, T. S., Robinson, J. L., and Visek, W. J., 1987, Influence of dietary orotic acid on hepatocarcinogenesis in Fischer-344 and Sprague–Dawley rats, *Fed. Proc.* **46**:746 (Abstr. 2508).

Enstrom, J. E., 1975, Colorectal cancer and consumption of beef and fat, *Br. J. Cancer* **32**:432–439.

Ernster, V. L., Selvin, S., Sacks, S. T., Austin, D. F., Brown, S. M., and Winklestein, W., Jr., 1978, Prostatic cancer: Mortality and incidence rates by race and social class, *Am. J. Epidemiol.* **107**(4):311–320.

Gaskill, S. P., McGuire, W. L., Osborne, C. K., and Stern, M. P., 1979, Breast cancer mortality and diet in the United States, *Cancer Res.* **39**:3628.

Graham, S., Levin, M., and Lilienfeld, A. M., 1960, The socioeconomic distribution of cancer of various sites in Buffalo, NY, 1948–1952, *Cancer* **13**:180–191.

Graham, S., Dayal, H., Swanson, M., Mittelman, A., and Wilkinson, G., 1978, Diet in the epidemiology of cancer of the colon and rectum, *J. Natl. Cancer Inst.* **61**:709–714.

Gray, G. E., Pike, M. C., and Henderson, B. E., 1979, Breast-cancer incidence and mortality rates in different countries in relation to known risk factors and dietary practices, *Br. J. Cancer* **39**:1.

Greenwald, P., Kirmas, V., Polan, A. K., and Dick, V. S., 1974, Cancer of the prostate among men with benign prostatic hyperplasia, *J. Natl. Cancer Inst.* **53**:335–340.

Gregor, O., Toman, R., and Prusova, F., 1969, Gastrointestinal cancer and nutrition, *Gut* **10**:1031–1034.

Gregor, O., Toman, R., and Prusove, F., 1971, Relation of gastrointestinal cancer mortality to cancer mortality in general, *Scand. J. Gastroenterol.* **9**[Suppl.]:79–85.

Haenszel, W., and Kurihara, M., 1968, Studies of Japanese migrants. I. Mortality from cancer and other disease among Japanese in the United States, *J. Natl. Cancer Inst.* **40**:43–68.

Haenszel, W., Berg, J. W., Segi, M., Kurihara, M., and Locke, F. B., 1973, Large-bowel cancer in Hawaiian Japanese *J. Natl. Cancer Inst.* **51**:1765–1779.

Haenszel, W., Locke, F. B., and Segi, M., 1980, A case–control study of large bowel cancer in Japan, *J. Natl. Cancer Inst.* **64**:17–22.

Hawrylewicz, E. J., 1986, Fat-protein interaction, defined 2-generation studies, in: *Dietary Fat and Cancer* (C. Ip, D. Birt, A. Rogers, and C. Mettlin, eds.), Alan R. Liss, New York, pp. 403–433.

Hawrylewicz, E. J., Huang, H. H., Kissane, J. Q., and Drab, E., 1982, Enhancement of 7,12-di-methylbenz(a)anthracene (DMBA) mammary tumorigenesis by high dietary protein in rats, *Nutr. Rept. Int.* **26**:793–806.

Hems, G., 1978, The contributions of diet and childbearing to breast-cancer rates, *Br. J. Cancer* **37**:974.

Hems, G. 1980, Associations between breast-cancer mortality rates, child-bearing and diet in the United Kingdom, *Br. J. Cancer* **41**:429.

Hevia, P., Truex, C. R., Imrey, P. B., Clinton, S. K., Mangian, H. J., and Visek, W. J., 1984, Plasma amino acids and excretion of protein end products by mice fed 10% or 40% soybean protein diets with or without dietary 2-acetyl-aminofluorene or*N-N*-dinitrosopiperazine, *J. Nutr.* **114**:555–564.

Higginson, J., and Oettle, A. G., 1960, Cancer incidence in the Banta and "Cape Colored" races of South Africa: Report of a cancer survey in the Transvaal (1935–1955), *J. Natl. Cancer Inst.* **24**:589–671.

Hill, A. B., 1965, The environment and disease: Association and causation, *Proc. R. Soc. Med.* **58**:295–300.

Hill, P., Wynder, E. L., Garbaczewski, L., Giarnes, H., and Walker, A. R. P., 1979, Diet and urinary steroids in black and white North American men and black South African men, *Cancer Res.* **39**:5101–5105.

Hill, P., Garbaczewski, L., Helman, P., Walker, A. R. P., Gurnes, H., and Wynder, E. L., 1981, Environmental factors and breast prostate cancer, *Cancer Res.* **41**:3817–3818.

Hill, P., Wynder, E. L., Garbaczewski, L., Games, H., and Walker, A. R., 1982, Response to leutinizing releasing hormone, thyrotropic releasing hormine, and human chronic genadotropin administration in healthy men at different risks for prostate cancer and in prostate cancer patients, *Cancer Res.* **42**:2074–2080.

Hirayama, T., 1977, Changing patterns of cancer in Japan with special reference to the decrease in stomach cancer mortality, in: *Origins of Human Cancer, Book A: Incidence of Cancer in Humans* (H. H. Hiatt, J. D. Watson, and J. A. Winsten, eds.), Cold Spring Harbor Laboratory, New York, pp. 55–75.

Hirayama, T., 1981, A large-scale cohort study on the relationship between diet and selected cancers of the digestive organs, in: *Gastrointestinal Cancer, Endogenous Factors; Banbury Report 7* (W. R. Bruce, P. Correa, M. Lipkin, S. R. Tannenbaum, and T. D. Wilkins, eds.), Cold Spring Harbor Laboratory, New York, pp. 409–429.

Howell, M. A., 1975, Diet as an etiological factor in the development of cancers of the colon and rectum, *J. Chronic Dis.* **28**:67–80.

Huang, H. H., Hawrylewicz, E. J., Kissane, J. Q., and Drab, E. A., 1982, Effect of protein diet on release of prolactin and ovarian steroids in female rats, *Nutr. Rep. Int.* **26**:807–820.

Hutchinson, G. B., 1976, Epidemiology of prostate cancer, *Semin. Oncol.* **3**:151–159.

Ishii, K., Nakamura, K., Ozaki, H., Yamada, N., and Takeuchi, T., 1968, [Epidemiological problems of pancreas cancer], *Jpn. J. Clin. Med.* **26**:1839–1842.

Jain, M., Cook, G. M., Davis, F. G., Grace, M. G., Howe, G. R., and Miller, A. B., 1980, A case–control study of diet and colorectal cancer, *Int. J. Cancer* **26**:757–768.

Jensen, O. M., 1986, The epidemiology of large bowel cancer, in: *Diet, Nutrition and Cancer: A Critical Evaluation* (B. S. Reddy and L. A. Cohen, eds.) CRC Press, Baca Raton, FL, Chapter 3.

Jose, D., 1979, Dietary deficiency of protein, amino acids and total calories on development and growth of cancer, *Nutr. Cancer* **1**:58–63.

Kappas, A., Anderson, K. E., Conney, H. H., and Alvares, A. P., 1976, Influence of dietary protein and carbohydrate on antipyrine and theophylline metabolism in man, *Clin. Pharmacol. Ther.* **20**:643–653.

Kari, F. W., Johnston, J. B., Truex, C. R., and Visek, W. J., 1983, Effect of dietary protein concentration on yield of mutagenic metabolites from 1,2-dimethylhydrazine in mice, *Cancer Res.* **43**(8):3674–3679.

Kelsey, J. L., 1979, A review of the epidemiology of human breast cancer, *Epidemiol. Rev.* **1**:74–109.

King, H., Diamond, E., and Lilienfeld, A. M., 1963, Some epidemiological aspects of cancer of the prostate, *J. Chronic Dis.* **16**:117–153.

Knox, E. G., 1977, Foods and diseases, *Br. J. Prev. Soc. Med.* **37**:71–80.

Kolonel, L. N., Hankin, J. H., Lee, J., Chu, S. Y., Nomura, A. M., and Hinds, M. W., 1981, Nutrient intakes in relation to cancer incidence in Hawaii, *Br. J. Cancer* **44**(3):332–339.

Kolonel, L. N., Nomura, A. M., Hinds, M. W., Hirohata, T., Hankin, J. H., and Lee, J., 1983, Role of diet in cancer incidence in Hawaii, *Cancer Res.* **43**:2397–2402.

Krain, L. S., 1974, Some epidemiologic variables in prostatic carcinoma in California, *Prev. Med.* **3**:154–159.

Laurier, C., Tatematsu, M., Rao, P. M., Rajalaksami, S., and Sarma, D. S. R., 1984, Promotion by orotic acid of liver carcinogenesis in rats initiated by 1,2-dimethylhydrazine, *Cancer Res.* **44**:2186–2191.

Lea, A. J., 1967, Neoplasms and environmental factors, *Ann. R. Coll. Surgeons Engl.* **41**:432.

Lennard-Jones, J. E., Morson, B. C., Ritchie, J. K., Shove, D. C., and Williams, C. B., 1977, Cancer in colitis: Assessment of individual risk by clinical and histological criteria, *Gastroentrology* **73**:1280–1289.

Lijinsky, W., and Shubik, P., 1964, Benzo(a)pyrene and other polynuclear aromatic hydrocarbons in charcoal broiled meat, *Science* **145**:53–55.

Lin, H. C., and Visek, W. J., 1988, Effect of dietary protein and fat on fecal ammonia and intracolonic pH in male Holtzman rats, *J. FASEB* **2**:A857 (abstr.).

Longnecker, D., Roebuck, B., Yager, J., Lilja, H., and Siegmund, B., 1981, Pancreatic carcinoma in azaserine-treated rats: Induction, classification, and dietary modulation of incidence, *Cancer* **47**:1562–1572.

Lorincz, A. B., and Kuttner, R. E., 1965, Response of malignancy to phenylalanine restriction; a preliminary report on a new concept of managing malignant disease, *Neb. State Med. J.* **50**:609–617.

Lubin, J. H., Burns, P. E., Blot, W. J., Ziegler, R. G., Lees, A. W., and Fraumeni, J. F., 1981, Dietary factors and breast cancer risk. *Int. J. Cancer* **28**:865–869.

MacMahon, B., 1982, Risk factors and cancer of the pancreas, *Cancer* **50**:2676–2680.

Madhavan, T. V., and Gopalan, C., 1965, Effect of dietary protein on aflatoxin liver injury in weanling rats, *Arch. Pathol.* **80**:123–126.

Madhavan, T. V., and Gopalan, C., 1968, The effect of dietary protein on carcinogenesis of aflatoxin, *Arch. Pathol.* **85**:133–137.

McLean, A. E., and Magee, P. N., 1970, Increased renal carcinogenesis by dimethylnitrosamine in protein deficient rats, *Br. J. Exp. Pathol.* **51**:587–590.

Meyer, F., 1977, Relationship between diet and carcinoma of the stomach, colon, rectum, and pancreas in France. *Gastroenterol. Clin. Biol.* **1**:971–982.

Miller, A. B., Kelly, A., Choi, N. W., Matthews, V., Morgan, R. W., Munan, L., Burch, J. D., Feather, J., Howe, G. R., and Jain, M., 1978, A study of diet and breast cancer, *Am. J. Epidemiol.* **107**(6):499–509.

Miyakawa, M., and Yoshida, O., 1973, DNA synthesis of the urinary bladder epithelium in rats with long term feeding of DL-tryptophane-added and pyridoxine-deficient diet, *Gann* **64**:411–413.

Moreschi, C., Beziehungen Zwischen Ernahrung und Tumorwachsten, *Zlmmunitatsforsch* **2**:651–685, 1909.

Muto, T., Bussey, H. J. R., and Morson, B. C., 1975, The evolution of cancer of the colon and rectum, *Cancer* **36**:2251–2270.

National Academy of Sciences, 1982, Committee on Diet, Nutrition, and Cancer, National Research Council, *Diet, Nutrition, and Cancer,* National Academy Press, Washington, DC.

National Research Council, 1978, *Nutrient Requirements of Laboratory Animals,* No. 10, 3rd rev. ed., National Academy of Sciences, Washington, DC.

Newberne, P., Bieri, J., Briggs, G., and Nesheim, M., 1978, Control of diets in laboratory animal experimentation. *Inst. Lab. Animals Res. New* **21**:A-1-A2.

O'Brian, J. G., Simsiman, R. C., and Boutwell, R. K., 1975, Induction of the polyamine-biosynthetic enzymes in mouse epidermis by tumor promoting agents, *Cancer Res.* **35**:1662–1670.

Phillips, R. L., 1975, Role of life-style and dietary habits in risk of cancer among Seventh-Day Adventists, *Cancer Res.* **35**:3513–3522.

Phillips, R. L., and Snowdon, D. A., 1985, Dietary relationships with fatal colorectal cancer among Seventh-Day Adventists, *J. Natl. Cancer Inst.* **74**:307–317.

Pour, P., and Birt, D., 1983, Modifying factors in pancreatic carcinogenesis in the hamster model. IV. Effects of dietary protein, *J. Natl. Cancer Inst.* **71**:347–353.

Pour, P., Birt, D., Salmasi, S., and Gotz, U., 1983, Modifying factors in pancreatic carcinogenesis in the hamster model. I. The effect of protein-free diet fed during early stages of carcinogenesis, *J. Natl. Cancer Inst.* **70**:141–146.

Preston, R. S., Hayes, J. R., and Campbell, T. C, 1976, The effect of protein deficiency on the *in vivo* binding of aflatoxin B_1 to rat liver macromolecules, *Life Sci.* **19**:1191–1197.

Radmoski, J. L., Glass, E. M., and Deichmann, W. B., 1971, Transitional cell hyperplasia in the bladders of dogs fed DL-tryptophan, *Cancer Res.* **31**:1690–1694.

Rao, P. M., Agamine, Y. N., Roomi, M. W., Rajalakshmi, S., and Sarma, D. S. R., 1984, Orotic acid, a new promoter for experimental liver carcinogenesis, *Toxicol. Pathol.* **12**:173–178.

Rao, P. M., Rajalakshimi, S., Alam, A., Sarma, D. S. R., Pala, M., and Parodi, S., 1985, Orotic acid, a promoter of liver carcinogenesis, induces DNA damage in rat liver, *Carcinogenesis* **6**:765–768.

Reddy, B. S., 1983, Experimental research on dietary lipids and colon cancer, in: *Dietary Fats and Health* (E. G. Perkins and W. J. Visek, eds.), Am. Oil Chemists' Society, Champaign, IL, pp. 741–760.

Reddy, B. S., 1986, Diet and colon cancer: Evidence from human and animal model studies, in: *Diet, Nutrition, and Cancer: A Critical Evaluation, Volume 1* (B. S. Reddy and L. A. Cohen, eds.), CRC Press, Boca Raton, FL, pp. 46–65.

Richardson, I. M., 1965, Prostate cancer and social class, *Br. J. Prev. Soc. Med.* **19**:140–142.

Roebuck, B., Yager, J., and Longnecker, D., 1981, Dietary modulation of azaserine-induced pancreatic carcinogenesis in rats. *Cancer Res.* **41**:888–893.

Roebuck, B., Longnecker, D., Baumgartner, K., and Thron, C., 1985, Carcinogen-induced lesions in the rat pancreas: Effects of varying levels of essential fatty acid, *Cancer Res.* **45**:5252–5256.

Roebuck, B. D., Kaplita, P. V., Edwards, B. R., and Praissman, M., 1987, Effects of dietary fats and soybean protein on azaserine-induced pancreatic carcinogenesis and plasma cholecystokinin in the rat, *Cancer Res.* **47**:1333–1338.

Ross, M. H., and Bras, G., 1973, Influence of protein under- and overnutrition on spontaneous tumor prevalence in the rat, *J. Nutr.* **103**:944–1963.

Ross, M. H., Bras, G., and Raybeer, M. S., 1970, Influence of protein and caloric intake upon spontaneous tumor incidence of the anterior pituitary gland of the rat, *J. Nutr.* **100**:177–189.

Ross, R. K., Shimizu, H., Paganini-Hill, A., Henda, G., and Henderson, B., 1987, Case–control studies of prostate cancer in blacks and whites in Southern California, *J. Natl. Cancer Inst.* **78**:869–874.

Rotkin, I. D., 1977, Studies in the epidemiology of prostatic cancer; expanded sampling, *Cancer Treat Rep.* **61**:173–180.

Rous, P., 1914, The influence of diet on transplanted and spontaneous mouse tumours, *J. Expl. Med.* **20**:433–451.

Russell, D. H., and Snyder, S. H., 1968, Amine synthesis in rapidly growing tissue: Ornithine decarboxylase activity in regenerating rat liver, chick embryo, and various tumors, *Proc. Natl. Acad. Sci. USA* **60**:1420–1427.

Sakata, T., Shirai, T., Fukushima, S., Hasegawa, R., and Ito, N., 1984, Summation and synergism in the promotion of urinary bladder carcinogenesis initiated by N-butyl-N-(4-hydroxy-butyl)nitrosamine in F344 rats, *Gann* **74**:950–956.

Sandford, E. J., Geder, L., Laychock, A., Rohner, J., and Rapp, F., 1977, Evidence for the association of cytomegalovirus with carcinoma of the prostate, *J. Urol.* **118**:789–792.

Shay, H., Gruenstein, M., and Shimkin, M. B., 1964, Effect of casein, lactalbumin, and ovalbumin on 3-methylcholanthrene-induced mammary carcinoma in rats, *J. Natl. Cancer Inst.* **33**:243.

Siegler, J. M., and Kazarinoff, M. N., 1983, Effects of acute and chronic protein deprivation on ornithine decarboxylase levels in rat liver and colon, *Nutr. Cancer* **4**:176–185.

Siegler, J. M., and Kazarinoff, M. N., 1984, The effect of a low protein diet on the response of rat colonic and hepatic ornithine decarboxylase activity to sodium deoxycholate and thioacetamide treatment, *J. Nutr.* **114**:574–580.

Silverberg, E., and Lubera, J., 1987, Cancer statistics, *Ca—A Cancer Journal for Clinicians,* **37**:2–19.

Silverstone, H., 1948, The levels of carcinogenic azo dyes in the livers of rats fed various diets containing *p*-dimethylamino-azobenzene: Relationship to the formation of hepatomas, *Cancer Res.* **8**:301–308.

Silverstone, H., and Tannenbaum, A., 1951, Proportion of dietary protein and the formation of spontaneous hepatomas in the mouse, *Cancer Res.* **11**:442–446.

Singletary, K. W., and Milner, J. A., 1987a, Influence of prior dietary protein intake on metabolism, DNA binding and adduct formation of 7,12-dimethylbenz(a)anthracene in isolated rat mammary epithelial cells, *J. Nutr.* **117**:587–592.

Singletary, K. W., and Milner, J. A., 1987b, Prior dietary protein intake and DNA-binding 7,12-dimethyl-benz(a)anthracene metabolites formed by isolated rat hepatocytes, *J. Natl. Cancer Inst.* **78**:727–733.

Singletary, K. W., Milner, J. A., and Martin, S. E., 1984, Effect of dietary protein concentration on rat-liver S-9 pioactivation of 7,12-dimethylbenz(a)anthracene in the salmonella/microsome assay, *Mutation Res.* **126**:19–24.

Staszewski, J., and Haenszel, W., 1965, Cancer mortality among Polish-born in the United States, *J. Natl. Cancer Inst.* **35**:291–297.

Steel, R., Lees, R. E. M., Kraus, A. S., and Rao, C., 1971, Sexual factors in the epidemiology of cancer of the prostate, *J. Chronic Dis.* **24**:29–37.

Swann, P. R., and McLean, A. E., 1971, Cellular injury and carcinogenesis: The effect of a protein-free high-carbohydrate diet on the metabolism of dimethylnitrosamine in the rat, *Biochem. J.* **124**:283–288.

Tabor, C. W., and Tabor, H., 1976, 1,4-Diaminobutane (putrescine), spermidine, and spermine, Annu. Rev. Biochem. **45**:285–306.

Takeda, Y., Tominaga, T., Tei, N., Kitamura, M., Taga, S., Murase, J., Taguchi, T., and Miwatani, T., 1975, Inhibitory effect of L-arginine on growth of rat mammary tumors induced by 7,12-dimethyl-benz(a)anthracene, *Cancer Res.* **35**:2390–2393.

Tannenbaum, A., 1959, Nutrition and cancer, in: *The Pathophysiology of Cancer* (F. Homburger, ed.), Hober and Harper, New York, pp. 517–562.

Tannenbaum, A., and Silverstone, H., 1949, The genesis and growth of tumors. IV. Effects of varying the proportion of protein (casein) in the diet, *Cancer Res.* **9**:162–173.

Temcharoen, P., Anukarahanonta, T., and Bhamarapravati, N., 1978, Influence of dietary protein and vitamin B_{12} on the toxicity and carcinogenicity of aflatoxins in rat liver, *Cancer Res.* **38**:2185–2190.

Topping, D. C., and Visek, W. J., 1976, Nitrogen intake and tumorigenesis in rats injected with 1,2-di-methylhydrazine, *J. Nutr.* **106**:1583–1590.

Visek, W. J., 1972, Effects of urea hydrolysis on cell life-span and metabolism, *Fed. Proc.* **31**:1178–1193.

Visek, W. J., 1978, Diet and cell growth modulation by ammonia. *Am. J. Clin. Nutr.* **31**:S216–S220.

Visek, W. J., Mangian, H., Elliott, T. S., Ruskin, B., Bragg, D. S. A., and Robinson, J. L., 1988, Renal damage and urinary lithiasis in mice fed orotic acid (OA), *J. FASEB* **2**:A863 (abstr.).

Walters, M. A., and Roe, F. J. C., 1964, The effect of dietary casein on the induction of lung tumours by the injection of 9,10-dimethyl-1,2-benzanthracene (DMBA) into newborn mice, *Br. J. Cancer* **18**:312–316.

Watt, B. K., and Merrill, A. L., 1975, *Composition of Foods,* Agriculture Handbook, No. 8, USDA, Washington, DC.

Wattenberg, L. W., 1975, Effects of dietary constituents on the metabolism of chemical carcinogens, *Cancer Res.* **35**:3526–3531.

Wells, P., Alftergood, L., and Alfin-Slater, R. B., 1976, Effect of varying levels of dietary protein on tumor development and lipid metabolism in rats exposed to aflatoxin, *J. Am. Oil Chem. Soc.* **53**:559–562.

Welsch, C. W., 1986, Interrelationship between dietary fat and endocrine processes in mammary gland tumorigenesis, in: *Dietary Fat and Cancer* (C. Ip, D. Birt, A. Rogers, and C. Mettlin, eds.), Prog. Clin. Biol. Res., Volume 222, Alan R. Liss, New York, pp. 623–654.

Woolf, C. M., 1960, An investigation of the familial aspects of carcinoma of the prostate, *Cancer* **13**:739–744.

Woteke, C. E., Briefel, R. R., and Sempos, C., 1987, Nutritional epidemiology and national surveys, *J. Nutr.* **117:**401–402.

Wynder, E. L., 1975, An epidemiological evaluation of the causes of cancer of the pancreas, *Cancer Res.* **35:**2228–2233.

Wynder, E. L., Mabuchi, K., Maruchi, N., and Fortner, J. G., 1973, Epidemiology of cancer of the pancreas, *J. Natl. Cancer Inst.* **50:**645–667.

Zaldivan, R., Wetterstrand, W. H., and Ghai, A. L., 1981, Relative frequency of mammary, colonic, rectal, and pancreatic cancer in a large autopsy series. Statistical Association between mortality rates from these cancers: Dietary fat intake as a common etiological variable, *Zentralbl. Bakteriol.* (*Naturwiss.*) **169:**474–481.

6

Fat and Cancer

David Kritchevsky and David M. Klurfeld

1. Introduction

In 1982 a committee of the National Academy of Sciences published a review of the state of knowledge pertinent to nutrition or diet and cancer (Committee on Diet, Nutrition and Cancer, 1982). The committee adduced a significant role for fat in cancer development and suggested, among other guidelines, that Americans reduce their intake of fats by 25% or from 40% of total calories to 30%. The data reviewed in drawing these conclusions were primarily international correlations. The most thorough correlation study was that of Armstrong and Doll (1975), who studied incidences for 14 cancers in 32 countries and for 27 cancers in 23 countries. Among environmental variables they studied in addition to foods were gross national product (GNP), physician density, population density, and use of solid and liquid energy. They found positive associations between breast and colorectal cancers and total fat consumption. They also observed strong positive associations between GNP and cancers of the colon, rectum, breast, and uterus, but not the ovary. Incidence of stomach cancer was inversely correlated with GNP, meat, animal protein, and total fat. In their conclusion they stated, ". . . it is clear that these and other correlations should be taken only as suggestions for further research and not as evidence of causation or as bases for preventive action."

2. Breast Cancer

Gray *et al.* (1979) examined breast cancer rates in 34 countries and compared those data with anthropomorphic measurements and food consumption. They found correlations with height, weight, and age at menarche as well as with total fat availability (Table I). Age at menarche was correlated inversely with intake of fat and animal protein. Hems (1978) studied 41 countries and found breast cancer correlated significantly with total fat

David Kritchevsky and David M. Klurfeld • The Wistar Institute of Anatomy and Biology, Philadelphia, Pennsylvania 19104.

Table I. Breast Cancer Rates, Anthropomorphic Measurements, and Fat Availability in Selected Countries[a,b]

Country	Breast cancer rates[c]		Anthropomorphic data			Total fat (g/day per person)
	Mortality	Incidence	Height (cm)	Weight (kg)	Menarche (years)	
Canada	49.9	116.5	159.0	56.2	14.0	141.4
Finland	27.6	64.1	161.8	56.8	16.0	114.4
Japan	8.8	29.7	154.3	48.9	15.0	41.3
Netherlands	50.1	95.6	162.8	60.0	14.1	153.5
Norway	35.1	89.8	164.6	60.2	14.5	131.8
United Kingdom	50.5	103.8	160.7	59.5	15.0	141.9
United States	45.5	134.9	163.8	58.6	13.4	148.0

[a]After Gray *et al.*, 1979.
[b]Countries listed were the only ones where data for all measures were available. From a total of 34 countries.
[c]Per 100,000 women aged 35–64 per year.

intake as well as intake of animal protein, animal fat, and refined sugar. Hill (1987) has pointed out that a major weakness of international comparisons is that, although the incidence data are reliable, the dietary data are soft. Furthermore, the populations under study differed by race, religion, and environment.

Kolonel *et al.* (1981) reported on nutrient intake and cancer incidence in 4657 Hawaiian adults. They found positive associations with fat and breast or uterine cancer and significant negative associations between these cancers and carbohydrate intake (Table II). Gaskill *et al.* (1979) found that breast cancer mortality in the United States was

Table II. Association of Age-Adjusted Mean Daily Nutrient Intakes and Average Annual Cancer Incidence per 100,000 for 10 Groups in Hawaii[a]

Cancer site	Fat	
	Component	r[b]
Lung	Cholesterol	0.94
Larynx	Cholesterol	0.76
Breast	Total	0.94
	Animal	0.89
	Saturated	0.95
	Unsaturated	0.90
Uterus	Total	0.98
	Animal	0.98
	Saturated	1.00
	Unsaturated	0.95
Prostate	Animal	0.90
	Saturated	0.87

[a]After Kolonel *et al.*, 1981.
[b]r = Partial correlation coefficient, adjusted for sex.

positively associated with milk, total calories, beef, fat, protein, butter, and margarine, and negatively associated with eggs. When the Southern states were eliminated or when age at first marriage or income was controlled, only the milk and egg association persisted (Table III).

Phillips (1975) compared diet data from 77 breast cancer cases and controls from among a Seventh Day Adventist population in California. The highest relative risk was associated with fried potatoes, and other risks were attributed to fried foods, frying in hard fat, and dairy products except milk and white bread. A case–control study in Canada (Miller *et al.*, 1978) with 400 cases and controls attributed high risk to ingestion of fat, saturated fat, linoleic acid, oleic acid, cholesterol, and total calories. Lubin *et al.* (1981) also carried out a case–control study in Canada examining dietary data from 577 cases and 82 controls and found positive associations with intakes of fat and meat. Graham *et al.* (1982) administered a food frequency questionnaire to 2024 cases and 1463 controls in Buffalo, New York, and found no association between consumption of animal fat and breast cancer.

The association between dietary fat and risk of breast cancer appears to be weakening (Byers, 1988). Goodwin and Boyd (1987) reviewed findings from international and national or regional studies. Seven (of 13) international studies that evaluated total fat and tested for association between fat and breast cancer risk all found a positive association. In seven regional studies, five found an association. However, when case–control studies were considered, only 1 of 14 found a significant association. Some of the data are presented in Table IV. Hirohata *et al.* (1987) studied diet and breast cancer in Japanese and Caucasian cases, hospital controls, and neighborhood controls in Hawaii. There were 183 subjects in each of the three Japaneses groups and 161 subjects in the Caucasian groups. No significant differences were found in mean intake of total fat, saturated fat, oleic acid,

Table III. Significance Levels of Correlations between Age-Adjusted Breast Cancer Mortality and Demand for Selected Foods[a]

Food	48 Contiguous states	32 Non-Southern states[b]
Milk	<0.001	0.005
Table Fats	0.009	0.764
Beef	0.050	0.017
Cheese	0.100	<0.001
Frozen desserts	0.071	0.526
Poultry	0.342	<0.001
Pork	0.357	0.196
Fish	0.292	<0.001
Eggs	<0.001	<0.001
Meat intake	0.181	0.248
Fat intake	0.008	0.385
Protein intake	0.002	0.810
Caloric intake	<0.001	0.667

[a]After Gaskill *et al.*, 1979.
[b]Southern states: Delaware, Maryland, West Virginia, Virginia, Kentucky, Tennessee, North Carolina, South Carolina, Georgia, Alabama, Florida, Mississippi, Arkansas, Louisiana, Oklahoma, Texas.

Table IV. Breast Cancer and Fat:
Case–Control Studies that Evaluated Total Fat[a]

Author	Cases	Controls	Significant association
Nomura *et al.*, 1978	86	6774	No
Graham *et al.*, 1982	2024	1463	No
Kolonel *et al.*, 1983	268	591	No
Nomura *et al.*, 1985	344	688	No
Sarin *et al.*, 1985	68	33	Yes
Hirohata *et al.*, 1985	212	424	No
Lubin *et al.*, 1986	818	1556	No

[a]After Goodwin and Boyd, 1987.

linoleic acid, animal protein or cholesterol. Hirohata *et al.* (1985) also found that Japanese subjects in Japan whose fat intake was in the lowest or highest quartile had identical relative risk. There were 212 cases and 424 controls in his study.

The NHANES I study reported on 99 cases of breast cancer and 5386 noncases (Jones *et al.*, 1987) and found no differences in fat intake (cases ingested 5% less) or in fat as percent of energy, saturated, monounsaturated, and polyunsaturated fatty acids, and cholesterol. The data of Rohan *et al.* (1988) also did not support a role for dietary fat in the etiology of cancer in an Australian cohort. In a study in Israel in which food containing more than 20% fat was the dietary factor studied, comparison of 318 cases and 607 controls younger than 50 years showed no increasing risk with increasing intake (by quartile). In 495 cases and 949 controls over 50, there was a slight difference in risk between the lowest and highest quartile of intake (Lubin *et al.*, 1986). In a recent study of 250 cases and 499 controls in Italy, a reduced risk was found for women who ingested 28% of calories from fat compared with those whose fat intake amounted to more than 36% of calories (Toniolo *et al.*, 1989).

Table V. Relative Risk of Breast Cancer in 89,538 Women
by Quintile of Fat Intake[a]

Quintile[b]		Total fat	Saturated fat	Linoleic acid	Cholesterol
1	CA[c]	1.00	1.00	1.00	1.00
	NCA	1.00	1.00	1.00	1.00
2	CA	0.80	0.80	0.83	1.11
	NCA	0.80	0.92	0.83	0.86
3	CA	0.88	0.89	0.73	1.01
	NCA	0.89	0.93	0.80	0.83
4	CA	0.80	0.74	0.80	1.10
	NCA	0.95	0.95	0.87	1.01
5	CA	0.82	0.78	0.84	0.89
	NCA	0.85	0.85	0.84	0.83

[a]After Willett *et al.*, 1987.
[b]Quintiles of approximately equal number of subjects.
[c]CA, Adjusted for calories; NCA, not adjusted for calories.

Willett *et al.* (1987) studied a cohort of 89,538 American women whose fat intake ranged from 32 to 44% of calories. The relative risk for the highest quintile of calorie-adjusted fat intake compared with the lowest quintile was 0.82 (Table V).

Factors other than diet exert an important influence in hormone-related cancers such as breast cancer. Epidemiologic data suggest that early menarche may put young women at greater risk for breast cancer (Staszewski, 1971; Apter and Vihko, 1983). Tall stature may also increase risk (DeWaard, 1975; Swanson *et al.*, 1988; Albanes *et al.*, 1988). Nutritional status affects age at menarche (Baanders-vanHalewijn and DeWaard, 1968; Apter and Vihko, 1983); Albanes (1987), in a review of caloric restriction, body weight, and cancer, summarized findings from 11 studies in which body weight, relative body weight, and body mass index at height was assessed for their effects on breast cancer. Nine of the eleven studies revealed a positive correlation.

3. Colon Cancer

Higginson (1966) searched for etiological factors in a group containing 93 subjects with stomach cancer, 340 with colorectal cancer, and 1020 controls. Cases used more fats and fewer dairy products, but the differences were not statistically significant. Graham *et al.* (1972) found no differences in fat intake between 168 cases and controls. Bingham *et al.* (1979) found no association between fat intake and mortality from colorectal cancer in England. Fat intake among residents of Utah is similar to that for the entire United States even though the former have a lower incidence of colon cancer (Lyon and Sorenson, 1978).

As in the case of breast cancer, the local studies show little correlations with fat intake, whereas international comparisons (Armstrong and Doll, 1975; Knox, 1977) show strong correlations. Rogers and Longnecker (1988), in their excellent review of diet and cancer, summarize 24 studies and find a small association between fat intake and cancer risk, but overall, the findings are inconsistent.

Stemmermann *et al.* (1984) examined 7074 Japanese men in Hawaii; of these, 106 had colon cancer, 59 rectal cancer, 490 other cancers, and 6419 acted as controls. The fat intake of the colon cancer patients (79.9 g/day) was slightly lower than that of the rectal cancer patients (88.4 g/day) or controls (86.5 g/day). Relative risk of colon cancer decreased with increasing intake of saturated fat, whereas risk of rectal cancer increased (Table VI). In contrast to Stemmermann's findings, Jain *et al.* (1980) and Stampfer *et al.* (1987) found risk to increase with increased intake of saturated fat. Jensen *et al.* (1982), in comparing colon cancer in Denmark and Finland, found saturated fat to be negatively correlated with risk. Stocks and Karn (1933), in an early epidemiologic study of colon cancer in England, found intake of dairy foods to be a negative risk factor. Manousos *et al.* (1983) found fat (as represented by meat) to be a risk for colon cancer, but Philipps and Snowdon (1983) did not. Fat was not found to be a risk factor for colon cancer in Belgium (Tuyns, 1986) or France (Marquart-Moulin *et al.*, 1986).

Lyon *et al.* (1987) studied colon cancer and diet in men and women in Utah. In men, eating less than 75 g of fat daily, more than 105 g, or being in between exerted the same relative risk. In women, however, relative risk for those ingesting less than 50 g/day was 1.0; ingestion of 50–70 g/day conferred a relative risk of 3.3, and in women eating more

Table VI. Saturated Fat Intake
and Risk of Colorectal Cancer in Men
of Japanese Ancestry[a,b]

Saturated fat intake (g/day)	Colon cancer RR[c]	Rectal cancer RR
>84.5	0.49	1.51
64.2–84.5	0.44	1.78
49.0–64.1	0.46	1.30
33.1–48.9	0.59	1.02
<33.1	1.00	1.00
	$p = 0.35$	$p = 0.222$

[a]After Stemmerman et al., 1984.
[b]106 cases of colon cancer; 59 cases of rectal cancer; 6419 controls.
[c]RR = relative risk.

than 70 g/day, risk rose to 4.7. The authors suggested total caloric intake to be the determining factor relative to risk. Two Australian studies present different findings with regard to fat intake and risk of colon cancer. In Adelaide, Potter and McMichael (1986) found increasing fat intake to confer a slight risk on men and a much higher risk on women. Kune et al. (1987), working in Melbourne, found a slightly elevated risk with increasing fat intake in men and a slightly reduced risk in women. A follow-up on the study of fat and breast cancer in 89,534 women found an increasing risk of colon cancer with increasing fat intake among the 106 cases (Stampfer et al., 1987).

A radically different view has been expressed recently by Tuyns and his co-workers (1987), who suggest that the nutritional culprit vis-à-vis colon cancer risk is not fat at all, but rather dietary oligosaccharides. They examined a Belgian cohort of 453 cases of colon cancer, 365 of rectal cancer, and 2851 controls. In examining trends by linear logistic regression, they found the risk for colon cancer to be significantly associated with mono-, di-, and polysaccharides and the risk for rectal cancer to be associated significantly with total carbohydrate, mono-, and disaccharides. They state, "By recommending that people eat less fat we cannot be sure, at the present state of knowledge in the field, that we are giving the right advice." Based on their experience in the Honolulu Heart Program, McGee et al. (1985) had come to a similar conclusion.

There are relatively few reports relating dietary fat to the risk of other tumors, but they all show small to moderate direct associations between fat intake and relative risk. The tumors studied have been lung cancer (Byers et al., 1987; Kvale et al., 1983); pancreatic cancer (Durbec et al., 1983); ovarian cancer (Byers et al., 1983; Cramer et al., 1984); and prostate cancer (Graham et al., 1983; Kolonel et al., 1983; Ross et al., 1987). In a more recent report from Hawaii, Severson et al. (1989) found no correlation between prostate cancer and total fat intake.

4. Animal Studies

The first experiment to show an influence of dietary fat on tumorigenesis was that of Watson and Mellanby (1930), who found that addition of 12.5–25.0% butter to a basal

(3% fat) diet increased incidence of skin tumors in coal-tar-treated mice from 34% to 57%. Lavik and Baumann (1941, 1943) found that addition of 15% shortening to a mouse diet enhanced the incidence of methylcholanthrene-induced skin tumors from 12% to 83%. The fat seemed to be most effective when added to the diet during the promotion phase of carcinogenesis. They also found that saturation of the fat exercised a slight effect since incidence of skin tumors in mice fed lard, coconut oil, or corn oil was 61, 66, and 76%, respectively.

The pioneering work in this area was carried out by Tannenbaum in the 1940s. Tannenbaum (1942a) was the first to show that spontaneous mammary tumors developed more rapidly in mice fed a high-fat diet. Another pioneer in this area is K. K. Carroll, who showed systematically that saturated fat was less cocarcinogenic than unsaturated fat (Gammal *et al.*, 1967; Carroll and Khor, 1971). He also showed first that addition of sufficient polyunsaturated fat (a source of essential fatty acids) to a diet rich in saturated fat enhanced tumor growth (Hopkins and Carroll, 1979). Carroll's experiments were carried out using 7,12-dimethylbenz(a) anthracene (DMBA) as a mammary carcinogen, but the difference in promoting effect between saturated and unsaturated fat has also been observed in 1,2-dimethylhydrazine (DMH)-induced colon cancer in rats (Reddy, 1975; Broitman *et al.*, 1977). The saturated—polyunsaturated fat difference has also been observed in pancreatic tumors (Roebuck *et al.*, 1981). The average survival time of leukemic mice fed 16% coconut oil was 7% greater than that of mice fed 16% safflower oil (Burns *et al.*, 1978).

The level of dietary fat is also important (Carroll and Khor, 1971) (Table VII). A 10-fold increase in fat (from 0.5 to 5.0% of diet) does not affect tumor incidence, multiplicity, or latency, but going from 5 to 10% fat increases incidence by 22% and multiplicity by 74% and reduces latency by 12%. Increasing dietary fat from 10 to 20% has no further effect.

The mechanism(s) by which unsaturated fat exerts its effect is unclear. Abraham *et al.* (1984) suggested that the effect might be mediated at the level of prostaglandin synthesis, but Ip *et al.* (1985), who titrated the optimum amount of essential fatty acid required for growth of DMBA-induced mammary tumors, found no changes in prostaglandin E levels. The possibility that peroxidized polyunsaturated fat might affect membrane function and risk of cancer was vitiated by the experiments of Lane *et al.* (1985). Based on their experiments with Chinese hamster cells, Aylsworth *et al.* (1984) suggested that polyunsaturated fat could promote tumorigenesis by inhibiting cellular communica-

Table VII. Influence of Dietary Fat (%) on DMBA-Induced Mammary Tumors in Rats[a]

Corn oil (% in diet)	Tumor incidence (%)	Multiplicity[b]	Latent period (days)
0.5	70	2.5 ± 0.40	78.4 ± 4.5
5.0	76	2.3 ± 0.39	77.4 ± 4.4
10.0	93	4.0 ± 0.48	68.0 ± 4.5
20.0	90	3.7 ± 0.58	68.2 ± 4.3

[a]After Carroll and Khor, 1971.
[b]Tumors/tumor-bearing rat.

Table VIII. Lack of Effect of Fat Level on Colon Tumors in Rats[a]

Fat (%)	Incidence (%)	Multiplicity	Mean size (mm ± SD)
Mix (5)[b]	55	1.64	6.19 ± 3.74
Beef (24)	63	1.44	5.56 ± 3.81
Corn oil (24)	55	1.23	7.00 ± 4.71
Shortening (24)	38	1.13	6.29 ± 3.26

[a]After Nauss et al., 1984. Tumors induced by N-nitrosomethyl urea.
[b]Equal parts of beef, corn oil, and shortening. Beef fat diet was 22 parts fat and 2 parts corn oil.

tion. Other possibilities are alterations in immune function, membrane composition, or enhanced production of bile acids (Hopkins and West, 1976; Carroll et al., 1981).

The difference in promotional activity between saturated and unsaturated fat is not a unanimous finding. Nauss et al. (1984) observed no significant effect of saturation or level of fat in rats given a colon carcinogen (N-nitrosomethylurea) and fed beef fat, corn oil, or a commercial shortening (Table VIII). The findings confirmed an earlier observation in an experiment using DMH (Nauss et al., 1983). Newberne and Nauss (1986) have suggested that the so-called fat effect is not a simple one and may involve interactions of a number of dietary components.

5. Fat Type

In most, but not all, naturally occurring unsaturated fats, the double bonds are in the *cis* configuration. However, partially hydrogenated fats, which are present to an appreciable extent in the American diet, also contain some double bonds in the *trans* configuration. The question of the effects of fat rich in fatty acids containing *trans*-unsaturated double bonds (*trans* fat) has been addressed. Selenskas et al. (1984) compared the effects of 5 and 20% *cis* fat, *trans* fat, and corn oil on incidence of DMBA-induced tumors in rats (Table IX). They found that *trans* fat feeding provided results similar to those obtained with saturated fat. The effects of *cis* and *trans* fat on colon cancer have also been studied in rats treated with DMH (Watanabe et al., 1985) and in a strain of rats (Wistar–Furth–Osaka) prone to develop colon cancer (Sugano et al., 1989), and no differences were observed.

Fats rich in omega-3 polyunsaturated fatty acids, which are found in fish and some plant oils, have gained nutritional prominence in the last few years. the compounds of particular interest are 5,8,11,14,17-eicosapentaenoic (EPA) and 4,7,10,13,16,19-docosahexaenoic (DHA) acids. Rats fed a fish oil supplement did not support growth of a transplanted tumor as well as rats fed corn oil (Karmali et al., 1984). Tumor weight was reduced by 32% ($p < 0.05$) and tumor volume by 40% ($p < 0.018$). A significant reduction in DMBA-induced colon tumors was seen in rats fed fish oil compared to those fed corn oil (Braden and Carroll, 1986). In rats treated with DMH and given corn or fish oil there was no difference in incidence of colorectal tumors, but there were fewer total

Table IX. Influence of Cis- and
Trans-Unsaturated Fat on DMBA-Induced
Mammary Tumors in Rats[a]

Fat	%	Incidence (%)	Multiplicity
Trans[b]	5	16	2.3 ± 0.5
	20	32	2.3 ± 0.4
Cis[c]	5	24	2.7 ± 0.9
	20	40	2.7 ± 0.4
Corn oil[d]	5	44	2.5 ± 0.3
	20	80	3.6 ± 0.5

[a]After Selenskas *et al.*, 1984.
[b]*Trans* fat: partially hydrogenated blend of soybean–cottonseed oil 1:1. Iodine value = 59. P/S = 0.17.
[b]*Cis* fat: mix of 58% olive oil, 40% cocoa butter, and 2% coconut oil. Iodine value = 65. P/S = 0.26.
[c]Corn oil: iodine value = 103. P/S = 4.81.

tumors and left colon tumors in rats fed fish oil (Nelson *et al.*, 1988). The mechanism by which fish oils exert their effects appears to involve, in part, the inhibition of arachidonic acid metabolism by EPA and DHA (Karmali *et al.*, 1984; Karmali, 1986). Studies need to be done in which animals fed fish oil are fed diets that meet the essential fatty acid (EFA) requirements of tumor growth before it can be concluded definitively that omega-3 fatty acids have a unique tumor-inhibiting effect.

6. Caloric Restriction

Tannenbaum's original studies were concerned with effects of underfeeding (Tannenbaum, 1940) and then caloric restriction (Tannenbaum, 1942b). He showed later that the degree of caloric restriction also influenced tumor growth (Tannenbaum, 1945). It is fair to speculate that the effect of fat on tumor growth is an effect of fat *per se* or is due, at least in part, to the caloric contribution from fat. Influence of caloric restriction on tumor growth is reviewed fully elsewhere in this volume, but a few words on the relation of caloric restriction vs. fat are in order. Lavik and Baumann (1943), in a study of methylcholanthrene-induced skin tumors in mice, found that a diet high in calories but low in fat led to almost double the tumor incidence seen when a diet low in calories but high in fat was fed. Kritchevsky *et al.* (1984) showed that a diet containing 4% fat fed *ad libitum* led to significantly more DMBA-induced mammary tumors than did a diet containing 13.1% fat but restricted in calories by 40%. The same observation was made in DMH-induced colon carcinogenesis (Klurfeld *et al.*, 1987). When the diet contained a saturated fat (coconut oil) augmented with enough corn oil to ensure against essential fatty acid deficiency, tumor incidence was lower than when the dietary fat was corn oil. To answer the criticism that the diets were too low in fat, an experiment in which both *ad libitum*-fed and caloric-restricted rats were fed high levels of fat and given DMBA confirmed the earlier findings (Klurfeld *et al.*, 1989) (Table X). Reduction of caloric intake at any stage of promotion will affect carcinogenicity. When DMBA-treated rats were subjected to

Table X. Influence of Fat Level and 25% Caloric Restriction
on DMBA-Induced Mammary Tumors in Rats[a]

Diet[b]	Incidence[c] (%)	Multiplicity[c] (± SEM)	Tumor burden[c,d] (g ± SEM)
Ad libitum			
5% corn oil	65	1.9 ± 0.3	4.2 ± 1.9
15% corn oil	85	3.0 ± 0.6	6.6 ± 2.7
20% corn oil	80	4.1 ± 0.6	11.8 ± 3.2
Restricted			
20% corn oil	60	1.9 ± 0.4	1.5 ± 0.5
26.7% corn oil	30	1.5 ± 0.3	2.3 ± 1.6

[a]After Klurfeld *et al.*, 1989.
[b]Calorically restricted rats fed 20 or 26.7% corn oil ate same amount of fat daily as
control rats fed 15 or 20% corn oil.
[c]$p < 0.001$.
[d]Total tumor weight/rat.

intermittent *ad libitum* feeding and caloric restriction over a 4-month period, the incidence of tumors correlated with total food intake, and it was shown that palpable tumor growth spurted when going from restricted to free feeding and slowed when freely fed rats were placed on a calorie-restricted diet (Kritchevsky *et al.*, 1989).

Davidson and Carroll (1982) compared effects of a fat-free and a 20% corn oil diet on DMBA-induced mammary tumors in rats. The fat-free diet provided 364 kcal/100 mg, and the corn oil diet provided 464 kcal/100 g. Tumor incidence was significantly lower on the fat-free diet. Switching rats fed the high-fat diet to the fat-free diet (22% reduction in calories) inhibited weight gain and slowed tumor growth; reversion to the high-fat diet caused a spurt in weight gain and tumor growth.

The data suggest that the caloric contribution from fat is the major component of the fat effect, although type of fat exerts some influence. Proper comparison of different studies suggests the needs for standardized protocols, which should include individual housing of animals and careful assessment of food intake as well as use of adequate numbers of experimental animals.

7. Conclusion

In conclusion, the epidemiologic data are inconsistent in that less rigorous ecological comparisons suggest large effects of dietary fat on cancer incidence while case–control studies indicate weak, if any, effects. Conflicting results have been derived from studies of different ethnic groups, nationalities, ages, genders, and place of residence. Since all these factors seem to modulate apparent effects of dietary fat on cancer, there remains much work to be done in developing more accurate instruments for assessment of current and past diet. Anthropomorphic indices in relation to diet at various stages of life need to be assessed better for effects on subsequent cancer risk. Experimental data show increasing dietary fat leads to greater tumor growth, but much of the effect can be attributed to provision of adequate EFA and excess calories. Dietary fat seems to be a promoter more in rats fed *ad libitum* than in those fed calorie-restricted diets. *Ad libitum* feeding and maximal growth rate in rodents is normal and desirable; it may be that these animals are the equivalent of obese humans who have higher incidence of many tumors, including those thought closely related to dietary fat. Animal studies may give clues to the degree and mechanism by which dietary fat affects tumor growth.

ACKNOWLEDGMENTS. This work was supported, in part, by Grant CA43856 and a Research Career Award (HL00734) from the National Institutes of Health, and by funds from the Commonwealth of Pennsylvania.

8. References

Abraham, S., Faulkin, L. J., Hillyard, L. A., and Mitchell, D. J., 1984, Effect of dietary fat on tumorigenesis in the mouse mammary gland, *J. Natl. Cancer Inst.* **72:**1421–1429.

Albanes, D., 1987, Caloric intake, body weight and cancer. A review, *Nutr. Cancer* **9:**199–217.

Albanes, D., Jones, D. Y., Schatzkin, A., Micozzi, M. S., and Taylor, P. R., 1988, Adult stature and risk of cancer, *Cancer Res.* **48:**1658–1662.

Apter, D., and Vihko, R., 1983, Early menarche, a risk factor for breast cancer, indicates early onset of ovulatory cycles, *J. Clin. Endocrinol. Metab.* **57:**82–86.

Armstrong, B., and Doll, R., 1975, Environmental factors and cancer incidence and mortality in different countries, with special reference to dietary practices, *Int. J. Cancer* **15:**617–631.

Aylsworth, C. F., Jone, C., Trosko, J. E., Meites, J., and Welsch, C. W., 1984, Promotion of 7,12-dimethylbenz(a) anthracene-induced mammary tumorigenesis by high dietary fat in the rat: Possible role of intracellular communication, *J. Natl. Cancer Inst.* **72:**637–645.

Baanders-vanHalewijn, E. A., and DeWaard, F., 1968, Menstrual cycles shortly after menarche in European and Bantu girls, *Hum. Biol.* **40:**314–322.

Bingham, S., Williams, D. R. R., Cole, T. J., and James, W. P. T., 1979, Dietary fibre and regional large-bowel cancer mortality in Britain, *Br. J. Cancer* **40:**456–463.

Braden, L. M., and Carroll, K. K., 1986, Dietary polyunsaturated fat in relation to mammary carcinogenesis in rats, *Lipids* **21:**285–288.

Broitman, S. A., Vitale, J. J., Vavrousek-Jakuba, E., and Gottlieb, L. S. 1977, Polyunsaturated fat, cholesterol and large bowel tumorigenesis, *Cancer* **40:**2453–2463.

Burns, C. P., Luttenegger, D. G., and Spector, A. A., 1978, Effect of dietary fat saturation on survival of mice with L1210 leukemia, *J. Natl. Cancer Inst.* **61:**513–515.

Byers, T., 1988, Diet and cancer. Any progress in the interim? *Cancer* **62:**1713–1724.

Byers, T., Marshall, J., Graham, S., Mettlin, C., and Swanson, M., 1983, A case–control study of dietary and non-dietary factors in ovarian cancer, *J. Natl. Cancer Inst.* **71:**681–686.

Byers, T. E., Graham, S., Haughey, B. P., Marshall, J. R., and Swanson, M. K., 1987, Diet and lung cancer risk: Findings from the Western New York diet study, *Am. J. Epidemiol.* **125:**351–363.

Carroll, K. K., and Khor, H. T., 1971, Effect of level and type of dietary fat on incidence of mammary tumors induced in female Sprague–Dawley rats by 7,12-dimethylbenz(a) anthracene, *Lipids* **6:**415–420.

Carroll, K. K., Hopkins, G. J., Kennedy, T. G., and Davidson, M. B., 1981, Essential fatty acids in relation to carcinogenesis, *Prog. Lipid Res.* **20:**685–690.

Committee on Diet, Nutrition and Cancer, 1982, *Diet, Nutrition and Cancer,* National Academy Press, Washington, DC.

Cramer, D. W., Welch, W. R., Hutchison, G. B., Willett, W., and Scully, R. E., 1984, Dietary animal fat in relation to ovarian cancer risk, *Obstet. Gynecol.* **63:**883–888.

Davidson, H. B., and Carroll, K. K., 1982, Inhibitory effect of a fat-free diet on mammary carcinogenesis in rats, *Nutr. Cancer* **3:**207–215.

DeWaard, F., 1975, Breast cancer incidence and nutritional status with particular reference to body weight and height, *Cancer Res.* **35;**3351–3356.

Durbec, J. P., Chevillotte, G., Bidart, J. M., Berthezene, P., and Sarles, H., 1983, Diet, alcohol, tobacco and risk of cancer of the pancreas: A case–control study, *Br. J. Cancer* **47**:463–470.

Gammal, E. B., Carroll, K. K., and Plunkett, E. R., 1967, Effects of dietary fat on mammary carcinogenesis by 7,12-dimethylbenz-(α)anthracene in rats, *Cancer Res.* **27**:1737–1742.

Gaskill, S. P., McGuire, W. L., Osborne, C. K., and Stern, M. P., 1979, Breast cancer mortality and diet in the United States, *Cancer Res.* **39**:3628–3637.

Goodwin, P. J., and Boyd, N. F., 1987, Critical appraisal of the evidence that dietary fat intake is related to breast cancer risk in humans, *J. Natl. Cancer Inst.* **79**:473–485.

Graham, S., Schotz, W., and Martino, P., 1972, Alimentary factors in the epidemiology of gastric cancer, *Cancer* **30**:927–938.

Graham, S., Marshall, J., Mettlin, C., Rzepka, T., Nemoto, T., and Byers, T., 1982, Diet in the epidemiology of breast cancer, *Am. J. Epidemiol.* **116**:68–75.

Graham, S., Haughey, B., Marshall, J., Priore, R., Byers, T., Rzepka, T., Mettlin, C., and Pontes, J. E., 1983, Diet in the epidemiology of carcinoma of the prostate gland, *J. Natl. Cancer Inst.* **70**:687–692.

Gray, G. E., Pike, M. C., and Henderson, B. E., 1979, Breast cancer incidence and mortality rates in different countries in relation to known risk factors and dietary practices, *Br. J. Cancer* **39**:1–7.

Hems, G., 1978, The contributions of diet and childbearing to breast-cancer rates, *Br. J. Cancer* **37**:974–982.

Higginson, J., 1966, Etiological factors in gastrointestinal cancer in man, *J. Natl. Cancer Inst.* **37**:527–545.

Hill, M., 1987, Dietary fat and human cancer (Review), *Anticancer Res.* **7**:281–292.

Hirohata, T., Shigematsu, T., Nomura, A. M. Y., Nomura, Y., Horie, A., and Hirohata, I., 1985, The occurrence of breast cancer in relation to diet and reproductive history. A case–control study in Fukuoka, Japan, *NCI Monogr.* **69**:187–190.

Hirohata, T., Nomura, A. M. Y., Hankin, J. H., Kolonel, L. N., and Lee, J., 1987, An epidemiological study on the association between diet and breast cancer, *J. Natl. Cancer Inst.* **78**:595–600.

Hopkins, G. J., and Carroll, K. K. 1979, Relationship between amount and type of dietary fat in promotion of mammary carcinogenesis induced by 7,12-dimethylbenz(a)-anthracene, *J. Natl. Cancer Inst.* **62**:1009–1012.

Hopkins, G. J. and West, C. E., 1976, Possible role of dietary fats in carcinogenesis, *Life Sci.* **19**:1103–1106.

Ip, C., Carter, C. A., and Ip, M. M., 1985, Requirement of essential fatty acid for mammary tumorigenesis in the rat, *Cancer Res.* **45**:1997–2001.

Jain, M., Cook, G. M., Davis, F. G., Grace, M., Howe, G. R., and Miller, A. B., 1980 A case–control study of diet and colorectal cancer, *Int. J. Cancer* **26**:757–768.

Jensen, O. M., Maclennan, R., and Wahrendorf, J., 1982, Diet, bowel function, fecal characteristics and large bowel cancer in Denmark and Finland, *Nutr. Cancer* **4**:5–19.

Jones, D. Y., Schatzkin, A., Green, S. B., Block, G., Brinton, L. A., Ziegler, R. G., Hoover, R., and Taylor, P. R., 1987, Dietary fat and breast cancer in the National Health and Nutrition Examination Survey. I. Epidemiologic Follow-up Study, *J. Natl. Cancer Inst.* **79**:465–471.

Karmali, R. A., 1986, Eicosanoids and cancer, *Prog. Clin. Biol. Res.* **222**:687–697.

Karmali, R. A., Marsh, J., and Fuchs, C., 1984, Effect of omega-3 fatty acids on growth of a mammary rat tumor, *J. Natl. Cancer Inst.* **73**:457–461.

Klurfeld, D. M., Weber, M. M., and Kritchevsky, D., 1987, Inhibition of chemically induced mammary and colon tumor promotion by caloric restriction in rats fed increased dietary fat, *Cancer Res.* **47**:2759–2762.

Klurfeld, D. M., Welch, C. B., Lloyd, L. M., and Kritchevsky, D., 1989, Inhibition of DMBA-induced mammary tumorigenesis by caloric restriction in rats fed high fat diets, *Int. J. Cancer* **43**:922–925.

Knox, E. G., 1977, Foods and diseases, *Br. J. Prev. Soc. Med.* **31**:71–80.

Kolonel, L. N., Hankin, J. H., Lee, J., Chu, S. Y., Nomura, A. M. Y., and Hinds, M. W. 1981, Nutrient intakes in relation to cancer incidence in Hawaii, Br. J. Cancer **44**:332–339.

Kolonel, L. N., Nomura, A. M. Y., Hinds, M. W., Hirohata, T., Hankin, J. H., and Lee, J., 1983, Role of diet in cancer incidence in Hawaii, *Cancer Res.* **43**:2397S–2402S.

Kritchevsky, D., Weber, M. M., and Klurfeld, D. M., 1984, Dietary fat versus caloric content in initiation and promotion of 7,12-dimethylbenz(a)anthracene-induced mammary tumorigenesis in rats, *Cancer Res.* **44**:3174–3177.

Kritchevsky, D., Welch, C. B., and Klurfeld, D. M., 1989, Response of mammary tumors to caloric restriction for different time periods during the promotion phase, *Nutr. Cancer* **12**:259–269.

Kune, S., Kune, G. A., and Watson, L. F., 1987, Case control study of dietary etiological factors: The Melbourne colorectal cancer study, *Nutr. Cancer* **9**:21–42.

Kvale, G., Bjelke, E., and Gart, J. J., 1983, Dietary habits and lung cancer risk, *Int. J. Cancer* **31**:397–405.

Lane, H. W., Butel, J. S., Howard, C., Shepherd, F., Halligan, R., and Medina, D., 1985, The role of high levels of dietary fat in 7,12-dimethylbenzanthracene-induced mammary tumorigenesis: Lack of an effect on lipid perioxidation, *Carcinogenesis* **3**:403–407.

Lavik, P. S., and Baumann, C. A., 1941, Dietary fat and tumor formation, *Cancer Res.* **1**:181–187.

Lavik, P. S., and Baumann, C. A., 1943, Further studies on tumor promoting action of fat, *Cancer Res.* **3**:749–756.

Lubin, F., Wax, Y., and Modan, B., 1986, Role of fat, animal protein and dietary fiber in breast cancer etiology: A case–control study, *J. Natl. Cancer Inst.* **77**:605–612.

Lubin, J. H., Burns, P. E., Blot, W. J., Ziegler, R. G., Lee, A. W., and Fraumeni, J. F., 1981, Dietary factors and breast cancer risk, *Int. J. Cancer* **28**:685–689.

Lyon, J. L., and Sorenson, A. W., 1978, Colon cancer in a low risk population, *Am. J. Clin. Nutr.* **31**:5227–5230.

Lyon, J. L., Mahoney, A. W., West, D. W., Gardner, J. W., Smith, K. R., Sorenson, A. W., and Stanish, W., 1987, Energy intake: Its relationship to colon cancer risk, *J. Natl Cancer Inst.* **78**:853–861.

Manousos, O., Day, N. E., Trichopoulous, D., Gerovassilis, F., Tzonou, A., and Polychronopoulou, A., 1983, Diet and colorectal cancer: A case–control study in Greece, *Int. J. Cancer* **32**:1–5.

Marquart-Moulin, G., Riboli, E., Cornee, J., Charnay, B., Berthezene, P., and Day, N., 1986, Case-control study on colorectal cancer and diet in Marseilles, *Int. J. Cancer* **38**:183–191.

McGee, D., Reed, D., Stemmermann, G., Rhoads, G., Yano, K., and Feinleib, M., 1985, The relationship of dietary fat and cholesterol to mortality in 10 years: The Honolulu Heart Program, *Int. J. Epidemiol.* **14**:97–105.

Miller, A. B., Kelly, A., Choi, N. W., Matthews, V., Morgan, R. W., Munan, L., Burch, J. D., Feather, J., Howe, G. R., and Jain, M., 1978, A study of diet and breast cancer, *Am. J. Epidemiol.* **107**:499–509.

Nauss, K. M., Locniskar, M., and Newberne, P. M., 1983, Effect of alteration in the quality and quantity of dietary fat on 1,2-dimethyl-hydrazine-induced colon tumorigenesis in rats, *Cancer Res.* **43**:4083–4090.

Nauss, K. M., Locniskar, M., Sondergaard, D., and Newberne, P. M., 1984, Lack of effect of dietary fat on *N*-nitrosomethyl urea (NMU)-induced colon tumorigenesis in rats, *Carcinogenesis* **5**:255–260.

Nelson, R. L., Tanure, J. C., Andrianopoulos, G., Souza, G., and Lands, W. E. M., 1988, A comparison of dietary fish oil and corn oil in experimental colorectal carcinogenesis, *Nutr. Cancer* **11**:215–220.

Newberne, P. M., and Nauss, K. M., 1986, Dietary fat and colon cancer: Variable results in animal models, *Prog. Clin. Biol. Res.* **222**:311–330.

Nomura, A., Henderson, B. E., and Lee, J., 1978, Breast cancer and diet among the Japanese in Hawaii, *Am. J. Clin. Nutr.* **31**:2020–2025.

Nomura, A. M., Hirohata, T., Kolonel, L. N., Hankin, J. N., Lee, J., and Stemmermann, G., 1985, Breast cancer in Caucasian and Japanese women in Hawaii, *NCI Monogr.* **69**:191–196.

Phillips, R. L., 1975, Role of life-style and dietary habits in risk of cancer among Seventh Day Adventists, *Cancer Res.* **35**:3513–3522.

Phillips, R. L., and Snowdon, D. A., 1983, Association of meat and coffee use with cancers of the large bowel, breast and prostate among Seventh Day Adventists: Preliminary results, *Cancer Res.* **43**:2403S–2408S.

Potter, J. D., and McMichael, A. J., 1986, Diet and Cancer of the colon and rectum: A case–control study, *J. Natl. Cancer Inst.* **76**:557–569.

Reddy, B. S., 1975, Role of bile metabolites in colon carcinogenesis, *Cancer* **36**:2401–2406.

Roebuck, B. D., Yager, J. D., Jr., Longnecker, D. S., and Wilpone, S. A., 1981, Promotion by unsaturated fat of azaserine-induced pancreatic carcinogenesis in the rat, *Cancer Res.* **41**:3961–3966.

Rogers, A. E., and Longnecker, M. P., 1988, Biology of disease. Dietary and nutritional influences on cancer: A review of epidemiological and experimental data, *Lab. Invest.* **59**:729–759.

Rohan, T. E., McMichael, A. J., and Baghurst, P. A., 1988, A population based case–control study of diet and breast cancer in Australia, *Am. J. Epidemiol.* **128**:478–489.

Ross, R. K., Shimizu, H., Paganini-Hill, A., Honda, G., and Henderson, B. E., 1987, Case–control studies of prostate cancer in blacks and whites in Southern California, *J. Natl. Cancer Inst.* **78**:869–874.

Sarin, R., Tandon, R. K., Paul, S., Ghandi, B. M., Kapur, B. M., and Kapur, K., 1985, Diet in the epidemiology of breast cancer, *Indian J. Med. Res.* **81**:493–498.

Selenkas, S. L., Ip, M. M., and Ip, C., 1984, Similarity between *trans* fat and saturated fat in the modification of rat mammary carcinogenesis, *Cancer Res.* **44**:1321–1326.

Severson, R. K., Nomura, A. M. Y., Grove, J. S., and Stemmermann, G. N., 1989, A prospective study of demographics, diet and prostate cancer among men of Japanese ancestry in Hawaii, *Cancer Res.* **49:**1857–1860.

Stampfer, M. J., Willett, W. C., Colditz, G. A., Rosner, B., Hennekens, C., and Speizer, F. E., 1987, A prospective study of diet and colon cancer in a cohort of women, *Fed. Proc.* **46:**883 (Abstract).

Staszewski, J., 1971, Age at menarche and breast cancer. *J. Natl. Cancer Inst.* **47:**935–940.

Stemmermann, G. N., Nomura, A. M. Y., and Heilbrun, K. L. 1984, Dietary fat and the risk of colorectal cancer, *Cancer Res.* **44:**4633–4637.

Stocks, P., and Karn, M. K., 1933, A cooperative study of the habits, homelife, dietary and family histories of 450 cancer patients and an equal number of control patients, *Ann. Eugen. (London)* **5:**237–280.

Sugano, M., Watanabe, M., Yoshida, K., Tomioka, M., Mayamoto, M., and Kritchevsky, D., 1989, Influence of dietary cis and trans fats on DMH-induced colon tumors, steroid excretion and eicosanoid production in rats prone to colon cancer, *Nutr. Cancer* **12:**177–187.

Swanson, C. A., Jones, D. Y., Schatzkin, A., Brinton, L. A., and Ziegler, R. G., 1988, Breast cancer risk assessed by anthropometry in the NHANES I epidemiological follow-up study, *Cancer Res.* **48:**5363–5367.

Tannenbaum, A., 1940, The initiation and growth of tumors. I. Effects of underfeeding, *Am. J. Cancer* **38:**335–350.

Tannenbaum, A., 1942a, The genesis and growth of tumors. II. Effects of caloric restriction *per se, Cancer Res.* **2:**460–467.

Tannenbaum, A., 1942b, The genesis and growth of tumors, III. Effects of a high-fat diet. *Cancer Res.* **2:**468–475.

Tannenbaum, A., 1945, The dependence of tumor formation on the composition of the calorie restricted diet as well as on the degree of restriction, *Cancer Res.* **5:**616–625.

Toniolo, P., Riboli, E., Protta, F., Charrel, M., and Cappa, A. P. M., 1989, Calorie-providing nutrients and risk of breast cancer, *J. Natl. Cancer Inst.* **81:**278–286.

Tuyns, A. J., 1986, A case–control study on colorectal cancer in Belgium: Preliminary results, *Med. Sociale Prevent.* **31:**81–82.

Tuyns, A. J., Haelterman, M., and Kaaks, R., 1987, Colorectal cancer and the intake of nutrients: Oligosaccharides are a risk factor, fats are not. A case–control study in Belgium, *Nutr. Cancer* **10:**181–196.

Watanabe, M., Koga, T., and Sugano, M., 1985, Influence of dietary cis- and trans-fat on 1,2-dimethylhydrazine-induced colon tumors and fecal steroid excretion in Fischer 344 rats, *Am. J. Clin. Nutr.* **42:**475–484.

Watson, A. F., and Mellanby, E., 1930, Tar cancer in mice. II. The condition of the skin when modified by external treatment or diet, as a factor in influencing the cancerous reaction, *Br. J. Exp. Pathol.* **11:**311–322.

Willett, W. C., Stampfer, M. J., Colditz, G. A., Rosner, B. A., Hennekens, C. H., and Speizer, F. E., 1987, Dietary fat and the risk of breast cancer, *N. Engl. J. Med.* **316:**22–28.

7

Serum Cholesterol and Human Cancer

Anthony John McMichael

1. Introduction

In the early 1980s, substantial interest centered on a series of epidemiologic observations indicating that individuals with low concentrations of serum cholesterol were at increased risk of cancer. In view of mounting advice from cardiovascular disease epidemiologists that the mean concentration of serum cholesterol within the community should be lowered, as an important means of primary and secondary prevention of coronary heart disease (Grundy *et al.*, 1982; World Health Organization, 1985), these cancer-related observations posed a potentially serious public health dilemma (Feinleib, 1982; McMichael *et al.*, 1984).

Detailed review of the available data, however, made clear that the apparent increase in cancer risk was essentially confined to individuals who, in observational (i.e., nonintervention) studies, had preexisting low serum cholesterol. With just one exception, experimental studies of the effect on risk of cardiovascular disease of deliberately lowered serum cholesterol revealed no associated change in cancer risk. Nevertheless, this latter category of study, carried out in predominantly older-age adults, cannot entirely dispel the possibility of an altered risk of cancer as a function of lifelong lowering of serum cholesterol in response to currently emerging public health policies.

An additional important element in the scientific debate has been the biological interpretation of the epidemiologic observations. Does a low concentration of serum cholesterol predispose to cancer? Or does the preclinical phase of carcinogenesis entail metabolic changes that cause a lowering of serum cholesterol? In relation to the latter possibility, it is of interest to note that in 1930 Muller reported that patients with leukemia commonly had hypocholesterolemia (Muller, 1930). Since then, several studies in patients with different newly diagnosed malignancies have shown an increased frequency of hypocholesterolemia unrelated to nutritional status (Bases and Krakoff, 1965; Nydegger and Butler, 1972).

Anthony John McMichael • Department of Community Medicine, University of Adelaide, Adelaide, South Australia 5000.

On current evidence, the more likely interpretation is that hypocholesterolemia is a consequence of, rather than a contributor to, carcinogenesis (McMichael *et al.*, 1984). However, these two alternatives are not mutually exclusive. Nor, in view of the biological heterogeneity of the many types of human cancer, does a general interpretation necessarily apply to all cancer types.

Before reviewing the evidence in detail, it is appropriate to summarize briefly what is known about the relationship between dietary cholesterol and fats and serum cholesterol.

1.1. Dietary Fat and Serum Cholesterol

Most of the cholesterol in blood, incorporated into the various lipoprotein fractions, derives from endogenous synthesis (predominantly in the liver). Some derives directly from the enteric absorption of dietary cholesterol, and the serum cholesterol level may be indirectly affected by cholesterol from this source (Nestel, 1989). However, the major dietary influence on serum cholesterol is that of dietary saturated fat intake—either in absolute terms or, more probably, relative to polyunsaturated fat intake. Indeed, the ratio of polyunsaturated fats to saturated fats (i.e., the P/S ratio) is the most consistently observed dietary influence on serum cholesterol concentration, and equations have been derived showing that saturated fatty acids are twice as effective in raising the serum cholesterol as are polyunsaturated fats in lowering it (Keys *et al.*, 1965).

These dietary fat parameters influence the endogenous synthesis of cholesterol. The endogenous synthesis and metabolism of cholesterol are also influenced by genetic factors, and by a variety of other "exogenous factors," including physical activity, alcohol consumption, administered sex steroid hormones (especially the oral contraceptive pill), and various other aspects of diet, such as dietary fiber and, perhaps, coffee consumption.

Thus, the relationship of dietary fat to serum cholesterol is neither simple nor constant. Nevertheless, despite the myriad influences on serum cholesterol and despite considerable interindividual variability in response to altered dietary fat intake, there is clear evidence from controlled trials and intervention studies in human populations that a reduction in dietary saturated fat intake (with or without an increase in polyunsaturated fat intake) will, on average, lower the serum cholesterol concentration (NIH Consensus Conference, 1985).

In examining the relationship of serum cholesterol to cancer risk it is therefore necessary to bear in mind that dietary fat, as partial determinant of plasma cholesterol, may be exerting other independent, potentially confounding, effects on the risk of cancer.

2. Serum Cholesterol and Cancer: Epidemiologic Data

2.1. Descriptive Studies

Descriptive studies show a strong correlation between the mean concentration of serum cholesterol in populations and their death rates from coronary heart disease (Keys, 1980). Since coronary heart disease is correlated with colon cancer mortality (Rose *et al.*, 1974), colon cancer and serum cholesterol are necessarily correlated at the population level. Seventh Day Adventists (Walden *et al.*, 1964) and Mormons (Enstrom, 1980) in California have serum cholesterol levels lower than those of the general U.S. population, and both groups have mortality rates for all combined cancers and colon cancer below that of the general U.S. population (Phillips, 1975; Lyon *et al.,* 1977). However, while population-based descriptive studies can suggest, they cannot confirm, causal relationships. Indeed, the correlated variables may not concur at the level of the individual.

2.2. Analytic Studies

Analytic epidemiologic studies entail the collection of data from or about sets of individuals—i.e., the data are individual-based, in contrast to measures made on groups or whole populations. Data are available from both experimental and observational analytic studies to examine the relationship of serum cholesterol to cancer risk. The experimental studies have investigated changes in cancer risk resulting from deliberate dietary or pharmacologic lowering of serum cholesterol levels. The observational studies have assessed the risk of cancer in individuals in relationship to their naturally occurring levels of serum cholesterol.

2.2.1. Experimental Studies

Seven experimental human studies have been reported in which the effect of lowering serum cholesterol by dietary or drug intervention on subsequent cancer risk has, in retrospect, been assessed. Each study was originally designed to assess the effect of the intervention upon risk of coronary heart disease (CHD).

2.2.1a. Dietary Lowering of Serum Cholesterol. The first report of an inverse relationship between serum cholesterol and cancer risk was from an 8-year CHD prevention trial on 846 men at the Veterans Administration Hospital, Los Angeles (Pearce and Dayton, 1971). A 12.7% difference in mean serum cholesterol was achieved between the two randomly allocated dietary groups. Although fatal CHD events were more common in controls (70 vs. 48 deaths, $p < 0.05$), a marked increase of fatal cancers occurred in the low-cholesterol group (31 vs. 17 deaths, $p = 0.06$). However, among the minority of subjects who closely adhered to their allocated diet, six (6.1%) of the cholesterol-lowering group and seven (5.5%) of the control group died from cancer.

Ederer *et al.* (1971) analyzed data from five dietary trials of CHD prevention performed during the 1960s, comprising the above-mentioned Los Angeles Veterans Trial, three other studies that had used randomization of individuals (in Oslo, London, and Minnesota), and the Finnish Mental Hospital Study referred to below. The pooled data from the four studies excluding the Los Angeles Veterans Trial indicated that the relative risks of cancer incidence and mortality were lower (0.75 and 0.62, respectively) in the serum-cholesterol-lowering diet group than in the control group, although this reduction was not statistically significant.

In a subsequent report of the Finnish Mental Hospital Study, in which 4000 institutionalized men had been followed for 12 years by means of a crossover design, the patients on a cholesterol-lowering diet achieved a 15% decrease in serum cholesterol relative to those on the control diet (Turpeinen, 1979). The total mortality rate was lower in the cholesterol-lowering diet group; however, there were no appreciable differences in the cancer mortality rates between the treatment and control groups.

2.2.1b. Pharmacologic Lowering of Serum Cholesterol. The Coronary Drug Project Research Group (1975) reported a CHD prevention trial of cholesterol lowering by drug therapy in men aged 30–64 years with a history of proven myocardial infarction. Groups that received niacin or clofibrate experienced significant lowering of serum cholesterol in comparison with the control group. Although case numbers were small, cancer mortality was not significantly different among the niacin (0.8%), clofibrate (0.9%), and placebo (0.9%) groups during an average of 6.2 years of treatment.

In a trial of primary prevention of CHD by clofibrate, based in three European centers (Edinburgh, Budapest, and Prague), three groups of approximately 5000 men aged 30–59 years at entry and free of manifest heart or other major disease were studied (Committee of Principal Investigators, 1978, 1980). After 9.6 years of follow-up, the total mortality rate was significantly higher in the clofibrate group than in either the high- or low-cholesterol control groups. However, no single cause of mortality, including cancer, accounted for this increase. Detailed data analysis not only suggested an increased overall hazard of mortality associated with use of clofibrate as a cholesterol-lowering agent, but also indicated that within the clofibrate group low serum cholesterol levels *per se* were not associated with an increased risk of total or cancer mortality. Further, the low-cholesterol control group demonstrated lower age-adjusted total mortality rates and virtually identical cancer mortality rates in comparison with the high-cholesterol control group.

Overall, of the various reports on dietary and drug trials of lowering serum cholesterol, only one (the Los Angeles Veterans Trial) indicated an increased cancer risk associated with the lowering of serum cholesterol *per se*. However, in that study, since the nonadhering subgroups within the two randomized groups (who, therefore, differed least in their subsequent diets) showed the greatest difference in cancer risk, interpretation is difficult.

2.2.2. Observational Studies

Most of the observational data relating serum cholesterol concentrations to subsequent cancer occurrence come from long-term prospective cohort studies in which cardiovascular disease was the outcome of primary interest. Therefore, while cancer mortality was usually well recorded, cancer morbidity often was not. For similar reasons, some confounding factors for cancer risk were often not measured; nevertheless, factors such as age, smoking, alcohol consumption, relative weight, and some index of social class were usually measured, and multivariate adjustment for these factors consistently made little difference to the results of the study.

In the published reports of 13 separate cohort studies (11 of which were originally designed to study the etiology, and one the preventability, of cardiovascular disease), an inverse relationship between serum cholesterol, as measured at entry into the study, and cancer is evident. Those studies, together with five case–control studies, and a study of colon cancer recurrence rates, each of which found an inverse relationship with serum cholesterol, are described below. The pooled data analysis of 11 individual studies conducted by the International Collaborative Group and an updated analysis of the Seven Countries Study are also presented. Subsequently, the seven cohort studies and three case–control studies in which no inverse relationship between serum cholesterol and cancer risk was found are considered, along with one cohort study that found serum cholesterol to be positively related to colon and rectal cancers.

2.2.2a. Studies Showing an Inverse Relationship to Cancer Risk. An early stimulus to epidemiologic research into the relationship between serum cholesterol and cancer came from the report of Rose *et al.* (1974). Those authors pooled the results of six cohort studies of coronary heart disease in men: the Seven Countries Study, the Framingham Study, the Chicago Gas Company Study, the London Whitehall Study, the Minnesota Businessmen Study, and the Western Electric Company Study. They found that the 90 subjects who had thus far died from colon cancer during these studies had mean serum cholesterol concentrations, measured at entry, about 5–7 mg/100 ml below the expected value ($p < 0.05$). Furthermore, this deviation was of similar size in those who died within 4 years of screening and in those who died later, suggesting that the presence of preclinical cancer at the time of entry into the study, with its possible metabolic consequences, did not explain the lowered serum cholesterol levels. (The proposition that the metabolic consequences of preexisting, undetected, cancer may be the cause of low serum cholesterol in those individuals at the time of their entry into the study is referred to, in the ensuing text, as the "preclinical cancer effect.")

Rose and Shipley (1980) reviewed the (updated) London Whitehall Study, one of the six cohort studies included in the above-mentioned report by Rose *et al.* (1974). Cancer mortality was 66% higher in those with the lowest serum cholesterol levels than in those with the highest levels. Site-specific analyses demonstrated an association between low serum cholesterol and cancers of the lung (143 deaths), stomach (35 deaths), and colon (28 deaths). The inverse relationship between serum cholesterol and cancer mortality was most evident during the first 1–2 years of follow-up. The authors concluded that this was probably a reflection of the preclinical cancer effect, wherein cancer caused low serum cholesterol rather than that low cholesterol contributed to cancer.

In the Paris Prospective Study of Coronary Heart Disease (Cambien *et al.*, 1980), 7603 French male government employees aged 43–52 years were followed for an average of 6.6 years. The mean serum cholesterol at entry was statistically significantly lower in the 134 persons who subsequently died of cancer than in the survivors. Among the cancer cases, the relative deficit in serum cholesterol was inversely related to time lapsed since entering the study ($p < 0.02$); initial mean serum cholesterol in cancer cases who died at least 7 years after entry into the study was not lower than that in the survivors. Furthermore, in those individuals who subsequently died from cancer and had also had serial cholesterol measurements, a mean decrease of 5 mg/100 ml in serum cholesterol occurred after an average of 3 years of follow-up. These findings are consistent with a preclinical cancer effect.

Analysis of the Framingham Study data (Williams *et al.*, 1981) with up to 24 years follow-up of 2336 men and 2873 women aged 35–64 years demonstrated, in men, a significant inverse association of the initial serum cholesterol levels with the incidence of cancer overall, and of colon cancer and of cancer of all sites other than colon. No such relationship was found in women. This inverse relationship was not attributable to the preclinical cancer effect since, first, of the 88 cases of colon cancer detected during follow-up, only five occurred during the first 4 years of follow-up, and, second, the excess overall cancer risk among those with initially low serum cholesterol was cumulative throughout the entire follow-up period.

A further analysis of the Framingham data (Sorlie and Feinleib, 1982) examined time trends in these cholesterol–cancer relationships across the succession of biennial follow-up examinations. The authors said of those cancer cases in which the serum cholesterol level was lower than expected as long as 16–18 years before cancer diagnosis: "most oncologists would be reluctant to accept that a metabolically active lesion would remain preclinical for 10 or more years." However, in some of these cancer cases serum cholesterol was reported to have progressively decreased at measurements made increasingly close to the time of cancer diagnosis.

An updated analysis of serum cholesterol and mortality in the Framingham cohort at 30 years of follow-up (Anderson *et al.,* 1987) showed an apparent weakening of the above-mentioned inverse relationship with cancer incidence. Curiously, there was now no tendency for those individuals (approximately one-sixth of the cohort) with a declining serum cholesterol over the follow-up period to be at above-average risk of cancer.

In the Honolulu Heart Study (Kagan *et al.,* 1981), 8006 Japanese–American men aged 45–68 years were followed for 9 years. Serum cholesterol level at entry was inversely related to total cancer mortality and to mortality from cancers of the esophagus, colon, liver, and lung and from malignancies of the lymphatic and hematopoietic systems. When deaths in the first 2 years of follow-up and cases of cancer present at intake were eliminated from the calculations, the inverse relationship persisted only for total cancers and cancers of the colon and lung.

Stemmermann *et al.* (1981), in a subsequent 5-year extension of the Honolulu Heart Study, found that the incidence of colon cancer was inversely associated with serum cholesterol measured at entry, and that this association was strongest for cancers of the cecum and ascending colon. The authors inferred from the lack of such an association with other site-specific cancer incidence (particularly stomach and lung) that the inverse association with cancer mortality reported earlier in the follow-up (Kagan *et al.,* 1981) may have reflected the preclinical cancer effect. However, for colon cancer, the inverse association persisted in cases diagnosed 5–9 years after entry, although not in those diagnosed 10–14 years after intake. Furthermore, the inverse association was independent of the clinical stage of colon cancer.

During 1970–1972, a sample of 2122 men from the abovementioned Honolulu Heart Study cohort of 8006 men of Japanese ancestry was selected for detailed blood lipid analysis (Reed *et al.,* 1986). Ten-year follow-up revealed no clear association of total cancer incidence with total serum cholesterol or with any other lipid or lipoprotein fraction. Cancer risk appeared to decrease with increasing concentration of high-density lipoprotein, but this was not statistically significant.

In an 8-year follow-up study in Puerto Rico of 9824 men aged 45–64 years, Garcia-Palmieri *et al.* (1981) found that serum cholesterol at entry was inversely related to total cancer mortality in those living in rural areas. Mortality was particularly increased in men with initial serum cholesterol levels less than 165 mg/100 ml. Furthermore, actuarial adjustment for any competing risk effect of cardiovascular disease mortality, as a function of serum cholesterol, did not eliminate this relationship. Initial serum cholesterol did not vary with proximity of time of cancer death to commencement of follow-up. No data were presented for specific cancer in relation to serum cholesterol.

In a much smaller cohort study of 630 male and female New Zealand Maoris aged 25–74 years, followed for 17 years, Salmond *et al.* (1985) reported that individuals with initially low serum cholesterol experienced increased death rates from all causes (women, but not men), from cancer (men and women combined), and from other noncardiovascular causes (both men and women). This inverse relationship with cancer mortality persisted when deaths within 2 years of intake were excluded.

In a 13-year follow-up study of 3102 males and females aged 15–74 years in Evans County, Georgia, the mean serum cholesterol level, measured at entry, in 166 individuals who subsequently developed cancer was 6.7 mg/100 ml lower than that in age- and sex-matched controls (Kark *et al.*, 1980). Serum cholesterol was 8 mg/100 ml lower in the "incident" group of 127 cancer cases, defined as those cancer cases diagnosed at least 1 year after the beginning of the study. This statistically significant inverse relationship was evident in both the earlier and later periods of follow-up, but only in men. Cancers of the colon, uterus, liver, skin (squamous cell), and prostate were associated with the lowest mean cholesterol levels; pancreas, ovary, and basal cell cancers were associated with increases in mean cholesterol level.

Because of the possibility of positive confounding between low serum cholesterol and low serum vitamin A, the latter factor was also examined, since retinol and carotenoids have been thought to be inversely associated with carcinoma risk (Peto *et al.*, 1981). Serum cholesterol and vitamin A (retinol) concentrations were strongly positively correlated in this population, and retinol levels were lower in cancer cases than in controls (Kark *et al.*, 1982). Independent data (Smith and Hoggard, 1981) from healthy adults have shown a statistically significant correlation between serum low-density-lipoprotein cholesterol and both serum retinol and β-carotene.

A 7-year follow-up study of 11,121 men aged 35–62 years in Yugoslavia (Kozarevic *et al.*, 1981) revealed an inverse relationship between initial serum cholesterol and total mortality. This relationship was statistically significant after multivariate confounder adjustment. While the inverse relationship of total cancer mortality to serum cholesterol was not statistically significant, that of colorectal cancer was (although the relevant data were not tabulated).

Preliminary data (mean follow-up of 2.5 years) from a prospective study of 10,000 men, initially aged 47–50 years, in Malmo, Sweden, showed an inverse relationship between serum cholesterol and cancer mortality (Peterson *et al.*, 1981). However, the short period of follow-up precludes discounting of the preclinical cancer effect.

The relation between serum cholesterol and cancer incidence was studied in the population of the Hypertension Detection and Follow-up Program (HDFP), in the United States (Morris *et al.*, 1983). In this multicenter trial, over 10,940 hypertensive participants, aged 30–69 years, and including blacks and whites of both sexes, were followed for five years. During follow-up, 286 new cancer cases were recorded. Within the four baseline serum cholesterol quartiles, age-adjusted cancer incidence rates showed a small, but statistically significant, inverse relationship with serum cholesterol. Multivariate analysis indicated that this relationship was not due to confounding by other known cancer risk factors. Nor was there evidence that it was attributable to a hypocholesterolemic effect of preclinical cancer: first, the inverse relationship was as strong in the latter three years of follow-up as in the first two years, and, second, there was no obvious correlation between baseline serum cholesterol and time from entry until cancer diagnosis. Where the numbers permitted, specific cancer sites were examined and the inverse relation was present for each site, except for breast cancer in women.

In a cohort comprising 16,711 members of the Northern California Kaiser Foundation Health Plan who had previously taken a multiphasic health examination, up to 16 years earlier, 7774 persons subsequently developed cancer (Hiatt *et al.*, 1983). The age-adjusted cancer incidence was the highest in the lowest quintile of cholesterol level

(< 185 mg/100 ml) for all cancer in men and women, for lung and stomach cancer in men, and for breast, lung, cervical, and ovarian cancer in women. The pattern of the incidence of other cancers by quintile of cholesterol level was erratic.

The National Health and Nutrition Examination Survey (NHANES I) was conducted during 1971–1975 on a probability sample of the civilian non-institutionalized population of the United States, and included measurement of serum cholesterol. Formal follow-up was carried out during 1981–1984, and included identification of cancer deaths and cancer hospitalizations (Schatzkin *et al.*, 1987). During this 10-year follow-up period, the 5125 men yielded 459 incident cancers and 258 cancer deaths, and the 7363 women yielded 389 incident cancers and 186 cancer deaths. In multivariate analysis adjusting for seven other cancer risk factors, men in the lowest serum cholesterol quintile had nearly double the cancer risk of those in the highest quintile, both for cancer incidence and mortality; the relationships were in the same direction but were much weaker for women. When the analysis of cancer incidence was stratified according to three intervals of follow-up (less than 2 years, 2–6 years, and 6-plus years) the inverse relationship was strongest in the third interval for men and in the first interval for women.

As a prelude to the Multiple Risk Factor Intervention Trial (MRFIT) in the United States 361,662 men aged 35–57 years were screened during 1973–1975. A subset of 12,866 of these men, all with high serum cholesterol, were subsequently entered into the trial. Mortality follow-up was carried out on the original large cohort of screenees (Sherwin *et al.*, 1987); during the seven-year follow-up 2,989 men were identified as having died from cancer. There was a statistically significant 40% excess of cancer mortality in the lowest decile of serum cholesterol (< 4.34 mmol/l) compared to the other nine deciles; cancer mortality in the three lowest deciles was 20% higher than in the other seven deciles. This general pattern was evident for several specific major cancer sites: lung, colon, stomach, and lymphohematopoietic. The overall cancer excess became attenuated over time of follow-up, being greatest for cancers occurring within 2 years of serum cholesterol screening, intermediate for cancers within 2–3 years, and least for cancers occurring after 4–7 years. Nevertheless, the risk in the lowest decile remained 20–30% higher than for the other nine deciles over this third, latest, stage of follow-up. No such change occurred in the positive association between high serum cholesterol and coronary heart disease. Among the trial participants, in whom annual measurements of serum cholesterol were made, 150 cancer deaths occurred. Serum cholesterol fell substantially more (0.59 mmol/l) in those 150 men than in the survivors over an equivalent period; this differential was clearly evident only in the 2 years immediately preceding cancer death.

In a different type of prospective study, colon cancer recurrence rates were examined in 279 surgically treated colon cancer patients in New York in relation to serum cholesterol concentration at initial treatment (Tartter *et al.*, 1984). The 141 patients with concentrations at or below the median had an 11% higher 5-year recurrence rate than did the 138 patients with concentrations above the median. For neither sex was this difference in recurrence rate statistically significant, although it approached significance ($p = 0.10$) for both sexes combined.

Three case-control studies have specifically examined the relationship between colon cancer and serum cholesterol.

In a matched case–control study of 133 patients in hospitalized Caucasian patients in

New York, Miller *et al.* (1981) found that, overall, the patients with colon cancer had serum cholesterol concentrations lower than those of the control subjects. When the comparison was stratified by tumor stage, statistically significant differences in serum cholesterol levels existed between cases with advanced tumors and their controls but not between early-stage cases and controls (although the same trend was noted).

Preliminary results from another case–control study of 76 colon cancer patients and 76 sex- and age-matched controls (all of whom had previously participated in annual cancer screening) show that serum cholesterol levels in cases had been consistently lower than in controls as far back as five or more years before cancer detection (Buchalter *et al.*, 1983). Furthermore, this difference increased nearer to the time of cancer diagnosis. The authors concluded that a low serum cholesterol may therefore be both a precursor and, subsequently, a metabolic response to colon cancer.

In a case–control study in New York (Neugut *et al.*, 1986), data on serum cholesterol measurements at admission were collected from 244 patients with adenomatous polyps of the colon, 182 patients with colon cancer, and 688 hospital controls with diseases thought to be unrelated to serum cholesterol and requiring elective surgery. The mean serum cholesterol concentrations were lower for patients with cancer (207.2 mg/dl) than for controls (219.5 mg/dl, $p < 0.003$), with patients with later-stage cancer accounting for most of the difference. Patients with adenomatous polyps had a mean serum cholesterol concentration similar to controls. After adjustments for nutritional status using the serum albumin level, there were no statistically significant differences among any of the groups. This study suggests that the low serum cholesterol level associated with malignancies, and colon cancer in particular, is a consequence rather than a cause of the cancer.

Two other case–control studies have examined cancer in general in relation to serum cholesterol. Both have paid particular attention to the interval between diagnosis and antecedent blood sampling.

Within a cardiovascular risk factor screening program in rural Iowa, 131 cancer cases occurred during six years of surveillance (Wallace *et al.*, 1982). Each case was matched with a cancer-free control. Antecedent plasma cholesterol levels were approximately 5 percent lower in male cases and 5 percent higher in female cases than in controls; these differences were not statistically significant. However, in males, the lower cholesterol levels occurred only in those with cancer developing within 2 years of screening. In younger women, a statistically significant positive association of plasma cholesterol was observed with cancers of the breast, endometrium, and ovary. Unfortunately, no analysis of both plasma cholesterol concentration and relative weight as covariates was carried out; such an analysis would help interpret the lipid profiles as part of a metabolic response to preclinical cancer.

A subsequent case–control study, reported from Stockholm (Gerhardsson *et al.*, 1986), sought explicitly to clarify whether low serum cholesterol concentrations occur prior to the onset of a malignancy or are an early metabolic effect of the malignancy. From a clinically registered population of 18,995 people (55% men and 45% women), 176 cases of cancer death were identified. A control group of 900 surviving subjects was randomly selected. Medical records, including results of repeated blood lipid determinations from up to 16 years earlier, were available for 100 cases and 393 controls. A statistically significant inverse association between serum cholesterol and cancer death was observed (particularly for cancers of the colon and rectum) for serum cholesterol measured within 6 years of death, but not for serum cholesterol measurements taken 7–16 years prior to death. Multivariate adjustment for potential confounders did not alter these findings. After excluding possible sources of bias, the authors concluded that low serum cholesterol concentrations were apparently a consequence of the preclinical stage of cancer.

Finally, there have been two reports from multicenter studies. The International Collaborative Group (1982) has analyzed the pooled data from 11 of their 15 independent prospective studies of cardiovascular disease. Five of the eleven studies have been discussed separately in this chapter, and they account for 975 of the total 1484 cancer deaths in the pooled data and 89 of the 105 colon cancer deaths. The International Collaborative Group found, among 61,567 men aged 40–69 years, followed for 5–10 years, that those dying of cancer within 1 year of cholesterol determination had mean cholesterol levels 24–35 mg/100 ml lower than the study population average. For follow-up during years 2–5 and 6–10, the inverse association diminished markedly, with differences in mean cholesterol levels of only 4–5 mg/100 ml and 2 mg/100ml, respectively. Both lung cancer and colon cancer mortality were inversely associated with cholesterol level in the first year after entry into follow-up, but not in later follow-up; the authors therefore attributed the findings to the preclinical cancer effect. However, it should be noted that while these pooled international data reveal no inverse association of serum cholesterol with colon cancer death in extended follow-up, the number of such deaths (105 deaths) is less than the combined number of 168 colon cancer cases in those two previously mentioned individual studies—in Honolulu and Framingham—in which an extended inverse association was observed.

In the Seven Countries Study, carried out in Finland, Greece, Italy, Japan, the Netherlands, the United States, and Yugoslavia, among 11,325 "healthy" men aged 40–59 years, there were 594 cancer deaths in 15 years of follow-up (Keys *et al.*, 1985). Among 477 cancer deaths occurring at least 5 years after serum cholesterol measurement, there was a significant excess of lung cancer deaths in the lowest 20% of the cholesterol distributions in the populations. Age, blood pressure, smoking habits, occupation, and relative body weight did not help explain this. Other cancer types did not display this inverse relationship. Trend analysis with various cutting points indicated an increasing risk of lung cancer death at cholesterol levels under 170 mg/dl. The 45 men who died from cancer in the first 2 years of follow-up had lower serum cholesterol levels than their compatriots who died from cancer later, but they did not differ in relative weight or fatness. The authors concluded that there is no evidence that any of the observed cancer–serum cholesterol relationships involve an effect of serum cholesterol concentration on carcinogenesis or cancer mortality.

2.2.2b. Studies Not Showing an Inverse Relationship to Cancer Risk. Westlund and Nicolaysen (1972) reported on the 10-year mortality and morbidity of 3751 Norwegian male workers aged 40–49 years. The serum cholesterol levels, measured at entry, of the 89 men who subsequently developed cancer did not differ from those of the remainder. However, very few men within the study population had low initial serum cholesterol concentrations; the study population mean was 271 mg/100 ml.

Dyer *et al.* (1981) examined data from three prospective studies of cardiovascular disease in the United States. Serum cholesterol at entry into the study was examined in relationship to death from cancer and from other noncardiovascular causes for 10,022 white men aged 40–64 years, followed for up to 18 years. In none of the three studies was there a significant association between initial serum cholesterol level and subsequent mortality from total cancer. When cancer deaths were examined by site, serum cholesterol level was not statistically significantly related to lung cancer, colorectal cancer, oral cancer, pancreatic cancer, or to all other cancers combined in any of the three studies, either in men or in women. There was, however, a positive association with breast cancer in women.

In 10,059 adult male civil servants and municipal employees aged 40–65 years and followed for 7 years in the Israel Ischaemic Heart Disease Study (Yaari *et al.*, 1981), an inverse relationship was found between levels of serum cholesterol concentrations measured at entry and total mortality. This association disappeared with multivariate confounder adjustment. No clear-cut association was demonstrated between either total serum cholesterol or high-density-lipoprotein cholesterol and cancer mortality.

Thomas *et al.* (1982) followed 1018 men aged 18–37 years from the time they entered medical school for 20–33 years. The 30 who subsequently developed cancer had not had low initial serum cholesterol levels. Indeed, the number of cancer cases among the 20% of men with the highest cholesterol levels was twice that expected. The four subjects who developed cancer less than 5 years after entering the study had the lowest initial cholesterol levels; this is consistent with a preclinical cancer effect.

Within a cohort of 95,179 women, who underwent a multiphasic health check-up and were then followed for an average of 9 years, the initial concentration of serum cholesterol was found to be unrelated to breast cancer incidence, both in univariate analysis and after multivariate confounder adjustment (Hiatt *et al.*, 1982).

Salonen (1982) reported results from the North Karelia project in eastern Finland. Random samples of the population aged 25–59 years (3745 men and 4221 women) were followed, and hospitalizations or deaths were recorded for the period between 8 months and 7 years after entry. There was no relationship between serum cholesterol at entry and subsequent development of cancer. Associations with individual sites were not examined, and it was not possible to examine the risk of very low serum cholesterol in this population, since only 3% had values of less than 180 mg/100 ml.

The relationship between plasma cholesterol concentration and 7-year cancer morbidity and mortality was assessed in a community of 4035 Californians aged 40–89 years (Wingard *et al.*, 1984). The age-adjusted cancer mortality rate showed a slightly U-shaped relationship with cholesterol levels in men. For women, little association was seen between cancer mortality and cholesterol levels. Age-adjusted cancer morbidity rates indicated no association with cholesterol for men or women. Mean cholesterol levels did not differ significantly by major cancer site (large bowel, lung, prostate, breast, uterus, cervix). In addition, analysis of cholesterol levels by length of time between cholesterol measurement and cancer occurrence showed no significant trends, suggesting the progression of subclinical cancer did not result in lower cholesterol levels.

Malarkey *et al.* (1977), in a small case–control study of women with benign and with malignant breast disease, found no difference in initial serum cholesterol concentrations between the breast cancer cases and the control women. A case–control study of primary brain cancers in Israel (Abramson and Kark, 1985) found that the 37 cases had, at the time of hospitalization, serum cholesterol concentrations that were approximately 15% higher than in the 74 matched hospital controls ($p < 0.025$).

A case–control study of the relationship of serum cholesterol concentration to colo-

rectal cancer incidence was performed for 245 cancer patients within the Kaiser Perma-
nente Medical Care Program in northern California, each with five cancer-free controls
matched for age, sex, race, and time of examination (Sidney *et al.,* 1986). The mean
serum cholesterol concentrations of cases were not significantly different from those of
controls for all colorectal cancers, proximal colon cancers, and distal colon cancers.
Analysis by quartiles of serum cholesterol suggested no relationship between serum
cholesterol and large bowel cancer, and there was no evidence of a threshold value below
which the risk of cancer increased.

The risk of colorectal cancer was studied in relation to serum cholesterol in a cohort
of 92,000 participants in a health screening program in Sweden (Tornberg *et al.*, 1986).
The cohort, aged 17–74 at intake during 1963–1965, comprised approximately equal
numbers of men and women. During follow-up via the Swedish Cancer Registry to 1979,
528 colon cancers and 311 rectal cancers developed. A positive association was observed
between serum cholesterol and rectal cancer in men, with a relative risk of 1.6 in men and
1.4 in women with levels over 6.5 mmol/l. Only small increases in colon cancer risk
occurred.

3. Discussion

3.1. Summary of Research Findings

Among the published observational studies indicating an inverse relationship between initial serum cholesterol and cancer, there have been reports of 12 large populations
followed for at least 5 years. Four of them (the Framingham, Evans County, Hypertension
Detection and Follow-up Program, and NHANES cohorts, each of which investigated
cancer incidence in men and women) demonstrate an inverse relationship between total
cancer risk and initial serum cholesterol that cannot readily be attributed to a preclinical
cancer effect. In each of these studies, the relationship was present in men only. This
relationship was clearly evident for colon cancer in the first two of these cohorts; data
were not presented for colon cancer in the other two cohort studies.

In the reports of seven other of these 12 studies, only male subjects were included. In
two such studies [Honolulu (incidence and mortality) and Yugoslavia (mortality)], an
inverse relationship with colon cancer is evident which cannot readily be explained by a
preclinical cancer effect; however, the inverse relationship with total cancer in those two
studies may largely reflect such preclinical effect (Honolulu) or is not presented very
clearly (Yugoslavia). In the Seven Countries Study an inverse relationship was evident for
lung cancer, but not for other types of cancer; overall, cancer deaths in the first 2 years of
follow-up were associated with lower serum cholesterol concentrations than were subsequent cancer deaths. In the Puerto Rican Study, the inverse relationship is evident for total
cancer mortality, after multivariate adjustment, and is not obviously attributable to a
preclinical cancer effect; site-specific data are not available. In each of the other three
studies (Whitehall, Paris, and MRFIT), the data indicate that a preclinical cancer effect
accounts largely or wholly for the apparent inverse relationship between initial serum
cholesterol and cancer risk.

The prospective data from the New Zealand and Maori Study and the Malmo Study
are insufficient to allow firm inferences. Three case–control studies of cancer and serum

cholesterol, two being confined to colon cancer while the other included all cancers, clearly support the preclinical cancer effect proposition. The follow-up study of colon cancer 5-year recurrence rate in surgically treated colon cancer patients showed a weak inverse relationship with initial serum cholesterol.

Nine published prospective studies in Norway, Israel, Finland, and the United States show no apparent relationship between serum cholesterol and total cancer risk. Three case–control studies (of breast cancer, brain cancer, and colorectal cancer, respectively) have shown no inverse relationship of cancer risk with serum cholesterol concentration. One large cohort study showed a positive association between serum cholesterol and cancers of the colon and rectum; this relationship was similar in men and women, albeit stronger in men.

3.2. Possible Biological Explanations

Several biological mechanisms have been proposed to account for an inverse relationship between serum cholesterol and cancer.

Low serum cholesterol may enhance carcinogenesis by means of cholesterol effects on cell membranes (Oliver, 1981). However, Marenah *et al.* (1983), in a study of 150 healthy adult males, have shown that cell membrane fluidity and lipid composition are unrelated to serum cholesterol. Furthermore, altered cell membrane fluidity *in vitro* occurred only at serum cholesterol levels well below the first percentile.

A second proposition is that an individual's innate (i.e., genetically determined) lipoprotein cholesterol profile is merely statistically associated with his/her predisposition to develop cancer, since both are expressions of some underlying shared (presumably genetic) factor. The observed cholesterol–cancer correlation is therefore not causal. Data from a cross-sectional study of 851 subjects in Cincinnati showed that, in general, low-density-lipoprotein (LDL) cholesterol was negatively correlated with a parental history of cancer (Laskarzewski *et al.*, 1982), leading the authors to conclude that the oft-reported familial aggregation of cancer risk may involve a shared lipoprotein cholesterol profile. The heritability of total and high-density-lipoprotein cholesterol has been estimated to be 50% and 37%, respectively (Dahlen *et al.*, 1983). Katan (1986) has stressed the distinction between apolipoprotein phenotype (predominantly determined by genotype) and serum cholesterol phenotype (partly determined by genotype) as one approach to elucidating the cholesterol–cancer relationship.

A third explanation has been proposed by Vitols *et al.* (1985), who studied 59 patients with acute leukemia to see if the hypocholesterolemia that commonly accompanies this malignancy is associated with a high activity of LDL receptors in leukemic cells. LDL-receptor activity (measured as the rate of *in vitro* degradation of radio labeled LDL by a sample of each patient's blood) was found to be inversely correlated with serum cholesterol concentration. During chemotherapy, cholesterol concentrations rose concomitantly with the disappearance of leukemic cells from the peripheral blood. Further, the authors calculated that the leukemic cells in peripheral blood would degrade and metabolize about 35% of the daily input of LDL into the blood. They therefore concluded that the high receptor-mediated uptake of LDL cholesterol by leukemic cells causes hypocholesterolemia in patients with acute leukemia. This interpretation represents a specific example of a malignancy causing a low serum cholesterol concentration, as has now been widely postulated to occur more generally as the posited "preclinical cancer effect," whereby occult cancer somehow depresses serum cholesterol concentration.

The repeated, albeit inconsistent, finding from various of these studies that a low concentration of serum cholesterol is associated with an increased risk of cancer of the colon in men warrants special consideration. The findings from the three cohort studies that presented data by serum cholesterol subrange—i.e., Framingham (Williams *et al.,* 1981), Honolulu (Stemmermann *et al.,* 1981), and Hiroshima–Nagasaki (Feinleib, 1982)—suggest a threshold effect, with increased risk consistently confined below a naturally occurring blood cholesterol of approximately 185 mg/100 ml. This is unlike the relationship between blood cholesterol and coronary heart disease risk, in which the risk increases progressively across the upper three quintiles (Grundy *et al.,* 1982). The relationship for colon cancer in men may therefore reflect the existence of a metabolically distinct subgroup, with naturally low blood cholesterol, and an associated increased susceptibility to colon cancer (McMichael *et al.,* 1984). In the two of those three studies that presented the equivalent data for women, there was no clear-cut or consistent relationship between blood cholesterol and colon cancer incidence.

In view of the hypothesis that bile constituents (acidic and/or neutral) and their intracolonic degradation products influence colon carcinogenesis (Zaridze, 1983), it may be that those individuals with a metabolic predisposition toward low serum cholesterol also have a raised secretion of bile (containing bile acids and cholesterol) or a higher excretion of nonabsorbed cholesterol in feces and are therefore at increased risk of colon cancer (McMichael *et al.,* 1984).

Since the data suggest that the inverse relationship with colon cancer applies particularly to men, it is of interest to note the evidence of the existence of intrinsic sex differences in large-bowel carcinogenesis (McMichael and Potter, 1985). The fact that women tend to have lower blood concentrations of total cholesterol and higher high-density-lipoprotein cholesterol concentrations than men, particularly before the age of female menopause, suggests, along with other epidemiologic, clinical, and animal experimental evidence, that bile in women differs in composition and amount from that in men. This could account for the consistently higher colon cancer incidence rates in women compared with men, before approximately age 55, if indeed bile constituents and metabolites influence colon carcinogenesis as has been generally suspected (Zaridze, 1983). Given these intrinsic sex differences in hepatic lipid metabolism and in bile composition, the biological significance (in both metabolic and disease risk terms) of having a naturally low blood cholesterol concentration may differ between the sexes.

Furthermore, the particular association of low serum cholesterol with cancer of the proximal colon in the Honolulu Study (other studies did not report details for colon subsites) accords with evidence from 10 of 14 recently published studies that, after cholecystectomy, any increased risk of colon cancer is maximal for the proximal colon (McMichael and Potter, 1985). However, the case–control study of Sidney *et al.* (1986) found no such association with cancer of the proximal colon.

A possible alternative explanation for the inverse association with colon cancer is that a low serum cholesterol is caused by some dietary factor (polyunsaturated fats, for example) that itself increases colon carcinogenesis. Furthermore, the only dietary trial to have indicated an increased cancer risk when serum cholesterol was lowered was that in which this effect was achieved by increasing the dietary polyunsaturated : saturated fat ratio (Pearce and Dayton, 1971).

Finally, it may be relevant that in the studies reporting an inverse association of antecedent serum cholesterol with colon cancer risk, and reporting that this association was not attributable to a preclinical cancer effect, cancer incidence, not mortality, was studied. Approximately one-third of colon cancer cases do not die from their cancer; furthermore, when death occurs from colon cancer, it does so, on average, 1–2 years after diagnosis (Axtell *et al.*, 1976). Thus, the incidence-based evidence from the Honolulu, Framingham, and Evans County studies refers to serum cholesterol levels measured several years earlier in the chronology of carcinogenesis than those measured in mortality-based studies and thus is more likely to predate any later-stage metabolic disturbance caused by cancer. This appears to strengthen the evidence against the inverse association with colon cancer being caused by a preclinical cancer effect (McMichael *et al.*, 1984).

Overall, the various observational studies differ in their design and in relationship to sex, age group, and cancer end point studied, and they show inconsistent relationships between serum cholesterol and both total and site-specific cancer risks. Colon cancer, however, displays a more clear-cut (although inconsistent) inverse association with serum cholesterol; the fact that this association has been reported in men only, and perhaps varies by colon subsite, appears to be biologically plausible.

Observational studies on serum cholesterol and cancer thus afford substantial evidence that preclinical cancer causes a lowering of serum cholesterol and limited, but biologically plausible, evidence that men with naturally low serum cholesterol levels may be at increased risk of colon cancer.

4. References

Abramson, S. H., and Kark, J. D., 1985, Serum cholesterol and primary brain tumours: A case–control study, *Br. J. Cancer* **52**:93–98.

Anderson, K. M., Castelli, W. P., and Levy, D., 1987, Cholesterol and mortality: 30 years of follow-up from the Framingham study, *JAMA* **257**:217–218.

Axtell, L. M., Asire, A. J., and Myers, M. H., 1976, Cancer patient survival, report no. 5, US Department of Health, Education and Welfare, Publication no. (NIH)77-992, Washington, DC.

Bases, R. E., and Krakoff, I. H., 1965, Studies of serum cholesterol levels in leukemia, *J. Reticuloendothel. Soc.* **2**:8–14.

Buchalter, J., Herbert, E., and Flehinger, B., 1983, A case–control study of time-trends in serum cholesterol levels prior to the detection of colon cancer (Abstract), *Gastroenterology* **84**:1403.

Cambien, F., Ducimetiere, P., and Richard, J., 1980, Total serum cholesterol and cancer mortality in a middle-aged male population, *Am. J. Epidemiol.* **112**:388–394.

Committee of Principal Investigators, 1978, A co-operative trial in the primary prevention of ischaemic heart disease using clofibrate, *Br. Heart J.* **40**:1069–1118.

Committee of Principal Investigators, 1980, WHO co-operative trial on primary prevention of ischaemic heart disease using clofibrate to lower serum cholesterol: Mortality follow-up, *Lancet* **2**:379–385.

Coronary Drug Project Research Group, 1975, Clofibrate and niacin in coronary heart disease, *JAMA* **231**:360–381.

Dahlen, G., Ericsson, C., de Faire, U., Iselius, L., and Lundman, T., 1983, Genetic and environmental determinants of cholesterol and HDL-cholesterol concentrations in blood, *Int. J. Epidemiol.* **12**:32–35.

Dyer, A. R., Stamler, J., Paul, O., Shekelle, R. B., Schoenberger, J. A., Berkson, D. M., Lepper, M., Collette, P., Shekelle, S., and Lindberg, H. A., 1981, Serum cholesterol and risk of death from cancer and other causes in three Chicago epidemiological studies, *J. Chronic Dis.* **34**:249–260.

Ederer, F., Leren, P., Turpeinen, O., and Frantz, I. D., 1971, Cancer among men on cholesterol-lowering diets, *Lancet* **2**:203–206.

Enstrom, J. E., 1980, Health and dietary practices and cancer mortality among California Mormons, in: *Cancer*

Incidence in Defined Populations (Banbury Report 4), (J. Cairns, J. L. Lyons, and M. Skolnick, eds.), Cold Spring Harbor Laboratory, Cold Spring Harbor, New York, pp. 69–92.

Feinleib, M., 1982, Summary of a workshop on cholesterol and noncardiovascular disease mortality, *Prev. Med.* **11**:360–367.

Garcia-Palmieri, M. R., Sorlie, P. D., Costas, R., and Havlik, R. J., 1981, An apparent inverse relationship between serum cholesterol and cancer mortality in Puerto Rico, *Am. J. Epidemiol.* **114**:29–40.

Gerhardsson, M., Rosenqvist, U., Ahlbom, A., and Carlson, L. A., 1986, Serum cholesterol and cancer—A retrospective case-control study, *Int. J. Epidemiol.* **15**:155–159.

Grundy, S. M., Bilheimer, D., Blackburn, H., Brown, W. V., Kwiterovich, P. O., Mattson, F., Schonfeld, G., and Weidman, W. H., 1982, Rationale of the Diet-Heart Statement of the American Heart Association. Report of Nutrition Committee, *Circulation* **65**:839A–854A.

Hiatt, R. A., Friedman, G. D., Bawol, R. D., and Ury, H. K., 1982, Breast cancer and serum cholesterol, *J. Natl. Cancer Inst.* **68**:885–889.

Hiatt, R., Fireman, B., and Friedman, G. D., 1983, Cholesterol and cancer (Abstract), *Am. J. Epidemiol.* **118**:438.

International Collaborative Group, 1982, Circulating cholesterol level and risk of death from cancer in men aged 40 to 69 years: Experience of an international collaborative group, *JAMA* **248**:2853–2859.

Kagan, A., McGee, D. L., Yano, K., Rhoads, G. G., and Nomura, A., 1981, Serum cholesterol and mortality in a Japanese–American population: The Honolulu Heart Program, *Am. J. Epidemiol.* **114**:11–20.

Kark, J. D., Smith, A. H., and Hames, C. G., 1980, The relationship of serum cholesterol to the incidence of cancer in Evans County, Georgia, *J. Chronic Dis.* **33**:311–322.

Kark, J. D., Smith, A. H., and Hames, C. G., 1982, Serum retinol and the inverse relationship between serum cholesterol and cancer, *Br. Med. J.* **284**:152–154.

Katan, M. B., 1986, Apolipoprotein E isoforms, serum cholesterol, and cancer, *Lancet* **1**:507–508.

Keys, A., 1980, *Seven Countries: A Multivariate Analysis of Death and Coronary Heart Disease,* Harvard University Press, Cambridge, MA.

Keys, A., Anderson, J. T., and Grande, F., 1965, Serum cholesterol response to changes in diet, *Metabolism* **14**:747–787.

Keys, A., Aravanis, C., Blackburn, H., Buzina, R., Dontas, A. S., Fidanza, F., Karvonen, M. J., Menotti, A., Nedeljkovic, S., Punsar, S., and Toshima, H., 1985, Serum cholesterol and cancer mortality in the Seven Countries Study, *Am. J. Epidemiol.* **121**:870–873.

Kozarevic, D. J., McGee, D., Vojvodic, N., Gordon, T., Racic, Z., Zukel, W., and Dawber, T., 1981, Serum cholesterol and mortality: The Yugoslavia Cardiovascular Disease Study, *Am. J. Epidemiol.* **114**:21–28.

Laskarzewski, P., Khoury, P., Morrison, J. A., Kelly, K., Mellies, M., and Glueck, C. J., 1982, Cancer, cholesterol, and lipoprotein cholesterols, *Prev. Med.* **11**:253–268.

Lyon, J. L., Gardner, J. W., Klauber, M. R., and Smart, C. R., 1977, Low cancer incidence and mortality in Utah, *Cancer* **39**:2608–2618.

Malarkey, W. B., Schroeder, L. L., Stevens, V. C., James, A. G., and Lanese, R. R., 1977, Twenty-four hour preoperative endocrine profiles in women with benign and malignant breast disease, *Cancer Res.* **37**:4655–4699.

Marenah, C. B., Lewis, B., Hassall, D., La Ville, A., Cortese, C., Mitchell, W. D., Bruckdorfer, K. R., Slavin, B., Miller, N. E., Turner, P. R., and Heduan, E., 1983, Hypocholesterolaemia and non-cardiovascular disease: Metabolic studies on subjects with low plasma cholesterol, *Br. Med. J.* **286**:1603–1606.

McMichael, A. J., and Potter, J. D., 1985, Host factors in carcinogenesis: Certain bile acid metabolic profiles that selectively increase the risk of proximal colon cancer, *J. Natl. Cancer Inst.* **75**:185–191.

McMichael, A. J., Jensen, O. M., Parkin, D. M., and Zaridze, D. G., 1984, Dietary and endogenous cholesterol and human cancer, *Epidemiol. Rev.* **6**:192–216.

Miller, S. R., Tartter, P. I., Papatestas, A. E., Slater, G., and Aufses, A. H., 1981, Serum cholesterol and human colon cancer, *J. Natl. Cancer Inst.* **67**:297–300.

Morris, D. L., Borhani, N. O., Fitzsimons, E., Hardy, R. J., Hawkins, C. M., Kraus, J. F., Labarthe, D. R., Mastbaum, L., and Payne, G. H., 1983, Serum cholesterol and cancer in the Hypertension Detection and Follow-up Program, *Cancer* **52**:1754–1759.

Muller, H. G., 1930, The cholesterol metabolism in health and anemia, *Medicine* **9**:119–174.

Nestel, P. J., 1989, Diet and hyperlipidaemia, in: *Clinical Biochemistry—Principles, Methods, Applications. Human Plasma Lipoproteins* (J. C. Fruchart and R. Shephard, eds.), Gruyler, New York, pp. 309–333.

Neugut, A. I., Johnsen, C. M., and Fink, D. J., 1986, Serum cholesterol levels in adenomatous polyps and cancer of the colon. A case–control study, *JAMA* **255**:365–367.

NIH Consensus Conference, 1985, Lowering blood cholesterol to prevent heart disease, *JAMA* **253**:2080–2086.

Nydegger, U. E., and Butler, R. E., 1972, Serum lipoprotein levels in patients with cancer, *Cancer Res.* **32**:1756–1760.

Oliver, M. F., 1981, Serum cholesterol—The knave of hearts and the joker, *Lancet* **2**:1090–1095.

Pearce, M. L., and Dayton, S., 1971, Incidence of cancer in men on a diet high in polyunsaturated fat, *Lancet* **1**:464–467.

Peterson, B., Trell, E., and Sternby, N. H., 1981, Low cholesterol level as a risk factor for noncoronary death in middle-aged men, *JAMA* **245**:2056–2057.

Peto, R., Doll, R., Buckley, J. D., and Sporn, M., 1981, Can dietary β-carotene materially reduce human cancer rates? *Nature* **290**:201–208.

Phillips, R. L., 1975, Role of life-style and dietary habits in risk of cancer among Seventh-Day Adventists, *Cancer Res.* **35**:3513–3522.

Reed, D., Yano, K., and Kagan, A., 1986, Lipids and lipoproteins as predictors of coronary heart disease, stroke, and cancer in the Honolulu Heart Program, *Am. J. Med.* **80**:871–878.

Rose, G., and Shipley, M. J., 1980, Plasma lipids and mortality, a source of error, *Lancet* **1**:523–526.

Rose, G., Blackburn, H., Keys, A., Taylor, H. L., Kannel, W. B., Paul, O., Reid, D. D., and Stamler, J., 1974, Colon cancer and blood-cholesterol, *Lancet* **1**:180–183.

Salmond, C. E., Beaglehole, R., and Prior, I. A. M., 1985, Are low cholesterol values associated with excess mortality? *Br. Med. J.* **290**:422–424.

Salonen, J. T., 1982, Risk of cancer and death in relation to serum cholesterol: A longitudinal study in an Eastern Finnish population with high overall cholesterol level, *Am. J. Epidemiol.* **116**:622–630.

Schatzkin, A., Hoover, R. N., Taylor, P. R., Ziegler, R. G., Carter, C. L., Larson, D. B., and Licitra, L. M., 1987, Serum cholesterol and cancer in the NHANES I Epidemiologic followup study, *Lancet* **ii**:298–301.

Sherwin, R. W., Wentworth, D. N., Cutler, J. A., Hulley, S. B., Kuller, L. H., and Stamler, J., 1987, Serum cholesterol levels and cancer mortality in 361622 men screened for the Multiple Risk Factor Intervention Trial, *JAMA* **257**:943–948.

Sidney, S., Friedman, G. D., and Hiatt, R. A., 1986, Serum cholesterol and large bowel cancer: A case–control study, *Am. J. Epidemiol.* **124**:33–38.

Smith, A. H., and Hoggard, B. M., 1981, Retinol, carotene, and the cancer/cholesterol association (Letter), *Lancet* **1**:1371–1372.

Sorlie, P. D., and Feinleib, M., 1982, The serum cholesterol–cancer relationship: An analysis of time trends in the Framingham Study, *J. Natl. Cancer Inst.* **69**:989–996.

Stemmermann, G. N., Nomura, A. M. Y., Heilbrun, L. K., Pollack, E. S., and Kagan, A., 1981, Serum cholesterol and colon cancer incidence in Hawaiian Japanese men, *J. Natl. Cancer Inst.* **67**:1179–1182.

Tartter, P. I., Slater, G., Papatestas, A. E., and Aufses, A. H., 1984, Cholesterol, weight, height, Quetelet's index, and colon cancer recurrence, *J. Surg. Oncol.* **27**:232–235.

Thomas, C. B., Duszynski, K. R., and Schaffer, J. W., 1982, Cholesterol levels in young adulthood and subsequent cancer: A preliminary note, *Johns Hopkins Med. J.* **150**:89–94.

Tornberg, S. A., Holm, L.-E., Carstensen, J. M., and Eklund, G. A., 1986, Risks of cancer of the colon and rectum in relation to serum cholesterol and beta-lipoprotein, *N. Engl. J. Med.* **315**:1629–1633.

Turpeinen, O., 1979, Effect of cholesterol-lowering diet on mortality from coronary heart disease and other causes, *Circulation* **59**:1–7.

Vitols, S., Gahrton, G., Bjorkholm, M., and Peterson, C., 1985, Hypocholesterolaemia in malignancy due to elevated low-density-lipoprotein-receptor activity in tumour cells: Evidence from studies in patients with leukaemia, *Lancet* **2**:1150–1154.

Walden, R. T., Schaefer, L. E., Lemon, F. R., Sunshine, A., and Wynder, E. L., 1964, Effect of the environment on the serum cholesterol–triglyceride distribution among Seventh-Day Adventists, *Am. J. Med.* **36**:269–276.

Wallace, R. B., Rost, C., Burmeister, L. F., and Pomrehn, P. R., 1982, Cancer incidence in humans: Relationship to plasma lipids and relative weight, *J. Natl. Cancer Inst.* **68**:915–918.

Westlund, K., and Nicolaysen, R., 1972, Ten-year mortality and morbidity related to serum cholesterol, *Scand. J. Clin. Lab. Invest.* **39**(Suppl. 127):3–24.

Williams, R. R., Sorlie, P. D., Feinleib, M., McNamara, P. M., Kannel, W. B., and Dawber, T. R., 1981, Cancer incidence by levels of cholesterol, *JAMA* **245**:247–252.

Wingard, D. L., Criqui, M. H., Holdbook, M. J., and Barrett-Connor, E., 1984, Plasma cholesterol and cancer morbidity and mortality in an adult community, *J. Chronic Dis.* **37**:401–406.

World Health Organization, 1985, Primary prevention of coronary heart disease: EURO Reports and Studies, 98, WHO Regional Office for Europe, Copenhagen.

Yaari, S., Goldbourt, U., Evan-Zohar, S., and Neufeld, N. H., 1981, Associations of serum high density lipoprotein and total cholesterol with total, cardiovascular, and cancer mortality in a 7-year prospective study of 10,000 men, *Lancet* **1**:1011–1014.

Zaridze, D. G., 1983, Environmental etiology of large bowel cancer, *J. Natl. Cancer Inst.* **70**:389–400.

8

Lipotropic Factors and Carcinogenesis

Paul M. Newberne and Adrianne E. Rogers

1. Introduction

The lipotropes (choline, methionine, vitamin B_{12}, and folic acid) have an interesting history with respect to their role in cancer causation, a part of which will be briefly reviewed here (Broad, 1982).

Frederick G. Banting, a practicing surgeon in London, Ontario, Canada, in 1920, came to J. J. R. Macleod, a distinguished physiologist, at the University of Toronto and described how the internal secretions of the pancreas might be isolated in order to further investigate certain aspects of diabetes. Macleod was persuaded and provided Banting with a room for surgery and a few dogs as experimental subjects. An assistant, Charles Best, was also available to help carry out the experimental work. After an intensive 2 months of labor, on Saturday, July 30, 1921, Banting and Best injected a depancreatized dog with a pancreatic extract. The dog's blood sugar level dropped 40% within an hour, and its clinical condition improved remarkably. On Monday, August 1, the experimenters gave an 8-ml injection of this extract to another depancreatized collie, then on the brink of death, and an hour later the dog came out of the coma, stood up, and walked around the room. The medical odyssey was thus initiated that led to the isolation, purification, and clinical use of "the elixir of life" for millions of humans, insulin. Daily injections of insulin were then given to a 14-year-old boy, in January 1922, the first diabetic human to receive the newly discovered hormone.

The linkage between these events and the lipotropes began while Banting, Best, and Macleod were conducting the studies that led to the discovery and purification of insulin. It was observed that the depancreatized dog receiving insulin failed to survive more than about a year when fed a diet of lean meat and sugar. At autopsy fat infiltration in the liver was extensive and the liver was the only organ seriously affected (Hershey, 1930). There was up to 35% fat, which had an iodine number of about 65. The addition of raw pancreas to the diet prevented the condition, including the fatty liver.

Paul M. Newberne and Adrianne E. Rogers • Department of Pathology, Boston University School of Medicine, Boston, Massachusetts 02118.

These observations were followed by a discovery that 10 g lecithin daily in the diet restored the animals to normal, the same as raw pancreas. Purified lecithin from egg yolk and fresh beef liver prevented the fatty liver, leading Best and associates (1932) to test effects of the components of lecithin on fatty liver (Best and Huntsman, 1932). Of the components tested, only choline chloride consistently inhibited the deposition of fat in the liver under the conditions of the experiments, demonstrating that the active principle of lecithin was choline.

Following these important observations, researchers in many laboratories demonstrated a relationship between choline deprivation and liver damage in a large number of species (Follis, 1958).

Numerous investigators documented the role of choline and other lipotropic agents in the homeostasis of the liver, particularly with respect to liver lipid and other organs and tissues. The choline-deficient liver exhibits fatty infiltration, fibrosis, cirrhosis, and, in extreme cases, hepatocellular carcinoma. Some of these changes will be illustrated in this chapter.

The lipotropes are essential to many metabolic processes, especially the synthesis of DNA, nucleoproteins, and membranes. All are required for cell proliferation and the maintenance of tissue integrity; they interact extensively with each other and with other nutrients in metabolism of one-carbon units. Choline and folic acid are plentiful, in both animal and plant foods, but plants are low in methionine and do not contain any vitamin B_{12}. Animal products and microorganisms are the sole dietary sources of vitamin B_{12}.

Only vitamin B_{12} is stored in the body for any length of time (from 3 to 6 years after intake of the vitamin ceases in humans). Methionine, an essential amino acid, is present in only relatively small amounts in its free state but exists as a structural unit of protein and, in its activated form, S-adenosylmethionine (SAM); it is also available from body protein during the catabolic phase of tissue and cell metabolism. Stores of folic acid last no more than a few months after intake ceases, and choline, as such, lasts only a few days or, at most, a few weeks. Like methionine, it can be derived from tissue breakdown, inasmuch as it is a major component of cell membranes and phospholipids. Thus a dietary deficiency of any or all of these nutrients is a potential continuous threat to health, and a deficit or imbalance may contribute to susceptibility to many diseases, including cancer.

Rats fed diets marginal or deficient in lipotropes are more susceptible to development of liver cancer induced by a wide variety of natural and synthetic carcinogens (Rogers and Newberne, 1980). Lipotrope deficiency influences the hepatic activation or detoxification of xenobiotics, including carcinogens, but the direction and magnitude of the effect vary (Newberne and Rogers, 1986). The deficiency also significantly increases hepatocyte cell proliferation (Newberne *et al.*, 1983b).

Lipotropes are essential to methylation of DNA and RNA and, by this mechanism, control of cell proliferation. It is not surprising, then, that a deficiency of lipotropes leads to impaired immunocompetence. The severity of impairment, however, depends on the age of the animal and the adequacy of other nutrients in the diet (Nauss and Newberne, 1981). Increased susceptibility to bacterial and parasitic infections has been observed in folate-deficient rats (Gross and Newberne, 1976) and guinea pigs (Gross and Newberne, 1980). Female rats fed diets deficient in methionine and choline during gestation and lactation give birth to young with hypoplastic and atrophic lymphoid tissue; there is diminished response of lymphocytes to mitogens, and susceptibility to infectious disease is increased (Newberne and Wilson, 1972; Gebhardt and Newberne, 1974).

Thus animal studies have established that lipotropes are involved in the activation or deactivation of carcinogens (Campbell *et al.*, 1978; Rogers and Newberne, 1973) and may alter immunosurveillance for tumor cells (Nauss and Newberne, 1981). These two areas of research related to susceptibility to cancer will be more fully explored in the following pages.

2. Lipotropes and Liver Injury

Rats maintained on choline-deficient diets for long periods develop hepatocellular carcinomas, an original observation that attracted widespread attention because it was the first report in which omission of a substance from the diet, rather than addition of one, resulted in neoplasia (Copeland and Salmon, 1946; Salmon and Copeland, 1954).

Salmon and colleagues reported a significant incidence of hepatocarcinomas in choline-deficient rats during many years of experimental work. Additional studies confirmed that choline deficiency was indeed associated with a significant incidence of hepatocellular carcinoma in rats. However, in some groups given the same diet supplemented with choline, significant numbers of animals had liver neoplasms without the injury of choline deficiency (Salmon and Newberne, 1963). This observation aroused further interest in the deficiency but also raised the question of dietary contamination as a contributing factor.

It was suggested that an alcohol-soluble contaminant in the peanut meal that served as the source of protein in the diet was probably responsible for the liver tumors and that deficient rats were simply more sensitive to the contaminant.

Shortly thereafter, our laboratory at the Massachusetts Institute of Technology identified aflatoxins in the peanut meal (Newberne, 1967), which strongly implied that these contaminants were the etiological agents for the hepatocellular carcinoma in choline-deficient rats. Furthermore (Newberne *et al.*, 1969a), diets with a protein source exclusively from purified amino acids, deficient in choline and low in methionine, did not result in hepatocellular tumors. Fatty, nodular, hyperplastic, cirrhotic livers resulted from uncomplicated choline deficiency, but in our hands at that time, tumors did not develop. However, we did not hold the rats until natural death, and the period of time probably was not long enough for the deranged liver to develop into hepatocellular carcinoma. We have continued research in this laboratory on the effects of lipotrope deficiency, other dietary insults, and surgical injury on the susceptibility of the liver to carcinogenesis (Rogers and Newberne, 1980; Newberne *et al.*, 1982, 1983a). Other laboratories have also worked with this model (Mikol *et al.*, 1983; Ghoshal and Farber, 1983) and confirmed our findings.

3. Lipotrope Deficiency, Cirrhosis, and Liver Tumors in Rats

All strains of rats used to date are sensitive to the deficiency and its enhancing effects on chemically induced cancer. Generally, the rats have been fed a choline-free diet such as that listed in Table I, from weaning until cirrhosis develops, which requires a period of time ranging from 200 to 500 days. The rats must be fed the diet continuously from weaning until the study is terminated; if the diet is started at a later period, cirrhosis is not induced but the liver is sensitized, even with marginal deficits (Rogers and Newberne,

Table I. Typical Diets Used in Lipotrope Studies[a]

Ingredient	Feed content (g/kg)	
	Diet 1	Diet 2 (deficient)
Casein	60	60
Peanut meal	250	250
Sucrose	467	470
Vitamin mix[b]	20	20
Mineral mix	50	50
Fat	150	150
Choline	3	0
Vitamin B_{12}	50 ug	0

[a]Amino acid diets have also been used for some studies. The diet listed here is a particularly good one because the combination of casein and peanut meal provides about 0.3% methionine, allowing for normal growth even in the choline-deprived group.
[b]Vitamin mix is complete except for folic acid (in folate deficiency studies), choline, and vitamin B_{12}, which were added at the time of diet preparation.

1980). Some deaths occur from the hemorrhagic kidney syndrome induced by choline deficiency, usually between days 8 and 10 following initiation of dietary treatment, but beyond that time, the clinical course is uneventful. However, renal injury may persist in some rats until they die or are sacrificed.

The earliest lesion in the liver of a choline-deficient animal is an accumulation of lipid in the centrilobular zone (Fig. 1) a few days after initiation of the diet. Lipid content continues to increase and within 2–3 weeks virtually all cells of the lobule are distended (Fig. 2). This is accompanied by the appearance of bizarre nuclei, many of which contain intranuclear inclusions, and single-cell necrosis is widespread throughout the lobe. It is at this point that mitotic figures (Fig. 3) and ^{3}H-thymidine labeling increase rapidly (Fig. 4). There is single-cell, as well as diffuse, labeling throughout the lobe, along with focal accumulations of hyperchromatic (basophilic) proliferating parenchymal cells (Fig. 5). The liver is pale and nodular (Fig. 6), with marked fibrosis and cirrhosis (Fig. 7). Nodules may or may not contain fat; in particular, those which are growing most rapidly have excluded it (Fig. 8). Some of the lesions progress through atypical nodular hyperplasia (Fig. 9), usually without lipid, to hepatocellular carcinoma (Fig. 10). Livers of such rats and mice are more susceptible to all hepatocarcinogens thus far tested (Rogers and Newberne, 1980). Figure 11 illustrates such increased sensitivity. These changes have been documented and illustrated in many publications (Best *et al.*, 1932; Salmon and Copeland, 1954; Newberne *et al.*, 1969b; Mikol *et al.*, 1983; Ghoshal *et al.*, 1984).

We and others have used the amino acid mixtures to replace the intact protein of choline-deficient diets. The livers of the choline-deficient animals had significant lipid accumulation after 10 weeks, and fibrosis, progressing to cirrhosis, began after they were on the diet for 4 months. Liver lipids reached a maximum of 69% of the dry weight, with triglyceride accounting for the bulk of the increase and cholesterol and phospholipids increased, but to a lesser degree. All three of the lipid fractions decreased in the serum of

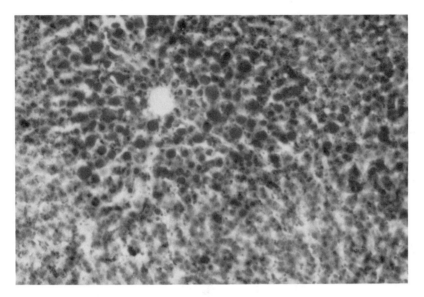

Fig. 1. Centrilobular lipid. Microscopic accumulation in liver of choline-deficient rat, 4 days after initiation of the dietary deficit. The dark-staining rounded globules are fat, identified by special staining of a frozen section of the liver.

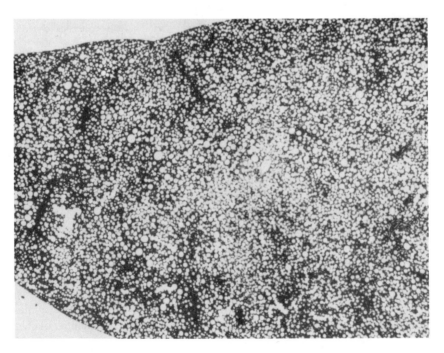

Fig. 2. Liver of rat fed choline-deficient diet for 3 weeks. The clear, rounded areas represent cells where fat had accumulated. The fat was dissolved during tissue preparation for paraffin section and embedding.

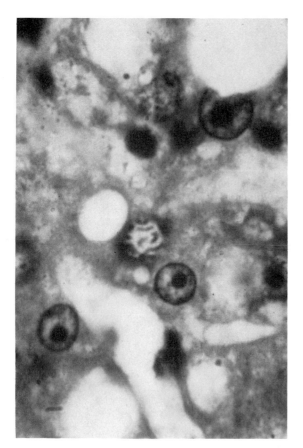

Fig. 3. Choline-deficient rat liver with bizarre nucleus containing chromosomes. Other nuclei at this stage of development have intranuclear and cytoplasmic inclusions.

the deficient rats, which is a characteristic finding in lipotrope deficiency, inasmuch as lipid secretion by the liver is abnormal under these conditions.

The chemical and morphological findings in studies using purified amino acids as a source of nitrogen indicated that fatty nutritional cirrhosis, characteristic of choline deficiency and identical to that induced with intact proteins, was induced with the purified L-amino acid diets eliminating much of the concern about contaminants in the peanut meal. This was confirmed by Mikol and co-workers (1983), and these investigators also found a significant incidence of hepatocarcinomas.

We have performed many experiments that have confirmed the increased susceptibility of the choline-deficient liver to hepatocarcinogenesis. We also observed that a marginal deficiency, which produces only a modest accumulation of fat without cirrhosis, sensitizes the liver to a number of carcinogens (Table II). We have followed these observations with experiments to determine the mechanism of increased sensitivity to a number of chemical carcinogens. Some of the data are given below.

As liver fat increases in the choline-deficient rat (Fig. 5), the number of cells labeled by [³H]-thymidine also increases (Newberne *et al.*, 1982). Choline deficiency alone

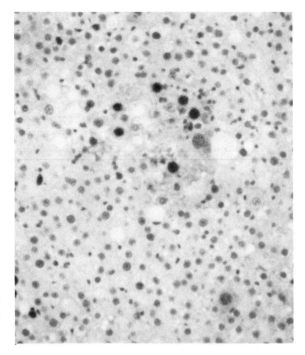

Fig. 4. Liver cell nuclei of choline-deficient rat that have taken up ^{3}H-thymidine, an indication of rapid cell proliferation. Lipid droplets (vacuoles) are nearby labeled nuclei.

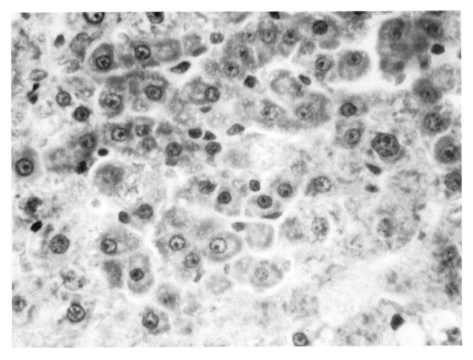

Fig. 5. Basophilic focus of hepatocytes, an early lesion indicative of cellular proliferation. These foci are considered by some to be precursor lesions of liver cell cancer.

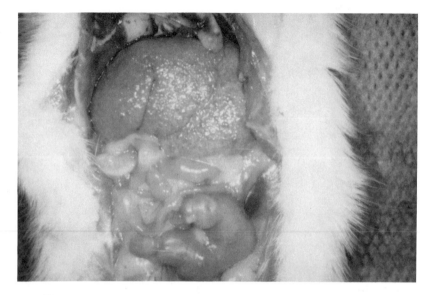

Fig. 6. Pale, fatty liver of choline-deficient rat with developing nodular cirrhosis.

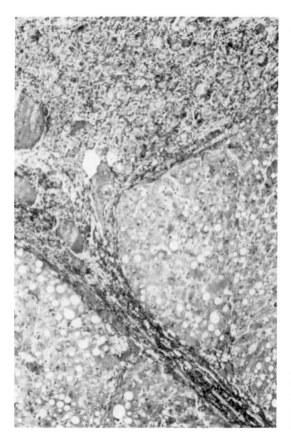

Fig. 7. Nodular, cirrhotic liver of choline-deficient rat. Note bridging fibrosis containing bile duct hyperplasia, reactive inflammatory cells, and cholangiofibrosis between proliferating nodules of hepatocytes.

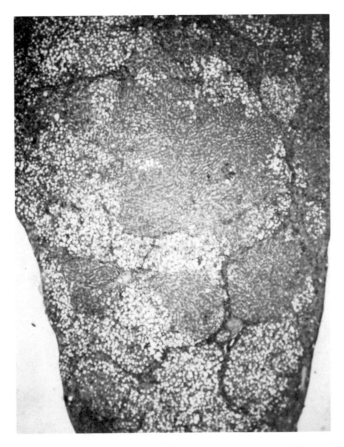

Fig. 8. Nodular, fibrotic fatty liver of choline-deficient liver of rat. The most rapidly growing nodules have excluded fat.

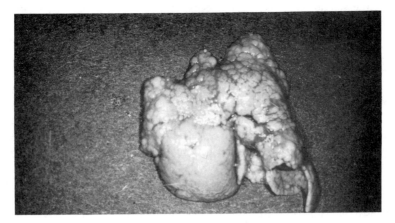

Fig. 9. Cirrhotic liver of choline-deficient rat with a large nodular liver cell carcinoma.

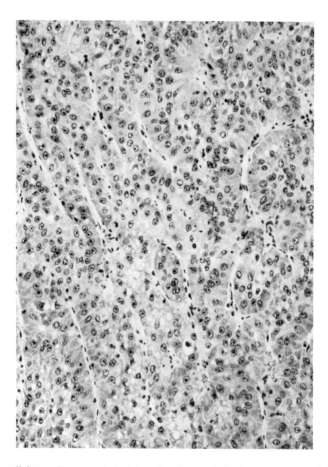

Fig. 10. Hepatocellular carcinoma, typical of those that develop in the liver of choline-deficient rats and mice.

causes a sharp increase in cell death. DNA synthesis is increased, as is cell turnover, both of which are essential components of liver parenchymal cell hyperplasia. Other studies (Newberne *et al.*, 1983a,b) provide evidence for a relationship between choline deficiency, fatty liver, and parenchymal cell proliferation (Table III). These data, taken from work done in collaboration with H.L. Leffert (Salk Institute), confirm a relationship between serum very-low-density-lipoprotein (VLDL) content and hepatic DNA synthesis. Partial hepatectomy and choline deficiency lower VLDL, and both "turn on" DNA synthesis and cell proliferation. The dietary effect is similar to that produced by a partial hepatectomy; however, a key difference is that cell death and compensatory hyperplasia of the parenchyma continue as long as the choline-deficient diet is fed, whereas partial hepatectomy results in a temporary wave of hyperplasia only; this returns to normal when the prehepatectomy liver volume is approximated.

More will be said later in this chapter about mechanisms, with respect to choline and experimental cancer. However, it seems appropriate at this point to illuminate certain key observations. Chemical induction of hepatocarcinoma is governed in part by the level of DNA synthesis in hepatocytes at the time of carcinogen exposure and also following

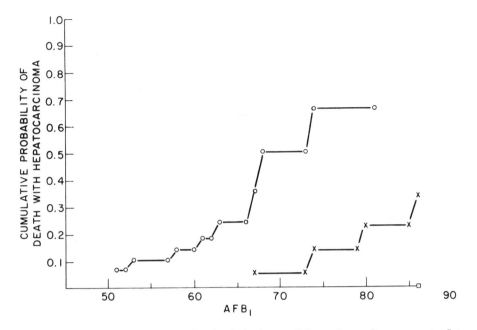

Fig. 11. Probability of choline-deficient rat liver developing hepatocellular carcinoma after exposures to aflatoxin B_1 (AFB$_1$). The open circles represent the choline-deficient group, the "x" lines represent the control choline-supplemented group, from 50 to 90 weeks on study.

exposure. Several models have been described, and investigators are using them to explore biochemical and morphological aspects of this relationship. Some aspects of these studies may explain at least the enhancement of hepatocarcinogenesis of choline deficiency. At this point, however, the nature of the effect is unclear. It must be involved in some way with the hepatic proliferation inhibitor (HPI) (Iype and McMahon, 1984), a chalone

Table II. Chemical Carcinogenesis in Rats Fed a Control Diet
or a Low-Lipotrope Diet[a]

Carcinogenic treatment	Tumor site	Tumor incidence (%)	
		Control	Low lipotrope
AFB$_1$, 350–375 μg, total intragastrically (3 experiments)	Liver	6–15	22–87
DENA, 40 mg/kg, in the diet			
18 weeks	Liver	70	88
12 weeks	Liver	24–43	60–86
DBN, 3.8 g/kg, total DMN			
100 mg/kg	Liver	28	27
25, 50 mg/kg	Liver	74	50
AAF, 0.0125%	Liver	19–61	41–91

[a]From Rogers and Newberne, 1980, abridged.

Table III. *Effect of Lipotrope Deficiency*
on Hepatocyte DNA Synthesis and Serum VLDL
in Weanling Rats[a]

Diet	DNA synthesis[b]	Serum VLDL[b]
Control	0.5–4	75
Marginal lipotrope	1–9	50
Low lipotrope	5–20	25

[a]From Newberne, 1986, abridged, by permission.
[b]Values are expressed in arbitrary units as an index of DNA synthesis and concentration of VLDL.

expressed by adult rat liver, or with hepatic stimulator substance (HSS) expressed by fetal and neonatal rat liver (LaBrecque and Dachur, 1982). Peroxidation and hypomethylation of DNA bases (cytosine), described later, are additional, alternative considerations (Ghoshal *et al.*, 1984; Newberne *et al.*, 1969b).

Lipoperoxidation has been considered by some to be related to the initiation of transformation of hepatocytes and promotion of hepatocarcinogenesis (Newberne *et al.*, 1969b; Perera *et al.*, 1984). We published in 1969 about such a relationship and confirmed the observations with more sophisticated techniques a few years later (Wilson *et al.*, 1973). The synthetic antioxidants butylated hydroxy anisole (BHA) and butylated hydroxy toluene (BHT) protected the kidney and liver from choline deficiency (Tables IV and V) and returned serum and tissue lipid concentrations to near-normal values. Furthermore, our later observations confirmed a relationship between lipid peroxidation and choline deficiency injury. Table VI indicates thiobarbituric acid values and the free radical index of the lipotrope-deficient liver. Further concurrence with these observations has derived from more recent unpublished studies; some of the results are shown in Table V.

The phospholipid changes in the above studies were of particular interest. The membrane phospholipids of the rat liver endoplasmic reticulum contain high levels of arachidonic acid (Rechnagel and Ghoshal, 1966); choline deficiency results in an increased requirement for arachidonate-containing phospholipids (Barker and Hamilton, 1968). Furthermore, choline deficiency is associated with a preferential decrease in he-

Table IV. *Antioxidants and Choline Deficiency Lesions*
in Weanling Rats[a]

Treatment	Mortality[b]	Liver injury
Control	0	0.0
Choline deficient	24	3.0
Choline deficient		
+ Tocopherol	18	2.6
+ Ascorbate	18	2.2
+ Tocopherol, ascorbate	18	2.5
+ BHA, BHT[c]	9	1.8

[a]See Newberne *et al.*, 1969b.
[b]Total number of rats was 45.
[c]BHA = butylated hydroxyanisole; BHT = butylated hydroxytoluene.

Table V. Antioxidants and Liver Lipids in Choline-Deficient Rats[a]

Treatment	Total[b]	Liver lipids (g/100 dry wt)	
		Cholesterol[b]	Phospholipids[b]
Control	30 ± 1	1.40 ± 0.07	10.5 ± 0.4
Choline deficient	54 ± 2	1.20 ± 0.05	6.5 ± 0.6
+ Tocopherol	48 ± 1	1.25 ± 0.06	8.1 ± 0.3
+ Ascorbate	59 ± 2	1.62 ± 0.11	5.9 ± 0.8
+ Tocopherol, ascorbate	46 ± 4	1.28 ± 0.04	7.4 ± 0.4
+ BHA, BHT[c]	43 −7	1.55 ± 0.08	9.4 ± 0.2

[a]See Newberne *et al.*, 1969b.
[b]Values are expressed as means ± SE (or SD).
[c]BHA = butylated hydroxyanisole; BHT = butylated hydroxytoluene.

patic output of longer chains and more unsaturated fatty acids (Tinoco et al., 1964). Although this effect is not explained, it may be due to an impairment of indirect synthesis of lecithin which could account in part for a higher rate of accumulation of longer-chain, more unsaturated fatty acids in the hepatic triglycerides of the choline-deficient rat, fatty acids that more easily undergo peroxidation.

Poirier and Whitehead (1973) and Mikol *et al.* (1981, 1983) have published important data relative to the effect of lipotrope deficiency on fundamental cellular metabolism. Table VII, abridged from Mikol and Poirier (1981), lists data that clearly indicate an effect of lipotrope deficiency on the concentration of SAM, the obligatory source of methyl groups essential to methylation of important bases in DNA, concerned with control of cell proliferation. A deficit of either choline or methionine or both resulted in decreased liver concentrations of SAM and increased ornithine decarboxylase (ODC) activity, the latter essential to polyamine synthesis and control of cell proliferation. Generally, SAM and ODC showed an inverse relationship, and this must bear on the induction of liver injury and, perhaps, promotion of carcinogenesis.

The data of Shank's laboratory (Becker *et al.*, 1981) clearly point to aberrant nucleic acid methylation in injured liver (Table VII) and support the view that such occurs and contributes to the cancer-prone liver of the choline-deficient rat. Additional data from Poirier's laboratory (Table VIII) and from our more recent investigations (Table IX) point

Table VI. Lipotrope Deficiency and Liver Lipids[a,b]

Parameter	Treatment		
	Chow diet	Choline deficient	Choline supplemented
Hepatic lipid, % dry weight	22.2 ± 0.5	44.6 ± 2.1	24.0 ± 1.8
Free radical index	464.0 ± 71.0	553 ± 85.0	303.0 ± 22.0
Liver TBA	129.0 ± 4.2	221 ± 9.6	6.2 ± 2.3

[a]See Wilson *et al.*, 1973.
[b]Values are mean ± SE, nine liver samples.

*Table VII. Lipotropes and Liver Levels of SAM
and ODC 4 Weeks on Diet[a]*

Treatment	SAM (μG/g liver)	ODC (pmol CO_2/mg protein per hr)
Control	44.5 ± 2.0	12.0 ± 8.0
Choline deficient	36.2 ± 1.9	37.9 ± 16.2
Methionine deficient	36.7 ± 2.1	206.0 ± 73.1
Choline/methionine deficient	35.5 ± 1.3	114.8 ± 26.5

[a]See Mikol and Poirier, 1981.

toward hypomethylation as a component of choline deficiency carcinogenesis. Wilson *et al.* (1984) observed a 10–15% decrease in the 5-methyldeoxycytidine in the deficient liver, but only after the animals were on the diet about 6 months. Our studies (P. Punyarit and P. M. Newberne, unpublished) and observations essentially confirm the data of Wilson *et al.* (Table IX), although our methods were slightly different. We maintained rats on the diet for up to 6 months, performed a partial hepatectomy to enhance the generation of new DNA (and accompanying methylation of DNA bases), and 2 weeks later killed the animals for DNA analyses. In agreement with Wilson *et al.* (1984), it was only after 6 months of continuous exposure to the lipotrope-deficient diet that we found a modest hypomethylation of cytosine. This indicates that it is a slow process, and if it is involved with carcinogenesis, hypomethylation most likely requires chronic derangement of liver genetic material over long periods of time.

It seems reasonable to assume that the lipotrope-deficient diet depresses normal methylation of DNA by lowering the pool of SAM, and when the cell prepares for normal division, methylation of the daughter strands of DNA after replication is diminished because of insufficient SAM. DNA thus produced has less 5-methylcytosine than the parent DNA. Because 5-methylcytosine is regarded as having a role in denying expression of genes ("turning off" genes), hypomethylation of DNA would be expected to increase the number of genes in a cell capable of being expressed. This then leads to a change in differentiation of the cell and its progeny (a neoplastic cell?). These alterations combined with modulation of xenobiotic metabolism of carcinogens, described below, and derangements resulting from peroxidation of hepatocyte lipids, referred to above, may account for

*Table VIII. Lipotrope Deficiency,
5'-Methyldeoxycytidine Content of Hepatic DNA[a]*

Treatment	Percent deoxycytidine residues as 5'-methyldeoxycytidine	
	8 weeks	22 weeks
Control	3.33 ± 0.03	3.27 ± 0.04
Deficient	3.13 ± 0.05	2.81 ± 0.04

[a]See Wilson *et al.*, 1984.

Table IX. Lipotropes and 5'-Methylcytosine in Liver DNA[a]

Time on diet	5'-Methylcytosine as percent of cytosine	
	Control	Deficient
3 weeks	4.8 ± 0.09	4.5 ± 0.11
3 months	4.4 ± 0.13	4.7 ± 0.20
6 months	4.5 ± 0.10	3.3 ± 0.06

[a]A two-thirds partial hepatectomy was performed 2 weeks before the animals were killed.

the association of choline deficiency with increased susceptibility to liver cancer. More will be said about this later.

4. Lipotrope Deficiency and Xenobiotic Metabolism

Microsomal oxidase activity of the liver is highly sensitive to lipotrope deficiency. A decrease in the activity of this enzyme system may be responsible for modification of carcinogenesis at a number of sites. Poirier and Whitehead (1973) demonstrated that diethylnitrosamine (DEN) induces tissue folate deficiency, even in the presence of adequate dietary folate. Table X contains data, abridged from the work of these investigators, that illustrate the marked abnormality of folate-dependent histidine metabolism when the animals were exposed to DEN. Studies in our laboratories have yielded similar evidence; DEN treatment increased the severity of lipotrope deficiency (Rogers and Newberne, 1980). It seems likely that cellular defects in one-carbon metabolism may be induced by carcinogens as well as by dietary deficiency and may be central to the dietary effects on carcinogenesis. A shifting of target organ from pancreas to the liver by the choline-deficient diet, probably associated with local tissue metabolism through microsomal enzymes, has been reported by other workers (Roebuck *et al.*, 1981). Shinozuka and co-

Table X. DEN and Folate Excretion[a]

	Urinary formiminoglutamic acid (moles/100 g body weight[b]) (95% confidence limits)		
	Mean	Lower	Upper
Control	2.0 ± 0.04	1.5 ± 0.60	2.6 ± 0.11
DEN	11.4 ± 1.20	8.8 ± 1.10	14.2 ± 1.90
DEN + 1.5% DL-methionine	1.8 ± 0.03	1.5 ± 0.10	2.2 ± 0.08
DEN + 1.5% choline chloride	3.5 ± 0.92	2.7 ± 0.40	4.5 ± 1.12

[a]See Poirier and Whitehead, 1973.
[b]Values are expressed as means ± SE.

workers (1978) have also reported that l-azaserine, a pancreatic carcinogen, induced liver as well as pancreatic carcinoma in lipotrope-deficient rats.

Lipotrope deficiency alters carcinogen metabolism *in vivo* (Newberne and Rogers, 1986). Metabolites and adducts are not the same in lipotrope-deficient rats as in control rats. In addition, rats fed the low-lipotrope diets were more sensitive to the toxicity of repeated doses of most hepatocarcinogens, including AFB_1. However, they were highly insensitive to toxicity of a single dose of AFB_1 (Rogers and Newberne, 1971). This suggests that metabolism of the chemical to its active, toxic form is decreased on first exposure, but induction of metabolism occurs following repeated exposures.

Liver SAM is decreased in lipotrope-deficient rats, but glutathione (GSH) content of liver does not appear to be affected (Poirier *et al.*, 1977). The reduction of SAM in rats fed the lipotrope-deficient diet is a direct result of the dietary treatment; this has been confirmed by Mikol and Poirier (1981) in rats fed diets deficient in one or more of the lipotropes. SAM would not likely influence carcinogenesis by serving as a trap for electrophilic carcinogens since it is an electrophile itself; however, it may play a role in alkylation. SAM is reduced by addition to the diet of ethionine or certain tumor promoters but not acetylaminofluorene (AAF) (Poirier *et al.*, 1977). Since hepatic SAM and folate are both decreased by carcinogens (Poirier and Whitehead, 1973), an indirect interaction may be occurring in one-carbon metabolism with depletion of SAM (Becker *et al.*, 1981).

Liver microsomal oxidases and NAD–NADH are diminished in rats fed lipotrope-deficient diets (Rogers and Newberne, 1971). The decreased activity of oxidases in livers of deficient rats observed by our laboratory staff was confirmed in another laboratory that also demonstrated the diminished content of cytochrome P-450. In the study of Campbell *et al.* (1978) and in some additional studies in our M.I.T. laboratory, rats fed the lipotrope-deficient diet bound about the same, or a slightly decreased, amount of AFB_1 to hepatic DNA as did rats fed the control diet. Higher exposure to AFB_1 depressed its binding to DNA in both control and lipotrope-deficient rats. The assay, like the bacterial assays, therefore indicated no enhancement of AFB_1 activation by the deficiency.

Most strains of mice are resistant to choline deficiency but the discovery that the hybrid B6C3F1 is susceptible not only to choline deficiency (Newberne *et al.*, 1982) but also to aflatoxin B_1 gave us an interesting additional model to investigate mechanisms for carcinogenesis. In recent studies, we have observed that the normal, supplemented control mice were not sensitive to AFB_1 (Table XI); if they were fed a choline-deficient diet, however, there was a significant incidence of liver tumors (80%). Furthermore, this relatively high incidence could be reduced to near the control levels by feeding the antioxidant, butylated hydroxyanisole (BHA). This suggested that, with choline deficiency, tissue peroxidation might be an important factor, interacting with AFB_1 as noted earlier in some of our rat studies. Acute, short-term studies were then conducted to evaluate this possibility. Other factors that might account for the susceptibility to AFB_1 were also examined. Table XII lists some of the results of the short-term studies.

Earlier studies had suggested that choline deficiency had little, if any, effect on liver concentration of GSH. However, as noted in Table XII, when AFB_1 was superimposed on the choline-deficient mouse, liver GSH levels were depressed. This decrease was in part moderated by BHA. Since a major route for detoxification of AFB_1 is by conjugation with GSH, we examined the livers of some of the mice in this study for GSH–AFB_1 conju-

Table XI. Influence of Choline Deficiency and
BHA on AFB_1-Induced Liver Tumors in Mice[a]

	Incidence of liver tumors	
Group treatment	No.	%
None—controls	3/25	12.0
Control + AFB_1	5/25	20.0
Choline deficient	7/25	28.0
Choline deficient + AFB_1	20/25	80.0
Choline deficient + AFB_1 + BHA	6/24	24.0

[a]Male mice, $B_6C_3F_1$, 9 weeks of age, given 6 mg/kg body weight in DMSO, by gavage. BHA was included in semisynthetic diet at 1% level. Sacrifice at 60 weeks.

gates. There was less conjugation of AFB_1 by GSH in the choline-deficient liver; this was reversed in animals fed BHA and the level of conjugation was significantly increased, compared to either control plus AFB_1 or choline-deficient plus AFB_1. Furthermore, this correlated well with the increased glutathione transferase (GSH-Tr), which was also depressed by choline deficiency but significantly increased by BHA.

The choline-deficient mouse model is an important tool for elucidating mechanisms for hepatocellular carcinogenesis. Table XII shows the effects of choline deficiency combined with AFB_1 on tumor induction. Only the deficient liver exposed to AFB_1 had a significant increase in liver tumors and this was inhibited by the antioxidant BHA. This

Table XII. Effects of AFB_1 on Lipid Peroxidation, Liver Necrosis, GSH, and AFB_1–GSH Conjugates in $B_6C_3F_1$ Male Mice[a]

	Control	Control + AFB_1	Choline deficient	Choline deficient + AFB_1	Choline deficient + AFB_1 + BHA
GSH (μmole/g liver)	8.11 ± 0.6	5.23 ± 1.4[b]	8.30 ± 0.8	4.1 ± 0.5[b]	6.0 ± 0.7
GSH–AFB_1 Conjugate (nmole/g per hr)	0	0.11 (0.07–0.14)	0	0.06 (0.04–0.08)	0.23[c] (0.12–0.32)
GSH-Tr	0.13 ± 0.02	0.18 ± 0.03	0.09 ± 0.02	0.05 ± 0.01	0.29 ± 0.04
SGPT (μ/liter)	93 ± 21	360 ± 36	342 ± 29	466 ± 42	206 ± 26
Necrotic index (mean no./10 fields)	0	6.3	2.4 ± 0.4	9.6 ± 1.1	2.6 ± 0.6
TBA reactants (μg MDA equiv/g dry fat-free liver)	8.3 ± 2.1	14.2 ± 3.1	210 ± 8.2	301 ± 14.1	29.4 ± 3.4

[a]Mice sacrificed 24 hr after exposure to i.g. dose AFB_1, 6 mg/kg, when acute injury has peaked.
[b]Significantly different from controls.
[c]Significantly different from controls or choline-deficient animals.

strongly suggests that peroxidation was in some manner involved with the development of tumors, a hypothesis supported further by the presence of TBA-reactive materials in high concentrations in those two groups with the increased tumor incidence (choline-deficient and choline-deficient plus AFB_1). It is not surprising, then, that tumors occurred in the choline-deficient mice; we have observed that previously (Newberne *et al.*, 1982). Evidence for necrosis serum glutamic pyruvic transaminase (SGPT) and necrotic index) and for peroxidation generally agrees with tumor appearance.

The role of GSH and other thiols in cellular toxicity has been demonstrated by many investigators (Jewell *et al.*, 1982; Orrenius *et al.*, 1983; Helliwell *et al.*, 1985; Stacey and Klassen, 1981; Jallou *et al.*, 1974; Casini *et al.*, 1985). There is little doubt that GSH, lipid peroxidation, and necrosis are important aspects of tissue injury, regeneration, and, in some cases, tumor formation in liver as well as in other organs and tissues. The significance of these factors, their interactions, and the relative importance of each, however, await further studies. It seems reasonable to assume that many factors, including liver lipid, cell injury, enzyme induction, beyond the capacity of the cell to sustain itself, availability of GSH or other biological antioxidants, can all play variable but, significant roles in hepatocellular necrosis and subsequent hyperplasia and neoplasia.

The relationship between cirrhosis and liver cell cancer in humans makes the animal model particularly interesting for investigations of interactions between diet and cancer. The ongoing hyperplasia of the lipotrope-deprived liver, apparently producing a high potential for malignant change, may be analogous to hyperplasia of skin and mucous membranes in response to chronic irritation that results also in greater potential for cancer.

The malignant change occurring in cirrhotic liver varies from one part of the world to another, but generally the coexistence is significant and the risk is high. In most series, 60–90% of hepatocarcinomas occur in cirrhotic livers, whereas the incidence of cirrhosis in the population tends to be about 10% (MacSween *et al.*, 1979). In Western countries, including the United States, chronic alcoholism seems to be the most common condition associated with the genesis of cirrhosis and liver cell cancer. The choline deficiency rat liver model for cirrhosis is histologically similar to alcoholic cirrhosis in human patients and, as such, provides us with a convenient means for exploring mechanisms for development of cirrhosis and hepatocellular carcinoma in humans.

5. Lipotropes and Immunocompetence

If one subscribes to an immunosurveillance over the carcinogenesis process, the established effects of lipotropes on the immune system must be taken into consideration. Hematopoietic cells, lymphoreticular tissues, and tumors that arise from them are sensitive to alterations in methyl group metabolism, a basis for antimetabolic chemotherapy of tumors arising in such tissues. Rapid cell turnover creates a need for methyl groups over and above the normal requirement, a condition characteristic of neoplastic tissues. The rapid cell turnover may result in cells with increased susceptibility to alkylating or other agents or conditions that modify the genetic material of the cell. A series of studies in our laboratory have shown that many animal species deprived of one or more of the major lipotropes have diminished immunocompetence.

5.1. Folic Acid

Aminopterin and methotrexate (MTX), antimetabolites of folic acid, were the first therapeutic agents used for temporary remission reported in acute leukemia in children (Farber *et al.*, 1948). Later, these chemicals were used to effect permanent cures of advanced choriocarcinoma of the uterus in women (Hertz *et al.*, 1963). Both drugs exert their effects against tumors by inducing a severe deficiency of the biologically active tetrahydrofolates. The suggestion that these antimetabolites of the folates decrease the risk of cancer has been challenged, and, in fact, they seem to make the normal cells more susceptible to neoplasia. That the antifolates do increase susceptibility to cancer has been shown in numerous studies (Table XIII). Whether these neoplasms were related in any way to immunosuppression by way of folate depletion is unknown, but the data listed in Table XIV strongly suggest that immunosuppression was involved. On the other hand, a deficiency of biologically active tetrahydrofolates induced by MTX may exert a cocarcinogenic effect that facilitates the other agents to which the host is exposed simultaneously.

Several studies (Nauss and Newberne, 1981) have demonstrated impaired humoral and cell-mediated immunity in folate-deficient humans and animals (Table XIV). A number of investigators have observed that guinea pigs deficient in folate are particularly susceptible to infectious disease (Haltalin *et al.*, 1970). Morbidity following *Shigella flexneria* infection in three groups of Hartley strain guinea pigs, fed either a control natural ingredient diet or a semisynthetic folate-supplemented or -deficient diet, was 0, 17, and 89%, respectively. Leukopenia marked the day after challenge with the organism; the increased susceptibility to infection could be reversed if the animals were supplemented with folic acid only a short time before exposure. The folate-deficient rat fails to transform lymphocytes adequately, compared to supplemented animals (Table XV).

The experiments referred to here and others with similar results established clearly that a significant defect occurred in young animals maintained on a folate-deficient diet from weaning. Rats fed a diet deficient in folate from 1 month through 1 year of age and examined sequentially for transformation response of lymphocytes from the thymus and lymph nodes to various mitogens exhibited a clear defect in response. The maximal response to mitogenic stimulation occurred in young animals about 7 weeks of age, 3 weeks after initiation of the diet, a postnatal period in the life of the rat when growth and

Table XIII. Neoplasms Observed in Patients Treated with MTX for Nonmalignant Disease

Disease	Neoplasm
Psoriasis	Lymphosarcoma
	Renal carcinoma
	Mammary cancer
	Lymphoma
	Cervical cancer
	Kaposi's sarcoma
Sarcoidosis	Leukemia

Table XIV. Effects of Folate Deficiency
on Immune Function[a]

Human studies
  Depressed peripheral lymphocyte response to PHA
  No change in neutrophil function
  Increased incidence of folate deficiency in patients with hyper-
    plastic candidiosis
  Depressed delayed cutaneous hypersensitivity
Animal studies
  Guinea pig
    Decreased white blood cell count
    Increased susceptibility to *Shigella* infection
  Rats
    Decreased: Leukocytes and granulocytes
               Hemagglutination titers
               Antibody-forming cells
               T-cells
    Depressed: Cytotoxicity
               Splenic PHA response
               Delayed cutaneous hypersensitivity
    Increased susceptibility to parasitic infection
  Chickens
    Decreased bacterial agglutination titers
    Increased susceptibility to viral infection

[a]From Nauss and Newberne, 1981, by permission.

Table XV. Folic Acid Deficiency in Rats[a]

Immune parameter tested	Control	Folate deficient
Delayed hypersensitivity (skin test response to PHA)	3.8 ± 0.4[b]	1.6 ± 0.4
Lymphocyte-mediated cytotoxicity (% killing)	29.1 ± 3.7[c]	5.2 ± 1.5
Spleen transformation (PHA response)	19,398 ± 1,014[d]	4,263 ± 579
[³H]uridine labeling of T cells		
Spleen	70 ± 2.4[e]	42 ± 1.9
Thymus	82 ± 1.5	73 ± 2.0
Blood	67 ± 1.7	44 ± 2.8

[a]From Gross and Newberne, 1976, abridged.
[b]Histological grading was based on degree of mononuclear cell infiltration: 0 = no response; 4 = severe response.
[c]Results are expressed as mean ± SE.
[d]Results are expressed as cpm ± SE.
[e]Results are expressed as percent cells labeled.

*Table XVI. Response of PHA before Treatment in Folic Acid–Deficient,
Iron-Deficient, and Control Patients[a]*

Group[b]	PHA stimulation of lymphocytes (dpm)[b]		Unstimulated lymphocytes (dpm)	
	Mean ± SD	Range	Mean ± SE	Range
Folate deficient, nonobstetric	8,800 ± 3,600	3,091–13,995	510±	219–1,200
Folate deficient, obstetric	6,800 ± 2,900	3,691–12,323	480±	176–1,250
Folate and iron deficient	6,000 ± 3,280	3,527–10,049	330±	130–510
Iron deficient	23,300 ± 5,470	15,005–28,896	390±	162–672
Control	26,340 ± 5,680	18,740–33,725	370±	130–719

[a]From Gross *et al.*, 1975.
[b]Values are uptake of [³H]dThd; results are expressed in mean ± SD and range.
[c]Values are uptake of [³H]dThd by lymphocytes in presence of saline; results are expressed as mean ± SE and range.

development of the total body and the lymphatic system are rapid. During this period, even a short-term folate deprivation caused a depressed mitogen transformation response. With aging, the amount of tritiated thymidine ([³H]dThd) incorporated into lymphocytes of deprived animals is decreased; the animals also demonstrated a reduction in the stimulation index of lymphocytes. However, after 12 months, no significant differences were seen between the control and experimental groups.

Folate deficiency is one of the common deficits found in protein–energy malnutrition in developing countries and in some subsets of populations of developed countries (i.e., women taking oral contraceptives; patients treated with anticonvulsants). Yet investigators have rarely singled it out for study in human clinical trials to determine its specific effects on immunity.

Our studies have shown a number of interesting correlates of cell-mediated immunity and megaloblastic anemia in human patients due to nutritional folate deficiency (Gross *et al.*, 1975). Cell-mediated immune response was determined in 23 Bantu patients in South Africa with normal levels of serum iron and vitamin B_{12}, except for two subgroups, one with iron deficiency and the other with combined folate–iron deficiency. Use of a Dinitrochlorobenzene (DNCB) skin test and peripheral lymphocyte response to PHA stimulation (Table XVI) produced data which demonstrated that before treatment, the depression in skin reaction to DNCB in the deficient group was highly significant compared with the group with pure iron deficiency or with control groups. Following folate supplementation, 80% of the patients in the first three groups had a positive skin test within about 3 weeks. The PHA response in the peripheral lymphocytes, one-third of the control or of the pure iron-deficient subjects, returned to normal values 7–14 days after therapy.

5.2. Vitamin B_{12}

Vitamin B_{12} can have long-term effects when the deficit is imposed in early life (Newberne and Young, 1973). In human cases of autoimmune phenomena associated with

Table XVII. Effect of Methionine on Immune Function

Dietary treatment	Species	Reported effect
Methionine deficient	Rat, monkey	None on primary or secondary antibody response
Methionine deficient	Chickens	None on resistance to *Salmonella gallinarum* infection
Marginal methionine–cystine	Mice	Depressed humoral immune, no change in cytotoxicity
Marginal methionine–choline	Rats, during gestation and weaning	Increased susceptibility to infection, decreased cell-mediated immunity, decreased lymphoid organ development

pernicious anemia, peripheral lymphocytes are sensitized to a variety of gastric antigens (Tai and McGuigan, 1969). Using the leukocyte migration test, other workers (Goldstone *et al.*, 1973; MacCuisk *et al.*, 1974) demonstrated *in vitro* a delayed hypersensitivity to these antigens.

5.3. Methionine and Choline

Conflicting reports have been made regarding the effect of methionine deficiency on immunocompetence in experimental animals, part of which can be explained on the basis of differences in species, age at time of initiation of the experimental diet, and other factors. Table XVII lists the effects of methionine on immune function drawn from

Table XVIII. Effect of Lipotropes on Response of Rats to Infection with Salmonella typhimurium 3 Months Postweaning

Dietary treatment		Average weight at infection (g)	Percent mortality[a]
Gestation and lactation	Postweaning		
Marginal methionine–choline minus B_{12}	Marginal methionine–choline minus B_{12}	233 ± 6	100
Marginal methionine–choline minus B_{12}	Control	240 ± 8	100
Marginal methionine–choline + B_{12}	Marginal methionine–choline + B_{12}	248 ± 5	91
Marginal methionine–choline + B_{12}	Control	285 ± 7	90
B_{12} deficient	B_{12} deficient	260 ± 3	71
B_{12} deficient	Control	308 ± 4	35
Control	Control	303 ± 4	25

[a]This value is as of 30 days postinfection.

literature references and from work conducted in our laboratories. Others (Gill and Gershoff, 1967; Jose and Good, 1973) have made similar observations.

In a series of studies, we have observed that the effect of specific nutrient deficiency on the immune system is dependent on a number of factors, including the age of the animal, length of time it is fed the experimental diet, adequacy of other nutrients, and time at which the immune system is challenged. It is important that these parameter be defined. For example (Table XVIII), lipotrope deprivation at different times during the prenatal and perinatal periods affects the response of offspring to the stress of infection. Clearly, the prenatal period is a time when the immune system of the developing embryo and fetus is subject to profound effects of deprivation, and these effects have long-range influences on immunocompetence later in life.

6. Discussion

The early discovery that choline was the constituent in lecithin that prevented fatty liver (Best and Huntsman, 1932) by inhibiting the accumulation of triacylglycerols and promoting the removal of excess fat from the liver initiated much fundamental research in lipid metabolism, liver homeostasis, and carcinogenesis. Short-term studies in choline-deficient rats clarified the interrelationships between choline and other lipotrops (methionine, folate, vitamin B_{12}) and led to elucidation of phospholipid biosynthesis and recognition of the significance of lipid metabolism in hepatocyte membrane integrity.

Reports of liver cancer in rats fed choline-deficient diet only (without added known carcinogen) provoked much excitement in the scientific community because this was a rare finding, that taking something out of the diet, rather than adding something to it, resulted in the development of hepatocellular carcinoma (Copeland and Salmon, 1946). During the 1940s and 1950s dietary liver injury from choline deficiency and hepatocarcinogenesis received considerable attention. However, questions arose about the true nature of choline deficiency cancer induction when it was discovered that peanut meal used in the diets was often contaminated with AFB_1, a potent liver carcinogen (Newberne, 1967). Following this discovery, the choline deficiency model was largely discarded, even though a continuing series of studies (Lombardi and Shinozuka, 1979; Rogers and Newberne, 1980) established that choline deficiency sensitized the liver to numerous hepatocarcinogens.

More recently, provocative results from several laboratories have reopened the choline deficiency question with respect to cancer induction. My associates and I (Newberne *et al.*, 1982, 1983a,b), Mikol *et al.* (1983), and Ghoshal and Farber (1983) reported the occurrence of liver cancer in rodents fed the choline-deficient diet only. Because it only require 1 part per billion of AFB_1 to induce rodent liver cancer (Wogan *et al.*, 1974), the nagging question in the minds of some investigators is whether the choline-deficient diets contain contaminants (e.g., AFB_1, nitrosamines, pesticides) that are below the level of detection but which, in concert, may contribute to the development of cancer. This is a reasonable apprehension, given the increased sensitivity of the choline-deficient liver to a number of hepatotoxic and hepatocarcinogenic agents. However, the use of the rigidly controlled semisynthetic diets should preclude such an exposure. Our more recent work indicates that chronic injury from the choline-deficient diet, hepatocellular necrosis, and cell renewal, together with tissue peroxidation and failure of some important enzyme systems, may be important factors.

7. Summary and Conclusions

As noted earlier, we do not know the mechanisms by which lipotropes exert their influence on carcinogenesis. We have postulated that the effect of a lipotrope deficiency is exerted early in the carcinogenesis process, and that effects on carcinogen metabolism, hepatocyte turnover, the induction of hyperplastic foci, secretion of alpha-fetoprotein, and aberrant nucleic acid methylation, among others, may contribute to cancer. Immunocompetence as it may relate to cancer induction has received attention only recently. Although a direct linkage is not currently obvious among lipotropes, chemical activation, deactivation, immunocompetence, and cancer, the observations are highly suggestive for interactions. it is clear from data presented here that lipotrope deficiency results in altered xeno biotic metabolism and increased risk for chemically induced cancer of several cites.

The effects on the liver of the choline-deficient diet (lipid accumulation, cell death, hepatocyte proliferation, with or without fibrosis or cirrhosis) are basic to the carcinogenic process. The similarity of effects of the choline-deficient diet and of partial hepatectomy is superficial; the diet is effective as long as it is fed, whereas partial hepatectomy is only effective for about 2 weeks, i.e., until the liver mass is restored.

One must consider also the effects of hepatocyte lipid peroxidation. In the choline-deficient liver, the highly reactive lipoperoxidases may cause alterations in the genome, as indicated by the occurrence of products of peroxidation in the liver of choline-deficient rats.

The question of hypomethylation or aberrant methylation of nucleic acid bases and an influence of cellular control mechanisms in the choline-deprived liver is important. Apparently, hypomethylation does occur under these conditions, but in our experiments, it occurs as a measurable event as a late phenomenon (6 months) and might be considered a promotional event. Currently, some believe that hypomethylation, persisting through more than one cycle of DNA replication, in some manner permanently modifies gene expression (Razin and Riggs, 1980; Felsenfeld and McGhee, 1982). In any case, the extent and pattern of DNA methylation are now considered to control expression of genetic information. Gene activity frequently correlates with hypomethylation (Doerfler, 1983). In addition to the data reported here, Wainfan and associates (1986) found that liver tRNA isolated from rats fed a lipotrope-deficient diet is hypomethylated and that the activity of guanine tRNA methyltransferase is increased, mimicking the effects of the liver carcinogen ethionine. Thus, not only is DNA hypomethylated, but tRNA, critical to normal cell proliferation, is hypomethylated in the choline-deficient liver.

We will probably have the means at hand soon for dissecting the basic role of diet-induced injury that contributes to the enhancing effect of lipotrope deficiency in hepatocellular carcinoma as more molecular biology techniques are utilized in our studies. This will move our efforts in understanding carcinogenesis considerably ahead and contribute to the ultimate goal of preventing liver cell neopalsia and perhaps other types of cancer. Lipotropes, natural components of our daily diet, deserve more attention from our oncology investigators.

8. References

Barker, M. O., and Hamilton, J. G., 1968, Incorporation of ^{14}C-methyl groups from methionine into subfractions of rat liver phosphatidyl choline, *Fed. Proc.* **27**:361.

Becker, R. A., Barrows, L. R., and Shank, R. C., 1981, Methylation of liver DNA guanine in hydrazine hepatotoxicity: Dose–response and kinetic characteristics of 7-methyl guanine and O-6-methylguanine formation and persistence in rats, *Carcinogenesis* **2**:1181–1188.

Best, C. H., and Huntsman, M. E., 1932, The effects of the components of lecithin upon deposition of fat in the liver, *J. Physiol.* **75**:405–412.

Best, C. H., Hershey, J. M., and Huntsman, M. E., 1932, The effect of lecithin on fat deposition in the liver of the normal rat, *J. Physiol.* **75**:56–66.

Broad, W. J., 1982, Toying with the truth to win a Nobel, *Science* **217**:1120–11122.

Campbell, T. C., Hayes, J. R., and Newberne, P. M., 1978, Dietary lipotropes, hepatic mixed function oxidase activities and in vivo covalent binding of aflatoxin B$_1$ in rats, *Cancer Res.* **38**:4569–4573.

Casini, A. F., Pompella, A., and Comporti, M., 1985, Liver glutathione depletion induced by bromobenzene iodobenzene and diethylmaleate poisoning and its relation to lipid peroxidation and necrosis, *Am. J. Pathol.* **118**:225–237.

Copeland, D. H., and Salmon, W. D., 1946, The occurrence of neoplasms in the liver, lungs and other tissues of rats as a result of prolonged choline deficiency, *Am. J. Pathol.* **22**:1059–1079.

Doefler, W., 1983, DNA methylation and gene activity, *Annu. Rev. Biochem.* **52**:93–124.

Farber, S., Diamond, L. K., and Mercer, R. D., 1948, Folate antimetabolites in leukemia therapy, *N. Engl. J. Med.* **238**:787–792.

Felsenfeld, G., and McGhee, J., 1982, Methylation and gene control, *Nature* **296**:602–608.

Follis, R. H., Jr., 1958, *Deficiency disease: The pathology of Nutritional disease; Physiological and Morphological Changes which Result from Deficiencies of the Essential elements, Amino Acids, Vitamins and Fatty Acids,* Charles C Thomas, Springfield, IL, pp. 251–262.

Gebhardt, B., and Newberne, P. M., 1974, Nutritional and immunological responsiveness: T-cell function in the offspring of lipotrope- and protein-deficient rats, *Immunology* **26**:489–496.

Ghoshal, A. K., and Farber, E., 1983, Induction of liver cancer by a diet deficient in choline and methionine, *Proc. Am. Assoc. Cancer Res.* **24**:98.

Ghoshal, A. K., Rushmore, T., Lim, Y., et al., 1984, Early detection of lipid peroxidation in the hepatic nuclei of rats fed a diet deficient in choline and methionine, *Cancer Res.* **25**:94.

Gill, T. J., and Gershoff, S. N., 1967, The effects of methionine and ethionine on antibody formation in primates, *J. Immunol.* **99**:883–893.

Goldstone, A. H., Calder, E., Barnes, E. W., and Irvine, W. J., 1973, The effect of gastric antigens on the *in vitro* migration of leukocytes from patients with atrophic gastritis and pernicious anemia, *Clin. Exp. Immunol.* **14**:501–508.

Gross, R. L., and Newberne, P. M., 1976, Malnutrition, the thymolymphatic system and immunocompetence, in: *The Reticuloendothelial System in Health and Disease* (H. Friedman, M. Escobar, and S. Reiehard, eds.), Plenum Press, New York, pp. 179–188.

Gross, R. L., and Newberne, P. M., 1980, Role of nutrition and immunologic function, *Physiol. Rev.* **60**:188–302.

Gross, R. L., Reid, J. V., Newberne, P. M., Burgess, B., Marston, R., and Hift, W., 1975, Depressed cell-mediated immunity in megaloblastic anemia due to folic acid deficiency, *Am. J. Clin. Nutr.* **28**:225–232.

Haltalin, K. C., Nelson, J. D., and Woodman, E. G., 1970, Fatal *Shigella* infection induced by folic acid deficiency in young guinea pigs, *J. Infect. Dis.* **121**:275–290.

Helliwell, T. R., Yeung, J. H. K., and Park, B. K., 1985, Hepatic necrosis and glutathione depletion in captopril-treated mice, *Br. J. Exp. Pathol.* **66**:67–78.

Hershey, J. M., 1930, Substitution of lecithin for raw pancreas in the diet of the depancreatized dog, *Am. J. Physiol.* **93**:657.

Hertz, R., Ross, G. T., and Lipsett, M. B., 1963, Primary chemotherapy of nonmetastatic trophoblastic disease of women, *Am. J. Obstet. Gynecol.* **86**:808–814.

Iype, P. T., and McMahon, J. B., 1984, Hepatic proliferation inhibitor, *Mol. Cell Biochem.* **59**:57–80.

Jallou, D. J., Mitchell, J. R., Zampaglione, N., and Gillette, J. R., 1974, Bromobenzene-induced liver necrosis.

Protective role of glutathione and evidence for 3,4-bromobenzene oxide as the heaptic metabolite, *Pharmacology* **11**:151–169.

Jewell, S. A., Bellows, G., Thor, H., Orrenius, S., and Smith, M. T., 1982, Bleb formation in hepatocytes during drug metabolism caused by disturbances in thiol and calcium ion homeostasis, *Science* **217**:1257–1259.

Jose, D. J., and Good, R. A., 1973, Quantitative effects of nutritional essential amino acid deficiency upon immune responses to tumors in mice, *J. Exp. Med.* **137**:1–9.

LaBrecque, D. R., and Dachur, N. R., 1982, Hepatic stimulator substance: Physico-chemical characteristics and specificity, *Am. J. Physiol.* **242**:G281–G288.

Lombardi, B., and Shinozuka, H., 1979, Enhancement of 2-AAF liver carcinogenesis in rats fed a choline-devoid diet, *Int. J. Cancer* **23**:565–572.

MacCuisk, A. C., Urbaniak, S., and Goldstone, A. H., 1974, PHA responsiveness and subpopulations of circulating lymphocytes in pernicious anemia, *Blood* **44**:849–855.

MacSween, R. N., Anthony, P. P., and Scheuer, P. J., 1979, *Pathology of The Liver*, Churchill Livingstone, Edinburgh, pp. 146–305.

Mikol, Y. B., and Poirier, L. A., 1981, An inverse correlation between hepatic ornithine decarboxylase and *S*-adenosylmethionine in rats, *Cancer Lett.* **13**:195–201.

Mikol, Y. B., Hoover, K. L., Creasia, D., and Poirier, L., 1983, Hepatocarcinogenesis in rats fed methyl-deficient, amino acid–defined diets, *Carcinogenesis* **4**:1619–1629.

Nauss, K. M., and Newberne, P. M., 1981, Effects of dietary folate, vitamin B_{12} and methionine/choline deficiency on immune function, in: *Diet and Resistance to Disease* (M. Phillips, and A. Baetz, eds.), Plenum Press, New York, pp. 63–91.

Newberne, P. M., 1967, Biological activity of the aflatoxins in domestic and laboratory animals, U.S. Fish Wildlife Serv. Res. Rep. **70**:131–144.

Newberne, P. M., 1986, Lipotropic factors and oncogenesis, in: *Essential Nutrients in Carcinogenesis* (L. Poirier, P. M. Newberne, and M. Pariza, eds.), Plenum Press, New York, pp. 223–251.

Newberne, P. M., and Rogers, A. E., 1986, The role of nutrients in cancer causation, in: *Diet, Nutrition, and Cancer* (Y. Hayashi, M. Nagao, and T. Sugimura, eds.), Japan Scientific Societies, Tokyo, pp. 205–224.

Newberne, P. M., and Wilson, R. B., 1972, Prenatal malnutrition and postnatal responses to infection, *Nutr. Rep.* **5**:151–160.

Newberne, P. M., and Young, V. R., 1973, Marginal maternal vitamin B_{12}: Long-term effects, *Nature* **242**:263.

Newberne, P. M., Bresnahan, M. R., and Kula, N. S., 1969a, Effects of two synthetic antioxidants, vitamin E and ascorbic acid on the choline deficient diet, *J. Nutr.* **97**:219–231.

Newberne, P. M., Rogers, A. E., Bailey, C., and Young, V. R., 1969b, The induction of liver cirrhosis in rats by purified amino acid diets, *Cancer Res.* **29**:230–235.

Newberne, P. M., deCamargo, J. L., and Clark, A. J., 1982, Choline deficiency, partial hepatectomy and liver tumors in rats and mice. *Toxicol. Pathol.* **2**:95–109.

Newberne, P. M., Rogers, A. E., and Nauss, K. M., 1983a, Choline, methionine and related factors in oncogenesis, in: *Nutritional Factors in the Induction and Maintenance of Malignancy* (C. E. Butterworth, and M. Hutchinson, eds.), Academic Press, New York, pp. 247–271.

Newberne, P. M., Nauss, K. M., and deCamargo, J. L., 1983b, Lipotropes, immunocompetence and cancer, *Cancer Res.* **43**:2426s–2434s.

Orrenius, S., Armstad, K., Thor, H., and Jewell, S. A., 1983, Turnover and functions of glutathione studied in isolated hepatic and renal cells, *Fed. Proc.* **42**:3177–3188.

Perera, M., Demetris, A., and Katyal, S., 1984, Lipid peroxidation as a possible underlying mechanism of liver tumor promotion by a choline deficient diet, *Cancer Res.* **25**:141.

Poirier, L. A., and Whitehead, V. U., 1973, Folate deficiency and formiminoglutamic acid excretion during chronic diethylnitrosamine administration to rats, *Cancer Res.* **33**:383–388.

Poirier, L. A., Grantham, P. H., and Rogers, A. E., 1977, The effects of a marginally lipotrope-deficient diet on the hepatic levels of *S*-adenosyl-methionine and on the urinary metabolites of 2-acetylaminofluorene in rats, *Cancer Res.* **37**:744–748.

Razin, A., and Riggs, A. D., 1980, DNA methylation and gene function, *Science* **210**:604–607.

Rechnagel, R. O., and Ghoshal, A. K., 1966, Quantitative estimation of peroxidative degeneration of rat liver microsomal and mitochondrial lipids after carbon tetrachloride poisoning, *Exp. Mol. Pathol.* **5**:413–426.

Roebuck, B. D., Yager, J. D., and Longnecker, D. S., 1981, Dietary modulation of azaserine-induced pancreatic carcinogenesis in the rat, *Cancer Res.* **41**:888–893.

Rogers, A. E., and Newberne, P. M., 1971, Diet and aflatoxin B_1 toxicity in rats, *Toxicol. Appl. Pharmacol.* **20**:113–121.

Rogers, A. E., and Newberne, P. M., 1973, Dietary enhancement of intestinal carcinogenesis by dimethylhydrazine in rats, *Nature* **246**:491–492.

Rogers, A. E., and Newberne, P. M., 1980, Lipotrope deficiency in experimental carcinogenesis, *Nutr. Cancer* **2**:104–112.

Salmon, W. D., and Copeland, D. H., 1954, Liver carcinoma and related lesions in chronic choline deficiency, *Ann. NY Acad. Sci.* **57**:664–667.

Salmon, W. D., and Newberne, P. M., 1963, Occurrence of hepatomas in rats fed diets containing peanut meal as a major source of protein, *Cancer Res.* **23**:571–576.

Shinozuka, H., Katyal, S. L., and Lombardi, B., 1978, Azaserine carcinogenesis: Organ susceptibility change in rats fed a diet devoid of choline, *Int. J. Cancer* **22**:36–39.

Stacey, N. H., and Klassen, C. D., 1981, Inhibition of lipid peroxidation without prevention of cellular injury in isolated rat hepatocytes, *Toxical. Appl. Pharmacol.* **58**:8–18.

Tai, C., and McGuigan, J. E., 1969, Immunologic studies in pernicious anemia, *Blood* **34**:63–71.

Tinoco, J., Shannon, A., and Lyman, R., 1964, Serum lipids in choline-deficient male and female rats, *J. Lipid Res.* **5**:57–62.

Wainfan, E., Diznik, M., and Hluboky, M., 1986, Alteration of tRNA methylation in rats fed lipotrope-deficient diets, *Carcinogenesis* **7**:473–476.

Wilson, M. J., Shivapurkar, N., and Poirier, L. A., 1984, Hypomethylation of hepatic nuclear DNA in rats fed with a carcinogenic methyl-deficient diet, *Biochem. J.* **218**:987–994.

Wilson, R. B., Kula, N. S., Newberne, P. M., and Connor, M. W., 1973, Vascular damage and lipid peroxidation in choline-deficient rats, *Exp. Mol. Pathol.* **18**:357–368.

Wogan, G. N., Paglialunga, A. S., and Newberne, P. M., 1974, Carcinogenic effects of low dietary levels of aflatoxin B_1 in rats, *Food Cosmet. Toxicol.* **12**:681–690.

9

The Effects of Caloric Restriction on Neoplasia and Age-Related Degenerative Processes

Bruce Ruggeri

1. Introduction

The role of diet in the etiology of cancer is a subject of ongoing controversy and continued research (for reviews, see Reddy and Cohen, 1986; Reddy, 1986; Ip *et al.*, 1986; Cohen, 1987). As noted by Brown (1983), a National Academy of Sciences 2-year study concluded that "although it is difficult to prove firmly a cause-and-effect relationship, the total evidence suggests that some type of dietary components tend to increase the risk of cancer and other types of diets or components tend to decrease the risk" (NAS, 1982). Wynder and Gori (1977) attributed approximately 40% of cancer incidence in men and 60% in women to dietary patterns. Similar estimates for the incidence of potentially preventable cancers in relation to dietary practices have been made by other workers (Bailar, 1979; Cimino and Demopoulous, 1980). Most animal studies indicate that dietary factors probably act at the promotional stage of carcinogenesis (Brown, 1983), although more recent studies (Kritchevsky *et al.*, 1984; Welsch, 1987; Albanes, 1987a,b; Hocman, 1988) suggest that dietary factors (i.e., high-fat, high-calorie intake) may influence both initiation and promotion of tumorigenesis.

The data suggesting a role of diet in the etiology of numerous cancers is largely based on epidemiologic studies in human populations, but has been substantiated by experimental animal studies. The promotional role of the level and type of dietary fat has been examined in colon cancer induced by a variety of carcinogenic agents and promoted by bile acid derivatives (Carroll, 1981, 1986); in murine melanoma growth and lymphocyte-mediated cytotoxicity (Erickson, 1984); and extensively in rodent mammary tumorigenesis induced by *N*-nitrosomethylurea (Chan *et al.*, 1977; Thompson *et al.*, 1985; Beth *et al.*, 1987; Cohen *et al.*, 1988) and 7,12-dimethylenz(a)anthracene (Hopkins and Carroll,

---

Bruce Ruggeri • Department of Pathology, The Fox Chase Cancer Center, Philadelphia, Pennsylvania 19117.

1979; Hopkins *et al.*, 1981; Welsch and Aylsworth, 1983; Clinton *et al.*, 1984; Kritchevsky *et al.*, 1984, 1986; Lane *et al.*, 1985). These findings and earlier studies have been reviewed and summarized (Kritchevsky, 1982; Erickson and Thomas, 1985; Welsch, 1987). In general, animals fed diets higher in polyunsaturated fats demonstrate greater tumor incidence and tumor growth rate than animals maintained on isocaloric diets in which saturated fats were the dominant dietary lipid. These results are due in part to an essential fatty acid (i.e., linoleic acid) requirement for mammary tumor growth (4–5% total calories) exceeding that required for the host animal (Ip *et al.*, 1985). With either type of dietary fat regimen, mammary tumor incidence is generally diminished in animals having a lower percentage of total fat in their diets (see Welsch, 1987; Hocman, 1988). Recent findings suggest that diets elevated in saturated fatty acids may play a critical role in the initiation of mammary tumorigenesis (see Welsch, 1987).

Studies by Carroll (1975, 1981) based on worldwide epidemiologic data suggested strong correlations between the mortality from breast, colon, and endometrial cancer and the consumption of neutral fats. Dietary recommendations to reduce fat intake to approximately 30% of calories (NAS, 1982) are based on these findings. As discussed by Willet *et al.* (1987) and others (Kelsey and Berkowitz, 1988), however, the relationship between dietary fat intake and breast cancer in particular has been examined in only a few case–control and prospective studies, with slight or no positive association ascertained. In many instances, the dietary assessment protocols were insufficiently comprehensive to provide accurate calculations of total fat intake (see Willet *et al.*, 1987). Willet *et al.* (1987), in a prospective study of 89,538 U.S. registered nurses between the age of 34 and 59 having no family history of breast cancer, found no evidence that total fat consumption or consumption of specific types of fat was positively correlated with breast cancer risk, in agreement with the findings of others (Graham *et al.*, 1982; Newman *et al.*, 1986; Hirohata *et al.*, 1985, 1987; Mills *et al.*, 1988). Goodwin and Boyd (1987) published a critical appraisal of human epidemiologic studies relating dietary fat to breast cancer risk. Their analyses and that of others (Kelsey and Berkowitz, 1988) indicated that the inconsistency of published evidence and weak association between dietary fat and breast cancer risk make it possible to conclude a causal relationship or appropriately apply the criteria for causal inference. Further, it was demonstrated that international correlation studies consistently demonstrated a strong positive association between dietary fat and breast cancer risk, but stronger study designs (case–control and cohort studies) failed to demonstrate a significant association, in agreement with the aforementioned studies (Graham *et al.*, 1982; Hirohata *et al.*, 1985, 1987; Willet *et al.*, 1987; Mills *et al.*, 1988). Methodologic limitations, particularly inaccurate or limited measurements of past dietary practices and the relatively small ranges of fat intake examined, may have been partly responsible for a weak association between dietary fat intake and cancer risk in humans (Goodwin and Boyd, 1987; Kelsey and Berkowitz, 1988). In this regard Willet *et al.* (1987) noted that the influence of dietary fat intake prior to adulthood or at levels below 30% of total caloric intake on breast cancer incidence was not evaluated in their study. Moreover, the possible implications of caloric intake during childhood or adolescence on the interpretation of international epidemiologic data relating per capita fat intake and cancer incidence warranted further evaluation, according to these investigators and others (see Albanes *et al.*, 1988; Swanson *et al.*, 1988). In summary, "the role of a high fat diet in breast cancer etiology is uncertain, but if it is a risk factor, it is unlikely to be a strong one" (Kelsey and Berkowitz, 1988).

2. Body Indices in Relation to Cancer Risk and Recurrence

The classic studies of Tannenbaum (1940a) suggested increased cancer mortality in relation to obesity in human populations. Similarly, in a review of experimental animal data during this period, a number of investigators (Bullough, 1950; Loeb *et al.*, 1942; Waxler, 1954, 1960) adduced a direct relationship between increased body weight in various strains of mice (e.g., from gold thioglucose–induced obesity) and the development of spontaneous mammary tumors. Similar findings from long-term animal studies have recently been addressed in detail (Wolff, 1987; Rao *et al.*, 1987; Albanes, 1987a). Albanes (1987a) examined the relationship between caloric intake, body weight, and murine tumorigenesis at various sites using data from 82 published experiments. The major results of these analyses indicated that the incidence of chemically induced and spontaneous tumors (primarily skin and mammary) in mice was proportional in an approximate dose-dependent manner to the level of caloric intake and resulting body weight over a wide range of macronutrient intakes, including moderate caloric restriction. Most important, this total calorie–body weight relationship with tumorigenesis was independent of the dietary fat intake in the experimental data analyzed (Albanes, 1987a). The magnitude of reduction in body weight required for a significant reduction in tumor incidence has been shown to vary with the neoplasm, with a 10–20% reduction inhibiting mammary tumorigenesis in mice, while weight reduction by 30–50% of *ad libitum*-fed controls was necessary for a significant reduction of hepatic or lymphoreticular tumors (Rao *et al.*, 1987; Hocman, 1988).

More recent human epidemiologic studies (Doll and Peto, 1981) have indicated that the incidence of several types of cancers, including stomach, colorectal, pancreatic, gallbladder, endometrial, and cervical, is significantly increased in those population groups having above-average body weight. Lew and Garfinkel (1979) and Garfinkel (1985) reported on a long-term prospective study by the American Cancer Society (1959–1972) on 750,000 men and women from the general population. Mortality for women from cancer of the breast, ovaries, uterus, endometrium, cervix, and gallbladder was increased by 55% but only among those individuals greater than or equal to 40% over their ideal body weight. Males demonstrated a greater than 30% increase in mortality for colorectal cancer among individuals in this higher-weight category, suggesting a possible threshold for body weight in relation to cancer risk and mortality.

A recent detailed review of human epidemiologic data by Albanes (1987b) revealed that cancer incidence and mortality at a number of sites (breast, colon, rectum, prostate, endometrium, kidney, cervix, ovary, thyroid, and gallbladder) increase with excess body weight and to a lesser extent caloric intake, although the influence of calories *per se* from dietary fat was difficult to discern. These collective epidemiologic data in humans thus corroborate observations based on animal data demonstrating the relationship of benign and malignant tumor incidence to caloric intake and body weight.

With regard to breast cancer risk specifically, Greenberg *et al.* (1985) and Hebert *et al.* (1988) reported findings from epidemiologic studies on pre- and postmenopausal breast cancer patients suggesting that increased body weight (to a greater extent than height or body mass index) is strongly related to increased recurrence and reduced survival from breast cancer, even after accounting for additional variables associated with elevated risk. Moreover, the effect of overweight on breast cancer risk recurrence was most pronounced among women with otherwise favorable prognostic indicators, e.g., those with early stage disease (Hebert *et al.*, 1988). Similarly, increased body weight in relation to increased breast cancer risk and or reduced survival time has been demonstrated in studies from Canada (Newman *et al.*, 1986), China (Yuan *et al.*, 1988; Tao *et al.*, 1988), the Netherlands, and Japan (DeWaard *et al.*, 1977). Further, several studies have reported an association of high body weight with axillary lymphy node involvement (DeWaard *et al.*, 1977; Greenberg *et al.*, 1985). In contrast, Williams and co-workers (1988) observed that body weight was not correlated with survival, progression of disease, or response to endocrine therapy in patients who either presented with or developed advanced cancer of the breast. Moreover, no correlation of high body weight and the estrogen receptor status of primary tumors was observed, although a positive association was noted between high body weight and progesterone receptor positivity, particularly among estrogen-receptor-positive tumors (Williams *et al.*, 1988). Among postmenopausal women, obesity may present a potentially greater risk for breast cancer due to an increased adipose tissue conversion of androstenedione to estrone and lower levels of circulating sex-hormone binding globulin, thus increasing the availability of circulating estrogens to peripheral tissues (Hebert *et al.*, 1988; Kelsey and Berkowitz, 1988).

In addition to body weight and body mass indices, adult height or stature has been implicated as a risk factor for breast cancer in some, but not all, studies (see Willet, 1987; Albanes *et al.*, 1988; Swanson *et al.*, 1988, and references within). Albanes *et al.* (1988) examined anthropomorphic data from the U.S. National Health and Nutrition Examination Survey and its follow-up study and deduced that for most cancer sites in men, particularly colorectal cancer, the lowest incidence was observed among those in the shortest quartile of stature. This relationship was stronger for men than women and appeared across subgroups of age, race, socioeconomic status, and body mass index (Albanes *et al.*, 1988). Analysis of the same anthropomorphic data by Swanson *et al.* (1988) revealed that the risk of breast cancer in pre- and postmenopausal women was increased in individuals who were taller and had a larger frame size. Body weight, relative weight, and skinfold measurements of adiposity were not associated with increased breast cancer risk (Swanson *et al.*, 1988; Kolonel *et al.*, 1986). These collective data suggest the importance of childhood and adolescent nutrition—a major influence in the determination of adult stature—in relation to future cancer risk in humans (Albanes *et al.*, 1988). As discussed by Willet (1987), the interpretation of data relating stature to cancer risk in case–control or cohort studies within a given setting is complex, as height and stature may largely reflect genetic factors in some populations and nutritional status during development in others. Hebert *et al.* (1988) postulated that stature may affect breast cancer risk but not survival, but given the relatively strong correlations between height and both body mass index and weight, the former may be related to prognosis as well.

Based on available epidemiologic data, a number of workers (Garfinkel, 1985; Albanes, 1987a,b; Hocman, 1988) concluded that the regularity with which obesity is found as a risk factor in a number of studies suggests that reducing caloric intake and relative body weight may lead to a considerable reduction in cancer risk in humans (see also Kelsey and Berkowitz, 1988; Rohan and Bain, 1987).

3. Caloric Restriction and Neoplasia

Of potentially greater importance than the influence of dietary fat on neoplastic promotion is the phenomenon of caloric restriction. Hocman (1988) has concluded that in both humans and rodents the restriction of energy intake from *all* dietary sources is more important in the prevention of carcinogenesis than dietary fat content, the latter playing a secondary role only (see also Lyon *et al.*, 1987). The effects of caloric restriction on reducing the onset and promotion of a variety of neoplastic and degenerative disease processes in rodents have been observed widely (for excellent reviews, see White, 1961; Pariza, 1986, 1987; Kritchevsky and Klurfeld, 1987). In this regard, while a wide range of chemical, hormonal, and pharmacological interventions have been examined for their potential to extend lifespan and life expectancy in laboratory animals (rodents) (see Schneider and Reed, 1985), the only consistent and reproducible method for achieving these effects has been caloric restriction. These observations were first reported by McCay and co-workers in the 1930s (McCay and Cromwell, 1934; McCay *et al.*, 1939) and have subsequently been verified by numerous workers (Weindruch *et al.*, 1979, 1986; Masoro *et al.*, 1982; Harrison *et al.*, 1984; Conner-Johnson *et al.*, 1986; Gajjar *et al.*, 1987; Kubo *et al.*, 1987). Reviews by Masoro (1985) and Hocman (1988) have examined in detail the scope and mechanistic basis of these findings with regard to the effects of caloric restriction delaying or preventing a host of age-associated physiological and biochemical aberrations, including neoplasia.

Among the earliest studies on caloric restriction and tumor growth were those of Moreschi (1909), who demonstrated that underfeeding could inhibit the growth of transplantable sarcomas in mice. Rous (1914) observed a reduction in spontaneous mammary tumor incidence in mice maintained on a calorically restricted regimen compared to *ad libitum*-fed controls. He further observed a growth-retarding effect on both the host animal and well-developed transplanted sarcomas in calorically restricted animals, but no effect on the development of the Flexner–Jobling rat carcinoma. Subsequent studies by Bischoff and co-workers (1935) demonstrated that a 50% reduction in caloric intake reduced the growth and development of the murine sarcoma 180, whereas less severe restriction produced little or no retardation of tumor growth.

The most extensive studies conducted on calorie restriction and spontaneous and carcinogen-induced tumor growth were those of Tannenbaum in the 1940s. Tannenbaum (1940b) examined the effects of *ad libitum* feeding and underfeeding one-half to one-third and the *ad libitum*-fed intake on the incidence of spontaneous mammary tumors in DBA mice. (The diet consisted of wheat, commercial dog chow, skim milk powder, and flour and was estimated to be 64% carbohydrate, 17% protein, 5% fat, and 3% ash.) Tumor incidence after 64 weeks of feeding the experimental diets was 30% and 7% in the *ad libitum*-fed and underfed groups, respectively. In examining the effects of 60% caloric restriction on benzo(a)pyrene-induced tumors in mice, Tannenbaum (1942) demonstrated that this intervention inhibited tumor growth to varying degrees in ABC, Swiss, or DBA strains. Subsequent studies (Tannenbaum, 1944, 1945a,b) confirmed earlier studies and those of others (Visscher *et al.*, 1942) regarding the inhibitory effect of caloric restriction on spontaneous mammary, lung, and hepatic tumors, as well as 3-methyl-cholanthrene- and 3,4-benzopyrene-induced epitheliomas and sarcomas. A hallmark of these collective studies was the finding that tumor incidence and latency were dependent on the degree of caloric restriction (as controlled by altering the proportion of cornstarch to a ration of fox chow and skimmed milk powder) and the composition of the diet; i.e., a high-fat diet was a stronger promoter than a low-fat diet at any degree of restriction. Thus, it was concluded that while *ad libitum*-fed animals demonstrated a higher tumor incidence, a specific action of fat, in addition to and independent of its net caloric effect, was influencing tumor growth. Furthermore, the most significant inhibition of tumor growth was observed when dietary restriction was imposed shortly after carcinogen treatment. Subsequent studies during this period further demonstrated the role of caloric restriction in inhibiting the development of spontaneous murine mammary tumors (White *et al.*, 1944), spontaneous lung tumors (Larsen and Heston, 1945), and murine leukemia (Saxton *et al.*, 1944).

The studies of Lavik and Baumann (1943) strengthened the case for a caloric influence on tumor promotion. It was observed that regardless of the level of dietary fat, the incidence of 3-methylcholanthrene-induced skin tumors was significantly higher on a high-calorie regimen compared to a low-calorie one. These observations suggested that at least part of the tumor-promoting action of fat was due to an accompanying increase in caloric consumption. Subsequent studies by Boutwell and co-workers (1949a,b) suggested that the difference in "net available energy" in high- versus low-fat diets may explain the promotional effects of dietary fat. Most convincing in this regard was a study (Boutwell *et al.*, 1949a) in which rats were maintained on isocaloric diets containing either 2% fat or 61% fat, yet did not demonstrate a highly significant increase in tumor incidence in the latter group despite their extremely high levels of dietary fat.

Despite the extensive observations made regarding caloric restriction and neoplastic growth, research in this field waned until the 1970s with the advent of more carefully controlled studies such as those of Ross and Bras (1971, 1973). These workers examined the effects of long- and short-term caloric restriction (and underfeeding) of varying duration in postweaned rats over their entire lifetime. Of the 25 taxonomic tumor types examined, tumors of hematopoietic and lymphoreticular origin were least responsive to caloric restriction. Benign tumors and tumors of epithelial and endocrine tissues were markedly affected, particularly by caloric restriction early in postweaning life; e.g., caloric restriction reduced tumor incidence even in animals restricted only 4 weeks (Ross and Bras, 1971). Significant was the observation that tumor incidence correlated with body weight of mature rats from the lightest to the heaviest animals, a finding subsequently confirmed in later studies (Ross *et al.*, 1983). As noted by Lagopoulous and Stalder (1987), the reduction in tumor incidence in calorically restricted animals is more closely correlated with the reduced body weight gain observed on such a regimen, rather than caloric restriction *per se*, since reducing body weight gain by elevating metabolism produced comparable reduction in tumor incidence despite normal food consumption (see Tannenbaum and Silverstone, 1949). With regard to these lifetime studies of Ross and Bras, Connor-Johnson and co-workers (1986) noted that dietary restriction of mice could be instituted as late as middle life or beyond and still exert its delaying effect on the onset of neoplastic disease and prolongation of lifespan (see Hocman, 1988).

During the mid-1970s, a number of reports appeared (Jose and Good, 1973; Gerbase-

DeLima *et al.*, 1975; Fernandes *et al.*, 1976) demonstrating that chronic protein–calorie or caloric restriction of rodents during postweaning life led to immunosuppression at an early age, but subsequently prolonged and heightened cell-mediated immune responsiveness and lifespan in these animals. Reduction in the incidence and growth of spontaneous mammary adenocarcinoma and mastocytoma was also observed in animals on these regimens (Jose and Good, 1973; Fernandes et al., 1976).

Tucker (1979) observed that spontaneous mammary, pituitary, and skin tumors were significantly reduced (and lifespan increased) in 20% underfed Wistar rats and Swiss albino mice maintained on such a regimen for 2 years.

A major flaw of many of the early and more recent studies of calorie restriction and tumorigenesis described here has been poor nutritional design. In a majority of early studies, the nutritional requirements of the rat were not fully known. Consequently, a "low fat" diet, e.g., 0.5 or 1% of calories, is not nutritionally adequate and may, in fact, result in essential fatty acid deficiency of both the host and the developing neoplasm (see Ip *et al.*, 1985). A second major flaw common to all but a few studies (Jose and Good, 1973; Fernandes *et al.*, 1976; Sarkar *et al.*, 1982; Masoro *et al.*, 1982; Reddy *et al.*, 1987) is the fact that caloric restriction was achieved by giving less food from an *ad libitum*-fed chow or standard dietary formulation; this potentially creates a malnourished condition and not an undernourished state in which the proportions of essential macro- and micronutrients in semipurified diets are varied, but absolute intakes maintained relatively constant (see Weindruch *et al.*, 1979; Masoro *et al.*, 1982; Kritchevsky *et al.*, 1984, 1986; Klurfeld *et al.*, 1987; Thompson *et al.*, 1985; Boissoneault *et al.*, 1986; Pariza, 1986, 1987; Cohen *et al.*, 1988). These flaws in experimental design complicate accurate interpretation of otherwise interesting studies.

In their studies on 7,12-dimethylbenzanthracene (DMBA)-induced mammary carcinogenesis and 1,2-dimethylhydrazine (DMH)-induced colon carcinogenesis, Kritchevsky and co-workers (1984, 1986; Klurfeld *et al.*, 1987) employed experimental designs in which the relative proportions of nutrients were similar and absolute amounts of macro- and micronutrients, except for carbohydrate, the same for all treatment groups. These workers observed (1984) that calorie intake may play a more paramount role than dietary fat in influencing DMBA-induced mammary tumorigenesis in Sprague–Dawley rats. Diets calorically restricted by 40%, yet providing 115% more fat than an *ad libitum*-fed diet, inhibited tumor incidence completely compared to *ad libitum*-fed rats (58% incidence). A similarly designed study using corn oil (at 15%) as the predominant dietary lipid resulted in a 20% tumor incidence in 40% restricted animals compared to 80% incidence in the *ad libitum*-fed animals; tumor weight, tumor burden, and tumors/tumor-bearing rats were likewise reduced in calorically restricted animals (Kritchevsky *et al.*, 1984). Subsequent studies (Klurfeld *et al.*, 1987) employing *ad libitum*-fed diets (at 5, 15, or 20% fat) and 25% calorically restricted diets (at 20 and 26.7% fat) further distinguished a fat-specific effect from an effect of overall calorie intake. Increasing dietary fat in the *ad libitum* diets caused an increase in tumor parameters examined, an effect inhibited in 25% calorically restricted animals despite their elevated fat intake. Similar findings have been reported by Thompson and co-workers (1985), who used a similar experimental approach to study *N*-methylnitrosurea-induced mammary tumorigenesis in rats over a 32-week period. This study in agreement with graded caloric restriction studies by Kritchevsky's group (Klurfeld *et al.*, 1989), concluded that the effects of dietary fat on the promotional stage of mammary tumorigenesis cannot be considered independent of the level of energy intake; i.e., a dietary intake approaching *ad libitum* is prerequisite for tumor promotion by dietary fat (Thompson *et al.*, 1985; Klurfeld *et al.*, 1989). These findings demonstrating an effect of caloric restriction independent of dietary fat on mammary tumorigenesis have been corroborated by Beth *et al.* (1987) and Cohen *et al.* (1988) in their methylnitrosourea (MNU)-induced mammary tumorigenesis studies in rats. Further, these collective findings provided further evidence that caloric restriction is effective against mammay tumorigenesis initiated by both indirect-acting (DMBA) and direct-acting (MNU) carcinogens.

The caloric restriction studies of Boissoneault *et al.* (1986) and Pariza (1986, 1987) have incorporated a concept initially described by Forbes *et al.* (1946), and most recently reevaluated by Donato and Hegsted (1985), that various dietary fuel sources are utilized with different levels of efficiency, with calories from fat being utilized more efficiently as indicated by less energy lost as heat from the animal and more energy retained in the carcass of the animal as fat (Donato, 1987). Pariza's findings, while substantiating the effects of caloric restriction on tumor growth, also suggest the importance of the complex interaction between energy intake, energy retention as lead body mass or adipose stores, and ultimate body size on tumor development (Pariza, 1986, 1987) rather than the amount or type of fat in the diet alone.

In contrast to these findings (Boissoneault *et al.*, 1986; Pariza, 1986, 1987), Cohen *et al.* (1988) demonstrated that body weight, percentage of body fat, and lean body mass were similar in *ad libitum*-fed sedentary rats independent of their dietary fat intake. Body fat, but not lean body mass, was significantly reduced by caloric restriction or moderate exercise concomitant with a marked inhibition of MNU-induced mammary tumorigenesis (Cohen *et al.*, 1988).

In addition to mammary tumorigenesis, caloric restriction has been examined with regard to a number of neoplasms common in Western societies. A limited body of data is available regarding caloric restriction and azaserine-induced pancreatic carcinomas in rats (Roebuck *et al.*, 1981a,b). These workers observed that a 10% caloric restriction caused a significant reduction in pancreatic neoplasms when administered during the initiation phase, but only a marginal effect in reducing tumor incidence during the promotional phase of tumorigenesis. Whether this marginal effect is a function of the azaserine carcinoma model *per se* or the result of only a moderate degree of caloric restriction is unclear at present.

Pollard and co-workers (1984, 1985) demonstrated an inhibition of methylazoxymethanol-induced intestinal tumorigenesis in 25% food-restricted rats, observing that restriction modified the tumorigenic response to an indirect-acting carcinogen (methylazoxymethanol acetate), but not a direct-acting one, the latter instilled intrarectally. More recently, Reddy *et al.* (1987) examined the effect of a high-fat (23.5%), semi-purified diet fed *ad libitum* and a 30% calorically restricted regimen on azoxymethane (AOM)-induced colon tumorigenesis in male F344 rats. Calorically restricted animals exhibited a 50% reduction in incidence of adenomas and 30% decrease in adenocarcinoma incidence. Tumor multiplicity and size were also reduced in restricted animals (Reddy *et al.*, 1987). A recent report by Klurfeld *et al.* (1987) demonstrated a 47% reduction in 1,2-dimethylhydrazine-induced color tumor incidence in 40% calorically restricted Fischer 344 rats, yet little or no alterations in tumor multiplicity compared to *ad libitum*-fed controls. An examination of colonic mucosal cytokinetics by these workers revealed that despite the significant reduction in colonic tumor incidence in calorically restricted rats, the latter displayed an increase in mucosal labeling index subsequent to [^{3}H]-thymidine autoradiography. This enhancement in mucosal cytokinetics was postulated to arise from the elevated fat consumption in the calorically restricted diet resulting in an increased level of colonic bile acids, the latter stimulating colonic epithelial cell turnover (Klurfeld *et al.*, 1987).

In addition to the studies just discussed, there have been reports regarding the effects of caloric or dietary restriction inhibiting radiation-induced tumors (Gross and Dreyfuss, 1984); virally induced leukemia (Ohno and Cardullo, 1983); murine B6 melanoma growth (Ershler *et al.*, 1986); diethylnitrosamine-induced hepatocarcinoma and adenoma incidence and growth in mice (Lagopoulos and Stalder, 1987); and the incidence, growth, and latency of DMBA-induced carcinomas in the cheek pouch epithelium of hamsters (Andreou and Morgan, 1981).

4. Potential Mechanisms by Which Caloric Restriction Inhibits Tumorigenesis

Despite decades of observations of the effects of caloric or dietary restriction on the inhibition of a broad spectrum of neoplasms in rodents, relatively little is known regarding mechanisms at the cellular and molecular level that might account for these pronounced effects. Table I lists a number of potential mechanisms or mediators by which dietary restriction may exert its effects on tumorigenesis. Evidence exists to support each of these, but in no instance, as yet, is any single mechanism fully explanatory (see also Hocman, 1988).

4.1. Activation of the Pituitary–Adrenocorticotropic Axis

With regard to a potential mechanism to explain the effects of caloric restriction on tumor growth, the early findings of Boutwell *et al.* (1949a,b) suggested the involvement of an activated pituitary–adrenocorticotropic axis. Boutwell *et al.* (1949b) reported that 40% caloric restriction of female rats resulted in a reduction in uterine and ovarian size, reduced gonadotropin secretion, and adrenal hypertrophy. These morphological changes accompany the increased production of adrenocorticotropic hormone (ACTH) and cortisol

Table 1. Potential Mechanisms by Which Caloric Restriction Inhibits Tumorigenesis

1. Active pituitary–adrenocorticotropic mechanism → elevated glucocorticoid levels → growth inhibition.
2. Reduced mitotic activity and cell proliferation.
3. Prolonged and heightened cell-mediated immune responsiveness.
4. Reduced nutrient availability to preneoplastic cells.
5. Alterations in mammotropic hormones and/or responsiveness in target tissues.
6. Alterations in nutritionally modulated peptide growth factors and/or receptor expression.
7. Modulation and repair of free radical–induced and carcinogen-mediated DNA damage.
8. Alterations in oncogene and protooncogene expression *in vivo*.

and reduced gonadotropin secretion consequent to caloric restriction (see Pariza, 1987). Similarly, Armario *et al.* (1987) reported that a 35% food restriction in adult male Sprague–Dawley rats caused alterations in ACTH and corticosterone circadian rhythms. These alterations were accompanied by elevated daily total corticosterone levels, but similar levels of total ACTH released daily compared to *ad libitum*-fed controls. Moreover, food restriction significantly depressed pulsatile growth hormone release, total growth hormone levels, and total thyroid-stimulating hormone levels in plasma (Armario *et al.*, 1987). Similar findings regarding ACTH and corticosterone circadian rhythms in 40% food-restricted Fischer rats have been reported by Stewart *et al.* (1988). These workers observed that the adrenocorticotropic response of rats subject to food restriction differs as a function of age. Young (5 month old) rats food restricted by 40% for 2 months displayed an elevated daily corticosterone level and normal adrenocortical response to stress. In contrast, aged rats (24 months) subjected to 1 month or lifelong 40% food restriction exhibited markedly reduced daily corticosterone levels and adrenal responsiveness to stress compared to *ad libitum*-fed animals of the same age (Stewart *et al.*, 1988). The influence of alterations in the pituitary–adrenocorticotropic axis on growth has been discussed by Loeb (1976), who noted the analogy between the effects of severe caloric deprivation in immature animals and children on depressing somatic growth and the physiological growth-depressing effects of a slight excess of circulating glucocorticoids (two to three times the average endogenous daily secretion). Moreover, the accelerated somatic growth observed upon restoration of calories resembles the accelerated growth and enhanced cell proliferation observed upon cessation of exogenous glucocorticoid therapy or management of clinical disorders (Cushing's syndrome) characterized by excess glucocorticoid secretion and growth suppression (Loeb, 1976). Based on these findings, Pariza (1987) and Hocman (1988) have alluded to a possible association between elevated glucocorticoid levels after moderate caloric restriction and a reduction in tumor incidence in experimental animals.

In support of a role for altered adrenal function and glucocorticoid status in tumorigenesis, Carter *et al.* (1988) demonstrated that adrenalectomy enhanced the carcinogenicity of DMBA in rats, increasing the incidence and multiplicity of mammary tumors and reducing tumor latency. These effects were enhanced synergistically upon grafting a prolactin-secreting pituitary transplant 6 days following carcinogen treatment. In contrast, administration of the synthetic corticosteroid methylprednisone during this time resulted in total inhibition of mammary tumorigenesis in both intact and adrenalectomized rats. These workers (Carter *et al.*, 1988; Carter and Carter, 1988) concluded that glucocorticoids have a direct inhibitory effect on the proliferation of initiated cells in the mammary gland, possibly by stimulating cellular differentiation. These findings are in agreement with those of Aylsworth and co-workers (1980), who demonstrated that daily injections of pharmacological levels (50 μg) of dexamethasone to rats reduced DMBA-induced mammary tumor growth and caused tumor remission in some cases, despite high serum prolactin levels in the animals.

In contrast to these tumor growth-inhibitory effects of glucocorticoids, Steffen and co-workers (1988) demonstrated that these effects may be specific only for particular cell populations. Fibroblastoid cells derived from stomal portions of DMBA-induced rat mammary tumors were mesenchymal in appearance; these cell strains exhibited reversible morphological changes and reduced fibrosarcoma growth *in vitro* and *in vivo* upon exposure to dexamethasone. In contrast, epithelioid cell strains derived from the same mammary tumors gave rise to adenocarcinomas and were unresponsive to glucocorticoids *in vitro* and *in vivo* (Steffen *et al.*, 1988). It appears that the *in vitro* and *in vivo* growth responsiveness of rat and human mammary tumor epithelial cells to glucocorticoids can vary widely—from inhibition to stimulation—depending on the specific properties of the cell population examined (see Steffen *et al.*, 1988, and references therein).

4.2. Effects on Cellular Proliferation

The early studies of Bullough (Bullough, 1950; Bullough and Eisa, 1950, and references therein) demonstrated the close dependence of both cellular proliferation and tumorigenesis to caloric intake (particularly carbohydrate nutriture), as both could be suppressed in a sigmoidal fashion by increasing caloric restriction. These studies did not suggest an absolute positive correlation between the proliferative rate of a tissue and its susceptibility to tumorigenesis, but rather that tissues having a higher rate of mitosis and cell proliferation had a correspondingly greater probability for latent or preneoplastic cells to proliferate. Moreover, increased cellular proliferation affects both the formation of DNA adducts (by reducing the time available for restorative DNA repair to occur) and the promotional phase of tumorigenesis (see Lok *et al.*, 1988). Since the initial studies of Bullough, dietary restriction at 50–75% of *ad libitum* intake has been shown to reduce cellular proliferation (as assessed by thymidine labeling and mitotic index) in a number of rodent tissues. Reductions in proliferation as a consequence of dietary restriction have been observed in murine crypt cells of the duodenum, jejunum, and colorectum (Koga and Kimura, 1979, 1980; Lok *et al.*, 1988); dermal and basal murine epithelial cells from the esophagus (Lok *et al.*, 1988); normal murine mammary epithelium (Sinha *et al.*, 1988) and alveolar cells (Lok *et al.*, 1988); and cheek pouch epidermal cells from hamsters (Andreou and Morgan, 1981). The studies of Koga and Kimura (1979, 1980) demonstrated that the effect of 40% food restriction on reducing mitotic activity of murine intestinal epithelium was accompanied by a prolongation of the cell cycle (particularly the GI phase) of jejunal and duodenal cells, as well as a reduced rate of migration of cells from crypts to villi in the small intestine.

This potential mechanism of action of dietary restriction awaits further investigation.

4.3. Enhanced Cell-Mediated Immunoresponsiveness

There is a considerable body of evidence that chronic protein–calorie, caloric, or dietary restriction of rodents early in life leads initially to immunosuppression, but subsequently prolongs and enhances cell-mediated immunity (Jose and Good, 1973; Gerbase-DeLima *et al.*, 1975; Fernandes *et al.*, 1976; Weindruch *et al.*, 1979, 1986).

Among the cell-mediated responses observed to be effected by such dietary regimens are increased mitogen-induced T-cell blastogenesis, enhanced T-cell-mediated cytotoxicity, increased protein synthesis, enhanced synthesis and responsiveness of T cells to interleukin 2, marked elevations in interleukin 3 production, macrophage activation, and enhanced NK cell activity (see Jose and Good, 1973; Richardson and Cheung, 1982; Weindruch *et al.*, 1983, 1986; Mutsuura *et al.* 1986; Fernandes *et al.*, 1987; Pahlavani and Richardson, 1987).

Enhanced immunoresponsiveness as a potential mechanism for the inhibition of tumor growth by caloric restriction is limited in its applicability in view of the diverse etiology of tumors inhibited by caloric restriction. Specific immune recognition and rejection of antigenically foreign tumor cells is largely restricted to virally induced neoplasms, particularly DNA viruses, and to some chemically induced tumors (Klein and Klein, 1985). Many carcinogen-induced mammary neoplasms contain tumor-specific or tumor-associated transplantation antigens on their cell surfaces; the immunological reactivity to these diverse antigens varies quantitatively and qualitatively over a wide range (Welsch, 1985). Further, the majority of spontaneous tumors are not highly antigenic and thus are unlikely targets for immunorejection (Klein and Klein, 1985).

A primary immunological mechanism to explain the inhibition of malignant tumor growth by caloric restriction is inconsistent with the findings of Giovanella *et al.* (1982). Human malignant tumors of the breast, colon, and lung were grown subcutaneously or subcapsularly as heterotransplants in nude mice subject to graded food restriction (25–75% of *ad libitum*). Food restriction of nude mice inhibited the growth of all four neoplasms differentially, but in proportion to the degree of restriction. Moreover, tumor growth inhibition was closely correlated with host body weight loss in both male and female mice (Giovanella *et al.*, 1982).

These collective findings suggest a limited role of cell-mediated immunoenhancement as a potential mediator of caloric restriction, but do not eliminate it entirely. In this regard, enhanced NK cell activity resulting from caloric or dietary restriction (Weindruch *et al.*, 1979, 1983, 1986) could provide a potential means of killing sensitive tumors without the host having been immunized against specific antigens on their cell surface. Moreover, NK cell action is not limited to virally or chemically induced neoplasms, although different tumors vary in their NK cell sensitivity (Klein and Klein, 1985).

4.4. Altered Nutrient Availability to Preneoplastic Cells

It has been suggested that as a result of dietary or caloric restriction, energy and nutrient availability to preneoplastic cells could be limited and so retard the promotion and progression of liver tumors (Lagopoulos and Stalder, 1987) and other neoplasms as well (see Hocman, 1988). Specifically, restriction of energy for cellular functions may result in enhanced cellular economy of utilization, thus depriving processes involved in tumorigenesis from sufficient substrates necessary for essential cellular activities (King and McCay, 1986). Indirect evidence exists to support the underlying premise of this hypothesis. Weindruch *et al.* (1986) demonstrated that hepatic mitochondria from 40% food-restricted mice exhibited increased state 3 rates of oxygen utilization, but normal state 4 rates compared to mitochondria from *ad libitum*-fed mice. These alterations resulted in an elevated respiratory control index in restricted mice indicative of a more effective coupling of oxidative phosphorylation to electron transport (Weindruch *et al.*, 1986). With regard to neoplastic tissues, Ruggeri *et al.* (1987) demonstrated that carcinogen-induced mammary tumors from rats subjected to graded caloric restriction exhibited biochemical alterations in carbohydrate metabolism compared to weight-matched tumors from *ad libitum*-fed animals. These alterations were suggestive of adaptive or compensatory changes in tumor carbohydrate metabolism in response to the altered nutritional state of the host (Ruggeri *et al.*, 1987).

4.5. Alterations in Mammotropic Hormones and/or Tissue Responsiveness

Alteration in circulating mammotropic hormones and/or tissue responsiveness to these agonists has been a major hypothesis to explain the inhibitory effects of caloric restriction on mammary tumorigenesis in rodents.

A considerable body of evidence suggests that estrogen and prolactin are the two most important endocrine influences involved in the development and growth of mammary tumors in rats (see Pearson *et al.* 1969; Meites, 1972; Leung and Sasaki, 1975; Manni *et al.*, 1977; Welsch and Aylsworth, 1983; Welsch, 1985). Administration of moderate doses of estrogens over a prolonged period early in life, or sustained elevated circulating prolactin levels, can result in spontaneous mammary tumorigenesis in rats. Conversely, ovariectomy and/or hypophysectomy of rodents can markedly inhibit mammary tumor development (Meites, 1972; Welsch, 1985). Moreover, ovariectomy or the administration of antiestrogens, aromatase inhibitors, or inhibitors of estrogen biosynthesis prior to, or shortly after, administration of a chemical carcinogen (e.g., 7,12-DMBA, 3-MCA) markedly inhibits tumor development and leads to growth stasis or regression of mammary tumors in rodents (see Lupulescu, 1985a,b; Welsch, 1985, and references within).

Despite the major influence of estrogens on mammary tumorigenesis, these growth-promoting effects are dependent on a functional pituitary gland (Pearson *et al.*, 1969; Meites, 1972; Welsch, 1985). Moreover, prolactin alone may have a limited capacity to induce and maintain mammary tumor growth in ovariectomized animals or those treated with antiestrogenic agents (see Meites, 1972; Manni *et al.*, 1977; Welsch, 1985). In this regard, estrogen administration to rodents has been shown to stimulate prolactin secretion *in vivo* (see Meites, 1972; Manni *et al.*, 1977) and *in vitro* (Pasqualini *et al.*, 1988) through a positive feedback mechanism. Similarly, evidence has been presented that the administration of DMBA mimics the acute effects of estrogens in stimulating pituitary prolactin release *in vivo* (Dao and Sinha, 1975) and *in vitro* (Pasqualini *et al.*, 1988), thus creating a hormonal milieu increasing the sensitivity of the mammary gland to tumorigenesis. Further, while moderate doses of estrogens are stimulatory to mammary tumor growth, larger doses are inhibitory *in vivo*, both by suppressing prolactin secretion and by interfering with prolactin action on mammary tissues. These inhibitory effects of pharmacological doses of estrogens can be partly alleviated by prolactin administration (Meites, 1972; Welsch, 1985).

Collectively, these findings suggest a salient influence of prolactin on mammary tumor growth and development surpassing that of estrogens. In summarizing the influence of prolactin on mammary tumorigenesis, Welsch (1985) has noted the positive correlation between serum prolactin levels and susceptibility to carcinogen-induced mammary tumorigenesis in various strains of rats. However, there does not appear to be a strong correlation between the magnitude of prolactin binding to carcinogen-induced rat mammary tumors and prolactin-induced tumor growth and/or serum prolactin levels (see Welsch, 1985). Moreover, the time period during which prolactin levels are altered in relation to mammary tumorigenesis appears to be critical. In both rats (Meites, 1972) and mice (Welsch and Aylsworth, 1983) elevating prolactin levels *in vivo* by pharmacological or surgical means prior to carcinogen administration inhibits mammary tumor development, while a stimulation of tumorigenesis is observed when such treatments are instituted following carcinogen exposure.

An influence of caloric restriction on mammotropic hormones in relation to mamma-ry tumor growth was suggested by the studies of Sylvester and co-workers (1981, 1982). These investigators demonstrated that a 66% reduction in the incidence and growth of DMBA-induced mammary tumors occurred in rats underfed by 50% 1 week prior and 1 month subsequent to carcinogen administration. These inhibitory effects of caloric re-striction could be prevented by treatments increasing circulating prolactin and estrogen levels 1 day prior and 7 days following DMBA administration (Sylvester *et al.*, 1981). A possible role for estrogens and prolactin in mediating the effects of caloric restriction (underfeeding 50% 2–4 weeks prior to and after DMBA administration) was further suggested by the finding that caloric restriction altered circulating levels of these mam-motropic hormones and disrupted estrus cycles (Sylvester *et al.*, 1982). However, only food restriction instituted 1 week prior, and subsequent to, DMBA administration was effective in reducing mammary tumorigenesis for the entire 5-month duration of the study. These findings suggested that alterations in mammotropic hormones by food restriction during the "critical period" 1 week prior and subsequent to carcinogen treatment may contribute to inhibition of mammary tumorigenesis (Sylvester *et al.*, 1981, 1982). Subse-quent work by Leung *et al.* (1983) demonstrated that administration of estradiol benzoate, and to a greater extent haloperidol (a prolactin secretagogue), could counter the inhibitory effects of 4 weeks of 50% underfeeding on the incidence and growth of DMBA-induced mammary tumors in Sprague–Dawley rats and restore serum prolactin levels to above normal levels. Atterwill and co-workers (1986) also observed a significant reduction in serum prolactin levels in female rats whose caloric intake was restricted by 20%. These collective findings suggested that alterations in prolactin levels by caloric restriction may be more important in inhibiting the growth and development of rat mammary tumors than alterations in estrogen levels, as less severe caloric restriction did not alter circulating estrogen levels (Sylvester *et al.*, 1981).

Sarkar and co-workers (1982) examined the influence of caloric restriction on the development of spontaneous mammary tumors in CH3 mice. Throughout the course of the 7- to 8-month study, calorically restricted animals (10 kcal/day) had a significant reduc-tion in tumor incidence (11%) compared to those on high-calorie diets (16 kcal/day) or *ad libitum*-fed animals (58–60% tumor incidence). Significant in these studies was the obser-vation that calorically restricted mice displayed significant reductions in serum prolactin levels, murine mammary tumor virus production, and mammary alveolar lesions (Sarkar *et al.*, 1982). Reduction in caloric intake, however, did not impair normal ovarian func-tion, estrogen production, or the growth and development of normal mammary epi-thelium; in addition, serum thyrotropin and growth hormone levels were not affected (Sarkar *et al.*, 1982). Holehan and Merry (1985) restricted food intake of female Sprague–Dawley rats from the time of weaning to a level that maintained their body weights to 50% that of *ad libitum*-fed animals. Underfed animals exhibited a highly significant delay in their onset of puberty (34–39 days vs. 63–189 days), but a significant delay in reaching reproductive senescence. Serum follicle-stimulating hormone (FSH) and progesterone were depressed in food-restricted animals, while 17B-estradiol levels were significantly elevated (Holehan and Merry, 1985). In contrast, Sinha *et al.* (1988) examined the effects of 20, 50, and 75% food restriction in female Sprague–Dawley rats treated with DMBA. The 20 and 50% food-restricted rats showed marked inhibition of tumor incidence, yet both groups underwent estrus cycles despite some irregularities in 50% food-restricted rats. Moreover, 20% food-restricted rats had normal estrogen levels, successful pregnan-cies, and normal litter weights, suggesting that alterations in circulating estrogen levels or estrus cycles are not requisite for inhibition of mammary tumor growth by food restriction (Sinha *et al.*, 1988).

At present, the role of specific steroid and/or peptide mammotropic hormones (and their interactions) in mediating the effects of caloric restriction on tumorigenesis is in-conclusive. A possible role of altered prolactin and/or glucocorticoid status in mediating the inhibitory effects of caloric restriction on mammary tumorigenesis is suggestive, given the body of experimental data just discussed. However, in view of the broad range of neoplasms responsive to caloric restriction, a mammotropic hormone(s) alone is unlikely to be the primary mediator of this phenomenon. In addition, the fact that alterations in circulating prolactin levels can have both marked inhibitory or stimulatory effects on mammary tumorigenesis relative to the time of carcinogen treatment is inconsistent with several studies demonstrating that alterations in circulating prolactin levels by food re-striction during the critical period prior and subsequent to carcinogen treatment can have marked inhibitory effects on mammary tumorigenesis (Sylvester *et al.*, 1981, 1982). Of peripheral relevance, a considerable body of evidence (reviewed by Welsch and Ayls-worth, 1983; Welsch, 1987) likewise suggests that the tumor-promoting properties of dietary fat in animal models are not mediated by alterations in circulating mammotropic hormone levels, specifically estrogen and progesterone.

4.6. Alterations in Peptide Growth Factors and/or Their Receptor Expression

A potential role for alterations in peptide growth factors, specifically insulin and the insulinlike growth factors, in mediating the effects of caloric restriction on tumor growth is suggestive in view of their nutritional modulation *in vivo* and their pronounced meta-bolic and mitogenic effects on numerous cell types *in vitro* and *in vivo* (for reviews see Kahn, 1985; Copinischi and Chatelain, 1985; Hill and Milner, 1985; Rosen, 1987).

With regard to rodent mammary tumor growth specifically, Heuson and Legros (1968, 1971) and Rudland *et al.* (1977) demonstrated that insulin stimulated cell prolifera-tion in explants and enzymatic digests of carcinogen-induced rat mammary tumors *in vitro*. These *in vitro* findings were extended to *in vivo* studies of the growth-stimulating properties of insulin on carcinogen-induced mammary tumors. Heuson and Legros (1972a,b) demonstrated that approximately 90% of DMBA-induced rat mammary car-cinomas were insulin dependent, as induction of diabetes by alloxan administration after carcinogen treatment caused a rapid regression in tumor growth similar to that observed following oophorectomy or hypophysectomy. Insulin administration stimulated tumor growth *in vivo* and reactivated growth of regressing tumors in hypophysectomized rats (Heuson *et al.*, 1972). Subsequent studies by Hilf and co-workers (Cohen and Hilf, 1974; Hilf *et al.*, 1978; Shafie and Hilf, 1978; Gibson and Hilf, 1980) demonstrated that the majority of DMBA-induced tumors are hormone-dependent, regressing in diabetic or ovariectomized animals. Further, diabetic rats exhibited an apparent adaptive increase in tumor insulin binding; treatment with insulin restored tumor growth with a concomitant increase in tumor estrogen receptors (Shafie and Hilf, 1978; Hilf *et al.*, 1978).

Despite extensive evidence for a role of insulin enhancing the growth and prolifera-tion of a variety of tumors *in vivo* (see Hill and Milner, 1985; Lupelescu, 1985b) and *in vitro* (see Furlanetto *et al.*, 1987; Taub *et al.*, 1987), the direct experimental evidence for a relationship between caloric or food restriction, tumor growth, and insulin status is limited. In their studies of the insulin dependency of DMBA-induced rat mammary carcinomas, Heuson and Legros (1972b) observed that induction of diabetes by alloxan or food restriction by approximately 60% several weeks following carcinogen treatment led to marked tumor regression and decreased tumor size. Moreover, regressing tumors in food-restricted, but not diabetic, rats were partially stimulated to grow by estrogen administration; tumors from both diabetic and food-restricted rats were highly insulin-dependent *in vitro* (Heuson and Legros, 1972b). Subsequent studies by McCumbee and Lebovitz (1981) demonstrated that caloric restriction, and to a greater extent, streptozotocin-induced diabetes, reduced chondrosarcoma growth in rats. Of significance was the insulin responsiveness of these tumors and the strong correlation of chondrosarcoma growth with serum somatomedin (IGF) activity (McCumbee and Lebovitz, 1981). These limited studies suggested that a reduction in circulating insulin and/or somatomedin levels *in vivo* may be a common factor in the inhibition of tumor growth in rodents by food restriction or chemically induced diabetes. In view of their range of target tissue specificity and the pleiotropic effects of these growth factors, this potential mechanism of tumor inhibition by caloric restriction warrants further study.

4.7. Alterations in Enzymatic Activities Involved in Modulating Free Radical– and Carcinogen-Mediated Damage and Enhancing DNA Repair from Carcinogen Insult

Koizumi and co-workers (1987) have examined the effects of long-term 40% caloric restriction on murine hepatic enzyme activities related to xenobiotic metabolism, superoxide production, free radical elimination, and lipid peroxidation. Long-term caloric restriction increased hepatic catalase activity by 42% and 64% at 12 and 24 months of age, respectively, but had no effect on superoxide dismutase (SOD) activity or β-oxidation in either age group of restricted mice. Moreover, long-term caloric restriction decreased hepatic lipid peroxidation by approximately 30% in 12-month-old mice and to a lesser extent in 24-month-old restricted animals. These results were in agreement with previous findings demonstrating that 50% food restriction of mice from weaning resulted in comparable reductions in hepatic lipid peroxidation, but no effect on SOD activity (Chipalkatti *et al.*, 1983). In contrast, Rao *et al.* (1988) demonstrated an increase in both hepatic catalase and SOD activities in food-restricted rats compared to *ad libitum*-fed controls.

These collective findings suggest that long-term dietary restriction, by selectively augmenting free radical scavenging enzymes (catalase and/or SOD) and reducing peroxidative damage, may provide increased protection against the carcinogenic insult of free radicals generated from normal oxidative processes in energy and xenobiotic metabolism, and from ionizing radiation as well (Koizumi *et al.*, 1987; Hocman, 1988). In contrast, virtually all of the hepatic xenobiotic metabolizing enzymes examined were not significantly enhanced by long-term caloric restriction (Kolzumi *et al.*, 1987), suggesting little, if any, effect of long-term restriction on the modulation of carcinogen (and cocarcinogen) metabolism *in vivo*.

There is a limited body of evidence indicating that dietary restriction may enhance cellular DNA repair capacity subsequent to mutational damage. Licastro and co-workers

(1986) measured ultraviolet (UV) light-induced DNA damage repair capacity in lymphocytes from mice maintained on 40% calorically restricted regimens. Lymphocytes from restricted mice exhibited a slightly enhanced capability to repair their damaged DNA (Licastro *et al.*, 1986). More recently, Weraarchakul and Richardson (1988) measured UV-induced unscheduled DNA synthesis in suspensions of hepatocytes and kidney cells obtained from rats fed *ad libitum* or 40% food-restricted regimens. Unscheduled DNA synthesis (as measured by [³H]-thymidine incorporation into DNA) was 20–30% higher in hepatocytes from restricted animals at 5 and 28 months of age compared to *ad libitum*-fed rats of the same age. Similarly, unscheduled DNA synthesis in kidney cells from restricted animals was likewise enhanced compared to the age-matched, *ad libitum*-fed counterparts (Weraardchakal and Richardson, 1988).

These collective studies, although limited, provide supportive evidence for the hypothesis that long-term caloric or dietary restriction may inhibit tumorigenesis and enhance lifespan both by augmenting host systems to prevent carcinogen- and free radical–mediated damage and by facilitating DNA repair mechanisms in the event of successful mutational events.

More detailed investigations of this potential mechanism are justified in view of its fundamental relevance and applicability both to tumor initiation from carcinogenic insult and to molecular aspects of cellular aging.

4.8. Alterations in Oncogene and Protooncogene Expression in Vivo

Recently, several reports have examined the role of caloric restriction in modulating oncogene expression *in vivo*. Khare *et al.* (1987) examined the effect of food restriction (underfeeding) on oncogene expression in various strains of autoimmune LPR mice. Reduced splenic mRNA levels for v-*raf*, v-*abl*, and v-*fos* were observed in most strains, as well as reduced c-*myc* mRNA levels in the lymph nodes of all strains examined (Khare *et al.*, 1987). Similarly, Fenandes *et al.* (1987) observed that male F344 rats maintained on a 40% calorically restricted regimen from 6 weeks of age demonstrated reduced splenic mRNA levels for v-*ras*, v-*raf*, and v-*src*, but no alterations in c-*myc* or c-*myb* transcripts compared to *ad libitum*-fed animals. Dietary regulation of hepatic c-*myc* oncogene expression in rats has been addressed by several workers (Corcos *et al.*, 1987; Horikawa *et al.*, 1986). Corcos *et al.* (1987) observed that hepatic c-*myc* mRNA levels remained relatively constant during the first 6 hr of starvation, but declined by approximately 10-fold by 12 hr and remained depressed at 5 days of starvation. This decline in c-*myc* expression was not the result of an overall decline in gene transcription with starvation and may have been attributable to an insulin dependency for the regulation of c-*myc* expression (Corcos *et al.*, 1987). In contrast, Horikawa *et al.* (1986) observed a fourfold elevation in hepatic c-*myc* mRNA levels induced by a 4-day administration of a protein-restricted diet to rats; c-*myc* mRNA levels were restored to basal levels upon restoration of protein intake.

In summary, this discussion reveals that dietary restriction results in diverse metabolic, endocrinologic, and immunological alterations, as well as marked affects on cellular proliferation, oncogene expression, and DNA repair capabilities. Each of these potential mechanisms or mediators of dietary restriction on tumorigenesis has been demonstrated in some, although not all, experimental systems examined. Moreover, specificity in the target tissue and particular cell populations affected by these potential mediators has been clearly demonstrated as well. In view of the diverse and complex effects of dietary restriction and the multifactorial nature of the entire process of tumorigenesis, a grand unifying mechanism of action of dietary restriction on tumor growth inhibition is unlikely. Suffice to say, each of the mechanisms discussed here both individually and collectively probably contributes to the pronounced inhibitory effects of dietary restriction on tumor growth. The magnitude and extent to which each of these mediators is acting may vary depending on the biology of the host organism and the tissue and cell populations under investigation.

5. References

Albanes, D., 1987a, Total calories, body weight, and tumor incidence in mice, *Cancer Res.* **47:**1987–1992.

Albanes, D., 1987b, Caloric intake, body weight, and cancer: A review, *Nutr. Cancer* **9:**199–217.

Albanes, D., Jones, D. Y., Schatzkin, A., Micozzi, M. S., and Taylor, P. R., 1988, Adult stature and risk of cancer, *Cancer Res.* **48:**1658–1662.

Andreou, K. K., and Morgan, P. R., 1981, Effect of dietary restriction on induced hamster cheek pouch carcinogenesis, *Arch. Oral Biol.* **26:**525–531.

Armario, A., Montero, J. L., and Jolin, T., 1987, Chronic food restriction and circadian rhythms of pituitary-adrenal hormones, growth hormone and thyroid-stimulating hormone, *Ann. Nur. Metab.* **31:**81–87.

Atterwill, C. K., Brown, C. G., Conybeare, G., and Meakin, J., 1986, Diet-restriction of rats decelerates age-related changes in serum prolactin levels and CNS dopamine receptor function, *Br. J. Pharmacol.* **89:**733.

Aylsworth, C. F., Sylvester, P. W., Leung, F. C., and Meites, J., 1980, Inhibition of mammary tumor growth by dexamethasone in rats in the presence of high serum prolactin levels, *Cancer Res.* **40:**1863–1866.

Bailar, J., 1979, The case for cancer prevention, *J. Natl. Cancer Inst.* **62:**727–730.

Beth, M., Berger, M. R., Aksoy, M., and Schmahl, D., 1987, Comparison between the effects of dietary fat level and of caloric intake on methylnitrosourea-induced mammary carcinogenesis in female S.D. rats, *Int. J. Cancer* **39:**737–744.

Bischoff, F., Long, M. L., and Maxwell, L. C., 1935, Influence of caloric intake upon the growth of sarcoma 180, *Am. J. Cancer* **24:**549–553.

Boissoneault, G. A., Elson, C. E., and Pariza, M. W., 1986, Net energy effects of dietary fat on chemically-induced mammary carcinogenesis in F344 rats, *J. Natl. Cancer Inst.* **76:**335–338.

Boutwell, R. K., Brush, M. K., and Rusch, H. P., 1949a, The stimulating effect of dietary fat on carcinogenesis, *Cancer Res.* **9:**741–746.

Boutwell, R. K., Brush, M. K., and Rusch, H. P., 1949b, Some physiological effects associated with chronic caloric restriction, *Am. J. Physiol.* **154:**517–524.

Brown, R. R., 1983, The role of diet in cancer causation, *Food Technol.* **37:**49–56.

Bullough, W. S., 1950, Mitotic activity and carcinogenesis, *Br. J. Cancer* **4:**329–336.

Bullough, W. S., and Eisa, E. A., 1950, The effects of a graded series of restricted diets on epidermal mitotic activity in the mouse, *Br. J. Cancer* **4:**321–328.

Carroll, K. K., 1975, Experimental evidence of dietary factors and hormone-dependent cancers, *Cancer Res.* **35:**3374–3383.

Carroll, K. K., 1981, Neutral fats and cancer, *Cancer Res.* **41:**3695–3699.

Carroll, K. K., 1986, Dietary fat and cancer: specific action or caloric effect? *J. Nutr.* **116:**1130–1132.

Carter, J. H., and Carter, H. W., 1988, Adrenal regulation of mammary tumorigenesis in female Sprague–Dawley rats: Histopathology of mammary tumors, *Cancer Res.* **48:**3808–3815.

Carter, J. H., Carter, H. W., and Meade, J., 1988, Adrenal regulation of mammary tumorigenesis in female Sprague–Dawley rates: incidence, latency, and yield of mammary tumors, *Cancer Res.* **48:**3801–3807.

Chan, P. C., Head, J. F., Cohen, L. A., and Wynder, E. L., 1977, Influence of dietary fat on the induction of rat mammary tumors by *N*-nitrosomethylurea: Associated hormone changes and differences between Sprague–Dawley and F-344 rats, *J. Natl. Cancer Inst.* **59**:1279–1283.

Chipalkatti, S., De, A. K., and Aiyar, A. S., 1983, Effect of diet restriction on some biochemical parameters related to aging in mice, *J. Nutr.* **113**:944–950.

Cimino, J. A., and Demopoulous, H. B., 1980, Introduction: Determinants of cancer relevant to prevention in the war on cancer, *J. Environ. Pathol. Toxicol.* **3**:1–10.

Clinton, S. K., Imrey, P. B., Alster, J. M., Simon, J., Truex, C. R., and Visek, W. J., 1984, The combined effects of dietary protein and fat on 7,12-dimethylbenzanthracene-induced breast cancer in rats, *J. Nutr.* **114**:1213–1223.

Cohen, L. A., 1987, Diet and cancer, *Sci. Am.* **257**:42–48.

Cohen, L. A., Keewhan, C., and Wang, C-X., 1988, Influence of dietary fat, coloric restrictor, and voluntary exercise on *N*-nitro-somethylurea-induced mammary tumorigenesis in rats, *Cancer Res.* **48**:4276–4283.

Cohen, N. D., and Hilf, R., 1974, Influence of insulin on growth and metabolism of 7,12-dimethylbenz(a) anthracene-induced mammary tumors, *Cancer Res.* **34**:3245–3252.

Connor-Johnson, B., Gajjar, A., Kubo, C., and Good, R. A., 1986, Calories versus protein in onset of renal disease in NZB x NZW mice, *Proc. Natl. Acad. Sci. USA* **83**:5659–5662.

Copinschi, G., and Chatelain, P. (eds.), 1985, Recent developments in the study of growth factors: GRF and somatomedins, *Hormone Res.* **24**:77–228.

Corcos, D., Vaulont, S., Denis, N., Lyonnet, S., Simon, M-P., Kitzis, A., Kahn, A., and Kruh, J., 1987, Expression of c-*myc* is under dietary control in rat liver, *Oncogene Res.* **1**:193–199.

Dao, T. L., and Sinha, D., 1975, Effect of carcinogen on pituitary prolactin release and synthesis, *Proc. Am. Assoc. Cancer Res.* **16**:28.

DeWaard, F., Cornelis, J. P., Aoki, K., and Yoshida, M., 1977, Breast cancer incidence according to weight and height in two cities of the Netherlands and in Aichi Prefecture, *Jpn. Cancer* **40**:1269–1275.

Doll, R., and Peto, R., 1981, The causes of cancer: quantitative estimates of avoidable risks of cancer in the U.S. today, *J. Natl. Cancer Inst.* **66**:1191–1308.

Donato, K., 1987, Efficiency of utilization of various energy sources for growth, *Am. J. Clin. Nutr.* **45**(Suppl.):164–167.

Donato, K., and Hegsted, D. M., 1985, Efficiency of utilization of various sources of energy for growth, *Proc. Natl. Acad. Sci.* **82**:4866–4870.

Erickson, K. L., 1984, Dietary fat influence on murine melanoma growth and lymphocyte-mediated cytotoxicity, *J. Natl. Cancer Inst.* **72**:115–120.

Erickson, K. L., and Thomas, I. K., 1985, The role of dietary fat in mammary tumorigenesis, *Food Technol.* **39**:69–73.

Ershler, W. B., Berman, E., and Moore, A. L., 1986, Slower B16 melanoma growth but greater pulmonary colonization in calorie-restricted mice, *J. Natl. Cancer Inst.* **76**:81–85.

Fernande, G., Yunis, E. J., and Good, R. A., 1976, Suppression of adenocarcinoma by the immunological consequences of caloric restriction, *Nature* **263**:504–506.

Fernandes, G., Khare, A., Langaniere, S., Yu, B., Sandberg, L., and Friedrichs, B., 1987, Effect of food restriction and aging on immune cell fatty acids, functions and oncogene expression in SPF Fischer 344 rats, *Fed. Proc.* **46**:567.

Forbes, E. B., Swift, R. W., Elliott, R. F., and James, W. H., 1946, Relation of fat to economy of food utilization. II. By the mature albino rat, *J. Nutr.* **31**:213–227.

Furlanetto, R. W., DiCarlo, J. N., and Wisehart, C., 1987, The type II insulin-like growth factor receptor does not mediate deoxyribonucleic ancid synthesis in human fibroblasts, *J. Clin. Endocrinol. Metab.* **64**:1142–1149.

Gajjar, A., Kubo, C., Johnson, B. C., and Good, R. A., 1987, Influence of extremes of protein and energy intake on survival of B/W mice, *J. Nutr.* **117**:1136–1140.

Garfinkel, L., 1985, Overweight and cancer, *Ann. Intern. Med.* **103**:1034–1036.

Gerbase-DeLima, M., Liu, R. K., Cheney, K. E., Michey, R., and Walford, R. L., 1975, Immune function and survival in a long-lived mouse strain subjected to undernutrition, *Gerontologia* **21**:184–202.

Gibson, S. L., and Hilf, R., 1980, Regulation of estrogen-binding capacity by insulin in 7,12-dimethylbenz(a)-anthracene-induced mammary tumors in rats, *Cancer Res.* **40**:2343–2348.

Giovanella, B. C., Shepard, R. C., Stehlin, J. S., Venditti, J. M., and Abbott, B. J., 1982, Calorie restriction: Effect on growth of human tumors heterotransplanted in nude mice, *J. Natl. Cancer Inst.* **68**:249–257.

Goodwin, P. J., and Boyd, N. F., 1987, Critical appraisal of the evidence that dietary fat intake is related to breast cancer risk in humans, *J. Natl. Cancer Inst.* **79**:473–485.

Graham, S., Marshall, J., Mettlin, C., Rzepka, T., Nemoto, T., and Byers, T., 1982, Diet in the epidemiology of breast cancer, *Am. J. Epidemiol.* **116**:68–75.

Greenberg, E. R., Vessey, M. P., McPherson, K., Doll, R., and Yeates, D., 1985, Body size and survival and premenopausal breast cancer, *Br. J. Cancer* **51**:691–697.

Gross, L., and Dreyfuss, Y., 1984, Reduction in the incidence of radiation-induced tumors in rats after restriction of food intake, *Proc. Natl. Acad. Sci. USA* **81**:7596–7598.

Harrison, D. E., Archer, J. R., and Astle, C. M., 1984, Effects of food restriction on aging: separation of food intake and adiposity, *Proc. Natl. Acad. Sci. USA* **81**:1835–1828.

Hebert, J. R., Augustine, A., Barone, J., Kabat, G. C., Kinne, D. W., and Wynder, E. L., 1988, Weight, height and body mass index in the prognosis of breast cancer: early results of prospective study, *Int. J. Cancer* **42**:315–318.

Heuson, J. C., and Legros, N., 1968, Study of the growth-promoting effect of insulin in relation to carbohydrate metabolism in organ culture of rat mammary carcinoma, *Eur. J. Cancer* **4**:1–7.

Heuson, J. C., and Legros, N., 1971, Effect of insulin on DNA synthesis and DNA oplymerase activity in organ culture of rat mammary carcinoma, and the influence of insulin pre-treatment and of alloxan diabetes, *Cancer Res.* **31**:59–65.

Heuson, J. C., and Legros, N., 1972a, Influence of insulin deprivation on growth of the 7,12-dimethylbenz(a)-anthracene-induced mammary carcinoma in rats subjected to alloxan diabetes and food restriction, *Cancer Res.* **32**:226–232.

Heuson, J. C., and Legros, N., 1972b, Influence of insulin deprivation on growth of the 7,12-dimethylbenz(a)-anthracene-induced mammary carcinoma in rats subjected to alloxan diabetes and food restriction, *Cancer Res.* **32**:226–232.

Heuson, J. C., Legros, N., and Heimann, R., 1972, Influence of insulin administration on growth of the 7,12-dimethylbenz(a)anthracene-induced mammary carcinoma in intact, oophorectomized, and hypophysec-tomized rats, *Cancer Res.* **32**:233–238.

Hilf, R., Hissin, P. J., and Shafie, S. M., 1978, Regulatory interrelationships for insulin and estrogen action in mammary tumors, *Cancer Res.* **38**:4076–4085.

Hill, D. J., and Milner, R. D. G., 1985, Insulin as a growth factor, *Pediatr. Res.* **19**:879–886.

Hirohata, T., Shigematsu, T., Nomura, A. M. Y., Normura, Y., Horie, A., and Hirohata, I., 1985, Occurrence of breast cancer in relation to diet and reproductive history: A case–control study in Fukuoka, Japan, *NCI Monogr.* **69**:187–190.

Hirohata, T., Nomura, A. M. Y., Hankin, J. H., Kolonel, L. N., and Lee, J., 1987, An epidemiologic study on the association between diet and breast cancer, *J. Natl. Cancer Inst.* **78**:595–600.

Hocman, G., 1988, Prevention of cancer: Restriction of nutritional energy intake (joules), *Comp. Biochem. Physiol.* **91A**:209–220.

Holehan, A. M., and Merry, B. J., 1985, The control of puberty in the dietary restricted female rat, *Mech. Ageing Dev.* **32**:179–191.

Hopkins, G. J., and Carroll, K. K., 1979, Relationship between amount and type of dietary fat in promotion of mammary carcinogenesis induced by 7,12-dimethylbenzanthracene, *J. Natl. Cancer Inst.* **62**:1009–1012.

Hopkins, G. J., Kennedy, T. G., and Carroll, K. K., 1981, Polyunsaturated fatty acids as promoters of mammary carcinogenesis induced in Sprague–Dawley rats by 7,12-dimethylbenzanthracene, *J. Natl. Cancer Inst.* **66**:517–522.

Horikawa, S., Sakata, K., Hatanaka, M., and Tsukada, K., 1986, Expression of c-*myc* oncogene in rat liver by a dietary manipulation, *Biochem. Biophys Res. Commun.* **140**:574–580.

Ip, C., Carter, C. A., and Ip, M. M., 1985, Requirement of essential fatty acid for mammary tumorigenesis in the rat, *Cancer Res.* **45**:1997–2001.

Ip, C., Birt, D. F., Rogers, A. E., and Mettlin, C., (eds.), 1986, Dietary fat and cancer, in: *Progress in Clinical and Biological Research, Volume 222*, Alan R. Liss, New York, 885 pp.

Jose, D. G., and Good, R. A., 1973, Quantitative effects of nutritional protein and calorie deficiency upon immune responses to tumors in mice, *Cancer Res.* **33**:807–812.

Kahn, C. R., 1985, The molecular mechanism of insulin action, *Ann. Rev. Med.* **36**:429–451.

Kelsey, J. L., and Berkowitz, 1988, Breast cancer epidemiology, *Cancer Res.* **48**:5615–5623.

Khare, A., Mountz, J., Fischbach, M., Talal, N., and Fernandes, G., 1987, Effect of dietary lipids and calories on oncogene expression in autoimmune LPR mice, *Fed. Proc.* **46**:441.

King, M. M., and McCay, P. B., 1986, Potentiation of carcinogenesis by dietary fat: Is it caused by high energy consumption or is it an effect of fat itself? *J. Nutr.* **116**:2313–2315.

Klein, G., and Klein, E., 1985, Evolution of tumors and the impact of molecular oncology, *Nature* **315**:190–195.

Klurfeld, D. M., Weber, M. M., and Kritchevsky, D., 1987, Inhibition of chemically induced mammary and colon tumor promotion by caloric restriction in rats fed increased dietary fat, *Cancer Res.* **47**:2759–2762.

Klurfeld, D. M., Welch, C. B., Davis, M. F., and Kritchevsky, D., 1989, Determination of degree of energy restriction necessary to reduce DMBA-induced mammary tumorigenesis in rats during the promotion phase, *J. Nutr.* **119**:286–291.

Koga, A., and Kimura, S., 1979, Influence of restricted diet on the cell renewal of the mouse small intestine, *J. Nutr. Sci. Vitaminol.* **25**:265–267.

Koga, A., and Kimura, S., 1980, Influence of restricted diet on the cell cycle in the crypt of mouse small intestine, *J. Nutr. Sci Vitaminol.* **26**:33–38.

Koizumi, A., Weindruch, R., and Walford, R. L., 1987, Influence of dietary restriction and age on liver enzyme activities and lipid peroxidation in mice, *J. Nutr.* **117**:361–367.

Kolonel, L. N., Nomura, A. M. Y., Lee, J., and Hirohata, T., 1986, Anthropometric indicators of breast cancer risk in postmenopausal women in Hawaii, *Nutr. Cancer* **8**:247–256.

Kritchevsky, D., 1982, Lipids and cancer, in: *Molecular Interrelations of Nutrition and Cancer* (N. S. Arnott, J. van Eys, and Y-M. Yang, eds.), Raven Press, New York, pp. 209–216.

Kritchevsky, D., and Klurfeld, D. M., 1987, Caloric effects of experimental mammary tumorigenesis, *Am. J. Clin. Nutr.* **45**:236–243.

Kritchevsky, D., Weber, M. M., and Klurfeld, D. M., 1984, Dietary fat versus caloric content in initiation and promotion of 7,12-dimethylbenzanthracene-induced mammary tumorigenesis in rats, *Cancer Res.* **44**:3174–3177.

Kritchevsky, D., Buck, C. M., Weber, M. M., and Klurfeld, D. M., 1986, Calories, fat and cancer, *Lipids* **21**:272–274.

Kubo, C., Johnson, B. C., Gajjar, A., and Good, R. A., 1987, Crucial dietary factors in maximizing life span and longevity in autoimmune-prone mice, *J. Nutr.* **117**:1129–1135.

Lagopoulous, L., and Stalder, R., 1987, The influence of food intake on the development of diethylnitrosamine-induced liver tumors in mice, *Carcinogenesis* **8**:33–37.

Lane, J. W., Bute, J. S., Howard, C., Shepherd, F., Halligan, R., and Medina, D., 1985, The role of high levels of dietary fat in 7,12-dimethylbenzanthracene-induced mouse mammary tumorigenesis. Lack of an effect on lipid peroxidation, *Carcinogenesis* **6**:403–407.

Larsen, C. D., and Heston, W. E., 1946, Effects of cystine and calorie restriction on the incidence of spontaneous pulmonary tumors in strain A mice, *J. Natl. Cancer Inst.* **6**:31–40.

Lavik, P. S., and Baumann, C. A., 1943, Further studies on the tumor-promoting action of fat, *Cancer Res.* **3**:739–756.

Leung, B. S., and Sasaki, G. H., 1975, On the mechanism of prolactin and estrogen action in 7,12-dimethylbenz(a)anthracene-induced mammary carcinoma in the rat. II. *In vitro* tumor responses and estrogen receptor, *Endocrinology* **97**:564–572.

Leung, F. C., Aylsworth, C. F., and Meites, J., 1983, Counteraction of underfeeding-induced inhibition of mammary tumor growth in rats by prolactin and estrogen administration, *Proc. Soc. Exp. Biol. Med.* **173**:159–163.

Lew, E. A., and Garfinkel, L., 1979, Variations in mortality by weight among 750,000 men and women, *J. Chronic Dis.* **32**:563–576.

Licastro, F., Weindruch, R., and Walford, R. L., 1986, Dietary restriction retards the age-related decline of the DNA repari capacity in mouse splenocytes, in: *Immunoregulation in Aging* (A. Facchini, J. J. Haaijman, and G. Labo, eds.)., Eurage, Rijswijk, The Netherlands, pp. 53–61.

Loeb, J. N., 1976, Corticosteroids and growth, *N. Engl. J. Med.* **205**:547–552.

Loeb, L., Suntzeff, V., Blumenthal, H. T., and Kirtz, M. M., 1942, Effect of weight on the development of mammary carcinoma in various strains of mice, *Arch. Pathol.* **33**:845–865.

Lok, E., Nera, E. A., Iverson, F., Scott, F., So, Y., and Clayson, D. B., 1988, Dietary restriction, cell proliferation and carcinogenesis: A preliminary study, *Cancer Lett.* **38**:249–255.

Lupelescu, A. P., 1985a, Effect of prolonged insulin treatment on carcinoma formation in mice, *Cancer Res.* **45:**3288–3295.

Lupelescu, A. P., 1985b, Enhancement of epidermal carcinoma formation by prolactin in mice, *J. Natl. Cancer Inst.* **74:**1335–1346.

Lyon, J. E., Mahoney, A. W., West, D. W., Gardner, J. W., Smith, K. R., Sorenson, A. W., and Stanish, W., 1987, Energy intake: Its relationship to colon cancer risk, *J. Natl. Cancer Inst.* **78:**853–861.

Manni, A., Trujillo, J. E., and Pearson, O. H., 1977, Predominant role of prolactin in stimulating the growth of 7,12-dimethylbenz(a)anthracene-induced rat mammary tumor, *Cancer Res.* **37:**1216–1219.

Masoro, E. J., 1985, Nutrition and aging: A current assessment, *J. Nutr.* **115:**842–848.

Masoro, E. J., Yu, B. P., and Bertrand, H. A., 1982, Action of food restriction in delaying the aging process, *Proc. Natl. Acad. Sci. USA* **79:**4239–4241.

McCay, C. M., and Crowell, M. F., 1934, Prolonging the lifespan, *Sci. Monthly* **39:**405–414.

McCay, C. M., Maynard, L. A., Sperling, G., and Barnes, L. L., 1939, Retarded growth, life span, ultimate body size and age changes in the albino rat after feeding diets in calories, *J. Nutr.* **18:**1–13.

McCumbee, W. D., and Lebovitz, H. E., 1981, Chondrosarcoma growth: influence of diabetes, caloric restriction and insulin treatment, *Am. J. Physiol. (Endocrinol. Metab.)* **4:**E129–E135.

Meites, J., 1972, Relation of prolactin and estrogen to mammary tumorigenesis in the rat, *J. Natl. Cancer Inst.* **48:**1217–1224.

Mills, P. K., Annegers, J. F., and Phillips, R. L., 1988, Animal product consumption and subsequent fatal breast cancer risk among Seventh-Day Adventists, *Am. J. Epidemiol.* **127:**440–453.

Moreschi, C., 1909, Beziehungern awischen ernahrung unt tumorwachstum, *Z. Immunitatforsch.* **2:**651.

Mutsuura, S., Sone, S., Tsubura, E., Tacibana, K., and Kishino, Y., 1986, Activation of antitumor properties in alveolar macrophages from protein–calorie malnourished rats, *Cancer Immunol. Immunother.* **21:**63–68.

NAS, 1982, *Committee on Diet, Nutrition and Cancer,* National Academy Press, Washington, DC., pp. 66–72.

Newman, S. C., Miller, A. B., and Howe, G. R., 1986, A study of the effect of weight and dietary fat on breast cancer survival time, *Am. J. Epidemiol.* **123:**767–774.

Ohno, T., and Cardullo, A. C., 1983, Effect of caloric restriction on neoplasm growth, *Mt. Sinai J. Med.* **50:**338–342.

Pahlavani, M. A., and Richardson, A., 1987, Influence of dietary restriction on the function of the immune system of rats, *Fed. Proc.* **46:**567.

Pariza, M. W., 1986, Calorie restriction, ad libitum feeding, and cancer, *Proc. Soc. Exp. Biol. Med.* **183:**293–298.

Pariza, M. W., 1987, Dietary fat, calorie restriction, *ad libitum* feeding, and cancer risk, *Nutr. Rev.* **45:**1–7.

Pasqualini, C., Bojda, R., and Kerdelhue, B., 1988, *In vitro* estrogen-like effects of 7,12-dimethylbenz(a)anthracene on anterior pituitary dopamine receptors of rats, *Cancer Res.* **48:**6434–6437.

Pearson, O. H., Llerena, O., Llerena, L., Molina, A., and Bulter, T., 1969, Prolactin-dependent rat mammary cancer: A model for man? *Trans. Assoc. Am. Physicians* **82:**225–238.

Pollard, M., and Luckert, P. H., 1985, Tumorigenic effects of direct- and indirect-acting chemical carcinogens in rats on a restricted diet, *J. Natl. Cancer Inst.* **74:**1347–1349.

Pollard, M., Luckert, P. H., and Pan, G-Y., 1984, Inhibition of intestinal tumorigenesis in methylazoxymethanol-treated rats by dietary restriction, *Cancer Treat. Rep.* **68:**405–408.

Rao, G. N., Piegorsch, W. W., and Haseman, J. K., 1987, Influence of body weight on the incidence of spontaneous tumors in rats and mice of long-term studies, *Am. J. Clin. Nutr.* **45**(Suppl.):252–260.

Rao, G., Heydari, A., Gu, M. Z., Waggoner, S., Marquardt, L., and Richardson, A., 1988, Effect of dietary restriction on gene expression, *FASEBJ.* **2:**A1209, #5307.

Reddy, B. S., 1986, Dietary fat and cancer: specific action or caloric effect? *J. Nutr.* **116:**1132–1135.

Reddy, B. S., and Cohen, L. A. (eds.), 1986, *Diet, Nutrition and Cancer: A Critical Evaluation. Vol 1. Macronutrients and Cancer,* CRC Press, Boca Raton, FL, 175 pp.

Reddy, B. S., Wan, C-X., and Maruyama H., 1987, Effect of restricted caloric intake on azoxymethane-induced colon tumor incidence in male F344 rats, *Cancer Res.* **47:**1226–1228.

Richardson, A., and Cheung, H. T., 1982, The relationship between age-related changes in gene expression, protein turnover, and the responsiveness of an organism to stimuli, *Life Sci.* **31:**605–613.

Roebuck, B. D., Yager, J. D., Jr., and Longnecker, D. S., 1981a, Dietary modulation of azaserine-induced pancreatic carcinogenesis in the rat, *Cancer Res.* **41:**888–893.

Roebuck, B. D., Yager, Jr., J. D., Longnecker, J. D., and Wilpone, S. E., 1981b, Promotion by unsaturated fat of azaserine-induced pancreatic carcinogenesis in the rat, *Cancer Res.* **41**:3961–3966.

Rohan, T. E., and Bain, C. J., 1987, Diet in the etiology of breast cancer, *Epidemiol. Rev.* **9**:120–145.

Rosen, O. M., 1987, After insulin binds, *Science* **237**:1452–1458.

Ross, M. H., and Bras, G., 1971, Lasting influence of early caloric restriction on prevalence of neoplasms in the rat, *J. Natl. Cancer Inst.* **47**:1095–1113.

Ross, M. H., and Bras, G., 1973, Influence of protein under- and overnutrition on spontaneous tumor prevalence in the rat, *J. Nutr.* **103**:944–963.

Ross, M. H., Lustbader, E. D., and Bras, G., 1983, Body weight, dietary practices, and tumor suspectibility in the rat, *J. Natl. Cancer Inst.* **71**:1041–1046.

Rous, P., 1914, The influence of diet on transplanted and spontaneous mouse tumors, *J. Exp. Med.* **20**:433.

Rudland, P. S., Hallowes, R. C., Durbin, H., and Lewis, D., 1977, Mitogenic activity of pituitary hormones on cell cultures of normal and carcingen-induced tumor epithelium from rat mammary glands, *J. Cell Biol.* **73**:561–577.

Ruggeri, B. A., Klurfeld, D. M., and Kritchevsky, D., 1987, Biochemical alterations in 7,12-dimethylbenz(a)-anthracene-induced mammary tumors from rats subjected to caloric restriction, *Biochem. Biophys. Acta.* **929**:239–246.

Sarkar, N. H., Fernandes, G., Telang, N. T., Kourides, I. A., and Good, R. A., 1982, Low calorie diet prevents the development of mammary tumors in C3H mice and reduces circulating prolactin level, murine mammary tumor virus expression, and proliferation of mammary alveolar cells, *Proc. Natl. Acad. Sci. USA* **79**:7758–7762.

Saxton, J. A., Boon, M. C., and Furth, J., 1944, Observations on the inhibition of development of spontaneous leukemia in mice by underfeeding, *Cancer Res.* **7**:401–409.

Schneider, E. L., and Reed, J. D., Jr., 1985, Life extension, *N. Engl. J. Med.* **312**:1159–1168.

Shafie, S. M., and Hilf, R., 1978, Relationship between insulin and estrogen binding to growth response in 7,12-dimethylbenz(a)anthracene-induced rat mammary tumors, *Cancer Res.* **38**:759–764.

Sinha, D. K., Gebhard, R. L., and Pazik, J. E., 1988, Inhibition of mammary carcinogenesis in rats by dietary restriction, *Cancer Lett.* **40**:133–141.

Steffen, M., Scherdin, V., Duvigneau, C., and Holzel, F., 1988, Glucocorticoid-induced alterations of morphology and growth of fibrosarcoma cells derived from 7,12-dimethylbenz(a)anthracene rat mammary tumor, *Cancer Res.* **48**:7212–7218.

Stewart, J., Meaney, M. J., Aitken, D., Jensen, L., and Kalant, N., 1988, The effects of acute and life-long food restriction on basal and stress-induced serum corticosterone levels in young and aged rats, *Endocrinology* **123**:1934–1941.

Swanson, C. A., Jones, D. Y., Schatzkin, A., Brinton, L. A., and Ziegler, R. G., 1988, Breast cancer risk assessed by anthropometry in the NHANES I epidemiological follow-up study, *Cancer Res.* **48**:5363–5367.

Sylvester, P. W., Aylsworth, C. F., and Meites, J., 1981, Relationship of hormones to inhibition of mammary tumor development by underfeeding during the "critical period" after carcinogen administration, *Cancer Res.* **41**:1383–1388.

Sylvester, P. W., Aylsworth, C. F., Van Vugt, D. A., and Meites, J., 1982, Influence of underfeeding during the "critical period" or thereafter on carcinogen-induced mammary tumors in rats, *Cancer Res.* **42**:4943–4947.

Tannenbaum, A., 1940a, Relationship of body weight to cancer incidence, *Arch. Pathol.* **30**:509–517.

Tannenbaum, A., 1940b, The initiation and growth of tumors. Introduction. I. Effects of underfeeding, *Am. J. Cancer* **38**:335–350.

Tannenbaum, A., 1942, The genesis and growth of tumors. II. Effects of calorie restriction *per se, Cancer Res.* **2**:460–467.

Tannenbaum, A., 1944, The dependence on the genesis of induced skin tumors on the fat content of the diet during different stages of carcinogenesis, *Cancer Res.* **4**:683–687.

Tannenbaum, A., 1945a, The dependence of tumor formation on the degree of caloric restriction, *Cancer Res.* **5**:609–615.

Tannenbaum, A., 1945b, The dependence of tumor formation on the composition of the calorie-restricted diet as well as on the degree of restriction, *Cancer Res.* **5**:616–625.

Tannenbaum, A., and Silverstone, H., 1949, Effect of low environmental temperature, dinitrophenol, or sodium fluoride on the formation of tumors in mice, *Cancer Res.* **9**:403–410.

Tao, S-C., Yu, M. C., Ross, R. K., and Xiu, K-W., 1988, Risk factors for breast cancer in Chinese women in Beijing, *Int. J. Cancer* **42**:495–498.

Taub, R., Roy, A., Dieter, R., and Koontz, J., 1987, Insulin as a growth factor in rat hepatoma cells, *J. Biol. Chem.* **262**:10893–10897.

Thompson, H. J., Meeker, L. D., Tagliaferro, A. R., and Roberts, J. S., 1985, Effect of energy intake on the promotion of mammary carcinogenesis by dietary fat, *Nutr. Cancer* **7**:37–41.

Tucker, M. J., 1979, The effect of long-term food restriction on tumors in rodents, *Int. J. Cancer* **23**:803–807.

Visscher, M. B., Ball, Z. B., Barnes, R. H., and Silvertsen, I., 1942, The influence of caloric restriction upon the incidence of spontaneous mammary carcinoma in mice, *Surgery* **11**:48–55.

Waxler, S. H., 1954, The effect of weight reduction on the occurrence of spontaneous mammary tumors in mice, *J. Natl. Cancer Inst.* **14**:1253–1256.

Waxler, S. H., 1960, Obesity and cancer susceptibility in mice, *Am. J. Clin. Nutr.* **8**:760–766.

Weindruch, R. H., Kristie, J. A., Cheney, K. E., and Walford, R. L., 1979, Influence of controlled dietary restriction on immunologic function and aging, *Fed. Proc.* **38**:2007–2016.

Weindruch, R. H., Devens, B. H., Raff, H. V., and Walford, R. L., 1983, Influence of dietary restriction on aging and natural killer cell activity in mice, *J. Immunol.* **130**:993–996.

Weindruch, R. H., Walford, R. L., Fligiel, S., and Guthrie, D., 1986, The retardation of aging in mice by dietary restriction: Longevity, cancer, immunity and lifetime energy intake, *J. Nutr.* **116**:641–654.

Welsch, C. W., 1985, Host factors affecting the growth of carcinogen-induced rat mammary carcinomas: A review and tribute to Charles Brenton Huggins, *Cancer Res.* **45**:3415–3443.

Welsch, C. W., 1987, Enhancement of mammary tumorigenesis by dietary fat: a review of potential mechanisms, *Am. J. Clin. Nutr.* **45**(Suppl.):192–202.

Welsch, C. W., and Aylsworth, C. F., 1983, The interrelationship between dietary lipids, endocrine activity, and the development of mammary tumors in experimental animals, in: *Dietary Fats and Health* (E. G. Perkins and W. J. Visek, eds.), AOCS Monograph 10, Champaign, IL, pp. 790–816.

Weraarchakul, N., and Richardson, A., 1988, Effect of age and dietary restriction on DNA repair, *FASEB J.* **2**:A1209, #5309.

White, F. R., 1961, The relationship between underfeeding and tumor formation, transplantation, and growth in rats and mice, *Cancer Res.* **21**:281–290.

White, F. R., White, J., Mider, G. B., Kelly, M. G., and Heston, W. E., 1944, Effect of caloric restriction on mammary tumor formation in strain C3H mice and on the response of strain DBA to painting with methylcholanthrene, *J. Natl. Cancer Inst.* **5**:43–47.

Willet, W. C., 1987, Implications of total energy intake for epidemiologic studies of breast and large-bowel cancer, *Am. J. Clin. Nutr.* **45**(Suppl.):354–360.

Willet, W. C., Stampfer, M. J., Colditz, G. A., Rosner, B. A., Hennekens, C. H., and Speizer, F. E., 1987, Dietary fat, and the risk of breast cancer, *N. Engl. J. Med.* **316**:22–28.

Williams, G., Howell, A., and Jones, M., 1988, The relationship of body weight to response to endocrine therapy, steroid hormone receptors and survival of patients with advanced cancer of the breast, *Br. J. Cancer* **58**:631–634.

Wolff, G. L., 1987, Body weight and cancer, *Am. J. Clin. Nutr.* **45**(Suppl.):168–180.

Wynder, E. L., and Gori, G. B., 1977, Contribution of the environment to cancer incidence: An epidemiologic exercise, *J. Natl. Cancer Inst.* **58**:825–832.

Yuan, J-M., Yu, M. C., Ross, R. K., Gao, Y-T., and Henderson, B. E., 1988, Risk factors for breast cancer in Chinese women in Shanghai, *Cancer Res.* **48**:1949–1953.

10

Dietary Fiber and Cancer

David Kritchevsky and David M. Klurfeld

1. Introduction

Fiber has been defined by Paul and Southgate (1978) as "the sum of the polysaccharides and lignin which are not digested by the endogenous secretions of the human gastrointestinal tract. This fraction has a variable composition as it is made up of several different types of polysaccharides (pectic substances, hemicelluloses, and celluloses) and the noncarbohydrate lignin." The description of fiber has been expanded to include plant gums, mucilages, and algal polysaccharides. It is convenient to classify these substances into insoluble fiber (cellulose, hemicellulose, lignin), which decreases intestinal transit time and increases fecal bulk, and soluble fiber (pectic substances, gums), which delays gastric emptying.

The "fiber hypothesis," which is based on overall lifestyle, owes its genesis to Burkitt (1971) and is based on observations of fiber intake and cancer incidence in African populations. Earlier, Cleave (1956) had related diseases of developed nations to diets rich in refined carbohydrates. Interest in diet as a factor in colon cancer was stimulated originally by the work of Higginson and Oettle (1960), who suggested that rarity of bowel cancer among African blacks might be due to diet and specifically to dietary bulk.

2. Epidemiologic Studies

The epidemiologic data relating diet and colon cancer date to the study of Stocks and Karn (1933), who studied the diets of 450 colon cancer patients and a like number of controls. They found negative correlations with intake of whole-meal bread, vegetables, and milk. The epidemiologic data have been reviewed (Byers and Graham, 1984; Willett and MacMahon, 1984; Klurfeld and Kritchevsky, 1986; Cummings and Bingham, 1987; Rogers and Longnecker, 1988) and provide no unanimity regarding a protective role for

David Kritchevsky and David M. Klurfeld • The Wistar Institute of Anatomy and Biology, Philadelphia, Pennsylvania 19104.

Table I. Correlation Coefficients between Environmental Variables[a]

Food	Total fat	Animal protein	Sugar	Gross national product
Cereals	−0.72	−0.76	−0.59	−0.71
Pulses, nuts, seeds	−0.55	−0.55	−0.67	−0.34
Potatoes, starch	0.34	0.28	0.43	0.09
Vegetables	−0.03	0.00	−0.28	0.03
Fruits	0.35	0.30	0.16	0.38

[a]After Armstrong and Doll, 1975.

fiber. Comparisons of fiber intake are really studies of intake of fiber-rich foods. Thus, other dietary components which may interact with fiber can play a role in determining efficacy of fiber. Alternatively, fiber may serve as a proxy nutrient in analysis and some minor component of fiber-rich food may have greater influence on colonic carcinogenesis. Colon cancer is more prevalent in affluent countries, where diets are generally lower in fiber than diets in underdeveloped countries. Armstrong and Doll (1975) (Table I) found intake of fiber-rich foods to be inversely correlated with gross national product. Mortality from colon cancer is, in general, positively correlated with gross national product (Kassira *et al.*, 1976). The five countries (of 37) with the highest colon cancer mortality rate in 1970 (21.4 ± 0.46 deaths/100,000 population) had a *per capita* gross national product in 1971 of $2556 ± 348, while the five countries with the lowest mortality rate (0.58 ± 0.16/100,000) had a *per capita* gross national product of $328 ± 69. There is a strong negative correlation ($r = -0.85$) between mortality rates from colon cancer and stomach cancer (Table II) (Gregor *et al.*, 1969). Hakama and Saxen (1967), surveying data from 16 countries, found a positive association between cereal consumption and stomach cancer mortality and a strong negative correlation between stomach cancer and *per capita* income. The data available relating fiber to colon cancer were such as to evoke the following conclusion from a committee of the National Academy of Sciences (Committee on Diet, Nutrition and Cancer, 1982): "The committee found no conclusive evidence to

Table II. Mortality Rates for Stomach
and Intestinal Cancer 1962–1963
(Rates/100,000 Males)[a]

Country	Stomach	Intestine
Greece	15.17	4.14
United States	14.87	12.25
Canada	18.69	13.88
Denmark	23.93	13.91
Italy	34.22	7.97
Finland	44.80	5.20
Chile	64.63	2.70
Japan	67.96	2.97

[a]After Gregor *et al.*, 1969.

*Table III. Large-Bowel Cancer and Diet
in Three Socioeconomic Groups in Hong Kong[a]*

	Income		
	Low	Median	High
Incidence of cancer			
Male	11.7	17.6	26.7
Female	11.2	16.2	no data
Calories (% total)			
Total	2163	2433	3183
Fat	711 (33)	837 (34)	1143 (57)
Protein	144 (7)	164 (7)	208 (7)
Carbohydrate	1308 (60)	1432 (59)	1832 (57)
Fiber rich foods (g)	520	573	672
g fiber-food/kcal	0.24	0.24	0.21

[a]After Hill *et al.*, 1979.

indicate that dietary fiber (such as present in fruits, vegetables, grains and cereals) exerts a protective effect against colorectal cancer in humans." Hill *et al.* (1979) compared diet and colon cancer incidence in three socioeconomic groups in Hong Kong. As can be seen from Table III, the highest socioeconomic group ate 29% more of fiber-rich foods than the lowest group; they ingested 47% more calories and exhibited a 128% greater incidence of colon cancer.

Jensen *et al.* (1982) examined diet, bowel function, fecal chemistry, and large-bowel cancer in Finland and Denmark. The incidence rates in rural and urban Denmark and Finland are presented in Table IV and fiber intakes in Table V. They analyzed 39 variables in relation to large-bowel cancer, including anthropometry (two), nutrients (14), foods (18), bowel habits (two) and fecal steroids (three). Six items were found to have a significantly negative correlation with risk. They were saturated fatty acids, carbohydrate, starch, protein, total dietary fiber, and cereals. Only two items were positively correlated with risk; they were fecal bile acids as mg/g dry weight of feces or mg/g wet weight of feces and alcohol. These findings are summarized in Table VI.

Cummings and Bingham (1987) summarized daily intake of nonstarch polysaccharides and cancer incidence in several populations (Table VII). Japan, whose intake is 61%

*Table IV. Incidence Rates (per 100,000) of Colorectal
Cancer among Men in Denmark and Finland[a]*

Country (period)	Site	Incidence rates	
		Colon	Rectum
Finland	Parikkala	6.7	7.5
(1970–1975)	Helsinki	17.0	8.7
Denmark	Them	12.9	15.0
(1968–1972)	Copenhagen	22.8	39.3

[a]After Jensen *et al.*, 1982.

Table V. Fiber Intake by 50- to 59-Year-Old Men
in Finland and Denmark[a]

Fiber	Intake (g)			
	Parikkala	Helsinki	Them	Copenhagen
Total fiber	18.4	14.5	18.0	13.2
Pentose	7.4	5.5	6.6	4.5
Hexose	5.3	3.7	5.5	3.6
Uronic acid	1.9	2.0	2.2	1.9
Cellulose	4.1	3.4	3.7	3.2

[a]After Jensen *et al.*, 1982.

that of rural Denmark, exhibits 40% lower cancer incidence. Walker *et al.* (1986) found fiber intakes of South African blacks, coloreds, Indians, and whites to be similar, but the incidence of colon cancer in these four groups is vastly different (Table VIII). Clearly, other factors in diet must be considered.

In 1988 Byers summarized findings relating to fiber and colon cancer in seven studies that had appeared since the interim dietary guidelines had been promulgated by the National Academy of Sciences (Committee on Diet, Nutrition and Cancer, 1982). In Greece, Manousos *et al.* (1983) had compared 100 cases and an equal number of controls using cereal as the paradigm for fiber and found no effects; high intake of vegetables reduced relative risk, however. Pickle *et al.* (1984) found increased relative risk associated with high intake of vegetables or high-fiber foods. They examined 86 cases and twice as many controls. In Belgium heavy intake of "fibers" conferred some reduction in relative risk (Tuyns, 1986). Comparison of fiber intake from vegetables in 399 cases and an equal number of controls in France showed reduced relative risk in the highest quartile (Marquart-Moulin *et al.*, 1986).

In a study among Mormons in Utah, Lyon *et al.* (1987) found that relative risk

Table VI. Variables Relating to Large-Bowel Cancer Trends in Denmark and Finland[a]

Positive	Negative	Not significant	
Fecal bile acids	Saturated fatty acids	Height	Vegetables
(mg/g)	Carbohydrates	Weight	Fruits, berries
Alcohol	Starch	Energy	Fats and oils
	Protein	Total fat	Milk
	Total fiber	Unsaturated fatty acids	Milk products
	Cereals	Vitamin A	Cheese
		Vitamin C	Meats
		Hexose (fiber)	Fish
		Pentose (fiber)	Eggs
		Cellulose	Coffee
		Rye	Transit time
		Wheat	Stool weight
		Other cereals	Fecal bile acids (24 hr)

[a]After Jensen *et al.*, 1982.

Table VII. Nonstarch Polysaccharide (NPS) Intake
(±SD) and Large-Bowel Cancer Incidence in Males
(per 100,000 per yr)[a]

		Cancer	
Country	NPS (g/day)	Colon	Colon plus rectum
Japan	10.9	7.8	17.3
Rural Finland	18.4 ± 7.8	6.7	14.2
Rural Denmark	18.0 ± 6.4	12.9	27.9
Helsinki	14.5 ± 5.4	17.0	25.7
Copenhagen	13.2 ± 4.0	22.8	42.1
United Kingdom	12.4	21.3	41.8

[a]After Cummings and Bingham, 1987.

increased as crude fiber intake increased. The finding held true for both male and female probands. This study encompassed 246 cases and 484 controls. Lyon *et al.* did find a strong positive correlation between colon cancer incidence and energy intake and concluded, "Total energy intake must be evaluated before attempting to assign a causal role to any food or nutrient that may be postulated to play a role in colon cancer." Table IX summarizes the relative risks as related to daily energy intake.

Two Australian studies offer interesting contrast. Kune *et al.* (1987) examined 388 male cases of colon cancer compared with 398 controls in Melbourne. Relative risk was halved in the third, fourth, and fifth quintiles of dietary fiber. Comparison of 327 female cases with 329 controls gave virtually the same result. Potter and McMichael (1986), on the other hand, examined 121 male cases and 241 controls and 99 female cases and 197 controls in Adelaide and found increasing risk with increasing fiber intake, especially in the women. They found increased dietary protein to be the most consistent risk factor. Total energy intake was also positively associated with risk. The increased risk associated with high-protein and high-energy intake was confined to subjects ingesting a diet low in fiber. Kune *et al.* suggest that their findings require a multifactorial hypothesis for satisfactory resolution.

Table VIII. Fiber Intake and Diet in Five South African Populations[a]

	Population				
	Rural black	Urban black	Indian	Colored	White
Proneness to colon cancer	0	±	+	+	+++
Fat (g/day)	38	66	99	85	82
Protein (g/day)	68	72	79	78	73
Total energy (kcal)	2045	2220	2330	2393	2010
Fiber (g/day)	25.2	18.1	20.5	21.3	22.6
Fecal pH	6.12	6.15	6.21	6.29	6.88

[a]After Walker *et al.*, 1986.

Table IX. Age-Adjusted Relative Risk (RR)
by Daily Energy Intake[a]

		RR at kcal/day	
Men	<1900	1900–2600	>2600
	1.0	2.5	2.5
Women	<1300	1300–1800	>1800
	1.0	2.0	3.6

[a]After Lyon *et al.*, 1987.

Slattery *et al.* (1988) reported on risk of colon cancer in Utah as a function of fiber source and food type. Crude fiber decreased risk consistently, but dietary fiber and neutral detergent fiber did not. Highest quartiles of intake of fruits and vegetables were associated with decreased risk of colon cancer but high intake of grains was not protective. The lowest risk for dietary fiber in males and females was in the second quartile of intake. This suggests the possibility that as dietary fiber intake increases, some other protective factor decreases. The data were analyzed for cancer in the ascending and descending colon and suggest that fiber components may exert their influence in different parts of the colon and that different risk patterns exist for males and females.

3. Effects of Dietary Fiber in the Human Colon

Table X lists the effects of dietary fiber in the human colon. It is of interest to see which of these may be operative vis-à-vis a possible protective role.

Fecal weight and transit time were not associated with cancer risk in the study of Danish and Finnish men cited earlier (Jensen *et al.*, 1982). A study of Japanese immigrants to Hawaii (Isei) and their Hawaiian-born sons (Nisei) showed that fathers and sons exhibited similar fecal transit times and fecal bulk. The transit times were shorter than those of Hawaiian Caucasians and the fecal bulk greater. However, the incidence of colon cancer in the Nisei and Caucasians was the same, being much higher than that of the Isei (Glober *et al.*, 1977). Thus, effects of fiber on some fecal characteristics do not appear to be important.

Table X. Effects of Dietary Fiber
in the Human Colon

Increases fecal weight
Increases frequency of defecation
Decreases transit time
Dilutes colonic contents
Increases microbial growth
Alters energy metabolism
Adsorbs organic and inorganic substances
Decreases dehydroxylation of bile acids
Produces H_2, CH_4, CO_2, and short-chain fatty acids

The increased fecal bulk that results from fiber ingestion may be regarded as dilution of colonic contents. The study by Jensen *et al.* (1982) showed high concentration of fecal bile acids to be a positive risk factor for colon cancer. Comparison of fecal bile acid concentrations in Finns (Kupio) and Americans (New York City) showed that while the two groups excreted the same amount of bile acids daily (275 mg) the concentration of bile acids was 4.6 mg/g feces in the Finns, who exhibit a relatively low incidence of colon cancer, and 12.3 mg/g feces in the Americans, in whom incidence of colon cancer is high (Reddy *et al.*, 1978).

Hill *et al.* (1971) found fecal acidic steroid concentrations in Uganda, Japan, and India to be 0.61 ± 0.13 mg/g feces, while in the United States, England, and Scotland they were 6.15 ± 0.66 mg/g.

Dietary fiber binds bile acids and bile salts, the extent of binding being a function of both the fiber and the particular bile salt or acid used (Eastwood and Hamilton, 1968; Story and Kritchevsky, 1976). However, when cholestyramine, a bile acid binding resin, was fed to rats given any one of three chemical carcinogens, colon carcinogenesis was enhanced significantly (Nigro *et al.*, 1973). Both the avidity of bile acid binding and stereochemical interactions between the binding agent and bile acid or bile salt may play a role in carcinogenesis. Effects of binding carcinogens or steroid hormones remain to be tested.

The liver produces cholic (3α, 7α, 12α-trihydroxycholanoic) and chenodeoxycholic (3α, 7α-dihydroxycholanoic) acids, which are dehydroxylated at the 7 position by intestinal flora to yield deoxycholic (3α, 12α-dihydroxycholanoic) and lithocholic (3α hydroxycholanoic) acid, respectively. Anerobic bacteria metabolize steroids more vigorously than aerobic bacteria, and the ratio of anaerobic to aerobic colonic bacteria in countries with a high incidence of colon cancer is about two and a half times that in countries with a low incidence of colon cancer (Hill *et al.*, 1971).

Efforts to correlate incidence of colon cancer with the ratio of primary (cholic and chenodeoxycholic acids) to secondary (deoxycholic and lithocholic acids) in feces have not been successful (Kritchevsky and Klurfeld, 1981).

Except for lignin, dietary fibers are fermented in the colon to yield short-chain fatty acids (SCFA), among other products. The principal SCFA in the large bowel are acetic, propionic, and butyric, which are formed in the approximate ratio of 3 : 1 : 1. Butyrate has been shown to alter the *in vitro* properties of human colorectal cell lines, slowing growth rate and prolonging doubling time (Kim *et al.*, 1982). Butyrate has also been shown to suppress proliferation of a variety of cells (Hagopian *et al.*, 1977). Butyrate is an important fuel for colon epithelial cells and may, indeed, be the preferred fuel for those cells. Thus, fiber might affect colon carcinogenesis by virtue of its conversion to butyric acid.

Production of SCFA may affect the pH of the intestine. Patients with bowel cancer exhibit higher fecal pH than controls (MacDonald *et al.*, 1978). Walker *et al.* (1986) found that fiber intakes of South African racial groups with different incidence of colon cancer were similar, but fecal pH was higher in the groups with higher incidence. These observations suggest interesting areas for further research.

Fiber enhances fecal energy loss. Young women fed diets low, medium, or high in fiber excreted an additional 83, 127, or 210 kcal/day respectively (Southgate and Durnin, 1970). Similar observations have been made by Kelsay *et al.* (1978) and Heaton *et al.* (1983). Caloric restriction inhibits spontaneous, transplanted, or induced cancer in rats

(Kritchevsky and Klurfeld, 1986). This particular topic is treated at length elsewhere in this volume. It is worth pointing out that 40% caloric restriction significantly reduced incidence of colon tumors in rats treated with 1,2-dimethylhydrazine (DMH) (Klurfeld *et al.*, 1987). The high ratio of fiber to calories could be one reason for the lower incidence of colon cancer in underdeveloped countries.

It is difficult to compare the effects of fiber on chemically induced cancers in rats because different strains of rats and genders are used, different carcinogens are administered by different routes, and diets vary in composition and fiber content. Protective effects, no effects, or enhancement of carcinogenicity have all been seen (Kritchevsky, 1983, 1985). Wheat bran most often shows a protective effect, but it is noteworthy that it protects male Sprague–Dawley rats but not female Sprague–Dawley rats against DMH-induced tumors (Barbolt and Abraham, 1978, 1980). Wheat bran enhances tumorigenesis when fed during carcinogen administration but reduces it when fed subsequent to carcinogen administration (Jacobs, 1983). Pectin enhances carcinogenicity when fed during DMH exposure (Bauer *et al.*, 1979). Corn bran also enhances carcinogenicity (Reddy *et al.*, 1983) as does undegraded carageenan (Watanabe *et al.*, 1978). Influences of fiber on experimental colon carcinogenesis have been reviewed by Jacobs (1986).

4. Conclusion

The question of dietary fiber effects on colon cancer remains unresolved. The epidemiologic data are inconsistent and tend not to support the original hypothesis. However, it may be that the original hypothesis was too simple; perhaps it is not the dietary fiber *per se* but the conditions governing its fermentation which determine its effects. The products of fermentation (SCFA, methane) may influence cell proliferation and may be, in turn, influenced by metabolic products of other nutrients. Other aspects of fiber nutriture, such as increased energy excretion, may also play a role. The relative contributions of the various effects of fiber are influenced by other aspects of diet and lifestyle. The interest in fiber effects on carcinogenesis has stimulated research and added much to our knowledge of the chemistry and physiology of fiber. Much work remains, however.

ACKNOWLEDGMENTS. Work described in this chapter is supported, in part, by Grant CA-43856 and a Research Career Award (HL-00734) from the NIH and by funds from the Commonwealth of Pennsylvania.

5. References

Armstrong, B., and Doll, R., 1975, Environmental factors and cancer incidence and mortality in different countries, with special reference to dietary practices, *Int. J. Cancer* **15**:617–631.

Barbolt, T. A., and Abraham, R., 1978, The effect of bran in dimethylhydrazine-induced colon carcinogenesis in the rat, *Proc. Soc. Exp. Biol. Med.* **157**:656–659.

Barbolt, T. A., and Abraham, R., 1980, Dose–response, sex differences and the effect of bran in dimethylhydrazine-induced intestinal carcinogenesis in rats, *Toxicol. Appl. Pharmacol.* **55**:417–422.

Bauer, H. G., Asp, N. G., Oste, R., Dahlqvist, A., and Fredlund, P. E., 1979, Effect of dietary fiber on the induction of colorectal tumors and fecal glucuronidase activity in the rat, *Cancer Res.* **39**:3752–3756.

Burkitt, D. P., 1971, Epidemiology of cancer of the colon and rectum, *Cancer* **28**:3–13.

Byers, T., 1988, Diet and cancer. Any progress in the interim? *Cancer* **62**:1713–1724.

Byers, T., and Graham, S., 1984, The epidemiology of diet and cancer, *Adv. Cancer Res.* **41**:1–69.

Cleave, T. L., 1956, The neglect of natural principles in current medical practice, *J. Roy. Nav. Med. Serv.* **42**:55–82.

Committee on Diet, Nutrition and Cancer, 1982, Diet, nutrition and cancer, National Academy Press, Washington, DC.

Cummings, J. H., and Bingham, S. A., 1987, Dietary fibre, fermentation and large bowel cancer, *Cancer Surveys* **6**:601–621.

Eastwood, M. A., and Hamilton, D., 1968, Studies on the adsorption of bile salts to non-absorbed components of diet, *Biochim. Biophys. Acta* **152**:165–173.

Glober, G. A., Nomura, A., Kamiyama, S., Shimoda, A., and Abba, B. C., 1977, Bowel transit time and stool weight in populations with different colon cancer risks, *Lancet* **2**:110.

Gregor, O., Toman, R., and Prusova, F., 1969, Gastrointestinal cancer and nutrition, *Gut* **10**:1031–1034.

Hagopian, H. K., Riggs, M. G., Swartz, L. A., and Ingram, V. M., 1977, Effect of *n*-butyrate on DNA synthesis in chick fibroblasts and HeLa cells, *Cell* **12**:855–860.

Hakama, M., and Saxen, E. A., 1967, Cereal consumption and gastric cancer, *Int. J. Cancer* **2**:265–268.

Heaton, K. W., Emmett, P. M., Henry, C. L., Thornton, J. R., Manhire, A., and Hartog, M., 1983, Not just fibre: the nutritional consequences of refined carbohydrate foods, *Hum. Nutr. Clin. Nutr.* **37C**:31–35.

Higginson, J., and Oettle, A. G., 1960, Cancer incidence in the Bantu and "Cape Coloured" races of South Africa: Report of a cancer survey in the Transvaal, *J. Natl. Cancer Inst.* **24**:589–671.

Hill, M. J., Drasar, B. S., Aries, V. C., Crowther, J. S., Hawksworth, G., and Williams, R. E. O., 1971, Bacteria and the aetiology of cancer of the large bowel, *Lancet* **1**:95–100.

Hill, M. J., Maclennan, R., and Newcombe, K., 1979, Diet and large bowel cancer in three socioeconomic groups in Hong Kong, *Lancet* **1**:436.

Jacobs, L. R., 1983, Enhancement of rat colon carcinogenesis by wheat bran consumption during the stage of 1,2-dimethylhydrazine administration, *Cancer Res.* **43**:4057–4061.

Jacobs, L. R., 1986, Modification of experimental colon carcinogenesis by dietary fibers, *Adv. Exp. Biol. Med.* **206**:105–118.

Jensen, O. M., Maclennan, R., and Wahrendorf, J., 1982, Diet, bowel function, fecal characteristics and large bowel cancer in Denmark and Finland, *Nutr. Cancer* **4**:5–19.

Kassira, E., Parent, L., and Vahouny, G. V., 1976, Colon cancer. An epidemiological survey, *Am. J. Dig. Dis.* **21**:205–214.

Kelsay, J. L., Behall, K. M., and Prather, E. S., 1978, Effect of fiber from fruits and vegetables on metabolic responses of human subjects. 1. Bowel transit time, number of defecations, fecal weight, urinary excretions of energy and nitrogen and apparent digestibilities of energy, nitrogen and fat, *Am. J. Clin. Nutr.* **31**:1149–1153.

Kim, Y. S., Tsao, D., Morita, A., and Bella, A., 1982, Effect of sodium butyrate on three human colorectal adenocarcinoma cell lines in culture, in: *Colon Carcinogenesis* (R. A. Malt, and R. C. N. Williamson, eds.), MTP Press, Lancaster, UK, pp. 317–323.

Klurfeld, D. M., and Kritchevsky, D., 1986, Dietary fiber and human cancer: Critique of the literature, *Adv. Exp. Med. Biol.* **206**:119–135.

Klurfeld, D. M., Weber, M. M., and Kritchevsky, D., 1987, Inhibition of chemically induced mammary and colon tumor promotion by caloric restriction in rats fed increased dietary fat, *Cancer Res.* **47**:2759–2762.

Kritchevsky, D., 1983, Fiber, steroids and cancer, *Cancer Res.* **43**(Suppl.):2491S–2495S.

Kritchevsky, D., 1985, Dietary fiber and cancer, *Nutr. Cancer* **6**:213–219.

Kritchevsky, D., and Klurfeld, D. M., 1981, Fat and cancer, in: *Nutrition and Cancer: Etiology and Treatment* (G. R. Newell and N. M. Ellison, eds.), Raven Press, New York, pp. 173–188.

Kritchevsky, D., and Klurfeld, D. M., 1986, Influence of caloric intake on experimental carcinogenesis: A review, *Adv. Exp. Med. Biol.* **206**:55–68.

Kune, S., Kune, G. A., and Watson, L. F., 1987, Case control study of dietary etiological factors: The Melbourne colorectal cancer study, *Nutr. Cancer* **9**:21–42.

Lyon, J. L., Mahoney, A. W., West, D. W., Gardner, J. W., Snuth, K. R., Sorenson, A. W., and Stanish, W., 1987, Energy intake: its relationship to colon cancer risk, *J. Natl. Cancer Inst.* **78**:853–861.

MacDonald, I. A., Webb, G. R., and Mahony, D. E., 1978, Fecal hydroxysteroid dehydrogenase activities in vegetarian Seventh-Day Adventists, control subjects and bowel cancer patients, *Am. J. Clin. Nutr.* **31:**S233–S238.

Manousos, O., Day, N. E., Trichopoulous, D., Gerovassilis, F., Tzonou, A., and Polychronopoulou, A., 1983, Diet and colorectal cancer: A case–control study in Greece, *Int. J. Cancer* **32:**1–5.

Marquart-Moulin, G., Riboli, E., Cornee, J., Charnay, B., Berthezene, P., and Day, N., 1986, Case-control study on colorectal cancer and diet in Marseilles, *Int. J. Cancer* **38:**183–191.

Nigro, N. D., Bhadrachari, N., and Chonichai, C., 1973, A rat model for studying colonic cancer: effect of cholestyramine on induced tumors, *Dis. Colon Rectum* **16:**438–443.

Paul, A. A., and Southgate, D. A. T., 1978, *McCance and Widdowson's The Composition of Foods,* 4th ed., Elsevier/North-Holland, Biomedical Press, Amsterdam.

Pickle, L. W., Greene, M. H., Ziegler, R. G., Toledo, A., Hoover, R., Lynch, H. T., and Fraumeni, J. F., Jr., 1984, Colorectal cancer in rural Nebraska, *Cancer Res.* **44:**363–369.

Potter, J. D., and McMichael, A. J., 1986, Diet and cancer of the colon and rectum: A case–control study, *J. Natl. Cancer Inst.* **76:**557–569.

Reddy, B. S., Hedges, A. R., Laakso, K., and Wynder, E. L., 1978, Metabolic epidemiology of large bowel cancer, *Cancer* **42:**2832–2838.

Reddy, B. S., Maeura, Y., and Wayman, M., 1983, Effect of dietary corn bran and autohydrolyzed lignin on 3,2-dimethyl-4-aminobiphenyl-induced intestinal carcinogenesis in male F344 rats, *J. Natl. Cancer Inst.* **71:**419–423.

Rogers, A. E., and Longnecker, M. P., 1988, Biology of disease. Dietary and nutritional influences on cancer: A review of epidemiological and experimental data, *Lab. Invest.* **59:**729–759.

Slattery, M. L., Sorenson, A. W., Mahoney, A. W., French, T. K., Kritchevsky, D., and Street, J. C., 1988, Diet and colon cancer: assessment of risk by fiber type and food source, *J. Natl. Cancer Inst.* **80:**1474–1480.

Southgate, D. A. T., and Durnin, J. V. G. A., 1970, Caloric conversion factors. An experimental reassessment of the factors used in the calculation of the energy value of human diets, *Br. J. Nutr.* **24:**517–535.

Stocks, P., and Karn, M. K., 1933, A cooperative study of the habits, homelife, dietary and family histories of 450 cancer patients and an equal number of control patients, *Ann. Eugen (London)* **5:**237–280.

Story, J. A., and Kritchevsky, D., 1976, Comparison of the binding of various bile acids and bile salts by several types of fiber, *J. Nutr.* **106:**1292–1294.

Tuyns, A. J., 1986, A case-control study on colorectal cancer in Belgium: Preliminary results, *Med. Sociale Preventive* **31:**81–82.

Walker, A. R. P., Walker, B. F., and Walker, A. J., 1986, Faecal pH, dietary fibre intake and proneness to colon cancer in four South African populations, *Br. J. Cancer* **53:**489–495.

Watanabe, K., Reddy, B. S., Wong, C. Q., and Weisburger, J. H., 1978, Effect of dietary undegraded carageenan on colon carcinogenesis in F344 rats treated with azoxymethane or methylnitrosourea, *Cancer Res.* **38:**4427–4430.

Willett, W. C., and MacMahon, B., 1984, Diet and cancer—An overview, *N. Engl. J. Med.* **310:**633–638, 697–703.

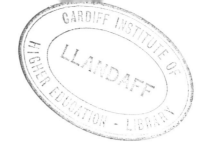

11

Chemoprevention by Nonnutrient Components of Vegetables and Fruits

Diane F. Birt and Edward Bresnick

1. Introduction

This chapter reviews data associating vegetable and fruit consumption with the inhibition of cancer. The next section deals with data on vegetables and fruits: epidemiologic studies, animal studies, and studies using whole vegetable or fruit extracts in metabolic or mutagenicity studies. The rest of the chapter reviews data on a variety of compounds and classes of compounds that have been identified in fruits and/or vegetables and have been studied for their potential as chemopreventive agents. The selection of potential inhibitors discussed in this chapter was not all inclusive because of the tremendous growth in this area of research in the past decade.

2. Studies Relating Vegetable and Fruit Consumption with Cancer Prevention

2.1. Relationship of Diet and Cancer Incidence

Considerable circumstantial evidence exists which implies a relationship between dietary intake and the incidence of cancer. This evidence derives from (1) epidemiologic data accumulated from humans and (2) experimental results obtained in animal model systems. The human epidemiologic data are considered in this section.

Graham *et al.* (1972) have reported an inverse relationship between the consumption of certain raw vegetables, e.g., red cabbage and cole slaw, and the incidence of gastric cancer in humans. Haenszel and colleagues (1972, 1976) have noted a lower risk of

Diane F. Birt • Eppley Institute for Research in Cancer and Allied Diseases and Department of Biochemistry, University of Nebraska Medical Center, Omaha, Nebraska 68105.   *Edward Bresnick* • Department of Pharmacology and Toxicology, Dartmouth Medical School, Hanover, New Hampshire 03756.

gastric cancer in Hawaiian Japanese, in consumers of several raw Western vegetables, and in native Japanese who consume substantial amounts of lettuce and celery. Bjelke has observed similar findings in case-controlled studies in Norway and Minnesota (Bjelke, 1978), with an inverse relationship existing between stomach cancer incidence and the consumption of vegetables. The confounding contribution of smoking to this relationship has been obviated in the study of Hirayama (1977), who reported a lower risk of gastric cancer in nonsmokers whose diets were enriched with green and yellow vegetables when compared to nonsmokers who did not routinely eat these vegetables. Consumption of allium vegetables, such as garlic and onions, was found to be associated with reduced gastric cancer risk in an area in China in which there was a high gastric cancer rate (You *et al.*, 1989). Individuals consuming large amounts of these vegetables had 40% of the risk of those people consuming limited qualities.

The incidence of colon and rectal cancers was compared in a population with a high dietary intake of vegetables and in hospital-based and neighborhood controls. An inverse relationship between the incidence of only colon cancer and the frequency of consumption of fiber-containing foods, including cabbage, was noted by Modan *et al.* (1975). A similar decreased risk for colon cancer was noted in a population from New York State who ingested large amounts of cabbage, broccoli, and/or brussels sprouts (Graham *et al.*, 1978).

In addition to gastrointestinal cancer, the incidence of other neoplasms has been shown to be affected by increased consumption of green and yellow vegetables. Thus, in a retrospective study, MacLennon *et al.* (1977) have reported the consumption of these vegetables to be inversely related to the incidence of lung cancer. A recent case–control study on the relationship between vegetable consumption and lung cancer in Hawaii indicated a strong negative association between lung cancer risk and intake of all vegetables, dark green vegetables, cruciferous vegetables, and tomatoes (Le Marchand *et al.*, 1989). A weaker inverse relationship was observed with beta-carotene intake. Bladder, breast, and prostate cancers were similarly negatively affected by increased vegetable consumption (Mettlin and Graham, 1979; Phillips, 1975; Armstrong and Doll, 1975; Correa, 1981).

The role of dietary habits as a risk factor for cancer has been evaluated using a very select population, the Seventh Day Adventists, by Phillips (1975). The Seventh Day Adventists are an evangelical religious group of approximately 2.5 million people of whom approximately 500,000 are located in North America. Of the latter number, almost 20% reside in California. The Seventh Day Adventists are generally a nonsmoking and nondrinking population, many of whom, i.e., 40–50%, adhere to a lactoovovegetarian diet. Virtually all of them abstain from consuming pork products and some refrain from imbibing caffeine-containing drinks. The population makes abundant use of fruits, vegetables, whole grains, and nuts. Consequently, this group serves as an excellent vehicle for assessing the contributions of several potential risk factors in cancer etiology.

Lemon and his colleagues (1964, 1966) have followed a group of more than 35,000 Seventh Day Adventists in California for 8 years. They observed that this group exhibited a cancer mortality rate that was ½ to ⅔ that of the general population. This decrease in cancer mortality was not simply caused by refraining from drinking or smoking, since sites such as the gastrointestinal tract and reproductive organs were affected.

Finally, in a prospective cohort study involving over 1200 Massachusetts residents 66 years and older, Colditz *et al.* (1985) examined the association between the consumption of green and yellow vegetables and the cancer mortality rates. They noted a considerable protection in those individuals who ingested more than one serving per day of these dietary components.

In summary, the daily consumption of vegetables appears associated with a reduced incidence of neoplasia in a number of regions of the world. Since vegetables contribute a variety of ingredients to our diet, e.g., fiber, vitamins, carotenes, it is difficult to dissect out the active component(s) that is(are) responsible for the effect on the incidence of neoplasia. It is also quite probable that this effect is due to the multiplicity of the ingredients and not to a single agent, e.g., carotenes. The evidence presented in the next section indicates that the effect of some cruciferous vegetables such as cauliflower or brussels sprouts has been observed under certain conditions in biological model systems in the laboratory.

2.2. Experimental Carcinogenesis Data

Relatively few studies have been conducted to test the ability of vegetables to prevent carcinogenesis in laboratory animals. This is somewhat surprising considering the interest generated by the epidemiologic data. The primary reason for the lack of such studies is the difficulty in conducting dietary experiments with laboratory animals when a large proportion of the diet must be replaced with a natural component. The importance of such studies, however, is evident from the observation that vegetables, or mixtures of agents, have generally been observed to have greater cancer inhibitory ability than single substances that have been isolated therefrom.

Studies by Boyd *et al.* (1982) indicated that incorporation of 25% beets into diets containing 1 ppm aflatoxin B1 (AFB) resulted in *elevated* liver tumor yield, while incorporation of cabbage in the diets inhibited liver tumor development. In addition, cabbage-containing diets reduced the α-fetoprotein elevation induced by AFB but beets elevated these levels. Urine from rats fed beets and AFB had more revertants with *Salmonella typhimurium* strain TA98 than did urine from control or cabbage-fed rats (Boyd *et al.*, 1982). Comparison of diets containing 25% green beans, beets, or squash in a similar study from the same laboratory (Boyd *et al.*, 1983) showed enhanced AFB-induced elevation of α-fetoprotein and hepatic foci staining positive for γ-glutamyl transpeptidase (GGT). Interestingly, more GGT-positive foci were observed in vegetable-fed rats in comparison with those animals that were fed non-vegetable-containing diets even if they were not treated with AFB, although the increase was greater in the AFB-treated rats. The glucosinolate-rich fraction from brussels sprouts exhibited the same ability as 20% dietary brussels sprouts in the inhibition of GGT-positive hepatic foci induced by AFB, while the non-glucosinolate-rich residue of brussels sprouts was inactive (Godlewski *et al.*, 1985). However, all three diets, 20% brussels sprouts and the diet containing the extract from this amount of brussels sprouts or the residue, induced high levels of hepatic glutathione sulfatransferase activity.

Diethylnitrosamine-induced hepatocarcinogenesis and death were delayed by feeding carrots only several days a week; the β-carotene content of the carrots did not account for the inhibition (Rieder *et al.*, 1983). This observation may have been related to a decrease in consumption of the control diet or the sporadic consumption of the control diet, since these factors were not controlled.

Several studies have indicated the inhibition of mammary cancer by vegetable-containing diets. Wattenberg (1983) noted a reduction in the incidence and the multiplicity (number of tumors per tumor-bearing animal) of 7,12-dimethylbenzanthracene (DMBA)-induced mammary neoplasms in rats fed diets containing 10% green coffee beans, cauliflower, cabbage, or 1 or 5% orange oil. Green coffee beans were effective when fed either before or after DMBA administration, while all others were studied only when fed following DMBA treatment. Mammary carcinogenesis induced by N-methylnitrosourea (NMU) was inhibited in rats fed 5% or 10% dried cabbage or cabbage residue throughout the carcinogenesis process (Bresnick et al., submitted for publication). Incorporation of 5% brown seaweed (Laminaria) into diets fed to rats also resulted in a reduction in DMBA-induced mammary adenocarcinomas (Teas et al., 1984). Scholar et al. (1989) found that pulmonary metastasis of mammary tumor cells (410.4 subline of Balb/c mammary tumor) were inhibited by 40–60% in mice fed diets containing 5% or 10% dried cabbage or collard greens. This suggests that vegetable components might be useful in preventing late stages of cancer.

In studies on skin tumorigenesis, onion oil applied topically three times per week at doses of 10–10,000 μg inhibited promotion by 12-O-tetradecanoyl phorbol-13-acetate (TPA) of DMBA-initiated skin tumors; garlic oil showed somewhat less inhibition at the same dosages (Belman, 1983).

In contrast with the studies described in the preceding paragraphs showing an inhibition of carcinogenesis in rodents fed cruciferous vegetables, results from our laboratory (Birt et al., 1987) and separate laboratories (Srisanganam et al., 1980; Temple and El-Khatib, 1987) indicated that addition of cabbage to the diet can actually enhance tumorigenesis. Diets containing 9% cabbage in a low- or high-fat formulation were fed to hamsters in studies on pancreatic carcinogenesis induced by bis(2-oxopropyl)nitrosamine (BOP). Cabbage feeding began 4 weeks prior to treatment with BOP and administration of the high-fat diet began 1 week following BOP treatment in the appropriate groups. The yield of pancreatic cancer was doubled in the group fed cabbage–high-fat diet in comparison with the groups fed the high-fat diet alone, or cabbage–low-fat diet. In two-stage mouse skin tumorigenesis experiments, cabbage was fed from 2 weeks before DMBA treatment and continued throughout TPA promotion. The number of skin papillomas was consistently elevated by about 15% throughout the study (Birt et al., 1987). Effects of 0, 10, 20, or 40% dietary cabbage on the tumorigenicity of 1,2-dimethylhydrazine (DMH) were assessed in C57BL/6 mice. Slightly elevated tumor yields were observed in groups fed 10 or 20% cabbage, but inhibition was seen in those receiving 40% cabbage (Srisanganam et al., 1980). Tumors of the spermatic cord were the most predominant. Colon tumors induced by DMH in Swiss mice increased in incidence and multiplicity in female animals fed diets diluted with 13% cabbage but decreased in incidence in male animals (Temple and El-Khatib, 1987). However, the number of animals was too low to make definitive conclusions.

These results suggest that although inhibitors of cancer are undoubtedly present in vegetables, some enhancing components may also be present and thus the active agents responsible for the enhancement need to be identified and isolated.

2.3. Mutagenesis Data

Evaluation of the ability of vegetable extracts or vegetable juices to inhibit the mutagenicity of known mutagenic compounds has been the objective of some research.

Barale *et al.* (1983) assessed the effects of various vegetable juices on the mutagenicity of nitrite combined with aminopyrine or methylurea. Aminopyrine combined with nitrite leads to the formation of dimethylnitrosamine. The mutagenicity of this combination was reduced by about 50% by the addition of juices from carrots, strawberries, or cauliflower and by a greater percentage by the juices of lettuce or spinach. Methylurea reacts with nitrite to form nitrosomethylurea, and the mutagenicity of this combination was reduced only slightly by carrot, strawberry, and lettuce juice and to a greater extent by spinach and cauliflower juices. It was not possible to determine how much the observed inhibitions were due to prevention of nitrosation and how much they were due to prevention of the mutagenicity of the nitrosated products.

Lai *et al.* (1980) evaluated the effects of aqueous and acetone extracts of various vegetables on the activation of 3-methylcholanthrene (3-MC) and benzo(a)pyrene (BP) in the Ames *Salmonella* assay; they observed that the potency of inhibition was well correlated with the chlorophyll content of the vegetables. In additional studies from this laboratory, chlorophyll was demonstrated to be the major active factor in wheat sprout extract, accounting for the antimutagenic effect of the latter in assays with 3-MC and BP (Lai, 1979). Mutagenicity of cigarette smoke condensate and BP was reduced by inclusion of chlorophyllin, chlorophyll a, and chlorophyll b in studies from another laboratory (Terwel and van der Hoeven, 1985).

2.4. Carcinogen/Drug Metabolism Data

Dietary effects on the drug metabolizing enzyme systems, particularly the mixed-function oxidase system, have been viewed as an important means for dietary modification of responses to the environment (Campbell, 1977). Vegetables and components from vegetables have been particularly effective in modifying drug and carcinogen metabolizing activities, and data of this nature were some of the first to suggest that vegetable consumption may alter carcinogenesis.

Elevated intestinal *in vitro* metabolism of hexobarbital, phenacetin, 7-ethoxycoumarin, and benzo(a)pyrene was observed in rats fed dried brussels sprouts or cabbage in semipurified diet (Pantuck, 1976). Pretreatment of the rats with indoles from brussels sprouts and cabbage also stimulated drug metabolism, but the effect was smaller than when the dried vegetables were fed. Studies with human subjects demonstrated an alteration of drug metabolism in those fed a brussels sprouts– and cabbage-containing diet (Pantuck, 1979). The plasma half-life of antipyrine was decreased by 13% and the mean metabolic clearance increased by 11% in humans fed vegetables. In addition, the plasma concentration of phenacetin decreased by 34–67% from 0.5–7.0 hr after drug administration in subjects supplemented with vegetables in comparison with those not fed these vegetables. Later investigations by Pantuck *et al.* (1984) observed glucuronidation and metabolic clearances of paracetamol increased in healthy subjects consuming cabbage and brussels sprouts.

Hepatic residues of polybrominated biphenyls and fatty liver induced by these compounds were reduced in rats fed diets containing 25% cauliflower (Stoewsand *et al.*, 1978). Cauliflower also reduced the toxicity of AFB and improved the survival of rats fed this carcinogen (Stoewsand *et al.*, 1978). This laboratory also reported that cabbage consumption increased the activity of aminopyrine *N*-demethylase and *p*-nitroanisole *O*-demethylase and that the apparent K_m of aryl hydrocarbon hydroxylase (AHH) was lower in the liver, kidney, and intestine; the V_{max} was higher in the intestine of cabbage-fed rats (Stoewsand *et al.*, 1978).

Increased glutathione *S*-transferase (GST) activity in small intestinal mucosa was observed in mice fed diets for 2 weeks which contained dried powdered brussels sprouts (20%), cabbage (20%), coffee beans (20%), or tea leaves (10–20%) (Sparnins *et al.*, 1982b). Increased activity was also observed in the livers of mice fed all of these diets except cabbage.

A series of studies from the laboratory of Bjeldanes (Hendrich and Bjeldanes, 1983; Bradfield and Bjeldanes, 1984; Bradfield *et al.*, 1985; Whitty and Bjeldanes, 1987) evaluated the addition of dried powdered vegetables to semipurified diets on hepatic and intestinal drug metabolism systems. Mice fed diets containing 20% cabbage, brussels sprouts, or alfalfa or 5% of two different Chinese herbs, in comparison with a chow or a control semipurified diet, demonstrated an induction in hepatic AHH activity by about 1.6- to 2.2-fold for the chow diet and the diets containing *Schizandra chinensis* or alfalfa and an induction of 1.4- to 2.1-fold in hepatic epoxide hydrolase (EH) in mice fed all of the diets except cabbage or alfalfa (Hendrich and Bjeldanes, 1983). In comparing the effects of diets containing 25% brussels sprouts with the level of indole-3-carbinol present in this amount of brussels sprouts, Bradfield and Bjeldanes (1984) found that sprouts appear to contain compounds other than indole-3-carbinol which account for effects on GST and EH. For example, brussels sprouts–containing diet elevated hepatic and intestinal GST by 1.9- and 1.6-fold, respectively, while indole-3-carbinol had no effect. Similarly, microsomal EH activity of the small intestine was increased by 2.0-fold in mice fed sprouts but not influenced by indole-3-carbinol; hepatic microsomal EH was elevated 1.3-fold for the sprouts diet but was elevated by only 1.1-fold with 500 ppm indole-3-carbinol. In these studies, 25% brussels sprouts fed for 10 days also elevated intestinal AHH by 3.6-fold and ethoxy-*O*-deethylase (ECD) by 3.2-fold (Bradfield and Bjeldanes, 1984). Effects on hepatic xenobiotic metabolism were compared in mice fed diets containing 20% freeze-dried, powdered kidney beans, soya beans, alfalfa, cauliflower, mustard greens, carrots, kale, brussels sprouts, beets, egg plant, onions, or sweet potatoes (Bradfield *et al.*, 1985). Hepatic ECD activity was significantly increased in mice fed kidney beans (1.5-fold), alfalfa (1.6-fold), cauliflower (2.2-fold), mustard greens (1.2-fold), carrots (1.2-fold), and kale (1.3-fold). Hepatic GST and EH were also significantly increased in mice fed soya beans (1.2- and 1.6-fold, respectively), brussels sprouts (2.0- and 1.6-fold), cauliflower (1.2- and 1.6-fold), alfalfa (1.3- and 2.0-fold), and onions (1.8- and 2.3-fold). In this study, cauliflower and brussels sprouts diets had no influence on hepatic AHH activity. The other vegetables were not tested.

3. Studies on Particular Compounds Found in Vegetables and Fruits

3.1. Indoles

For many years, indole and its derivatives have been examined for their effects on carcinogenesis. Early studies were conducted primarily with indole, but in more recent work indole-3-carbinol, indole-3-acetonitrile, and other derivatives of the indole ring structure have been employed. Some representative structures are shown in Fig. 1. A variety of indole derivatives occur naturally in cruciferous vegetables (Loub *et al.*, 1975)

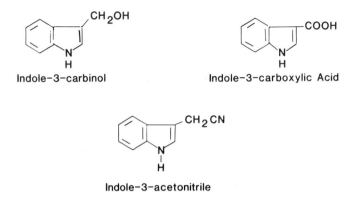

Fig. 1. Structures of selective indole compounds.

and indole is synthesized by the gut bacteria from dietary precursors (Sims and Renwick, 1985).

Indole supplementation was shown to increase 2-acetylamino-fluorene (AAF)-induced urinary bladder cancer in Fischer 344 rats when the indole and AAF were administered simultaneously in the diet (Dunning and Curtis, 1958). Studies by Oyasu *et al.* (1963) indicated that Wistar rats given 1.6% or 3.25% indole lived longer when given the higher indole level and developed more urinary bladder tumors, but these tumors developed late in the study. In addition, 3.2% indole inhibited malignant tumor development in comparison with 1.6% indole, but the high-indole-fed animals had more benign tumors. Further studies by Oyasu *et al.* (1972) with hamsters showed that indole addition increased the development of AAF-induced urinary bladder tumors when a low dose of carcinogen was administered, but indole or DL-tryptophan had no effect when a high dose of carcinogen was used. In this study, both indole and tryptophan protected against liver injury from AAF, but indole was more effective. The indole-fed hamsters had reduced body weights and thus the reduced tumorigenesis may have been due to reduced food and carcinogen consumption.

Prefeeding 1.6% dietary indole was found by Hopp *et al.* (1976) to reduce the 24-hr biliary excretion of N-hydroxy-2-acetylaminofluorene (N-OH-AAF)-glucuronide by rats at 2 and 4 weeks after AAF administration. At 2 weeks, the biliary excretion was reduced in the indole-fed rats to 8% of the amount excreted by the groups not receiving indole. These results indicated a suppression of the activation of AAF in indole-fed rats. This group also found that indole could prevent the enhanced toxicity of AAF in Na_2SO_4-treated rats (Hopp *et al.*, 1976).

When urinary bladder cancer was induced in hamsters by dibutylnitrosamine (DBN), indole supplementation inhibited the development of carcinomas when diet consumption was *ad libitum* and when consumption was rigorously controlled (Matsumoto *et al.*, 1977). In the first experiment, a diet containing 1.6% indole was offered *ad libitum* and the hamsters decreased food consumption in comparison with the controls. The experiment was repeated using pair-fed hamsters. In both studies, urinary bladder tumor incidence was suppressed, but tumors at sites such as the nasal sinuses, trachea, esophagus, and forestomach were not influenced (Matsumoto *et al.*, 1977). In studies of DBN-treated rats, supplementation with 1.6% dietary indole extended survival and reduced papillary esophageal carcinogenesis (Kitajima *et al.*, 1975).

Studies on indole-3-carbinol, indole-3-acetonitrile, and 3,3'-diindolylmethane were initiated when these components were found to account for much of the induction of the mixed-function oxidase (MFO) system by cruciferous vegetables (Loub *et al.*, 1975). These indole derivatives are produced during hydrolysis by myrosinase of indoylmethyl glucosinolate (Virtanen, 1965). Oral administration of indole-3-carbinol and 3,3'-diindolylmethane 8 hr before treatment with DMBA resulted in a reduction in the mammary tumor incidence and in the number of tumors per rat, but treatment with indole-3-acetonitrile did not affect these parameters (Wattenberg and Loub, 1978). Dietary administration of indole-3-carbinol also inhibited DMBA mammary carcinogenesis. In addition, feeding each of these three compounds inhibited the BP-induced forestomach tumor incidence (Wattenberg and Loub, 1978). The effects of indole-3-carbinol on AFB hepatic carcinogenesis in trout differed depending on the time of administration of indole-3-carbinol (Nixon *et al.*, 1984; Bailey *et al.*, 1987). When indole-3-carbinol was fed in the diet for 8 weeks prior to 2 weeks of AFB treatment, the *in vivo* AFB DNA binding was reduced and carcinogenesis was inhibited by as much as 90% (Nixon *et al.*, 1984). *In vitro* kinetic studies with trout hepatic microsomes indicated that reaction products of indole-3-carbinol inhibited the microsome activated binding of AFB with DNA (Fong *et al.*, 1990). However, feeding indole-3-carbinol *following* AFB resulted in a strong promotion of hepatocarcinogenesis (Bailey *et al.*, 1987). Similarly, studies by Pence *et al.* (1986) indicated that feeding indole-3-carbinol in diets high in cholesterol and beef tallow *following* DMBA treatment resulted in an elevation in mammary cancer yield.

Other biological effects of indole-3-carbinol have been extensively studied. The effects of indole-3-carbinol on MFO activities have varied depending on the experimental design employed. Studies on trout liver indicated no effect of this agent on hepatic MFO activities (Nixon *et al.*, 1984; Bailey *et al.*, 1987). Feeding lower doses of indole-3-carbinol induced intestinal AHH activity and ethoxycoumarin-*O*-deethylase in rats but did not alter hepatic activities of these enzymes (Bradfield and Bjeldanes, 1984). In work by Shertzer (1983), indole-3-carbinol administration by gavage to mice resulted in a 90% inhibition of covalent binding of BP metabolites to hepatic cellular macromolecules at a dosage where hepatic AHH activity was not influenced.

The effects of indole-3-carbinol on hepatic GST have also been investigated with somewhat divergent results. Sparnins *et al.* (1982b) reported that GST activity was induced in the liver and small intestine of mice fed 0.04 mmole indole-3-carbinol or indole-3-acetonitrile/g diet for 2 weeks. In contrast, Bradfield and Bjeldanes (1984) saw no influence of indole-3-carbinol on hepatic GST and suggested that *Brassica oleracea* contained other components responsible for the GST-inducing effects of this vegetable.

Indole-3-carbinol decreased the rate of hepatic metabolism of *N*-nitrosodimethylamine (NDMA) and the covalent binding of its oxidation products to DNA and protein in mouse liver (Shertzer, 1984). The administration of indole-3-carbinol by gavage in *in vivo* studies and pretreatment with indole-3-carbinol in *in vitro* experiments resulted in a 60–90% decrease in covalent binding of oxidative products to DNA or protein. However, pretreatment of mice with indole-3-carbinol did not alter the activity of AHH (Shertzer, 1984). In studies from another laboratory, indole-3-carbinol, indole-3-acetonitrile, and indole were all found to induce demethylation of NDMA and 4-(methylnitrosamino)-1-(3-

pyridyl)-1-butanone (Chung *et al.*, 1985). Since demethylation of these nitrosamines is an important step in their activation, enhancement of this step could potentially result in increased activation, depending on the effects of the compounds on other steps in the metabolism of the compounds.

Reddy *et al.* (1983) assessed the effect of indole-3-carbinol or indole-3-acetonitrile on DMBA-induced mutagenicity in *Salmonella* TA100 or TA98 systems. Indole-3-carbinol enhanced mutagenicity in TA100 cultures but had no effect on the TA98 system. Indole-3-acetonitrile had little effect on either strain. Birt *et al.* (1986) found that indole-3-carbinol had little effect on the mutagenicity of methylnitrosourea or methyl-*N*-nitro-*N*-nitrosoguanidine in a TA100 bacterial system or on the mutagenicity of BP tested in a TA98 culture supplemented with an S9 preparation. In addition, indole-3-carbinol was not mutagenic when tested alone. Studies on the effects of indole-3-carbinol on the induction of epidermal ornithine decarboxylase (ODC) activity by TPA were conducted to assess potential effects on tumor promotion. Indole-3-carbinol pretreatment of mouse skin at dosages of 25–50 μmoles resulted in an enhancement of ODC induction by TPA, while pretreatment with 50 or 100 μmoles resulted in ODC induction in the absence of TPA (Birt *et al.*, 1986). These results are consistent with the observed enhancement of tumorigenesis in animals treated with indole-3-carbinol (Bailey *et al.*, 1987; Pence *et al.*, 1986).

3.2. Thiocyanates and Isothiocyanates

Isothiocyanates are derived from the enzymatic decomposition of glucosinolates which are present in a number of plants eaten as vegetables and spices (Fenwick *et al.*, 1982). Cruciferous vegetables are particularly noteworthy for their high content of isothiocyanates; phenethyl isothiocyanate is present in cabbage, brussels sprouts, cauliflower, kale, and turnips; watercress contains benzyl isothiocyanate (Virtanen, 1962; Kjaer, 1961; Miller, 1973; Josephsson, 1967).

In early studies, a number of isothiocyanic esters were studied for their ability to inhibit the growth of Ehrlich ascites carcinoma cells in mice (Daehnfeldt, 1968). In studies reported by Sasaki (1963), treatment with alpha-naphthyl isothiocyanate resulted in proliferation of bile ductules and increased bile secretion, and feeding this agent before and during feeding of 3-methyl-4-diaminoazobenzene inhibited liver carcinogenesis. However, in studies where alpha- or beta-naphthyl isothiocyanate was fed in low-protein- or low-riboflavin-containing diet, no alteration in hepatic carcinogenesis by *p*-dimethylaminoazobenzene was observed (Lacassagne *et al.*, 1970).

In extensive studies, Wattenberg's laboratory has assessed the inhibition of carcinogenesis by isothiocyanates and related compounds in the mammary gland, forestomach, and lung of rodents (Wattenberg, 1974, 1977, 1980, 1981). Benzyl thiocyanate was found to inhibit DMBA-induced mammary cancer in rats by nearly 90% when fed in the diet at 0.03 mmole/g diet from 1 week before DMBA treatment until the termination of the study (Wattenberg, 1974). Later, benzyl isothiocyanate and phenethyl isothiocyanate were investigated because of their natural occurrence and a synthetic analog, phenyl isothiocyanate, was evaluated because of a similar structure (Wattenberg, 1977). All three compounds inhibited DMBA-induced mammary tumorigenesis in female rats when administered orally 4 hr before DMBA treatment. Benzyl isothiocyanate was effective if given 2 hr before DMBA, while the other two compounds were less effective at this time. In separate experiments, benzyl isothiocyanate was more effective at 4 hr before DMBA than was benzyl thiocyanate, but it was ineffective when administered 24 hr before or 4 hr after DMBA (Wattenberg, 1977). In addition, BP- and DMBA-induced forestomach tumors were inhibited by dietary benzyl isothiocyanate, DMBA-induced forestomach tumors were inhibited by phenethyl isothiocyanate, and DMBA-induced pulmonary tumors were inhibited by both compounds, but forestomach tumors induced by DMBA were not influenced by benzyl thiocyanate (Wattenberg, 1977).

The effects of sodium cyanate on DMBA-induced mammary carcinogenesis and BP-induced tumors were assessed because of its chemical relationship to the isothiocyanates, although humans are not exposed to this compound in their diets (Wattenberg, 1980). Dietary sodium cyanate inhibited DMBA-induced mammary and BP-induced forestomach and pulmonary tumors when fed from 8 days before until 1–3 days after carcinogen treatment. A separate report compared sodium cyanate, tert-butyl isocyanate, and benzyl isothiocyanate on DMBA- and DMH-induced tumorigenesis when the agents were fed following carcinogen exposure (Wattenberg, 1981). All three compounds were effective in reducing the incidence and multiplicity of mammary neoplasms, while sodium cyanate inhibited large-bowel tumors induced by DMH. The author speculated that the effects of sodium cyanate may be related to the inhibition of protein and DNA synthesis.

The inhibition of carcinogenesis by benzyl isothiocyanate was associated with a 78–182% increase in GST activity in the forestomach of mice and a decrease in acid soluble sulfhydryl levels (Sparnins and Wattenberg, 1981). In the esophagus, benzyl isothiocyanate increased GST activity and sulfhydryl levels (Sparnins *et al.*, 1982a). Similar results were observed in the liver and small intestine after the consumption of this agent (Sparnins *et al.*, 1982b). These authors suggested that an enhancement of GST activity by greater than 70–80% is generally observed with compounds capable of inhibiting carcinogenesis.

The influence of a number of thiocyanates or isothiocyanates on carcinogen metabolism was reported by Chung *et al.* (1984, 1985). *In vitro* alpha hydroxylation of *N*-nitrosopyrrolidine or *N*-nitrosonornicotine by liver microsomes or cultured esophagus, respectively, was studied in rats that had been gavaged 2 hr before sacrifice or prefed for 2 weeks with benzyl isothiocyanate, allyl isothiocyanate, phenethyl isothiocyanate, phenyl isothiocyanate, benzyl thiocyanate, or sodium thiocyanate (Chung *et al.*, 1984). Alpha-hydroxylation of both compounds was inhibited with all compounds except sodium thiocyanate when the compounds were given by gavage. In rats pretreated by dietary administration, only phenyl isothiocyanate and sodium thiocyanate inhibited carcinogen alpha hydroxylation. Similar studies were conducted on the *in vitro* demethylation of NDMA and 4-(methylnitrosamine)-1-(3-pyridyl)-1-butanone (Chung *et al.*, 1985). Phenethyl isothiocyanate and phenyl isothiocyanate inhibited demethylation of both compounds in acute and chronic studies, benzyl isothiocyanate had little inhibitory action in acute studies and showed some potential for enhancement in chronic studies, and allyl isothiocyanate was less effective than phenethyl isothiocyanate or phenyl isothiocyanate in the inhibition of demethylation. In *in vivo* studies, the formation of 7-methylguanine and O[6]-methylguanine in hepatic DNA from rats treated with these carcinogens was inhibited in animals treated with phenethyl isothiocyanate or phenyl isothiocyanate in an analogous manner to the *in vitro* assays (Chung *et al.*, 1985).

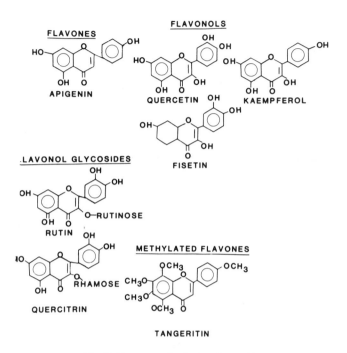

Fig. 2. Structures of selective flavonoids.

3.3. Flavonoids

The flavonoids are a group of carbon-, hydrogen-, and oxygen-containing organic molecules that are ubiquitously distributed in vascular plants. Approximately 2000 individual members of the flavonoid class have been described (e.g., see Harborne *et al.*, 1975). The structure of some of the members of this class are indicated in Fig. 2.

The flavonoids are composed of flavones, flavonols, flavonones, *O*-glycosides of the flavonols and flavonones, and methylated flavones. Most of the flavonols and flavonones occur as glycosides of which only about 70% have been fully characterized. Specific examples of each of these groups are presented in Table I. The flavonoids are consumed in rather large amounts through dietary fruits and vegetables. For example, the flavonols (generally as the *O*-glycosides) may be present in soft fruits and in their juices at a concentration of 100 mg/kg fresh weight (Pierpoint, 1986). In the outer skins of certain onions, i.e., *Allium cepa*, the flavonols may occur between 2.5 and 6.5% of the fresh weight. In one cup of brewed black Indian tea, over 40 mg of the flavonols and their glycosides might be found, while in green tea, 30% of the dry matter may be phenolic compounds including 3–4% of kaempferol and guercetin. The average daily intake of the flavonoids by the U.S. population is indicated in Table II. As is apparent from this table, the average individual might consume over 1 g of flavonoids per day. The flavonoids, however, unlike *N*-containing plant alkaloids, are generally conceded to be nontoxic. In fact, they are often found in health stores, where they are sold as food supplements.

Table I. The Flavonoids

Category	Examples
Flavones	Apigenin, diosmetin
Flavonols	Flavonol, galangin, kaempferol, fisetin, morin, quercetin, rhamnetin, robinetin, myricetin
Flavonol glycosides	Quercitrin, rutin, robinin
Flavonones	Taxifolin, hesperetin
Flavonone glycosides	Hesperidin, naringin
Methylated flavones	Tangeretin, nobeletin

The flavonoid glycosides are generally cleaved in the gastrointestinal tract by intestinal enzymes and may undergo more significant degradation in the large bowel through the bacterial flora (cited in Brown and Dietrich, 1979).

3.3.1. Function of the Flavonoids

These agents fulfill a variety of functions for the vegetable and plant (reviewed in Swain, 1986). As typical phenolic compounds, they act as potent antioxidants and metal chelators. Because of their conjugated ring structure, they serve as ultraviolet light screens, they attenuate visible light in the 350- to 450-nm range, and they provide for the dispersion of visible color signals for such processes as pollen dispersal. The flavonoids interfere with the feeding on the plant of certain viruses, fungi, and animals. Some of the flavonoids actually serve as feeding attractants, e.g., morin for the silkworm, *Bombyx mori.* Finally, they provide some structural strength to the plant cell wall.

3.3.2. Biosynthesis of the Flavonoids

The flavonoids are synthesized from relatively simple substances in the plant. The general biosynthetic scheme is presented in Fig. 3 (this information comes from Swain, 1986). The amio acid L-phenylalanine is the precursor for this class of compounds, with naringenin providing the bridge to most of the other important ingredients. Although not

Table II. Daily Intake of the Flavonoids[a]

Foodstuff	mg/day (average serving)
Potatoes, bulbs, roots	79
Peanuts, nuts	45
Cereals	44
Vegetable, herbs	162
Fruits, fruit juices	290
Cocoa, cola, coffee, beer, wine	420
All foodstuffs	1040

[a]Pierpoint, 1986.

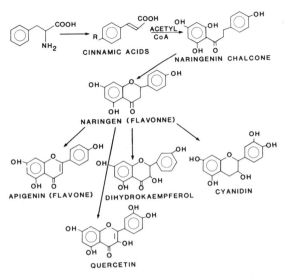

Fig. 3. Biosynthesis of flavonoids.

indicated in this figure, the glycosides of the flavonoids, e.g., rutin or quercitrin, result from the action of the plant glycosyltransferases.

3.3.3. Genotoxicity and Carcinogenicity of the Flavonoids

Prior to discussing the chemopreventive effects of certain of the flavonoids, a presentation of the evidence for their mutagenicity in nonmammalian and mammalian systems and for their carcinogenicity is germane to this section.

A number of investigators have reviewed the mutagenicity of the flavonoids in the *Salmonella* test system (e.g., MacGregor and Gurd, 1978; Brown and Dietrich, 1979; MacGregor, 1984). We will use the data of Brown and Dietrich (1979) to illustrate this biological activity. The data are presented in Table III.

The two most common flavonols, quercetin and kaempferol, do exhibit some mutagenicity in the Ames assay using several strains of *Salmonella*. With these organisms, they have been shown to be frameshift mutagens (Bjeldanes and Chang, 1977; Sugimura *et al.*, 1977). Kaempferol requires activation by a rat liver microsomal preparation, while quercetin is slightly active in the absence of the latter. The microsomal preparation does, however, enhance the mutagenic activity of quercetin.

The active mutagenic flavonoids are all hydroxyflavones with free hydroxyl groups at positions 3 and 5. The 7-hydroxyl does not appear to be required for this mutagenic property. Compounds without 3',4'-hydroxyl groups, e.g., kaempferol, are activated by rat microsomal preparations, while compounds with hydroxyls at these positions exhibit direct-acting mutagenicity; enhancement does occur in its presence. If a methyl (or other) group is substituted at the 3',4'-hydroxyls, then the mutagenicity is blocked. Finally, reduction of the unsaturated bond at position 2,3 results in a complete loss of mutagenic activity.

Table III. *Mutagenicity of the Flavonoids in the Ames Assay*[a]

Compound	His[+] revertants/nmole	Microsomal activation
Flavones		
Apigenin	0	Not required
Flavone	0	Not required
Flavonols		
Galangin	2	Required
Kaempferol	7	Required
Morin	0.1	Required
Fisetin	0.1	Enhanced
Quercetin	12	Enhanced
Rhamnetin	0.5	Enhanced
Robinetin	0.1	Required
Myricetin	0.1	Required
Flavonol glycosides		
Quercitrin	3	Required
Rutin	1	Required
Flavonones		
Hesperetin	0	Not required
Flavonone glycosides		
Hesperidin	0	Not required

[a]From Brown and Dietrich, 1979.

The mutagenic effects in systems other than the Ames assay have been reviewed (MacGregor, 1984, 1986; Bjeldanes and Chang, 1977; Sugimura *et al.*, 1977). Quercetin effected an increase in gene conversion frequency in *Saccharomyces cerevisiae* and in the reversion frequency at the *nad* locus in *E. coli* at concentrations in excess of 1 mg/ml. Therefore, these organisms were not as sensitive as the *Salmonella* to this flavonoid. Quercetin was not effective in *Bacillus subtilis* as a mutagen. In *Drosophila melanogaster,* both quercetin and kaempferol increased the frequency of sex-linked recessive lethal mutations at dietary levels between 0.04 and 0.17 M. The data on other flavonoids are not available. Structure–activity relationships among the flavonids in various mammalian cell screens for mutagensis are also very sketchy. These have been reviewed by MacGregor (1984, 1986).

In regard to mutagenicity in mammalian systems, sufficient data have only been accumulated for quercetin. This flavonoid increased the frequency of genetic damage in several lines of cultured mammalian cells. For example, the number of mutations at the hgprt locus in V79 hamster fibroblasts was significantly increased by both quercetin and kaempferol (Maruta *et al.*, 1982). The frequency of chromosomal aberrations and of sister chromatid exchanges in human and Chinese hamster cells is increased by quercetin (Yoshido *et al.*, 1980; MacGregor *et al.*, 1983a). The frequency of chromosomal aberrations, of mutations at four loci, and of sister chromatid exchanges has been measured in cells that were exposed to either galangin, kaempferol, or quercetin. All three flavonoids increased chromosomal aberrations but exerted no effect on the incidence of mutations at the hgprt, aprt, or Na/K-ATPase loci. In all instances, the genotoxicity could be classified as weak at best (Carver *et al.*, 1983).

The effects of administration of quercetin *in vivo* have been determined using sister chromatid exchange in lymphocytes obtained from treated rabbits (MacGregor *et al.*, 1983b). No change in frequency was reported. On the other hand, two reports have been published in which some of the flavonoids induced bone marrow micronuclei (Sahu *et al.*, 1981; Cea *et al.*, 1983). Finally, feeding a diet containing as much as 4% quercetin to mice did not result in any change in the frequency of nuclear anomalies in colonic epithelium (Wargovich and Newmark, 1983).

3.3.4. Mechanism of Action as a Mutagen

Early studies (reviewed in MacGregor and Gurd, 1978) suggested that flavonols, such as quercetin, were activated to DNA-reactive intermediates by an oxidative pathway, as indicated in Fig. 4. The observation of Ochiai *et al.* (1984) that the mutagenicity of quercetin is heavily dependent on oxygen is consistent with this proposed pathway. Furthermore, the dependence on the presence of an excision-repair deficiency in the test organism is suggestive of a bulky DNA adduct (reviewed in MacGregor, 1986). Compounds II and III of Fig. 4 would be very reactive and would attack macromolecular nucleophiles such as DNA.

Ochiai *et al.* (1984) noted that enhancement of mutagenic effects of quercetin on *Salmonella* occurs when rat cytosol is added to the incubation medium. They have been able to separate four factors from this cytosolic fraction that are responsible for the enhancement. One of these factors has been identified as superoxide dismutase (SOD). Additional work by Ueno *et al.* (1986) has suggested that SOD may play a direct role in the activation of quercetin for mutagenesis since the addition of diethyldithiocarbamate, an inhibitor of this enzyme, reduces the mutagenic enhancement. Furthermore, the addition of Mn-SOD or Fe-SOD increased the mutagenicity of quercetin in the *Salmonella* (Ueno *et al.*, 1986). These data imply that superoxide–SOD complex may function in the oxidative activation of flavonols, yielding an intermediate that is capable of interacting with DNA and generating a bulky DNA adduct.

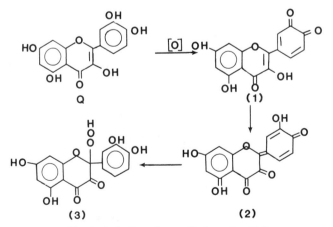

Fig. 4. Activation of quercetin through oxidation.

3.3.5. Carcinogenicity of the Flavonoids

The testing of the flavonoids for carcinogenicity is very incomplete although some data do exist for quercetin and its derivatives. Because of the positive finding in regard to mutagenicity in the Ames assay, this flavonoid was suspected as a potential carcinogen. Although tested in several biological model systems by several groups of investigators, only one positive report of quercetin's carcinogenicity has been published (Pamucku *et al.*, 1980). In this study, Norwegian rats were fed a basal diet containing 0.1% quercetin of 33% bracken fern until the termination of the experiment at 58 weeks. In the quercetin-fed animals, 75–85% of both females and males showed intestinal cancer and 20–30% were positive for transitional-cell carcinoma of the bladder. This was extraordinarily high for such a limited amount of quercetin.

All other reported studies on quercetin proved negative. For example, Hirono *et al.* (1981) tested the carcinogenicity of 5 and 10% quercetin-containing diets in ACI rats and found this agent to be negative. Morino *et al.* (1981) tested quercetin and its rhamnose derivative, rutin, in golden hamsters; this study also proved negative. Saito *et al.* (1980) fed ddY mice diets containing 2% quercetin for life and did not observe any statistically significant difference from control tumor incidence. Quercetin has also been tested in a two-stage carcinogenesis rat urinary bladder model (Hirose *et al.*, 1983). Fischer 344 rats were fed 5% quercetin as a potential initiator for 4 weeks, which was then followed by a nitrosamine as a promoter. In another series, the rats were given the nitrosamine as an initiator and quercetin as a promoter. No increased tumorigenesis due to the flavonoid was observed in either model. Finally, Takanashi *et al.* (1983) fed Fischer rats 0.1% quercetin for 540 days; no significant difference was observed in the tumor incidence between the experimental and control groups.

As indicated in the preceding paragraphs, some controversy exists as to whether or not quercetin (and other flavonoids) are truly carcinogenic, although some of them have yielded positive Ames assays. The activity of quercetin as a promoter has been tested in several studies, one of which has already been described, the two-stage bladder tumorigenesis model (Hirose *et al.*, 1983). In an earlier investigation by Van Duuren and colleagues (1968), quercetin, rutin, and quercitrin were examined for promoter activity. The results were negative.

The question arises: why are quercetin and other flavonoids negative as carcinogens but positive as bacterial mutagens? Several investigators have suggested that perhaps these agents are initiators but also possess antipromotion activity, thus negating any potential role as a carcinogen. This aspect will be discussed in the next section.

3.3.6. Anticarcinogenic and Antipromotion Activity of the Flavonoids

A number of investigators have tested the ability of these agents, particularly quercetin, to inhibit the promotion phase of carcinogenesis. Recall that in the two-stage model for skin tumorigenesis, both an initiator (generally a genotoxin) and a promoter are required for cancer development. Nishino *et al.* (1984b) have determined the antipromoter activity of quercetin. After topical application of DMBA to the backs of mice, the promoter teleocidin was administered twice weekly beginning 1 week after initiation. Quercetin was applied either 40 min before the teleocidin or concurrently. Potent inhibition of the tumor incidence and prolongation of the latency period were observed after administration of the flavonoid. For example, in this study, the first tumor appeared in the positive controls at week 8, while in the quercetin-treated group, the first tumor was observed at week 16. By week 20, an 83% reduction in papillomas per mouse was noted in the treated group. Nishino *et al.* (1983) also noted that luteolin, a flavonoid that does not exhibit any mutagenic activity, proved a potent inhibitor of promotion. Indeed, this inhibition was even greater than that observed with quercetin.

The antipromoter activity of topically administered quercetin is not limited to tele-ocidin action. For example, Kato *et al.* (1983) observed a similar effect of quercetin in initiated mice that received TPA as the promoter. In addition, recent studies (Wei *et al.*, 1990), demonstrated an inhibition of skin papillomas and carcinomas initiated by DMBA and promoted by TPA in SENCAR mice treated topically with apigenin 30 min before TPA. The number of papillomas or carcinomas was inhibited by 60–70% or 60–100%, respectively, in the apigenin-treated groups in two different experiments.

The antipromoter activity of quercetin has been determined in initiated and promoted mice that receive the flavonoid in the diet (Fujiki *et al.*, 1986). In these experiments, however, 1–4% dietary quercetin exerted little effect on the promoter activity of tele-ocidin. These results suggest that the flavonoid may not be absorbed sufficiently well or reach the epidermis in sufficient amount to alter promotion.

The application of promoters to mouse skin results in a number of changes in the biochemistry of the epidermal cells. These have been thoroughly reviewed by Blumberg (1981) and Diamond *et al.* (1980). Several of the major biochemical alterations accompanying promoter action are a very dramatic and prompt increase in the activity of ODC; a profound increase in the incorporation of ^{32}P-inorganic phosphate into membranal phospholipids of the cell; a substantial increase in the incorporation of labeled thymidine in epidermal cell DNA; an increase in the uptake of sugars, e.g., 2-deoxy-D-glucose, into cells; and an activation of Ca^{2+}-dependent phospholipid-activated protein kinase C.

Several flavonoids, including quercetin, kaempferol, and luteolin, were concomitantly applied to mouse skin with the promoter teleocidin by Fujiki *et al.* (1986). The promoter itself caused a substantial increase in ODC activity in the epidermis. This increase was blocked by kaempferol and luteolin to the extent of 62 and 48%, respectively; quercetin was without any effect. Nakadate *et al.* (1984) have reported that morin, fisetin, and kaempferol reduced TPA-stimulated increase in ODC substantially in epidermis; morin was the most effective in this regard. Similarly, Birt *et al.* (1986) reported that pretreatment of mouse skin with apigenin or robinetin inhibited TPA-induced ODC by approximately 70–80%.

The effects of some of the flavonoids on ^{32}P incorporation into phospholipids have been determined by several groups. Quercetin blocked the teleocidin-stimulated incorporation in a dose-dependent manner (Nishino *et al.*, 1984b). The overall effectiveness in this regard was luteolin > quercetin > chrysin > hesperetin. Nishino *et al.* (1984a) noted that TPA stimulates the incorporation of ^{32}P-phosphate into the phospholipids of human embryonic fibroblasts; this stimulation was inhibited by quercetin.

As indicated earlier, another early change after administration of tumor promoters is stimulation of the transport of sugars and other nutrients. Quercetin blocked this stimulation of deoxyglucose uptake as a result of TPA exposure (Nishino *et al.*, 1984a) or teleocidin administration (Fujiki *et al.*, 1986).

The current belief in regard to promoter action is that many of the biochemical alterations occur as a result of the activation of protein kinase C. Furthermore, evidence has indicated that this enzyme is, in fact, the phorbol ester receptor with which TPA and some other promoters interact in specific and high-affinity manner. The phorbol receptor or protein kinase C is a Ca^{2+}-stimulated and phospholipid-dependent protein. Fujiki *et al.* (1984) have used the increase in phosphorylation of H1 histone mediated by protein kinase C as an expression of the promoter stimulation of this enzyme. They have reported that quercetin, kaempferol, morin, and luteolin significantly inhibited the teleocidin and TPA-induced increase in this parameter. A similar effect of quercetin on TPA-stimulated increase in protein kinase C activity has been reported by Gschwendt *et al.* (1983) using mouse brain cytosolic fractions.

The effect of myricetin and similar flavonoids on tyrosine protein kinases and serine/threonine protein kinases were investigated by Hagiwara *et al.* (1988). Myricetin competitively inhibited pp130[fps] tyrosine kinase, myosin light chain kinase, casein kinase I and II with ATP, but did not inhibit several other protein kinases. Structure activity studies indicated that inhibition of tyrosine protein kinases by flavonoids correlated with the number of hydroxyl residues on the flavone ring, but inhibition of serine/threonine protein kinase was less influenced by hydroxylation of the flavonoid.

All in all, there appears to be a good, but not exact, relationship between the ability of some of the flavonoids to inhibit certain promoter-stimulated biochemical processes and their activity as antipromoters. The latter action may explain, at least in part, why quercetin (and perhaps some of the other flavonoids) is a mutagen in the *Salmonella* system, but is not carcinogenic in rodents.

Flavonoids were also found to influence activation of carcinogens. AFB is a potent mycotoxin that must be activated to the 2,3-oxide prior to eliciting its carcinogenic effects. The rainbow trout, *Salmo gairdneri,* is extraordinarily sensitive to this agent. The combination of tangeretin and nobeletin has been treated as an inducer of cytochrome P450 and of ethoxyresorufin *O*-deethylase by Nixon and colleagues (1984). Although no change was observed in the concentration of the hemoprotein in the livers of trout that had been fed diets containing tangeretin–nobeletin, AHH and *O*-deethylase activities were elevated by 2- and 2.5-fold, respectively. The combined flavonoids also increased aflatoxicol but not aflatoxin M1 formation from the parent mycotoxin. Finally, the combined flavonoids suppressed the incidence of hepatocellular carcinoma in the trout that received 20 ppb of the mycotoxin from 38% in the positive controls to 25%. Quercetin reduced this incidence to 28%, while flavone itself was ineffective.

Several flavonoids were tested for their effects on tumorigenicity induced by BP and its diol epoxide-2 derivative, by Chang and his colleagues (1985). The carcinogens were administered to newborn mice intraperitoneally and the flavonoids were given 10 min before this treatment. Quercetin, robinetin, and myricetin were ineffective in preventing the incidence of lung tumors in these mice when treated with BP. On the other hand, these agents were quite effective in reducing the tumor incidence with the diol epoxide-2 as the carcinogen. The most potent of the inhibitors proved to be robinetin, which, at 1400 nmoles total dose, reduced the percentage of mice with lung tumors after administration of 15 and 30 nmoles of diol epoxide from 63 and 93% to 41 and 50%, respectively. The number of lung tumors per mouse after 15 and 30 nmoles diol epoxide was reduced from 1.25 and 5.23 to 0.76 and 1.29, respectively, in the robinetin-treated mice. The next most efficacious inhibitor was myricetin, which at the highest dose of carcinogen reduced the percentage of mice with tumors and the numbers of tumors per mouse from 93% to 65% and from 5.23 to 2.59, respectively. No reason was given for the lack of any effect of the flavonoids upon BP-induced tumorigenesis.

3.3.7. Mechanism of Action of the Flavonoids

Many carcinogens require metabolic activation prior to eliciting their pharmacological effects in the host. In some instances, this activation proceeds through the NADPH-mediated cytochrome P450-dependent monooxygenase system. Some reports have appeared indicating that certain flavonoids can exert marked effects on this activating mechanism. Wattenberg *et al.* (1968) have found that the parent compound, flavone, as well as two methylated derivatives, tangeretin and nobiletin, increase AHH activity in lung and liver after their administration. A similar finding has been published by Buening *et al.* (1981). These substances have also been tested (Buening *et al.*, 1978) on the activation of AFB to mutagenic components using *Salmonella typhimurium* TA98 as the test organism. The three flavonoids increased the metabolic activation of this fungal toxin to mutagenic components.

Although some of the flavonoids, as indicated earlier, do induce a cytochrome P450-mediated reaction, i.e., AHH, the addition of these components *in vitro* results in inhibition. Thus, Sousa and Marletta (1985) have noted that quercetin profoundly inhibited cytochrome P450 activity in rat liver microsomes, while Wiebel *et al.* (1974) have reported the inhibition of AHH in both control and induced microsomes by tangeretin and nobiletin. In the study of Sousa and Marletta (1985), the hydroxylation of BP catalyzed by human liver microsomes was inhibited by a series of polyhydroxylated flavonoids; myricetin was most active. In regard to the deethylation of ethoxyresorufin by microsomes obtained from 5,6-benzoflavone-induced rats, the inhibitory efficacy was in the following order: galangin > kaempferol > quercetin > dihydroquercetin > morin. Beyeler *et al.* (1988) studied the inhibition of rat liver microsome aminopyrine N-demethylation, biphenyl 4-hydroxylation, and biphenyl 2-hydroxylation by flavanone and several flavonoid derivatives. Their results suggest different types of inhibition (competitive, noncompetitive, or mixed) depending upon the inhibitor and the enzyme system. They suggested a dual cytochrome P-450 binding mode involving electrostatic and lipophilic interactions.

Huang *et al.* (1983) have determined the effect of certain flavonoids on mutagenesis in *Salmonella typhimurium* TA100 with BP and the proximal mutagen BP-7,8-dihydrodiol as the test substances. Myricetin, robinetin, and luteolin depressed the mutagenesis by both of the polycyclic hydrocarbons in a dose-dependent manner. The flavonoids appeared more effective with the dihydrodiol as the promutagen. These authors also tested the effects of these flavonoids on the metabolism of BP; a 50% inhibition of the formation of phenolic derivatives was observed with 50 nmoles of the flavonoids. In contrast, only 1.3–5 nmoles of the latter were required to block the mutagenicity of BP diol epoxide 2, purportedly the ultimate mutagen of the polycyclic hydrocarbon. The ID_{50} for a large group of flavonoids as inhibitors of the mutagenicity of the diol epoxide as abstracted from the published data (Huang *et al.*, 1983) is presented in Table IV. These results suggest that the polyhydroxylated flavonoids may exert their inhibitory efficacy by reacting with ultimate electrophilic forms of at least this mutagen. Furthermore, in order to exhibit this antimutagenic activity, the flavonoid must have at least three hydroxyl groups.

Birt *et al.* (1986) reported the effects of apigenin and robinetin on methylnitrosourea

Table IV. Inhibition of the Mutagenic
Activity of BP 7,8-Diol-9,10-Epoxide-2
by Flavonoids[a]

Flavonoid	ID_{50} (nmoles)
Myricetin	2
Robinetin	2.5
Luteolin	5
Quercetin	5
Rutin	5
Quercitrin	5
Morin	10
Kaempferol	10
Apigenin	10
Fisetin	10
Chrysin	>100
Tangeretin	>100 ·
Nobiletin	>100

[a]From Huang *et al.*, 1983.

(MNU) and N-methyl-N'-nitro-N-nitrosoguanidine (MNNG) mutagenicity with TA100 and BP, and 2-aminoanthracene (2-AA) mutagenicity with TA98. Little inhibition of MNNG or MNU mutagenicity was observed. But, both flavonoids inhibited 2-AA mutagenicity, and apigenin inhibited BP mutagenicity by 43–87%. Inhibiting MNNG mutagenicity in TA100 NR was examined with a series of flavonoids. Although several of the flavonoids were effective, the most striking inhibition was observed with naringin (Francis *et al.*, 1989).

Flavonoids also have been shown to be immunomodulative, which may be important in their ability to interfere with tumor development (reviewed by Wiltrout and Hornung, 1988). This effect has been studied more with respect to the ability of some flavonoids in the therapy of cancer, but it should be considered in carcinogenesis also, particularly in the later stages of carcinogenesis. Flavone acetic acid, for example, has been found to augment natural killer cell activity and induce interferon-alpha and act synergistically with interlukin-2.

3.3.8. Flavonoids as Antioxidants

As indicated in Section 3.3.7., the topical application of a tumor promoter such as TPA results in a number of phenotypic alterations. Indeed, some of these biochemical alterations may comprise an integral component of the action of promoters.

The arachidonate cascade mechanism for the biosynthesis of the prostanoids, i.e., prostaglandins, thromboxanes, and leukotrienes, represents an important reaction sequence in regard to carcinogenesis. During the course of this cascade, e.g., the transformation of prostaglandin G2 to prostaglandin H2, a radical is generated which may contribute to the activation of procarcinogens to carcinogens. Thus, it has been reported that the 7,8-dihydrodiol of BP may be converted to the carcinogenic diol epoxide in a cooxygenation mechanism involving the utilization of arachidonate. Consequently, the cooxygenation pathway can contribute to the process of initiation.

Nakadate and colleagues (1982a,b) have suggested that lipoxygenase products from arachidonic acid may contribute to some of the effects seen after the topical application of TPA during the process of promotion. Arachidonate-5-lipoxygenase catalyzes the oxidation of arachidonic acid at the C5 position, yielding 5-hydroperoxy-6,8,11,14-eicosatetraenoic acid. The latter compound ultimately contributes to the formation of the leukotrienes (LT).

LT-C4 and LT-D4 are responsible for the biological activity of the slow-reacting substance of anaphylaxis (Samuelson, 1983). Mediation of anaphylactic-like reactions may form part of the mechanism of promotion. Consequently, a number of flavonoids have been tested as inhibitors of this pathway and, in particular, of the lipoxygenase enzyme. Several of the flavonoids, including quercetin, have shown inhibitory efficacy against lipoxygenase (Nakadate *et al.*, 1982a,b; Baumann *et al.*, 1980; Hope *et al.*, 1983; Yoshimoto *et al.*, 1983; Wheeler and Berry, 1986). Both quercetin and its rhamnose derivative, rutin, have demonstrated antiallergic actions in concert with the inhibition of this system. Of a series of flavonoids, Yoshimoto *et al.* (1983) demonstrated that cirsiliol was the most effective inhibitor of 5-lipoxygenase and quercetin was less effective. Both compounds also inhibited the 12-lipoxygenase but to a lesser extent. The cyclooxygenase that catalyzes the conversion of arachidonic acid to prostaglandin G2 was not affected by the flavonoids.

Wheeler and Berry (1986) have purified lipoxygenase from mouse epidermal cells and tested the potency of several flavonoids as inhibitors. Inhibition of this enzyme was observed with luteolin, flavonol, and quercetin. The most potent inhibitors of this enzyme contained a 3-hydroxyl group and maintained unsaturation at the 2,3 position in the flavone ring.

In summary, the flavonoids have shown some promising anticarcinogenic activity, but the mutagenic property of some of these substances in *Salmonella* has prevented further exploitation of this group. This is unfortunate since little genotoxicity is manifested by the flavonoids in nonbacterial systems and, with the exception of a single report, these compounds do not exhibit any carcinogenicity. The flavonoids deserve a more thorough testing as potential chemopreventive agents.

3.4. Ellagic Acid and Other Phenols

The flavonoids are not the only phenolic compounds present in fruits and vegetables that are able to affect carcinogenesis. These foodstuffs contain a group of phenols consisting of hydroxycinnamic acid and its derivatives (Mosel and Hermann, 1974; Schmidtlein and Hermann, 1975). The hydroxycinnamic acids have been evaluated as potential chemopreventive agents by Wattenberg *et al.* (1980) and Shugar and Kao (1984).

The incidence and the numbers of BP-induced forestomach tumors developing in mice that had been pretreated with either *o*-hydroxycinnamic acid, 3,4-dihydroxycinnamic acid (caffeic acid), or 4-hydroxy-3-methoxy cinnamic acid (ferulic acid) have been investigated (Wattenberg, 1980). Only weak inhibition was observed with these agents administered in the diet. A similar lack of effect of caffeic acid on the covalent binding of the diol epoxide of BP to mouse skin DNA in organ cultures has been observed (Shugar and Kao, 1984).

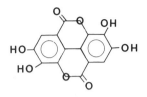

Fig. 5. Structure of ellagic acid.

Ellagic acid is a naturally occurring plant phenol that can be found in high concentration in grapes and nuts (Fig. 5). It had previously been found (Wood *et al.*, 1982) that ellagic acid is a potent inhibitor of the mutagenic activity of the diol epoxide of BP. Ellagic acid apparently exerted this inhibitory action by accelerating the disappearance of the diol epoxide from the aqueous medium. This was accomplished by its covalently adducting to the diol epoxide as proposed by Sayer *et al.* (1982).

Chang *et al.* (1985) have determined the effects of topical ellagic acid on the incidence of skin tumors in mice that received the diol epoxide-2 of BP as the initiator and TPA as the promoter. A dose-dependent decrease in tumorigenesis was observed with a 60% inhibition by 2500 nmoles of ellagic acid. They also determined the effects of this polyhydroxylated compound on the incidence of lung tumors in mice that, as newborns, had received BP diol epoxide-2 or another polycyclic hydrocarbon, dibenz(a,h)pyrene diol epoxide. In both instances, tumorigenesis was significantly reduced. At 300 nmoles of ellagic acid and a total dose of BP diol epoxide-2, the percentage of mice with tumors and the numbers of tumors per mouse decreased from 86 to 76% and from 3.41 to 1.76, respectively. An interesting aspect of this study was the lack of any effect of ellagic acid on the induction of lung tumors in this model by the parent hydrocarbon, BP (Chang *et al.*, 1985). This contrasts with the findings of Lesca (1983), although in the latter, the plant phenol was administered to A/J mice in the diet for 5 days prior to intraperitoneally administered polycyclic aromatic hydrocarbon.

The effects of ellagic acid have been studied in some detail in Mukhtar's laboratory. He found that this phenol protects against 3-MC-induced skin tumorigenesis in Balb/c mice (1984a). This laboratory has also studied the effects of this agent on a number of enzymes of biotransformation and on the metabolism of BP (Mukhtar *et al.*, 1984b; Das *et al.*, 1985). Using cultured mouse keratinocytes, they (Mukhtar *et al.*, 1984b) have found a depression by ellagic acid of the activities of AHH and 7-ethoxycoumarin *O*-deethylase and a reduction in the amount of BP metabolism. As a consequence, the amount of adduction of the polycyclic hydrocarbon to DNA was significantly depressed.

In a similar series of experiments (Das *et al.*, 1985) mice administered ellagic acid in the drinking water for 16 weeks or injected i.p., showed comparable reductions in these enzymes in the liver and lung. Epoxide hydrolase activity of the liver was unaffected, while glutathione *S*-transferase was significantly elevated in this tissue. After oral feeding, the hepatic and pulmonary metabolism of BP was markedly depressed in these mice. found to be effective in the inhibition of murine subcutaneous and intravenous benzo(rst)pentaphene (DBP) carcinogenesis (Homburger *et al.*, 1971). Comparison of pure d-

Teel and colleagues (1985) have studied the effects of ellagic acid on the metabolism of BP in lung explants obtained from the sensitive mouse A/J. As noted by Mukhtar's group, the metabolism of this polycyclic hydrocarbon was depressed by ellagic acid, as was the binding to DNA. They also noted a significant increase in the amount of BP and its metabolites remaining associated with the total lipids, suggesting that ellagic acid may increase the persistence of the polycyclic hydrocarbon but not alter its uptake. Teel (1986) also showed that ^{3}H-ellagic acid binds to the DNA in rat explants with the decreasing order of binding as indicated: esophagus > trachea > bladder > colon > forestomach. Teel proposed that this binding may, in fact, contribute to the antimutagenic and anticarcinogenic activities of ellagic acid.

Modulation of N-nitrosobenzylmethylamine (NBMA) induced esophageal carcinogenesis in rats by ellagic acid was reported by Mandal and Stoner (1990) and by Barch and Fox (1988). Mandal and Stoner conducted tumorigenesis studies with rats fed 0.0, 0.4, or 4 g ellagic acid/Kg diet and treated with 20 weekly doses of NBMA. Tumor incidence was 100% in most groups but the number of tumors was reduced in the ellagic acid groups by 21–55%. Barch and Fox (1988) found that dietary ellagic acid reduced the *in vivo* formation in NBMA treated rats of the potentially cancer-inducing, esophageal O^6-methylguanine, but ellagic acid did not influence formation of 7-methylguanine, a lesion not believed to be related to tumor induction. Further *in vitro* studies supported this observation (Barch and Fox, 1988).

Additional studies bearing on the action of ellagic acid have been conducted by Dixit and Gold (1986). They have studied the effects of this phenolic compound on *N*-methyl-*N*-nitrosourea-induced mutagenesis and the methylation of DNA. Ellagic acid at low concentrations *selectively* blocked the methylation of the O^6 position of guanine in DNA. Comparable reduction in the methylation at the N^7 position of guanine was achieved at much higher concentrations of ellagic acid. Furthermore, the DNA had to be double-stranded. Although, as found by Teel (1986), ellagic acid covalently adducted to DNA, the binding occurs to *both* single- and double-stranded polynucleotides. However, the amount of binding to poly(dA.dT) exceeds that to poly(dG.dC), suggesting a preference of ellagic acid for A.T sites. These studies suggest that the effects of ellagic acid as an anticarcinogen and antimutagen are much more complicated than proposed by Sayer *et al.* (1982), i.e., that they involve interaction with the diol epoxide. The selective inhibition of the alkylation of specific sites of the DNA may also play a role in these properties.

The preceding studies on ellagic acid indicate its potential effectiveness as a chemopreventive agent. Furthermore, the compound appears to be well tolerated, at least by rodents. Consequently, more extensive studies in biological models employing additional carcinogens might be in order.

3.5. Terpenes

The terpene most extensively studied for its ability to prevent cancer is d-limonene (Fig. 6). d-Limonene, which is found naturally in citrus oils (Shaw, 1977), was investigated early for its chemotherapeutic properties (Leiter *et al.*, 1959). A mixture of essential oils (menthone, menthol, camphor, alpha-pinene, beta-pinene, borneol, and cineol) high in terpenes inhibited skin carcinomas induced by benzo(a)pyrene when mice were treated with the essential oils on alternate days with the BP (Benko *et al.*, 1963). Citrus oils were

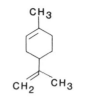

Fig. 6. Structure of limonene.

limonene, a mixture of d-limonene with its hydroperoxide, and orange oil indicated that the three agents were similar in their ability to prevent subcutaneous tumors induced by DBP (Homburger *et al.*, 1971). In contrast, both spontaneous and DBP-induced lung adenoma yield was reduced by pure limonene, but not by orange oil or the hydroperoxide of limonene (Homburger *et al.*, 1971).

In studies reported by Van Duuren and Goldschmidt (1976), d-limonene partially inhibited BP-induced skin carcinogenesis in mice. In this study, 5 µg BP was applied topically three times weekly with 10 mg d-limonene, and four squamous cell carcinomas arose in 13 mice in the limonene group, while 13 carcinomas developed in 16 mice in the control group.

More recent studies indicated that feeding diet containing 1000 or 10,000 ppm d-limonene from 1 week before treatment with DMBA until the end of the experiment resulted in decreased incidence, increased latency, and increased regression of frank mammary tumors in Sprague–Dawley rats (Elegbede *et al.*, 1984). A further report from this laboratory indicated that d-limonene was effective in increasing the latency only when fed during initiation. In addition, feeding d-limonene during initiation caused the greatest reduction in total tumor incidence, and a small reduction was observed in animals fed d-limonene during promotion/progression (Gould *et al.*, 1986). A combination of d-limonene (95%), myrcene (1.86%), and a-pinene (0.42%) was shown to have somewhat greater chemopreventive ability than limonene alone, but was not as effective as 5% orange peel oil in the inhibition of mammary carcinogenesis (Maltzman *et al.*, 1986). Limonine and orange oil also were effective in the inhibition of mammary carcinogenesis induced by the direct-acting carcinogen MNU. In this model inhibition of promotion was observed but no inhibition of initiation was apparent (Maltzman *et al.*, 1989).

In studies designed to test the effects of d-limonene on the regression of mammary tumors, 10% dietary d-limonene was compared with 10% cellulose (Elegbede *et al.*, 1986a). Dietary d-limonene increased the regression of the first tumors and inhibited the formation of subsequent multiple tumors.

Two other citrus liminoids, limonin and nomilin, were examined for their effects on DMBA-induced, buccal pouch epidermoid carcinogenesis in Syrian hamsters (Miller *et al.*, 1989). Buccal pouches were treated topically with 2.5% solutions of the liminoids with or without alternate day treatments of 0.5% DMBA. Limonin treatment reduced the tumor burden 60% in comparison with the DMBA group while nomilin caused only a small reduction.

Earlier investigations had indicated promoting activity of citrus oils in skin tumorigenesis (Roe and Pierce, 1960), but more recent work suggested that this activity was not due to d-limonene (Elegbede *et al.*, 1986b). Studies with humans demonstrated the absence of toxicity of a single 20-g dose of d-limonene (Igimi *et al.*, 1976). The low apparent toxicity of d-limonene, coupled with its effectiveness in the inhibition of carcinogenesis, provides promise of a potentially useful agent for the prevention of cancer in humans, and further studies on this compound will be of considerable interest.

3.6. Sulfides

Sulfur-containing compounds have a long history of use as agents to protect against toxicity. Naturally occurring dietary sulfur-containing compounds are abundantly found in the garlic and onion genus, *Allium* (Brodnitz *et al.*, 1969). As indicated in Section 2.2 studies have demonstrated inhibition of skin tumor promotion by TPA on mice treated topically with onion and garlic oils (Belman, 1983). Onion oil was effective when given at dosages of 0.1–10 mg 30 min after three times per week treatment with TPA. Garlic oil was less effective and 1-mg dosages were necessary in the same protocol. In addition, the growth of Ehrlich ascites tumor cells implanted in mice was inhibited in animals fed garlic supplements (Choy *et al.*, 1983). When garlic was homogenized and fed by gastric intubation at a daily dosage of 0.6 or 1.2 g, the number of tumor cells recovered from these mice was reduced by approximately 40% and 60%, respectively, in comparison with the non-garlic-fed group.

The principal form of the sulfur compounds in garlic is as allyl sulfide. Several milligrams of sulfide are present in an average clove of garlic. Brodnitz *et al.* (1969) identified several methyl and allyl sulfides, disulfides, and trisulfides. Garlic is particularly rich in diallyl disulfide and diallyl sulfide.

The potential for diallyl sulfide as a chemopreventive agent was assessed by Wargovich and Goldberg (1985) using the nuclear aberration assay. The nuclear aberration assay measures morphological evidence of genotoxic damage in the proliferating cells of the gastrointestinal epithelium. This assay has been shown to be useful for assessing chemopreventive agents for colon carcinogenesis. Diallyl sulfide was administered orally at a dose of 200 mg/g body weight 1.5 hr before carcinogenic dosages of MNU, N'-nitro-N-nitrosoguanidine (MNNG), or DMH, and mice were killed 24 hr later. Diallyl sulfide treatment caused a 70% inhibition in the induction of nuclear aberrations by DMH, a colon carcinogen requiring metabolic activation, but did not influence the damage caused by the direct-acting carcinogens MNU or MNNG, thus suggesting the involvement of diallyl sulfide in metabolic activation. Subsequent studies verified that orally administered diallyl sulfide was effective in the inhibition of colon carcinogenesis induced by DMH in rats (Wargovich, 1987) and in esophageal carcinogenesis induced by NBMA (Wargovich *et al.*, 1988). The hepatic microsomal metabolism of NBMA was also reduced in rats administered diallyl sulfide (Wargovich *et al.*, 1988).

The effects of diallyl sulfide on hepatic metabolism of nitrosamines and isozymes of cytochrome P-450 were studied by Brady *et al.* (1988). Diallyl sulfide was found to be a competitive inhibitor of N-dimethylnitrosamine demethylase activity. It was most effective in the inhibition of demethylation of dimethylnitrosamine, less effective against NBMA, and ineffective against benzphetamine or ethylmorphine. Immunoblot studies indicated an elevation of P45OIIB1 and a suppression of P450IIE1 in hepatic microsomes treated with diallyl sulfide. Because P450IIE1 is important in the oxidative metabolism of

DMH, this observation possibly explains some of the chemopreventive effects of diallyl sulfide.

Studies from the laboratory of Sparnins (1986) indicated that allyl methyl trisulfide, another garlic oil constitutent, enhanced GST activity in several tissues and inhibited forestomach tumorigenesis by BP. GST activity was elevated by a single low dose (3.0 μmoles) of allyl methyl trisulfide in the forestomach and small-bowel mucosa, but liver and lung GST were less responsive and dosages of 15.0–22.5 μmoles were required for consistent elevation. For tumorigenesis studies, 15.0 μmoles allyl methyl trisulfide was administered at 48 and 96 hr preceding BP treatment; this protocol was repeated after 1 week, and forestomach tumor induction was inhibited by 70%, but lung tumorigenesis was not influenced.

These studies indicate the need for further studies on the chemopreventive potential of sulfur-containing compounds from *Allium*.

3.7. Protease Inhibitors

Shortly after usage in the United States as a source of a vegetable oil, soybeans were demonstrated by Osborne and Mendel (1917) to support the growth of rats only if they were heated. Subsequently, Kunitz (1945) demonstrated that soybeans contained a potent inhibitor of some proteases such as trypsin. The trypsin inhibitor was heat-labile, which explains the inability of raw soybean to uphold growth. Further evidence in this regard was provided by the finding of Liener *et al.* (1949) that the significant growth reduction seen when animals were placed on a raw soybean-containing diet could almost (but not quite) be duplicated by supplementing the heated soybean diet with purified soybean inhibitor at the same level as would be present in the uncooked vegetable. The growth inhibition was, therefore, due in part to a reduction in the digestion of dietary protein by proteolytic enzymes present in the intestinal tract and which would be sensitive to the inhibitor occurring in raw soybean. That this was not the complete story was shown by the studies of Liener *et al.* (1949) and Westfall *et al.* (1948). They reported that incorporation of the trypsin inhibitor into the diets that contained already predisgested protein or free amino acids as the nitrogen sources also resulted in a significant growth reduction.

A most significant observation was provided by Chernick *et al.* (1948), who reported the occurrence of pancreatic hypertrophy in animals fed either raw soybeans or the trypsin inhibitor. It was subsequently postulated that at least some of the growth inhibition would occur as a result of the endogenous loss of essential amino acids secreted by hyperactive pancreas (Lyman and Lepkovsky, 1957).

The preceding paragraphs are not to be interpreted as indicating that only *one* proteinase inhibitor exists in legumes. In fact, a number of such inhibitors may be found in these plants. An excellent review of this area may be found in Laskowski and Kato (1980). Many of these proteinase inhibitors function naturally to prevent proteolysis that could yield injury, e.g., alpha$_1$-antitrypsin, which prevents the destructive action of the proteinase upon lung tissue, thus avoiding emphysema. Indeed, the inhibitor concentration can be significantly reduced in heavy smokers (Carp and Janoff, 1978; Janoff *et al.*, 1979), thus contributing to lung injury in the latter.

Protease inhibitors are widely distributed in plants (Richardson, 1977), particularly in seed foods. At least five different inhibitors that interact with serine proteases have been reported (Ikenate *et al.*, 1974). These agents may serve as protective agents against insect infestation by inhibiting insect proteases, as suggested by Ryan (1973).

3.7.1. Proteinase Inhibitors as Inhibitors of Carcinogenesis

Soybean preparations, purified proteinase inhibitors, and synthetic inhibitors have proven effective in the reduction of cancer incidence in biological model systems. As originally proposed by Berenblum and Shubik (1947), mouse skin tumorigenesis can be characterized in terms of two phases, initiation and promotion. The effects of certain proteinase inhibitors have been tested on the promotion phase of mouse skin tumorigenesis by Troll and his colleagues (1970).

In these experiments, DMBA was applied as an initiator to the ears of mice, and the promoting agent, croton oil or TPA, was topically administered. As proteinase inhibitors, the chlormethylketones of tosyllysine (TLCK) and phenylalanine (TPCK), which inhibit trypsin and chymotrypsin, respectively, were employed. In addition, the competitive inhibitor of trypsin and papain, tosylarginine methyl ester (TAME), was also tested. All agents were topically applied to the mouse ears along with either the croton oil or TPA.

Troll and colleagues (1970) observed that TLCK reduced the TPA-promoting activity by about 90%; the effectiveness of croton oil as a promoter was impaired by approximately 50%. TAME exhibited an efficacy similar to that of croton oil, as an antipromoter, while TPCK suppressed all tumor formation in the DMBA, croton oil-promoted system. A profound effect of all the synthetic proteinase inhibitors upon the immediate inflammatory response to both croton oil and TPA was also observed.

The Troll laboratory (1972) has also tested the inhibitory efficacy of a naturally occurring proteinase inhibitor from *Actinomycetes,* leupeptin. Leupeptin effectively countered the promoting effect of either croton oil or TPA when applied to the backs of DMBA-initiated mice.

Soybean-containing diets, partially purified preparations, as well as protease inhibitors have been tested in models for other than skin tumorigenesis systems. In a study from Troll's laboratory (1980), raw soybean was contrasted with casein and Purina chow in supporting mammary carcinogenesis in rats. In these experiments, rats were placed on diets consisting of raw soybean (50% of the components), or casein (32%), or Purina chow. The animals were X-irradiated with 300 rad of total body irradiation and then palpated weekly. The contents of protease inhibitors in the soybean diet, casein diet, and Purina chow were 4.75%, 0.23%, and 0%, respectively. The percentage of rats exhibiting mammary fibroadenomas and adenocarcinomas on these three diets were 44, 70, and 74%, respectively. Consequently, the soybean-containing diet significantly reduced the incidence of mammary tumors in X-irradiated rats.

Becker (1981) has determined the effects of EdiPro A, an isolated soybean protein with high protease inhibitor activity, on the incidence of spontaneous hepatocarcinogenesis in a strain of mouse, the C3H/HeN, that exhibits a high incidence of this type of tumor. The mice were fed semipurified diets containing casein as the protein source. EdiPro A was incorporated into this diet in place of casein at from 0 to 5.2%; i.e., casein levels were reduced from 26 to 20.8%, respectively. A dose-dependent reduction in the incidence of liver tumors was observed from 100% (no EdiPro A) to 0% (5.2% of the soybean derivative in the diet). Even at 2.6% EdiPro A, a 75% reduction in tumor incidence was seen.

Aprotinin, a broad-spectrum inhibitor of a variety of proteases, has also been tested as a potential chemopreventive agent (Ohkoshi, 1980). Aprotinin has been administered intraperitoneally into mice that had been treated with the potent carcinogen 3-MC. A dramatic effect on the incidence of squamous cell carcinoma was observed.

In addition to the protein inhibitors, some small-molecular-weight compounds that affect certain proteases have also been tested as to their effectiveness as anticancer agents. Previous work (Corasanti *et al.*, 1980) has shown that human colon tumors have a higher level of plasminogen activator activity than the corresponding normal intestinal mucosa. Plasminogen activator is a serine protease that catalyzes the conversion of plasminogen to plasmin, the active fibrinolytic protein. In order to further assess the importance of this process to carcinogenesis, Corasanti *et al.* (1982) administered dimethylhydrazine to mice to induce colonic tumors. The latter exhibited 10-fold more extractable plasminogen activator activity than the normal colon. The treated mice also received a potent inhibitor of plasminogen activator activity, epsilon-aminocaproic acid, in the drinking water. The treated tumor-bearing group exhibited 10-fold fewer tumors per mouse and a number demonstrated complete prevention of the disease. It was concluded that the use of a specific protease inhibitor proved most efficacious in the prevention of colon cancer.

Protease inhibitors have been tested as protectors against radiation damage as well as against radiation-induced tumorigenesis. In the syndrome induced by radiation, death may occur from hematopoietic damage in the host, from gastrointestinal damage in animals receiving larger doses, or from central nervous system damage in animals receiving very large doses. In certain fowl given in excess of 800 rads, Stearner *et al.* (1955) observed that death was preceded by increased vascular permeability, plasma leakage, hemoconcentration, and degeneration of the endothelium, all of which accounted for the vascular collapse. A trypsinlike enzyme has been implicated in this syndrome, particularly since protection was afforded by soybean trypsin inhibitor (Stearner and Azuma, 1968).

Palladino *et al.* (1982) have examined the effects of several protease inhibitors on gamma-irradiation-induced mortality in mice and also in the chicken. They observed that soybean trypsin inhibitor, lima bean inhibitor, antipain, leupeptin, and alpha-*N*-benzoyl-L-arginine ethyl ester, a synthetic inhibitor of proteases, protected against the mortality in chickens of acute gamma-irradiation. Certain other synthetic protease inhibitors, such as *p*-tosyl-L-arginine-methyl ester, α-tosyl-lysyl chloromethyl ketone, and ε-aminocaproic acid, had little effect. In certain mouse strains that were given gamma-irradiation, soybean trypsin inhibitor and antipain served as protectants. These patterns were suggestive of a kallikrein-like enzyme contributing to radiation damage in the chicken and mouse.

The effects of various protease inhibitors on radiation-induced malignant transformation of C3H10T1/2 cells *in vitro* have been examined by Kennedy and Little (1978, 1981). These investigators have reported focus formation of these cells as a result of their exposure to 400 or 600 rads of radiation. Furthermore, at the lower dose, promoters such as TPA increase the numbers of foci, in an apparent initiation–promotion manner. The incorporation of antipain or leupeptin into the medium very effectively reduced the radiation-induced foci formation (Kennedy and Little, 1978). In the later publication (1981), this effect was studied in more detail.

Three different protease inhibitors were employed in the same two-stage C3H10T1/2 model system. Soybean trypsin inhibitor, of molecular weight 24,000, inhibits trypsin, chymotrypsin, thromboplastin, plasmin, and elastase (Kunitz, 1947). Antipain, molecular weight 500–600 and isolated from *Actinomycetes,* is active against papain, trypsin, plasmin, cathepsin B, and plasminogen activator (Aoyagi and Umezawa, 1975). Leupeptin, molecular weight 500–600 and also isolated from *Actinomycetes,* inhibits papain, trypsin, plasmin, cathepsin B, and plasminogen activator (Aoyagi and Umezawa, 1975). Leupeptin, molecular weight 500–600 and also isolated from *Actinomycetes,* inhibits papain, trypsin, plasmin, cathepsin B, and plasminogen activator (Aoyagi and Umezawa, 1975). All three protease inhibitors were employed at nontoxic concentrations. The inhibitors were most effective in preventing focus formation when given immediately after the X-ray irradiation. When treatment was delayed for 4 days, a lesser effect was noted.

Radiation transformation has been divided into the following three phases: phase 1, the fixation phase, which occurs up to 24 hr after radiation; phase 2, the expression phase, which occurs up to 6 weeks following X-ray; and phase 3, the promotion phase, which consists of an enhancement of transformation occurring during the 6-week expression period. As indicated above, the fixation phase was significantly affected by the protease inhibitors *except* soybean trypsin inhibitor. The expression phase was markedly impaired by antipain and leupeptin. The promotion phase was inhibited by soybean trypsin inhibitor and antipain. As is apparent, antipain was active in all three phases. Its mechanism of action, however, is unknown.

Another purified protease inhibitor, the Bowman–Birk trypsin inhibitor, has been isolated from soybeans (Birk, 1961) and tested for antitransformation properties using the cell culture model. The Bowman–Birk inhibitor reduces the activity of both trypsin and chymotrypsin and causes enlargement of the pancreas and increased secretion of pancreatic proteolytic enzymes. Yavelow *et al.* (1983) have studied whether, in fact, the protease inhibitor is absorbed after its administration by gavage. Virtually all of the protein was found in the feces, indicating its lack of absorption. Using the C3H10T1/2 cell model, Yavelow *et al.* (1983) have not seen any effects on either the fixation phase of radiation transformation or the subsequent expression and promotion phases. These results indicate that at least this purified soybean trypsin inhibitor has no antitransformation activity.

3.7.2. Mechanism of Action of the Protease Inhibitors

From the bulk of the available evidence, it appears unlikely that the protease inhibitors exerted their effects on carcinogenesis or on radiation injury solely through inhibition of the action of some proteinase (Desikachar and De, 1949). This is particularly true in those examples where absorption was required as well as distribution to some peripheral organ in appropriate amounts to block the proteinase effectively. Some results have subsequently been published that suggest an involvement of the protease inhibitors on the production of oxygen radicals, e.g., superoxide anion radical.

It has previously been reported that phagocytosis of bacteria by polymorphonuclear leukocytes (PMN) is accompanied by a burst in oxygen consumption and the generation of superoxide anion radical through the NADPH oxidase system (Curnatte *et al.*, 1974). Superoxide dismutase would then catalyze the formation of hydrogen peroxide from some of the superoxide anion radical, and the hydrogen peroxide could subsequently interact with superoxide anion radical as catalyzed by trace amounts of iron-containing compounds, e.g., transferrin, to yield hydroxyl radical. All three agents, superoxide anion radical, hydrogen peroxide, and hydroxyl radical, would then be involved in the digestion of the endocytosed bacteria.

An increase in oxygen consumption by PMN has also been reported to occur when these cells are exposed to promoters, such as TPA (Goldstein *et al.*, 1979). Indeed, Witz *et al.* (1980) have postulated that tumor promoters may exert some of their action as a result of the stimulation of superoxide anion radical formation (and other oxygen radicals).

Goldstein *et al.* (1979) have determined the effect of soybean trypsin inhibitor and other protease inhibitors on the oxygen burst in human PMN as a result of their exposure to TPA. They found that this burst was completely eliminated by soybean trypsin inhibitor, while trasylol and e-aminocaproic acid had little effect. They also measured the effects of several protease inhibitors on superoxide anion radical production by measuring the reduction of cytochrome c. Soybean trypsin inhibitor, lima bean trypsin inhibitor, antipain, and elastatinol were effective suppressors of the formation of this radical, while chymostatin was much less effective. Without any effect were Σ-aminocaproic acid, TAME, pepstatin, and leupeptin.

In a more thorough study of the efficacy of protease inhibitors on superoxide anion radical production, Troll's laboratory (Yavelow *et al.*, 1982) has blended a variety of canned foods, soybeans, bean curd, and soybean milk powder and determined the protease inhibitor activity of the clarified extracts.

Antichymotrypsin activity was present in the following order: canned chickpea $<$ kidney beans $<$ bean curd. On the other hand, antitrypsin activity was observed in the following order: kidney beans $<$ chickpeas $<$ bean curd. The ability to inhibit the production of superoxide anion radical fell into the following order: kidney bean $<$ chickpea $<$ bean curd. They also tested the efficacy of the Bowman–Birk inhibitor and the Kunitz soybean trypsin inhibitor in regard to their ability to reduce superoxide anion radical formation caused by the exposure of human PMN to TPA. The former was much more efficacious.

In summary, a number of the protease inhibitors appear to inhibit mouse skin tumorigenesis effectively, probably by interfering with the promotion phase. In addition, these agents are able to interfere with the expression and promotion phases of radiation-induced transformation of certain cell cultures. Finally, some of these protease inhibitors can interfere with the formation of colon cancer and some other cancers in biological model systems. The exact mechanism for these actions is unknown, but at least some of their effects may be due to the reduction in the generation of radicals, particularly oxygen radicals.

4. Summary and Conclusions

Epidemiologic studies have provided circumstantial evidence for cancer prevention by dietary vegetables and fruits. Numerous studies have shown inverse relationships between gastrointestinal tract cancer and vegetable consumption, and some reports have suggested that the incidence of cancer of the lung, bladder, breast, and prostate was lower in people consuming diets rich in vegetables and fruits. These reports have led to recommendations that individuals increase their consumption of fruits and vegetables. Carotene-rich fruits and vegetables, citrus fruits, and cruciferous vegetables were given special recognition in these recommendations because of their content of nutrients suspected in the prevention of cancer and because of the results from epidemiologic studies.

Few studies have been conducted on the inhibition of cancer in animals fed vegetables. The primary reason for this is the difficulty in designing and interpreting such studies. First, it is impossible to formulate diets such that animals will receive equivalent nutrient levels in vegetable-containing and control diets. Vegetables are generally added to the diets at a rate of 5–20% and thus a major dilution is made of the basal diet. Second, vegetables usually must be dried prior to addition to the diet since rodent diets are generally fed in a dry form to maintain homogeneity. This drying process certainly alters the composition of the vegetable. Third, it is impossible to have a uniform vegetable supplement for an entire carcinogenesis study. If a large quantity of vegetable is obtained at the beginning of a study and stored, there is a problem of changes during storage, or if vegetable is obtained at intervals throughout the study, there is a problem of seasonal differences in quality. These difficulties make investigations on the influence of vegetable consumption on carcinogenesis in animals difficult to interpret and to relate to human studies.

In the studies that have been conducted, results have been inconsistent; vegetable supplements can inhibit, enhance, or not influence carcinogenesis. Different results are probably due to differences in the type of cancer being studied, the manner of treating with the vegetable supplement, the handling of the supplement, and as yet unidentified experimental factors.

Several studies have demonstrated potential antimutagenic properties of vegetable and fruit extracts. These studies suggest that vegetables contain components which influence the activation and/or detoxication of chemical carcinogens. In this regard, a tremendous body of literature describes effects of vegetable extracts on MFO activities and GST. It is apparent that vegetables and fruits contain inducers for enzymes in these drug/carcinogen metabolizing systems.

A number of chemical components of vegetables and fruits have been studied for their effects on cancer. This chapter reviewed those compounds which have been most extensively studied and/or have shown the most promise as potential inhibitors. The classes of compounds covered were indoles, isothiocyanates, flavonoids, ellagic acid and other phenols, terpenes, sulfides, and protease inhibitors.

Several of the indoles were shown to influence metabolism of drugs and carcinogens. The most extensively studied compound in this class has been indole-3-carbinol. Indole-3-carbinol inhibits initiation of several forms of cancer but it also appears to enhance the promotion of cancer in some model systems. Other natural indoles should receive more attention.

Isothiocyanates have been studied as inhibitors of initiation. Available evidence suggests that they may function by enhancing conjugation through inducing elevations in GST. Few studies have been conducted on these compounds and the need for additional work is apparent.

Large quantities of flavonoids are consumed by people because of the ubiquitous occurrence of these compounds in plants. A diverse group of flavonoid classes has been described but little work has been conducted on the influence of these compounds on carcinogenesis. Most of the work relating flavonoid intake with cancer has followed from the observation that quercetin and kaempferol are mutagenic in the *Salmonella* assay. However, although a number of carcinogenesis studies have been reported, only one showed evidence of carcinogenicity for quercetin. In addition, there is evidence that some flavonoids may actually inhibit promotion and possibly inhibit initiation through alteration of carcinogen metabolism. More work needs to be done with this diverse group of interesting chemicals.

Several compounds have been studied as chemopreventive agents because of their presence in fruits and/or vegetables and promising results were obtained, but other members of these classes of compounds have generally not been investigated. Ellagic acid has been extensively studied for its ability to block DNA damage by carcinogens and thus inhibit initiation. D-Limonene also shows potential as an inhibitor of initiation, but its mechanism has not been pursued. Allyl sulfides were found to inhibit initiation and they are being studied for their effects on metabolism. Studies on these compounds have provided promising results and these areas should be vigorously pursued.

Protease inhibitors appear to interfere with the promotion of skin cancer and the expression and promotion stages of radiation-induced transformations. Inhibition of free radical generation may account for some of these effects.

Plants are complex chemical mixtures. The potential for finding new chemopreventive agents in plants is high. Studies are underway to identify new agents in plants with chemopreventive potential. The effects of these agents on carcinogenesis should be rigorously studied to assist in the discovery and development of new chemopreventive agents.

5. References

Aoyagi, T., and Umezawa, H., 1975, Structure and activities of protease inhibitors of microbial origin, *Cold Spring Harbor Conference of Cell Proliferation* 2:429–454.

Armstrong, B., and Doll, R., 1975, Environmental factors and cancer incidence and mortality in different countries, with special reference to dietary practices, *Int. J. Cancer* 15:617–631.

Bailey, G. S., Hendricks, J. D., Shelton, D. W., Nixon, J. E., and Pawlowski, N. E., 1987, Enhancement of carcinogenesis by the natural anticarcinogen indole-3-carbinol, *J. Natl. Cancer. Inst.* 78:913–917.

Barale, R., Zucconi, D., Bertani, R., and Loprieno, N., 1983, Vegetables inhibit, *in vivo,* the mutagenicity of nitrite combined with nitrosable compounds, Istituto di Biochimica, Biofisica e Genetica, Universita di Pisa, Italy, *Mutat Res.* 120:145–150.

Barch, D. H., and Fox, C. C., 1988, Selective inhibition of methylbenzylnitrosamine-induced formation of esophageal O[6]-methylguanine by dietary ellagic acid in rats[1], *Cancer Res.* 48:7088–7092.

Baumann, J., Buichhausen, F. V., and Wurm, G., 1980, Flavonoids and related compounds as inhibitors of arachidonic acid peroxidation, *Prostaglandins* 20:627–639.

Becker, F. F., 1981, Inhibition of spontaneous hepatocarcinogenesis in C3H/HeN mice by Edi Pro A, an isolated soy protein, *Carcinogenesis* 2:1213–1214.

Belman, S., 1983, Onion and garlic oils inhibit tumor promotion, *Carcinogenesis* 4:1063–1665.

Benko, A., Tiboldi, T., and Bardos, J., 1963, The effect of painting with cyclical terpenes on the skin of white mice and on the skin carcinoma developed by benzopyrene painting, *Acta Un. Int. Cancer* 19:786–788.

Berenblum, I., and Shubik, P. A., 1947, A new quantitative approach to the study of the stages of chemical carcinogenesis in the mouse's skin, *Br. J. Cancer* 1:383–391.

Beyeler, S., Testa, B., and Perrissoud, D., 1988, Flavonoids as inhibitors of rat liver monooxygenase activities, *Biochem. Pharmacol.* **37:**1971–1979.

Birk, Y., 1961, Purification and some properties of a highly active inhibitor of trypsin and chymotrypsin from soybeans, *Biochim. Biophys. Acta* **54:**378–381.

Birt, D. F., Walker, B., Tibbels, M. G., and Bresnick, E., 1986, Anti-mutagenesis and antipromotion by apigenin, robinetin and indole-3-carbinal, *Carcinogenesis* **7:**959–963.

Birt, D. F., Pelling, J. C., Pour, P. M., Tibbels, M. G., Schweickert, L., and Bresnick, E., 1987, Enhanced pancreatic and skin tumorgenesis in hamsters and mice, *Carcinogenesis* **8:**913–917.

Bjeldanes, L. F., and Chang, G. W., 1977, Mutagenic activity of quercetin and related compounds, *Science* **197:**577–578.

Bjelke, E., 1978, Dietary factors and the epidemiology of cancer of the stomach and large bowel, *Aktuel. Ernehrangsmed. Klin. Prax. Suppl.* **2:**10–17.

Blumberg, P. M., 1981, *In vitro* studies on the mode of action of the phorbol ester potent tumor promoters, *CRC Crit. Rev. Toxicol.* **9:**199–234.

Boyd, J. N., Babish, J. G., and Stoewsand, G. S., 1982, Modification by beet and cabbage diets of aflatoxin B_1-induced rat plasma α-foetoprotein elevation, hepatic tumorigenesis, and mutagenicity of urine, *Food Chem. Toxicol.* **20:**47–52.

Boyd, J. N., Missubeck, N., and Stoewsand, G. S., 1983, Changes in preneoplastic response to aflatoxin B_1 in rats fed green beans, beets or squash, *Food Chem. Toxicol.* **21:**37–40.

Bradfield, C. A., and Bjeldanes, L. T., 1984, Effect of dietary indole-3-carbinal on intestinal and hepatic mono-oxygenase glutathione *S*-transferase and epoxide hydrolase activities in the rat, *Food Chem. Toxicol.* **22:**977–982.

Bradfield, C. A., Chang, Y., and Bjeldanes, L. F., 1985, Effects of commonly consumed vegetables on hepatic xenobiotic-metabolizing enzymes in the mouse, *Food Chem. Toxicol.* **23:**899–904.

Brady, J. F., Li, D., Ishizaki, H., and Yang, C. S., 1988, Effect of diallyl sulfide on rat liver microsomal nitrosamine metabolism and other monooxygenase activities, *Cancer Res.* **48:**5937–5940.

Brodnitz, M. H., Pollock, C. L., and Vallon, P. P., 1969, Flavor components of onion oil, *J. Agr. Food Chem.* **17:**760–763.

Brown, J. P., and Dietrich, P. S., 1979, Mutagenicity of plant flavonols in the *Salmonella*/mammalian microsome test, *Mutat. Res.* **66:**223–240.

Buening, M. K., Fortner, J. G., Kappas, A., and Conney, A. H., 1978, 7,8-Benzoflavone stimulates the metabolic activation of aflatoxin B_1 to mutagens by human liver, *Biochem. Biophys. Res. Commun.* **82:**348–355.

Buening, M. K., Chang, R. L., Huang, M-T., Fortner, J. G., Wood, A. W., and Conney, A. H., 1981, Activation and inhibition of benzo(a)pyrene and aflatoxin B_1 metabolism in human liver microsomes by naturally-occurring flavonoids, *Cancer Res.* **41:**67–72.

Campbell, T. C., 1977, Nutrition and drug-metabolizing enzymes, *Clin. Pharm. Ther.* **22:**699–706.

Carp, H., and Janoff, A., 1978, Possible mechanisms of emphysema in smokers. *In vitro* suppression of serum elastase-inhibitory capacity by fresh cigarette smoke and its prevention by antioxidants, *Am. Rev. Respir. Dis.* **118:**617–621.

Carver, J. H., Carrano, A. V., and MacGregor, J. T., 1983, Genetic effects of the flavonols, galangin, kaempferol, and quercetin on Chinese hamster ovary cells *in vitro*, *Mutat. Res.* **113:**45–60.

Cea, G. F. A., Etcheberry, K. F. C., and Dulout, F. N., 1983, Induction of micronuclei in mouse bone marrow by the flavonoid 5,3′,4′-trihydroxy-3,6,7,8-tetramethoxyflavone (THTMF), *Mutat. Res.* **119:**339–342.

Chang, R. L., Huang, M-T., Wood, A. W., Wong, C-Q., Newmark, H. L., Yagi, H., Sayer, J. M., Jerina, D. M., and Conney, A. H., 1985, Effect of ellagic acid and hydroxylated flavonoids on the tumorigenicity of benzo(a)pyrene on mouse skin and in the newborn mouse, *Carcinogenesis* **6:**1127–1133.

Chernick, S. S., Lepkovsky, S. S., and Chaikoff, I. L., 1948, A dietary factor regulating the enzyme content of the pancreas: Changes induced in size and proteolytic activity of the chick pancreas by the ingestion of raw soy-bean meal, *Am. J. Physiol.* **155:**33–41.

Choy, Y. M., Kwok, T. T., Fung, K. P., and Lee, C. Y., 1983, Effect of garlic, Chinese medicinal drugs and amino acids on growth of Erhlich ascites tumor cells in mice, *Am. J. Chinese Med.* **11:**69–73.

Chung, F. L., Juchatz, A., Vitarius, J., and Hecht, S. S., 1984, Effects of dietary compounds on hydroxylation of *N*-nitrosopyrrolidine and *N*-nitrosonornicotine in rat target tissues, *Cancer Res.* **44:**2924–2928.

Chung, F. L., Wang, M., and Hecht, S. S., 1985, Effects of dietary indoles and isothiocepanate on *N*-

nitrosodimethylamine and 4(methylnitrosamino)-1-(3-pyridyl)-1-butanone α hydroxylation and DNA methylation in rat liver, *Carcinogenesis* **6**:539–543.

Colditz, G. A., Branch, L. G., Lipnick, R. J., Willett, W. C., Rosner, B., Posner, B. M., and Hennekens, C. H., 1985, Increased green and yellow vegetable intake and lowered cancer deaths in an elderly population, *Am. J. Clin. Nutr.* **41**:32–36.

Corasanti, J., Celik, C., Camiolo, S. M., Mittelman, A., Evers, J. L., Barbasch, A., Hobika, G. H., and Markus, G., 1980, Plasminogen activator content of human colon tumors and normal mucosae: Separation of enzymes and partial purification, *J. Natl. Cancer Inst.* **65**:345–351.

Corasanti, J. G., Hobika, G. H., and Markus, G., 1982, Interference with dimethylhydrazine induction of colon tumors in mice by e-aminocaproic acid, *Science* **216**:1020–1021.

Correa, P., 1981, Epidemiological correlation between diet and cancer frequency, *Cancer Res.* **41**:3685–3690.

Curnatte, J. T., Whitten, D. M., and Babior, B. M., 1974, Defective superoxide production by granulocytes from patients with chronic granulomatous disease, *N. Engl. J. Med.* **290**:593–597.

Daehnfeldt, J. L., 1968, Cytostatic activity and Metabolic effects of aromatic isothiocyanic acid esters. Fibiger Lab., Kongens Lyngby, Denmark, *Biochem. Pharm.* **17**(4):511–518.

Das, M., Bickers, D. R., and Mukhtar, H., 1985, Effect of ellagic acid on hepatic and pulmonary xenobiotic metabolism in mice: Studies on the mechanism of its anticarcinogenic action, *Carcinogenesis* **6**:1409–1413.

Desikachar, H. S. R., and De, S. S., 1949, Role of inhibitors in soybean, *Science* **106**:421–422.

Diamond, L., O'Brien, T. H., and Baird, W. M., 1980, Tumor promoters and the mechanism of tumor promotion, *Adv. Cancer Res.* **32**:1–74.

Dixit, R., and Gold, B., 1986, Inhibition of N-methyl-N-nitrosourea-induced mutagenicity and DNA methylation by ellagic acid, *Proc. Nat. Acad. Sci. USA* **83**:8039–8043.

Dunning, W. F., and Curtis, M. R., 1958, The nole of indole in incidence of 2-acetylamino fluorene-induced bladder cancer in rats, *Proc. Soc. Exp. Biol. Med.* **99**:91–95.

Elegbede, J. A., Elson, C. E., and Qureshi, A., 1984, Inhibition of DMBA-induced mammary cancer by the monoterpene d-limonene, *Carcinogenesis* **5**:661–664.

Elegbede, J. A., Elson, C. E., Tanner, M. A., Qureshi, A., and Gould, M. N., 1986a, Regression of rat primary mammary tumors following d-limonene, *J. Natl. Cancer Inst.* **76**:323–325.

Elegbede, J. A., Maltzman, T. H., Verma, A. K., Tanner, M. A., Elson, C. E., and Gould, M. N. (1986b), Mouse skin tumor promoting activity of orange peel oil and d-limonene: A reevaluation, *Carcinogenesis* **7**:2047–2049.

Fenwick, G. R., Heaney, R. K., and Mullin, W. J., 1982, Glucosinulates and their breakdown products in foods and food plants, *CRC Crit. Rev. Food. Sci. Nutr.* **18**:123–201.

Fong, A. T., Swanson, H. I., Dashwood, R. H., Williams, D. E., Hendricks, J. D., and Bailey, G. S., 1990, Mechanisms of anti-carcinogenesis by indole-3-carbinol. Studies of enzyme induction, electrophile-scavenging, and inhibition of aflatoxin B_1 activation, *Biochem. Pharmacol.* **39**:19–26.

Francis, A. R., Shetty, T. K., and Bhattacharya, R. K., 1989, Modulating effect of plant flavonoids on the mutagenicity of N-methyl-N'-nitro-N-nitrosoguanidine, *Carcinogenesis* **10**:1953–1955.

Fujiki, H., Tanaka, Y., Miyake, R., Kikkawa, U., Nishizuka, Y., and Sugimura, T., 1984, Action of calcium-activated, phospholipid-dependent protein kinase (protein kinase C) by new classes of tumor promoters; Teleocidin and debromoaplysiatoxin, *Biochem. Biophys. Res. Commun.* **120**:339–343.

Fujiki, H., Horiuchi, T., Yamashita, K., Hakii, H., Suganuma, M., Nishino, H., Iwashima, A., Hirata, Y., and Sugimura, T., 1986, Inhibition of tumor promotion by flavonoids, in: *Plant Flavonoids in Biology and Medicine* (V. Cody, E. Middleton, Jr., and J. B. Marbone, eds.), Alan R. Liss, New York, pp. 429–440.

Godlewski, C. E., Boyd, J. N., Sherman, W. K., Anderson, J. L., and Stoewsand, G. S., 1985, Hepatic glutathione S-transferase and aflectoxin B_1-induced enzyme altered foci in rats fed fractions of brussels sprouts, *Cancer Lett.* **28**:151–157.

Goldstein, B. D., Witz, G., Amoruso, M., and Troll, W., 1979, Protease inhibitors antagonize the activation of polymorphonuclear leukocyte oxygen consumption, *Biochem. Biophys. Res. Commun.* **88**:854–860.

Gould, M. N., Maltzman, T. H., Boston, J. L., Tanner, M. A., Sattler, C. A., and Elson, C. E., 1986, The anticarcinogenic action of d-limonene at initiation and promotion/progression in the rat mammary gland, *Proc. Am. Assoc. Cancer Res.* **27**:131.

Graham, S., Schotz, W., and Martino, P., 1972, Alimentary factors in the epidemiology of gastric cancer, *Cancer* **30**:927–938.

Graham, S., Dayal, H., Swanson, M., Mittelman, A., and Wilkinson, G., 1978, Diet in the epidemiology of cancer of the colon and rectum, *J. Natl. Cancer Inst.* **51**:709–714.

Gschwendt, M., Horn, F., Lottstein, W., and Marks, F., 1983, Inhibition of the calcium and phospholipid dependent protein kinase activity from mouse brain cytosol by quercetin, *Biochem. Biophys. Res. Commun.* **117**:444–447.

Haenszel, W., Kurihara, M., Segi, M., and Lee, R. K. C., 1972, Stomach cancer among Japanese in Hawaii, *J. Natl. Cancer Inst.* **49**:969–988.

Haenszel, W., Kurihara, M., Locke, F. B., Shimuzu, K., and Segi, M., 1976, Stomach cancer in Japan, *J. Natl. Cancer Inst.* **56**:265–274.

Hagiwara, M., Inoue, S., Tanaka, T., Nunoki, K., Ito, M., and Hidaka, H., 1988, Differential effects of flavonoids as inhibitors of tyrosine protein kinases and serine/threonine protein kinases, *Biochem. Pharmacol.* **37**:2987–2992.

Harborne, J. B., Mabry, T. J., and Mabry, H., 1975, *The Flavonoids,* Academic Press, New York, pp. 1011–1014, 1033–1036.

Hendrich, S., and Bjeldanes, L. F., 1983, Effects of dietary cabbage, brussels sprouts, *Illicium verum, schizandra, chinensis* and alfalfa on the benzo(a)pyrene metabolic system in mouse liver, *Food Chem. Toxicol.* **21**:479–486.

Hirayama, T., 1977, Changing patterns of cancer in Japan with special reference to the decrease in stomach cancer mortality, in: *Origins of Human Cancer. Book A: Incidence of Cancer in Humans* (H. H. Hiatt, J. D. Watson, and J. H. Winston, eds.), Cold Spring Harbor Laboratory, Cold Spring Harbor, NY, pp. 55–75.

Hirono, I., Ueno, I., Hosaka, S., Takanashi, H., Matsushima, T., Sugimura, T., and Natori, S., 1981, Carcinogenicity examination of quercetin and rutin in ACI rats, *Cancer Lett.* **13**:15–21.

Hirose, M., Fukushima, S., Sakata, T., Inui, M., and Ito, N., 1983, Effect of quercetin on two-stage carcinogenesis of the rat urinary bladder, *Cancer Lett.* **21**:23–27.

Homburger, F., Treger, A., and Boger, E., 1971, Inhibition of murine subcutaneous intravenous benzo(rjt)pentaphene carcinogenesis by sweet orange oils and d-limonene, *Oncology* **25**:1–10.

Hope, W. C., Welton, A. F., Fielder-Nagy, C., Batula-Bernardo, C., and Coffey, J. M., 1983, *In vitro* inhibition of the biosynthesis of slow reacting substance of anaphylaxis (SRS-A) and lipoxygenase activity by quercetin, *Biochem. Pharmacol.* **32**:367–371.

Hopp, M. L., Matsumoto, M., Wendell, B., Lee, C., and Oyasu, R., 1976, Suppressive role of indole on 2-acetylaminofluorene hepatotoxicity, *Cancer Res.* **36**:234–239.

Huang, M-T., Wood, A. W., Newmark, H. L., Sayer, J. M., Yagi, H., Jerina, D. M., and Conney, A. H., 1983, Inhibition of the mutagenicity of bay-region diol-epoxides of polycyclic aromatic hydrocarbons by phenolic plant flavonoids, *Carcinogenesis* **4**:1631–1637.

Igimi, H., Hisatsuge, T., and Nishimu, M. M., 1976, The use of d-limonene preparation as a dissolving agent of gallstones, *Dig. Dis.* **21**:926–939.

Ikenate, T., Odani, S., and Kende, T., 1974, Chemical structure and inhibitory activities of soybean proteinase inhibitors, in: *Proteinase Inhibitors* (J. Fritz, H. Tschesche, L. H. Greene, and E. Truscheit, eds.), Springer-Verlag, New York, pp. 325–343.

Janoff, A., Carp, H., Lee, D. K., and Drew, R. T., 1979, Cigarette smoke inhalation decreases alpha-antitrypsin activity in rat lung, *Science* **206**:1313–1314.

Josephsson, E., 1967, Distribution of thioglucoside in different parts of *Brassica* plants, *Phytochemistry* **5**:1617–1627.

Kato, R., Nakadate, T., Yamamoto, S., and Sugimura, T., 1983, Inhibitor of 12-*O*-tetradecanoyl phorbol-13-acetate-induced tumor promotion and ornithine decarboxylase activity by quercetin: Possible involvement of lipooxygenase inhibition, *Carcinogenesis* **4**:1301–1305.

Kennedy, A. R., and Little, J. B., 1978, Protease inhibitors suppress radiation-induced malignant transformation *in vitro, Nature* **276**:825–826.

Kennedy, A. R., and Little, J. B., 1981, Effects of protease inhibitors on radiation transformation *in vitro, Cancer Res.* **41**:2103–2108.

Kitajima, T., Murakami, Y., and Morii, S., 1975, Effect of indole on rat esophageal carcinoma induced by *N*-nitrosodibutylamine (DBN), Dept. Path., Kansai Med. Univ., Moriguchi, Japan Gann, *Proc., Jpn. Cancer Assoc.,* 33rd annual meeting, October 1974, Japanese Cancer Association, Tokyo, p. 66.

Kjaer, A., 1961, Naturally occurring isothiocyanates and their parent gly-cosides, in: *Chemistry of Organic Sulfur Compounds,* Volume 1 (N. Kharasch, ed.), Pergamon Press, Elmsford, NY, pp. 409–420.

Kunitz, M., 1945, Crystallization of a trypsin inhibitor from soybean, *Science* **101**:668–669.

Kunitz, M., 1947, Crystalline soybean trypsin inhibitor, *J. Gen. Physiol.* **30**:291–310.

Lacassagne, A., Hurst, L., and Xuong, M. D., 1970, *p*-Dimethylaminoazobenzene (DAB) hepatocacinogenesis in rats: Inhibition by two naphthylisothiocyanates, Inst. Radium, Paris, France, *CR Soc. Biol. (Paris)* **164**(2):230–233.

Lai, C. N., 1979, Chlorophyll: the active factor in wheat sprout extract inhibiting the metabolic activation of carcinogens *in vitro, Nutr. Cancer* **1**(3):19–21.

Lai, C. N., Butler, M. A., and Matney, T. S., 1980, Antimutagenic activities of common vegetables and their chlorophyll content, *Mutat. Res.* **77**:245–250.

Laskowski, M., Jr., and Kato, I., 1980, Protein inhibitors of proteinases, *Annu. Rev. Biochem.* **49**:593–626.

Le Marchand, L., Yoshizawa, C. N., Kolonel, L. N., Hankin, J. H., and Goodman, M. T., 1989, Vegetable consumption and lung cancer risk: A population- based case-control study in Hawaii, *JNCI* **81**:1158–1164.

Leiter, J., Wodinsky, I., and Bourke, A. R., 1959, Screening data from the cancer chemotherapy National Service Center Screening laboratories, *Cancer Res.* **51**(Suppl.):309–396.

Lemon, F. R., and Walden, R. T., 1966, Death from respiratory system disease among Seventh-day Adventist men, *JAMA* **198**:117–126.

Lemon, F. R., Walden, R. T., and Woods, R. W., 1964, Cancer of the lung and mouth in Seventh-day Adventists, *Cancer* **17**:486–497.

Lesca, P., 1983, Protective effects of ellagic acid and other plant phenols on benzo(a)pyrene-induced neoplasia in mice, *Carcinogenesis* **12**:1651–1653.

Liener, I. E., Deuel, H. J., Jr., and Fevold, H. L., 1949, The effect of supplemental methionine on the nutritive value of diets containing concentrates of soybean trypsin inhibitor, *J. Nutr.* **39**:325–339.

Loub, W. D., Wattenberg, L. W., and Davis, D. W., 1975, Arylhydrocarbon hydroxylase induction in rat tissues by naturally occurring indoles of cruciferous plants, *J. Natl. Cancer Inst.* **54**:985–988.

Lyman, R. L., and Lepkovsky, S. S., 1957, The effect of raw soybean meal and trypsin inhibitor diets on pancreatic enzyme secretion in the rat, *J. Nutr.* **62**:269–284.

MacGregor, J. T., 1984, Genetic and carcinogenic effects of plant flavonoids: An overview, in: *Nutritional and Toxicological Aspects of Food Safety* (M. Friedman, ed.), Plenum Press, New York, pp. 499–526.

MacGregor, J. T., 1986, Mutagenic and carcinogenic effects of flavonoids, *Prog. Clin. Biol. Res.* **213**:411–424.

MacGregor, J. T., and Gurd, L., 1978, Mutagenicity of plant flavonoids: Structural requirements for mutagenic activity in *Salmonella typhimurium, Mutat. Res.* **54**:297–309.

MacGregor, J. T., Carrano, A. V., and MacGregor, J. T., 1983a, Genetic effects of the flavonols, galangin, kaempferol, and quercetin on Chinese hamster ovary cells *in vitro, Mutat. Res.* **113**:45–60.

MacGregor, J. T., Wehr, C. M., Manners, G. D., Gurd, L., Minkler, J. L., and Carrano, A. V., 1983b, *In vivo* exposure to plant flavonols: Influence on frequencies of micronuclei in mouse erythrocytes and sister-chromatid exchange in rabbit lymphocytes, *Mutat. Res.* **124**:255–270.

MacLennon, R., DeCosta, J., Day, N. E., Law, C. H., Ng, Y. K., and Shanmugaratnam, K., 1977, Risk factors for lung cancer in Singapore Chinese, a population with high female incidence rates, *Int. J. Cancer* **20**:854–860.

Maltzman, T. H., Tanner, M. A., Elson, C. E., and Gould, M. N., 1986, Anticarcinogenic activity of specific orange peel oil monotrepenes, *Fed. Proc.* **45**:970.

Maltzman, T. H., Hurt, L. M., Elson, C. E., and Tanner, M. A., and Gould, M. N., 1989, The prevention of nitrosomethylurea-induced mammary tumors by *d*-limonene and orange oil, *Carcinogenesis* **10**:781–783.

Mandal, S., and Stoner, G. D., 1990, Inhibition of *N*-nitrosobenzylmethylamine-induced esophageal tumorigenesis in rats by ellagic acid, *Carcinogenesis* **11**:55–61.

Maruta, A., Ishei, T., and Uyeta, M., 1982, Mutagenicity of quercetin and kaempferol on cultured mammalian cells, *Gann* **70**:273–276.

Matsumoto, M., Oyasu, R., Hopp, M. L., and Kitajimat, 1977, Supression of dibutylnitrosamine-induced bladder carcinomas in hamsters by dietary indole, *J. Natl. Cancer Inst.* **58**:1825–1829.

Mettlin, C., and Graham, S., 1979, Dietary risk factors in human bladder cancer, *Am. J. Epidemiol.* **110**:255–263.

Miller, E. G., Fanous, R., Rivera-Hidalgo, F., Binnie, W. H., Hasegawa, S., and Lam, L. K. T., 1989, The effect of citrus limonoids on hamster buccal pouch carcinogenesis, *Carcinogenesis* **10**:1535–1537.

Miller, L. P., 1973, Glycosides, in: *Phytochemistry* (L. P. Miller, ed.), Van Nostrand Reinhold, New York, pp. 197–375.

Modan, B., Barrell, V., Lubin, F., Modan, M., Greenberg, R. A., and Graham, S., 1975, Low-fiber intake as an etiologic factor in cancer of the colon, *J. Natl. Cancer Inst.* **55**:15–18.

Morino, K., Matsukura, N., Kawachi, T., Ohgaki, H., Sugimura, T., and Hirono, I., 1981, Carcinogenicity test of quercetin and rutin in golden hamster by oral administration, *Carcinogenesis* **3**:93–98.

Mosel, H., and Hermann, K., 1974, The phenolics of fruit. III. The contents of catechins and hydroxycinnamic acids in pome and stone fruits, *Z. Lebensm. Unters. Forsch.* **154**:6–11.

Mukhtar, H., Dason, M., DelTito, Jr., B. J., and Bickers, D. R., 1984a, Protection against 3-methylcholanthrene-induced skin tumorigenesis in Balb/c mice by ellagic acid, *Biochem. Biophys. Res. Commun.* **49**:751–757.

Mukhtar, H., DelTito, Jr., B. J., Marcelo, C. L., Das, M., and Bickers, D. R., 1984b, Ellagic acid: A potent naturally-occurring inhibitor of benzo(a)pyrene metabolism and its subsequent glucuronidation, sulfation and covalent binding to DNA in cultured Balb/c mouse keratinocytes, *Carcinogenesis* **5**:1565–1571.

Nakadate, T., Yamamoto, S., Ishii, M., and Kato, R., 1982a, Inhibition of 12-O-tetradecanoyl-13-acetate induced epidermal ornithine decarboxylase activity by phospholipase A2 inhibitors and lipoxygenase inhibitors, *Cancer Res.* **42**:2841–2845.

Nakadate, T., Yamamoto, S., Ishii, M., and Kato, R., 1982b, Inhibition of 12-O-tetradecanoyl-13-acetate-induced epidermal ornithine decarboxylase activity by lipoxygenase inhibitors: Possible role of product(s) of lipoxygenase pathway, *Carcinogenesis* **3**:1411–1414.

Nakadate, T., Yamamoto, S., Aizu, E., and Kato, R., 1984, Effects of flavonoids and antioxidants on 12-O-tetradecanoyl phorbol-13-acetate-caused epidermal ornithine decarboxylase induction and tumor promotion in relation to lipoxygenase inhibition by these compounds, *Gann* **75**:214–222.

Nishino, H., Nagao, M., Fujiki, H., and Sugimura, T., 1983, Role of flavonoids in suppressing the enhancement of phospholipid metabolism by tumor promoters, *Cancer Lett.* **21**:1–8.

Nishino, H., Nishino, A., Iwashima, A., Tanaka, K., and Matsuura, T., 1984a, Quercetin inhibits the action of 12-O-tetradecacoyl phorbol-13-acetate, a tumor promoter, *Oncology* **41**:120–123.

Nishino, H., Iwashima, A., Fujiki, H., and Sugimura, T., 1984b, Inhibition by quercetin of the promoting effect of teleocidin on skin papilloma formation in mice initiated with 7,12-dimethylbenz(a)anthracene, *Gann* **75**:113–116.

Nixon, J. E., Hendricks, J. D., Pawlowski, N. E., Pereira, C. B., Sinnhuber, R. O., and Bailey, G. S., 1984, Inhibition of aflatoxin B_1 carcinogenesis in rainbow trout by flavone and indole compounds, *Carcinogenesis* **5**:615–619.

Ochiai, M., Nagao, M., Wakabayashi, K., and Sugimura, T., 1984, Superoxide dismutase is one enhancing factor for quercetin mutagenesis in rat liver cytosol by preventing its decomposition, *Mutat. Res.* **129**:19–24.

Ohkoshi, M., 1980, Effect of aprotinin on growth of 3-methylcholanthrene-induced squamous cell carcinoma in mice, *Gann* **71**:246–250.

Osborne, T. B., and Mendel, L. B., 1917, The use of soybean as food, *J. Biol. Chem.* **32**:369–387.

Oyasu, R., Miller, D. A., McDonald, J. H., and Hass, G. M., 1963, Neoplasms of rat urinary bladder and liver: Rats fed 2-acetylaminofluorene and indole, *Arch. Pathol.* **75**:184–190.

Oyasu, R., Kitajima, T., and Hopp, M. L., 1972, Enhancement of urinary bladder tumorigenesis in hamsters by coadministration of 2 acetylaminofluorene and indole, *Cancer Res.* **32**:2027–2033.

Palladino, M. A., Galton, J. E., Troll, W., and Thorbecke, J. J., 1982, Gamma irradiation-induced mortality: Protective effect of protease inhibitors in chickens and mice, *Int. J. Radiat. Biol.* **41**:183–191.

Pamucku, A. M., Yalciner, S., Hatcher, J. F., and Bryan, G. T., 1980, Quercetin, a rat intestinal and bladder carcinogen present in bracker fern (*Pteridium aquilinum*), *Cancer Res.* **40**:3468–3472.

Pantuck, E. J., 1976, Stimulatory effect of vegetables on intestinal drug metabolism in the rat, *J. Pharm. Exp. Ther.* **198**:278–283.

Pantuck, E. J., 1979, Stimulatory effect of brussels sprouts and cabbage on human drug metabolism, *Clin. Pharm. Ther.* **25**:88–95.

Pantuck, E. J., Pantuck, C. B., Anderson, K. E., Wattenberg, L. W., and Conney, A. H., 1984, Effect of brussels sprouts and cabbage on drug conjugations in humans, *Clin. Pharmacol. Ther.* **35**:161–169.

Pence, B. C., Buddingh, F., and Yang, S. P., 1986, Multiple dietary factors in the enhancement of dimethylhydrazine carcinogenesis: Main effect of indole-3-carbinol, *J. Natl. Cancer Inst.* **77**:269–276.

Phillips, R. L., 1975, Role of life-style and dietary habits in risk of cancer among Seventh-day Adventists, *Cancer Res.* **35**:3513–3522.

Pierpoint, W. S., 1986, Flavonoids in the human diet, in: *Plant Flavonoids in Biology and Medicine. Biochemical, Pharmacological, and Structure-Activity Relationships* (V. Cody, E. Middleton, Jr., and J. B. Harborne, eds.), Alan R. Liss, New York, pp. 125–140.

Reddy, B. S., Hanson, D., Mathews, L., and Sharma, C., 1983, Effect of micronutrients, antioxidants and related compounds, mutagenicity of 3,2′-dimethyl-4-aminobiphenyl, a colon and carcinogen, MEDL/ 83/12372, *Food Chem. Toxicol.* **21**(2):129–132.

Richardson, J., 1977, The proteinase inhibitors of plants and microorganisms, *Phytochemistry* **16**:159–169.

Rieder, A., Adamek, M., and Wrba, H., 1983, Delay of diethylnitrosamine-induced hepatoma in rats by carrot feeding, *Oncology* **40**:120–123.

Roe, F. J. C., and Pierce, W. E. H., 1960. Tumor promotion by citrus oils: Tumors of the skin and urethral orfice in mice, *J. Natl. Cancer Inst.* **24**:1289–1403.

Ryan, C. A., 1973, Proteolytic enzymes and their inhibitors in plants, *Annu. Rev. Plant Physiol.* **24**:173–199.

Sahu, R. K., Basu, R., and Sharma, A., 1981, Genetic toxicological testing of some plant flavonoids by the micronucleus test, *Mutat. Res.* **89**:69–74.

Saito, D., Shirai, A., Matsushima, T., Sugimura, T., and Hirono, I., 1980, Test of carcinogenicity of quercetin, a widely distributed mutagen in food, *Terat. Carc. Mutagen* **1**:213–221.

Samuelsson, 1983, Leukotrienes: Mediators of immediate hypersensitivity reactions and inflammation, *Science* **220**:568–575.

Sasaki, S., 1963, Inhibitory effects of alpha-naphthylisothiocyanate on the development of hepatoma in rats treated with 3′methyl 4 dimethylaminoazobenzene, *J. Nara Med. Assoc.* **14**:101–115.

Sayer, J. M., Yagi, H., Wood, A. W., Conney, A. H., and Jerina, D. M., 1982, Extremely facile reaction between the ultimate carcinogen benzo(a)pyrene 7,8-diol 9,10-epoxide and ellagic acid, *J. Am. Chem. Soc.* **104**:5562–5564.

Schmidtlein, H., and Hermann, K., 1975, On phenolic acids of vegetables. Hydroxycinnamic acids and hydroxybenzoic acids of *Brassica* species and leaves of other Cruciferae, *Z. Lebensm. Unters. Forsch.* **159**:139–148.

Scholar, E. M., Wolterman, K., Birt, D. F., and Bresnick, E., 1989, The effect of diets enriched in cabbage and collards on murine pulmonary metastasis, *Nutr. Cancer* **12**:121–126.

Shaw, P. E., 1977, Essential oils, in: *Citrus Science and Technology* (S. Nagy, P. E. Shaw, and M. K. Veldhuis, eds.), AVI Publ., Westport, CT, pp. 427–478.

Shertzer, H. G., 1983, Protection by indolel-3-carbinol against covalent binding of benzo(a)pyrene metabolites to mouse liver DNA and protein, ICDB/83/12418, *Food Chem. Toxicol.* **21**(1):31–35.

Shertzer, H. G., 1984, Indole-3-carbinol protects against covalent binding of benzo(a)pyrene and *N*-nitrosodimethylamine metabolites to mouse liver macromolecules, MEDL/83/50733, *Chem. Biol. Interact.* **48**(1):81–90.

Shugar, L., and Kao, J., 1984, Effect of ellagic and caffeic acids on covalent binding of benzo(a)pyrene to epidermal DNA of mouse skin in organ culture, *Int. J. Biochem.* **16**:571–573.

Sims, J., and Renwick, A. G., 1985, The microbial metabolism of tryptopran in rats fed a diet containing 7.5% saccharin in a two-generation protocal, *Food Chem. Toxicol.* **23**:437–444.

Sousa, R. L., and Marletta, M. A., 1985, Inhibition of cytochrome P_{450} activity in rat liver microsomes by the naturally-occurring flavonoid, quercetin, *Arch. Biochem. Biophys.* **240**:345–357.

Sparnins, V. L., and Wattenberg, L. W., 1981, Enhancement of glutathione *S*-transferase activity of the mouse forestomach by inhibitors of benzo(a)pyrene-induced neoplasia of the forestomach, *J. Natl. Cancer Inst.* **66**:769–771.

Sparnins, V. L., Chean, J., and Wattenberg, L. W., 1982a, Enhancement of glutathione *S*-transferase activity of the esophagus by phenols, lactones and benzyl isothiocyanate, *Cancer Res.* **42**:1205–1207.

Sparnins, V. L., Venegas, P. L., and Wattenberg, L. W., 1982b, Glutathione *S*-transferase activity: Enhancement by compounds inhibiting chemical carcinogenesis and by dietary constituents, *J. Natl. Cancer Inst.* **68**:493–496.

Sparnins, V. L., Mott, A. W., Barany, G., and Wattenberg, L. W., 1986, Effects of allyl methyl trisulfide on glutathione *S*-transferase activity and BP-induced neoplasia in the mouse, *Nutr. Cancer* **8**:211–215, 1986.

Srisanganam, C., Hendricks, D. G., Sharma, R. P., Salunkhe, D. K., and Mahoney, A. W., 1980, Effects of dietary cabbage (*Brassica oleraces L.*) on the tumorigenicity of 1,2-dimethylhydrazine in mice, ICDB/ 81/16469, *J. Food Safety* **2**:235–245.

Stearner, S. P., and Azuma, S. A., 1968, Early radiation lethality: Enzyme release and the protective action of soybean trypsin inhibitor, *Proc. Soc. Exp. Biol. Med.* **128**:913–917.

Sterarner, S. P., Brues, A. M., Sanderson, M., and Christian, E. J., 1955, Role of hypotension in the initial response of X-irradiated chicks, *Am. J. Physiol.* **182**:407–410.

Stoewsand, G. S., Babish, J. B., and Wimberly, H. C., 1978, Inhibition of hepatic toxicity from polybrominated biphenyls and aflatoxin B_1 in rats fed cauliflower, *J. Envir. Path. Toxicol.* **2**:399–406.

Sugimura, T., Nagao, M., Matusushima, T., Yahagi, T., Seino, Y., Shirai, A., Sawamura, M., Natori, S., Yoshihira, K., Fukuoka, M., and Kuroyanagi, M., 1977, Mutagenicity of flavone derivatives, *Proc. Jpn. Acad., Ser. B.* **53**:194–197.

Swain, T., 1986, The evolution of flavonoids, *Prog. Clin. Biol. Res.* **213**:1–14.

Takanishi, H., Aiso, S., Hirono, I., Matsushima, T., and Sugimura, T., 1983, Carcinogenicity test of quercetin and kaempferol in rats by oral administration, *J. Food Safety* **5**:55–60.

Teas, J., Harbison, M. L., and Gelman, R. S., 1984, Dietary seaweed (*Laminaria*) and mammary carcinogenesis in rats, *Cancer Res.* **44**:2758–2761.

Teel, R. W., 1986, Ellagic acid binding to DNA as a possible mechanism for its antimutagenic and anticarcinogenic action, *Cancer Lett.* **30**:329–336.

Teel, R. W., Dixit, R., and Stoner, G. D., 1985, The effect of ellagic acid on the uptake, persistence, metabolism and DNA-binding of benzo(a)pyrene in cultured explants of strain A/J mouse lung, *Carcinogenesis* **6**:391–395.

Temple, Norman, J., and El-Khatib, Shukri M., 1987, Cabbage and vitamin E: Their effect on colon tumor formation in mice, *Cancer Lett.* **35**:71–77.

Terwel, L., and van der Hoeven, J. C. M., 1985, Antimutagenic activity of some naturally occurring compounds towards cigarette smoke condensate and benzo(a)pyrene in the *Salmonella* microsome assay, *Mutat. Res.* **152**:1–4.

Troll, W., Klassen, A., and Janoff, A., 1970, Tumorigenesis in mouse skin: Inhibition by synthetic inhibitors of proteases, *Science* **169**:1211–1213.

Troll, W., Hozumi, M., Ogawa, M., Sugimura, T., Takeuichi, T., and Umezawa, H., 1972, Inhibition of tumorigenesis in mouse skin by leupeptin, a protease inhibitor from Actinomycetes, *Cancer Res.* **32**:1725–1729.

Troll, W., Wiesner, R., Shellabarger, C. J., Holtzman, S., and Stone, J. P., 1980, Soybean diet lowers breast tumor incidence in irradiated rats, *Carcinogenesis* **1**:469–472.

Ueno, I., Haraikawa, K., Kohno, M., Hinomoto, T., Ohya-Nishiguchi, H., Tomatsuri, T., and Yoshihara, K., 1986, Possible involvement of superoxide dismutase in Salmonella typhimurium strain TA98, *Prog. Clin. Biol. Res.* **213**:425–428.

Van Duuren, B. L., and Goldschmidt, B. M., 1976, Cocarcinogenic and tumor promoting agents in tobacco carcinogenesis, *J. Natl. Cancer Inst.* **56**:1237–1242.

Van Duuren, B. L., Sivak, A., Langseth, L., Goldschmidt, B. M., and Segal, A., 1968, Initiators and promoters in tobacco carcinogenesis, *NCI Monogr.* **28**:173–180.

Virtanen, A., 1962, Some organic sulfur compounds in vegetables and fodder plants and their significance in human nutrition, *Angew Chem.* **1**:299–306.

Virtanen, A., 1965, Studies on organic sulphyr compounds and other labile substances in plants, *Phyto. Chem.* **4**:207–228.

Wargovich, M. J., 1987, Diallyl sulfide, a flavor component of garlic (allium sativum), inhibits dimethylhydrazine-induced colon cancer, *Carcinogenesis* **8**:487–489.

Wargovich, M. J., and Goldberg, M. T., 1985, Diallyl sulfide. A naturally occurring thioether that inhibits carcinogen-induced nuclear damage to colon epithelial cells in vivo, *Mutat. Res.* **143**:127–129.

Wargovich, M. J., and Newmark, H. L., 1983, Inability of several mutagen-blocking agents to inhibit 1,2-dimethylhydrazine-induced DNA-damaging activity in colonic epithelium, *Mutat. Res.* **121**:77–80.

Wargovich, M. J., Woods, C., Eng, V. W. S., Stephens, L. C., and Gray, K., 1988, Chemoprevention of *N*-nitrosomethyl-benzylamine-induced esophageal cancer in rats by the naturally occurring thioether, diallyl sulfide, *Cancer Res.* **48**:6872–6875.

Wattenberg, L. W., 1974, Inhibition of carcinogenic and toxic effects of polycyclic hydrocarbons by several sulfur-containing compounds, *J. Natl. Cancer Inst.* **52**:1583–1587.

Wattenberg, L. W., 1977, Inhibiton of carcinogenic effects of polycyclic hydrocarbons by benzyl isothiocyanate and related compounds, *J. Natl. Cancer Inst.* **58**:395–398.

Wattenberg, L. W., 1980, Inhibition of polycyclic aromatic hydrocarbon-induced neoplasia by sodium cyanate, *Cancer Res.* **40**:232–234.

Wattenberg, L. W., 1981, Inhibition of carcinogen-induced neoplasia by sodium cyanate, tert-butyl isocyanate, and benzyl isothrocyanate administered subsequent to carcinogen exposure, *Cancer Res.* **41:**2991–2994.

Wattenberg, L. W., 1983, Inhibition of neoplasia by minor dietary constituents, *Cancer Res.* **43:**2448S–2453S.

Wattenberg, L. W., and Loub, W. D., 1978, Inhibition of polycyclic aromatic hydrocarbon-induced neoplasia by naturally occurring indoles, *Cancer Res.* **38:**1410–1413.

Wattenberg, L. W., Page, M. A., and Leong, J. L., 1968, Induction of increased benzpyrene hydroxylase activity by flavones and related compounds, *Cancer Res.* **28:**934–937.

Wattenberg, L. W., Coccia, J. B., and Lam, L. K. T., 1980, Inhibitory effects of phenolic compounds on benzo(a)pyrene-induced neoplasia, *Cancer Res.* **40:**2820–2823.

Wei, H., Tye, L., Bresnick, E., and Birt, D. F., 1990, Inhibitory effect of apigenin, a plant flavonoid, on epidermal ornithine decarboxylase and skin tumor promotion in mice, *Cancer Res.* **50:**499–502.

Westfall, R. J., Bosshardt, D. K., and Barnes, R. H., 1948, Incidence of crude trypsin inhibitor on utilization of hydrolyzed protein, *Proc. Soc. Exp. Biol. Med.* **68:**498–500.

Wheeler, E. L., and Berry, D. L., 1986, *In vitro* inhibition of mouse epidermal cell lipoxygenase by flavonoids: Structure–activity relationships, *Carcinogenesis* **7:**33–36.

Whitty, J. P., and Bjeldanes, L. F., 1987, The effects of dietary cabbage on xenobiotic-metabolizing enzymes and the binding of aflatoxin B1 to hepatic DNA in rats, *Fd. Chem. Toxic.* **25:**581–587.

Wiebel, F. D., Gelboin, H. V., Buu-Hoi, N. P., Stout, M. G., and Burnham, W. S., 1974, Flavones and polycyclic hydrocarbons as modulators of aryl hydrocarbon hydroxylase, in: *Chemical Carcinogenesis* (P. O. P. Ts'o and J. A. DiPaolo, eds.), Marcel Dekker, New York, pp. 249–270.

Wiltrout, R. H., and Hornung, R. L., 1988, Natural products as antitumor agents: Direct versus indirect mechanisms of activity of flavonoids, *J. Natl. Cancer Inst.* **80:**220–222.

Witz, G., Goldstein, B. D., Amoruso, M., Stone, D. S., and Troll, W., 1980, Retinoid inhibition of superoxide anion radical production by human polymorphonuclear leukocytes stimulated with tumor promoters, *Biochem. Biophys. Res. Communs.* **97:**883–888.

Wood, A. W., Huang, M-T., Chang, R. L., Newmark, H. L., Lehr, R. E., Yagi, H., Sayer, J. M., Jerina, D. M., and Conney, A. H., 1982, Inhibition of the mutagenicity of bay-region diol epoxides of polycyclic aromatic hydrocarbons by naturally occurring plant phenols: Exceptional ability of ellagic acid, *Proc. Natl. Acad. Sci. USA* **79:**5513–5517.

Yavelow, J., Gidlund, M., and Troll, W., 1982, Protease inhibitors from processed legumes effectively inhibit superoxide generation in response to TPA, *Carcinogenesis* **3:**135–138.

Yavelow, J., Finlay, T. H., Kennedy, A. R., and Troll, W., 1983, Bowman–Birk soybean protease inhibitor as an anticarcinogen, *Cancer Res.* **43:**2454s–2459s.

Yoshido, M. A., Sasaki, M., Sugimura, K., and Kawachi, T., 1980, Cytogenetic effects of quercetin on cultured mammalian cells, *Proc. Jpn. Acad.* **56B:**443–447.

Yoshimoto, T., Furukawa, M., Yamamoto, S., Horie, T., and Watanabe-Kohno, S., 1983, Flavonoids. Potent inhibitors of arachidonate 5-lipoxygenase, *Biochem. Biophys. Res. Commun.* **116:**612–618.

You, W.-C., Blot, W. J., Chang, Y.-S., Ershow, A., Yang, Z. T., An, Q., Henderson, B. E., Fraumeni, J. F., Jr., and Wang, T.-G., 1989, Allium vegetables and reduced risk of stomach cancer, *JNCI* **81:**162–164.

12

Vitamins and Cancer

Alfred H. Merrill, Jr., Ann T. Foltz, and Donald B. McCormick

The requirement of vitamins for growth and development, as well as their central role in carcinogen metabolism, has called the attention of many investigators toward their potential involvement in tumor induction and growth. Vitamins A, C, and E have been most associated with cancer (Committee on Diet, Nutrition, and Cancer, 1982), and the consumption of foods rich in these nutrients has been encouraged in public information brochures by major cancer organizations (e.g., the American Institute for Cancer Research and the American Cancer Society), and most recently, *The Surgeon General's Report on Nutrition and Health* (Nutrition Policy Board, 1988) and *Diet and Health* (National Research Council, 1989).

It warrants emphasis that the course of action consistently recommended is consumption of foods rich in these vitamins rather than use of supplements.

In fact, unlike the fairly convincing evidence linking an imbalanced diet with some neoplasias, there is little solid evidence that vitamin supplementation at levels much above the current recommendations prevents cancer. Discretion appears in order here since these compounds are not without risks: several fat-soluble vitamins are toxic at levels just above their usual requirement, and reports of side effects of megadoses of water-soluble vitamins are becoming common. In some models, megadoses of vitamins appear to be tumor promoters rather than inhibitors of carcinogenesis. Furthermore, there is concern that overemphasis on megavitamin supplements may be disadvantageous if it leads to complacency toward controlling other risk factors for cancer.

Nonetheless, vitamin supplements have always been perceived by the public as an ideal form of dietary self-therapy, and they continue to be so regarded (however correctly or incorrectly) in the prevention and cure of cancer. They are relatively inexpensive and easily obtained without a doctor's prescription, and they are convenient to take with little modification of one's dietary habits and lifestyle. This underscores the importance of

Alfred H. Merrill, Jr., Ann T. Foltz, and Donald B. McCormick • Departments of Biochemistry and Medicine, Emory University School of Medicine, Atlanta, Georgia 30322.

well-designed studies of their benefits and risks in cancer. This chapter presents an overview of the major relationships between vitamins and cancer, with emphasis on recent studies (at the time of writing this review). Earlier literature is included for clarity or because interesting findings have not been followed up. Several sources are available for more complete descriptions of earlier work (e.g., Committee on Diet, Nutrition, and Cancer, 1982; Shamberger, 1984; Prasad, 1984; Meyskens and Prasad, 1986).

1. Vitamin A

The essential requirement of vitamin A for normal growth and cellular development was recognized in the early 1900s. The relationship between vitamin A and cancer was first noted by Fujimaki in 1926, when he found that vitamin A–deficient rats developed stomach cancer. Interest in the role of vitamin A in cancer prevention, promotion, and treatment has grown since that time.

1.1. Background

Vitamin A refers, in general, to compounds that reverse the effects of vitamin A deficiency. Vitamin A consists of a carbocyclic (beta-ionone) ring, a polyene side chain, and a polar end group. The natural retinoids vary both in the nature of the beta-ionone ring, e.g., 3-dehydro, and in the polar end group, which can be an alcohol (retinol, vitamin A), an aldehyde (retinal), or an acid group (retinoic acid) (Mills, 1983).

Vitamin A usually occurs in the diet as retinol and its esters (milk, organ meats) and as β-carotene (yellow and green leafy vegetables). β-Carotene is cleaved in the intestine to retinal molecule(s) which are convertable to retinol. Retinol is the source for both retinal and retinoic acid. Retinal is required for the visual cycle of the rod and cone cells, retinol for reproduction, growth promotion, and epithelial cell differentiation and maintenance. For an excellent review of carotenoid compounds, see Goodwin (1986).

The considerable toxicity of vitamin A (reviewed by Howard and Willhite, 1986) has led to careful assessment of body stores and needs (Olson, 1987). Whereas β-carotene is a relatively plentiful and safe source of retinoid equivalents, studies using the other naturally occurring retinoids (retinal, retinol) in animal and human experiments resulted in a hypervitaminosis syndrome before full therapeutic effects could be obtained. This led to the development of a large number of synthetic retinoids, including retinyl palmitate, all-*trans*-retinoic acid, 13-*cis*-retinoic acid, and the aromatic retinoids (Bollag and Matter, 1981), with lesser toxicity. These have undergone extensive testing (as will be discussed in Section 1.4); however, the question of toxicity must be raised continuously as new protocols and combinations of agents are tried. For instance, McCormick *et al.* (1986) found that combined administration of retinoic acid and butylated hydroxytoluene (BHT) was more effective in mammary cancer chemoprevention than either alone; however, chronic exposure resulted in a hepatic fibrosis and bile duct hyperplasia. Hence, they caution that chemopreventive compounds may interact not only to inhibit carcinogenesis, but also to induce toxicity.

Although the role of retinoids in the visual cycle has been well described, the mechanisms by which retinoids control cellular differentiation and growth, particularly in relation to malignant changes, are not completely understood. A review of specific effects is beyond the scope of this chapter and the interested reader is referred to other treatments (Roberts and Sporn, 1984; Sherman, 1986). Two mechanisms are currently accepted. One is based on the similarity of vitamin A activity on basal epithelial layers to that of hormonal activity. Ong and Chytil (1983) have suggested that the retinoids act like steroids and form a retinoid–protein complex within the cell. The complex can then translocate to the cell nucleus and alter gene expression. Another, less established, mechanism is for retinoids to affect glycoprotein and glycoconjugate synthesis. This process could also affect the genome and indirectly lead to changes in intercellular recognition, adhesion, and aggregation properties.

Because the mechanisms by which vitamin A affects normal cells are unknown, those activities that have a protective or therapeutic role in neoplasia are also unclear. Specific mechanisms that have been proposed as effective in altering neoplastic formation have included suppression of phorbol-ester–induced ornithine decarboxylase activity, antioxidant activity on singlet oxygen, or deactivation of free radicals. More global approaches to the role of retinoids in prevention or reversal of neoplasia suggest an effect through direct influences on epithelial differentiation, inhibition of promotion, stimulation of immune activity, repression of protein transforming factors, delay in cancer phenotypic expression, or interference with carcinogen activation or binding.

1.2. Epidemiologic Evidence Relating Cancer and Vitamin A

The influence of vitamin A intake on carcinogenesis has been studied in several epidemiologic surveys. Some of these have not been focused on particular disease entities, while others have evaluated retinoid intake in specific tumors of epithelial origin. Before any discussion of the epidemiologic studies, a few general points should be mentioned which affect interpretation of the research findings.

1.2.1. Comments Regarding Epidemiologic Surveys

A central area of importance in all studies of vitamin A and retinoid levels is the index of foods included in the dietary survey. There is, at this time, no consistent listing of food items used by all researchers. Consequently, the vitamin A intake may be determined from as few as 25 food items (Bjelke, 1975) or as many as 84 (Hinds *et al.*, 1984). Moreover, the foods listed may vary significantly in the source of vitamin A. Bjelke (1975) and Mettlin and others (1979), for example, quantified primarily milk and green and yellow vegetables. Other sources of vitamin A, such as cheese, butter, and organ meats, were not included. These studies, therefore, are more accurately termed assessments of β-carotene (provitamin A) intake and cancer, rather than of vitamin A or retinoids and cancer. There is hope that greater consistency will be maintained by the expanded use of the "Health Habits and History Questionnaire" recently prepared and distributed by the National Cancer Institute; however, much more research is needed on the food composition and bioavailability of all of the vitamins.

A related problem with accurate determination of vitamin A intake is the absence of identifying vitamin supplementation among the subjects. Gregor *et al.* (1980) noted that the primary difference in vitamin A intake in their study was derived from vitamin supplementation. A concern related to both the index chosen and adequate documentation of vitamin supplementation is the quality assurance supplied by the persons obtaining the dietary information. Adequate training for dietary probing for details, e.g., portion size, recipe determination, and preparation details, is important in complete and valid dietary documentation. It should also be noted that retrospective studies, which rely on recalled dietary data, must be viewed with caution, even when well-trained nutritional personnel are obtaining the information.

Another area of evaluation in epidemiologic studies is the statistical control of known risk factors: e.g., smoking, socioeconomic factors, and gender in lung cancer patients; alcohol, smoking, race, and gender in esophageal cancer patients. Some researchers were able to supply matched controls on all risk factors, while others were not. The relationships between cancer and high consumption of other nutrients (e.g., fat and protein) as well as total caloric intake also pose complications. Vitamin intakes that accrue from general "overeating" are less likely to prove beneficial than those that arise as part of a more prudent diet.

1.2.2. Epidemiologic Studies

Discussed in the following sections are some of the major epidemiologic studies concerning vitamin A and cancer (updated from Hill and Grubbs, 1982). Points regarding diet index size, vitamin supplementation documentation, and risk factor consideration have been included. The more general surveys are presented first and are followed by studies of site-specific cancers. A large number of epidemiologic studies identify an inverse relationship between various types of cancer and low serum retinol or carotene levels and/or low vitamin A or carotene dietary intake. However, not all surveys support this association.

1.2.2a. General Studies. Wald *et al.* (1980): Serum rational levels in 86 clients of a medical center who subsequently developed cancer were compared in a prospective study to those of 172 healthy controls matched for age, smoking history, and date of venipuncture. Cancer patients had significantly lower retinol levels than controls; 14 lung cancer patients had the lowest levels; gastrointestinal, skin, and kidney cancers were all lower than controls; and other cancers were not different from the controls.

Kark *et al.* (1981): Serum retinol levels in 85 participants in a screening study who subsequently developed cancer were compared to serum levels in 174 healthy screened participants, matched for age, sex, and race, but not adjusted for smoking. Retinol levels were significantly lower in cancer patients. The 12 lung cancer patients averaged 9.1 $\mu g/dl$ lower than controls.

Willett *et al.* (1984): Serum retinol, retinol-binding protein, and carotenoids in 111 participants in a hypertensive program, who subsequently developed cancer of the breast, lung, or prostate, were compared in a prospective study to serum levels in 210 healthy controls, adjusted for age, sex, smoking history, date of venipuncture, and blood pressure. There were no significant differences in serum retinol, retinol-binding protein, or carotinoids for the cancers chosen.

Pelej *et al.* (1984): In a follow-up to Kark's study, serum retinol was determined for 135 participants in an earlier health survey who developed cancer, and compared with 237 healthy controls matched for race, sex, age, and date of venipuncture. No significant differences were found. There was a nonsignificant trend to lower retinol levels in colon and breast cancer, and sex and socioeconomic factors appeared to be important.

Nomura *et al.* (1985): Serum carotene and vitamin A levels in 280 Hawaiian males who subsequently developed cancer were compared to 302 controls matched for age and sex. There was no significant difference in serum retinol, and there was a negative association between lung cancer and carotene.

Byers *et al.* (1986): A retrospective case–control study of vitamin A and relative cancer risk with controls for age, alcohol consumption, and smoking exposure found that among men, dietary vitamin A is associated with lower risk for cancers of the tongue and mouth, pharynx, larynx, esophagus, and lung, but with higher risk for Hodgkin's disease and leukemia. For women, there was less of an association, but there appeared to be a lower risk for bladder cancer.

Paganini-Hill *et al.* (1987): Food consumption and vitamin supplement data were collected for a cohort of 10,473 residents of Leisure World, Laguna Hills, California, with a cancer incidence of 56 lung, 110 colon, 59 bladder, 93 prostate, 123 female breast, and 202 cancers of other sites. There was little indication that increased intake of vitamin A or β-carotene from the diet or supplements protects against the development of cancer overall; among men who never smoked there was some indication (not statistically significant) that cancer rates decreased with increasing vitamin A intake.

1.2.2b. Lung Cancer. Bjelke (1975): A prospective study of diet histories in 19 survey participants who developed lung cancer compared with the diets of healthy participants, adjusted for smoking. The risk appeared highest in those who had lower vitamin A intake.

Basu *et al.* (1976): Plasma vitamin A was compared in 28 lung cancer patients, nine noncancer lung patients, and 10 healthy controls; all were smokers but were not matched for age, sex, or socioeconomic status. Patients with oat cell or squamous cancers had lower serum vitamin A levels.

Cohen *et al.* (1977): Serum vitamin A was compared in 67 newly diagnosed lung cancer patients vs. laboratory normals; the intake of vitamin A was determined in 43 subjects. Serum vitamin A was within the normal range for 66 of 67 subjects; 18 of 43 had intakes < 5000 IU/day and 25 of 43 had intakes > 5000 IU/day.

MacLennon *et al.* (1977): Diet was compared by interview and food frequency analyses for 233 lung cancer patients and 300 controls matched for age, sex, and area in Singapore. Multivariate analysis indicated higher risk related to lower vegetable intake.

Atukorala *et al.* (1979): Data from 26 lung cancer patients were compared with data from 10 subjects with noncancer lung diseases and 11 controls with nonpulmonary disease—not matched for age, sex, smoking history, or socioeconomic status. Serum vitamin A and retinol-binding protein levels were lower in lung cancer; carotene was not significantly different.

Mettlin *et al.* (1979): A retrospective study of diet interview data on 292 white male lung cancer patients compared to 801 noncancer controls adjusted for age and sex. The relative risk factor was higher with lower vitamin A intake.

Gregor *et al.* (1980): The current diet and recalled diet were compared in 104 lung cancer patients and 175 noncancer controls matched for age; supplementation was documented. The current vitamin A intake was lower in male cancer patients owing to supplementation; women had higher, but nonsignificant, levels than controls.

Hirayama (1979): The dietary intakes of various foods were compared among 807 subjects who participated in a diet survey and subsequently developed cancer; age, smoking, and socioeconomic status were standardized. Mortality was less in each smoking category for those with higher intake of green and yellow vegetables.

Shekelle *et al.* (1981): Date from a study of 33 men who participated in a diet frequency survey of 195 foods over 28 days were compared for subsequent development of cancer, adjusted for age and smoking history. Highest cancer risks were related to lowest carotene intake.

Lopez *et al.* (1981): Serum vitamin A, retinol-binding protein, carotene, and recalled intakes were compared in lung cancer patients and controls (25 of each). Lung cancer patients tended to have higher intakes of retinol and lower intakes of carotene; however, the differences were not significant.

Lopez and LeGardeur (1982): Serum retinol and carotene were compared in 29 lung cancer patients and 29 noncancer controls and 122 healthy controls, matched for age, race, sex, and area. Serum carotene was significantly lower in lung cancer patients than controls; no difference was found in retinol.

Stahelin *et al.* (1982): Vitamin A and carotene were compared in 121 participants who later developed lung cancer vs. 308 noncancer participants; controls were randomly chosen. Carotene levels were significantly lower in lung cancer participants; there was no difference in vitamin A level.

Kvale *et al.* (1983): The diet histories of 153 lung cancer patients were compared with those of case controls. A difference in vitamin A intake was noted in small-cell and squamous histologies, but not adenocarcinomas.

Hinds *et al.* (1984): The diet histories of 364 lung cancer patients were compared with those of 364 healthy controls matched for sex, age, and season of interview; supplementation was noted. Multiple regression analyses revealed vitamin A from food and supplements, vitamin A from food only, and carotene were inversely associated with lung cancer in men, but not women.

Ziegler *et al.* (1984, 1986): A case–control study of 763 lung cancer patients and 900 controls matched for age, race, area, and smoking. Increased intake of vegetable carotenoids was a beneficial risk factor; there was little association with retinol or total vitamin A.

Pastorino *et al.* (1987): Plasma and dietary levels of retinol and β-carotene were evaluated for 47 women with primary lung cancer and 159 nonneoplastic hospital controls. The age-adjusted plasma values for retinol and carotene were lower for cases, as was dietary intake of both.

Byers *et al.* (1987): The 450 lung cancer cases (296 men, 154 women) were compared with 902 controls (587 men, 315 women). The intake of vitamin A from fruits and vegetables (carotene) was associated with reduced cancer risk for men (the relative risks by quartiles for the lowest intake to highest intake were 1.8, 1.8, 1.0, 1.0); there was a much weaker association for women.

Bond *et al.* (1987): A case–control study of vitamin A and lung cancer among chemical manufacturing employees (308 former male employees who had died of lung cancer) and controls individually matched to the cases indicated an association.

Colditz *et al.* (1987): A review of the human epidemiologic studies concludes that "beta carotene has strong potential as a protective agent, though constituents of green and yellow vegetables other than carotene may account for the reduced cancer incidence observed in many studies."

1.2.2c. Breast Cancer. Wald *et al.* (1984): Serum retinol and carotene were compared in 39 patients with breast cancer and 78 controls matched for age, menopausal status, family history, and parity. There were no differences in either parameter.

Katsouyanni *et al.* (1988): A case–control study conducted in Athens, Greece, with 120 patients with breast cancer and an equal number of hospital controls found significantly less frequent consumption of vitamin A, even after controlling for total caloric intake, potential external confounding variables, and other nutrients associated with breast cancer risk.

Marubini *et al.* (1988): A study at the National Cancer Institute of Milan involving 214 previously untreated individuals with breast cancer and 215 hospital controls (both groups 30–65 years of age) found no association between dietary (or plasma) β-carotene and the risk of breast cancer. There even appeared to be an increasing risk with higher levels of serum retinol.

1.2.2d. Head and Neck Cancer. Marshall *et al.* (1982): The vitamin A intake of 425 oral cancer patients was compared with that of 588 controls chosen randomly, using dietary frequency with 27 items in the vitamin index. There was an inverse relationship between vitamin A intake and the risk of cancer.

1.2.2e. Gastric Cancer. Stehr (1983): Results from retrospective diet interviews of 111 gastric cancer patients and next of kin were compared to those of a control group who died of heart disease, matched for age, sex, race, and area. The interview noted vitamin supplementation. Stomach cancer patients had significantly lower total vitamin intake than heart patients.

1.2.2f. Bladder Cancer. Mettlin and Graham (1979): A retrospective study of diet data obtained from 569 bladder cancer patients and 1025 controls matched for age, smoking, and occupational risks. Cancer was associated with lower vitamin A intake, especially below 75,000 IU/week.

Mahmoud and Robinson (1982): Comparison of serum carotene and vitamin A in 10 bladder cancer patients and 20 patients with schistosomiasis and 10 controls. Serum vitamin A and carotene were significantly lower in the cancer patients.

1.2.2g. Prostate Cancer. Whelen *et al.* (1983): Serum vitamin A and retinol-binding protein levels were compared in 19 prostate cancer patients with those of 20 controls with benign prostatic hypertrophy. No differences were noted.

Kolonel *et al.* (1987): Diet histories were used to assess vitamin A among 452 men with prostate cancer and 899 population controls in Hawaii. In the men less than 70 years of age, there were no significant associations of vitamin A with prostate cancer; however, among older men the risk increased with the amount of vitamin A consumed. The association was somewhat stronger for total carotenes than for retinol.

Ohno *et al.* (1988): A Japanese study of 100 patients with prostate cancer and two matching controls [100 each with benign prostatic hyperplasia (BPH) and general hospital patients] found that the smaller the dietary intake of β-carotene and vitamin A, the higher the risk. The β-carotene and vitamin A in green/yellow vegetables were significantly protective, and in seaweeds and kelp were suggestively protective. In contrast, that in fruits appeared to enhance the risk.

1.2.2h. Colon. Potter and McMichael (1986): Dietary analyses of 419 patients with colon and rectal cancer and 732 controls residing in metropolitan Adelaide, Australia, found association with vitamin A.

1.3. Experimental Evidence Relating Cancer and Vitamin A

The possible association of vitamin A deficiency and cancer was first described by Wolbach and Howe, in their 1925 study of histological changes in vitamin A–deprived rats. Alteration in epithelial structures was noted in the respiratory tract, salivary glands, eye structures, and genitourinary tract. It was of interest that increased numbers of mitotic figures were especially evident in the renal pelvis, ureters, and bladder. Later studies incorporated vitamin A deficiency in the presence of carcinogens. Cohen and others (1976) found that vitamin A deficiency in rats resulted in squamous metaplasia of the bladder; administration of a known carcinogen accelerated cancer formation. Nettlesheim and Williams (1976) reported similar findings in their study of vitamin A–deprived rats and pulmonary carcinogens. In a project comparing aflatoxin-exposed rats with low and adequate vitamin A intake, Newberne and Rogers (1973) noted that the vitamin A–deprived rats developed tumors in both colon and liver, while the adequately nourished rats developed liver tumors only. The relationship of vitamin A deficiency and colon cancer is not clarified by the additional two studies available. Rogers *et al.* (1973) reported a slightly increased incidence of bowel tumors in rats on low-vitamin diets compared to rats with adequate vitamin A diet. Narisawa and co-workers (1976) found that rats fed a vitamin A–free diet developed fewer tumors than those fed an adequate diet.

The majority of studies indicate that vitamin A deficiency increases the susceptibility of animals to chemically induced cancers in a variety of sites. The application of these findings to clinical tumors in humans, as with all animal studies, must be done with caution.

1.4. Retinoid Activity in Tumor Prevention and Enhancement

The epidemiologic evidence that low serum vitamin A, serum carotene, or dietary intake exists in some cancer patients (as well as the activity of retinoids in normal cellular differentiation) led to the investigation of these products in cancer prevention. A large number of studies have used various animal models, carcinogenic agents, and retinoids. A few studies have investigated the use of retinoids in humans with preneoplastic diseases as well as frankly malignant cancers. The animal experiments will be listed briefly; the clinical trials in human cancers will be discussed more fully. For recent discussions of the design and interpretation of intervention trials, consult Mettlin (1986) and Moon *et al.* (1986b).

1.4.1. Experimental Evidence for the Usefulness
of Retinoids as Chemotherapeutic Agents

Skin papillomas in rabbits and mice (Epstein and Grenkin, 1981; Bollag, 1974, 1975; Ito, 1981; Davies, 1967), tongue cancers in hamsters (Shklar *et al.*, 1980), skin cancers in rats (Schmaehl and Habs, 1978), and mammary tumors in rats (Moon *et al.*,

1977; McCormick *et al.,* 1980) have all been prevented or reduced by retinoids. However, other studies have been less consistent in supporting the role of retinoids as cancer-preventive agents.

For example, the protective effect of retinyl palmitate in hamster respiratory tracts, originally reported by Saffiotti and others (1967) and also noted by Sporn and Newton (1979), was not reproduced by Smith (1975a,b), who performed two replicative investigations with larger numbers of animals. In an investigation by Nettlesheim (1980), hamsters treated with Rospoull-1340 had a lower rate of lung cancer development, while those treated with 13-*cis*-retinoic acid had a reduced survival period.

Ward and others (1978) employed three retinoids in rats exposed to chemically induced colon cancers; no inhibitory effect was seen. A promoting effect for retinoids was noted following topical applications of 10% retinyl palmitate or 0.3% retinoic acid, which increased the tumorogenic response of the skin to UV light (Levij and Pollack, 1968; Epstein, 1977). Although there is evidence to suggest that the response to retinoid may have some relationship to dosage, Schroder and Black (1980) note that dose effects and application methods do not adequately explain the difference between tumor prevention and enhancement. Thus, the role of retinoid therapy as a chemopreventive agent in cancer is not clearly established in the animal studies available.

The use of vitamin A preparations as a sole therapeutic agent has been tested in a number of animal models. Induced cancers included oral (cheek pouch), bladder, colon, lung, breast, and limb (wing) sites. A variety of retinoids have been used; the effects have been either negligible (Schmaehl and Habs, 1978; Silverman *et al.,* 1981; Wenk *et al.,* 1981) or deleterious (Smith *et al.,* 1975a,b; Welsch *et al.,* 1981; Polliack and Sasson, 1972). Interestingly, there has been some suggestion of activity of retinoids in transplantable tumors (Brandes *et al.,* 1966; Patek *et al.,* 1979; Paveic *et al.,* 1980; Trown *et al.,* 1976), although several of those trials indicate that retinoid therapy does not alter tumor growth.

Retinoids have also been used in conjunction with standard chemotherapeutic agents in mouse models of leukemia, adenocarcinoma, and sarcoma. Retinol and retinyl palmitate have been the retinoids usually employed. The results have been variable: improved responses have been noted with adenocarcinoma (Brandes *et al.,* 1966), some leukemias (Stewart *et al.,* 1979; Cohen, 1972), and lung cancer (Paveic *et al.,* 1980), but other investigations of leukemias (Patek *et al.,* 1979; Cohen, 1972; Cohen and Carbone, 1972) and sarcomas (Patek *et al.,* 1979) revealed no improvement from the addition of the retinoids to the standard treatment regimen. The question of specific synergistic effects between retinoids and given chemotherapeutic agents, which might explain some of the differences in responses, has not been explored to any great extent.

1.4.2. Evidence of the Effect of Retinoids on Preneoplastic or Nonmetastasizing Lesions in Humans

A variety of retinoids have been used to control or reverse the cellular dysplasia which can be a precursor to cancer (Moon *et al.,* 1986a). The studies are presented by site and include skin, respiratory tract epithelium, oral mucosa, and uterine cervix.

Human studies of the effects of retinoids on skin lesions have included evaluation of growth changes of actinic keratoses, keratoacanthomas, errdermodysplasia verruciformis, and frankly malignant basal cell carcinomas. Bellog and Ott (1971) used 0.1% or 0.3% vitamin A ointment in 60 patients with actinic keratoses and 16 patients with basal cell carcinomas. They noted that in 3–10 weeks, 24 of 51 patients had complete disappearance of the keratoses, 20 had a 50% reduction in the keratotic lesions, and seven had no change. Five of the sixteen patients with basal cell cancers had complete regression of tumors, 10 had a partial reduction in tumor size, and one had no change. Unfortunately, both keratoses and basal cell carcinomas recurred in several patients with complete responses. Bellog and Ott noted that the results obtained using vitamin A were inferior to the methods currently used in treating keratoses and basal cell cancers.

Peck and others (1979) treated 11 patients with 248 basal cell carcinomas. The retinoid used was 13-*cis*-retinoic acid, with an average dose of 4.7 mg/kg per day. Thirty-nine of the lesions completely regressed, 162 decreased in size, and 47 tumors were stable.

Haydey *et al.* (1980) and Meyskens *et al.* (1982) used 2 mg/kg 13-*cis*-retinoic acid to treat keratoacanthomas. Haydey reported good regression of tumor size, but rapid recurrence of the tumor. Haydey then put the case study patient on maintenance therapy at 2 mg/kg, with good resolution of the disease. The patient did have mild cheilosis. Meyskens noted only partial response in five patients with keratoacanthoma, multiple basal cell carcinomas, or epidermal dysplasia eruciformis. The keratoacanthomas and multiple basal cell carcinoma patients had responses lasting more than 12 months; however, treatment with surgery and radiation, respectively, was also administered. The patient with epidermal dysplasia had difficulty with skin toxicity and discontinued therapy after 2 months, with rapid recurrence of disease.

Lutzner and Blanchet-Bardon (1980) also reported the use of retinoids in a patient with epidermodysplasia, using an aromatic compound, RO-10-9359, at 1 mg/kg per day. Significant regression of all tumors occured in 2 months. The patient remained on the retinoid at the time of the report.

Saccomanno and others (1982) studied the effect of 13-*cis*-retinoic acid on 26 patients with varying degrees of cytological abnormalities in their sputum. The dose began at 1 mg/kg and increased to 2.5 mg/kg. Saccomanno noted that the sample was too small for statistical analysis; however, a trend toward prevention of progression of the abnormalities was seen.

Gouveia and others (1982) also studied persons at risk for lung cancer. Seventy volunteers with a smoking history of at least 15 pack-years (range, 15–100 pack-years; mean, 40.75 pack-years) underwent bronchoscopic biopsy. Thirty-four had a metaplastic index of above 15 and were given 6 months of etretinate, 25 mg daily. There was no control group. Only 12 had completed the 6-month course at the time of the report, and endosopic reports were available for 11. Ten had significant reductions and one had no change in the metaplastic index. The 11 subjects denied any change in smoking pattern. The only major toxicity from the retinoid was noted in a person with preexisting liver disease; therapy was discontinued early in that individual because of biochemical evidence of compromised liver function.

Stitch *et al.* (1984) used an index similar to that of Gouveia in their study of betel nut and tobacco chewers. The number of micronucleated exfoliated cells obtained from a buccal mucosal scraping was noted in 36 betel nut and tobacco chewers. All participants were given vitamin A (50,000 IU) and β-carotene (150,000 IU) twice weekly for 3 months. The frequency of exfoliated cells was significantly reduced bilaterally in 30 of the subjects, unilaterally in three subjects, and not reduced in three others. No increase was noted in the frequency of cellular abnormalities.

Koch (1978) studied the effects of three different retinoids in 75 patients with leukoplakia of at least 6 months' duration. All-*trans*-retinoic acid, 13-*cis*-retinoic acid, and an aromatic retinoid were each used for an 8-week period. Ninety-one of the subjects responded to treatment with the aromatic retinoid; the *cis*-retinoic acid was helpful to 87% of that group of patients, while only 59% of the patients receiving all-*trans*-retinoic acid had remission of leukoplakia. Remission has been maintained at 50%, 44%, and 43%, respectively. Relapse occurred as early as 30–60 days after treatment was discontinued. Half of all patients had some toxicity.

Munoz and others (1985) used a combination of 50,000 IU of vitamin A, 200 mg of riboflavin, and 50 mg of zinc or placebo in a randomized, double-blind study of 610 subjects in a high-risk area for esophageal carcinomas. Endoscopic examination was performed at the end of the study period of 13.5 months. No significant difference in the number of esophageal lesions was noted between the treatment and placebo groups. Unfortunately, no endoscopy was performed prior to the initiation of therapy.

Surwit *et al.* (1982) used *trans*-retinoic acid (0.5%) applied to the cervices of 18 women with moderate to severe dysplasia or carcinoma *in situ* by colposcopic examination. The concentration of retinoid was increased until symptoms of toxicity appeared. One-third of the subjects had at least a 25% regression and two women had a complete response. All women noted some vaginal irritation, which was the dose-limiting factor.

1.5. Effect of Retinoids Used as Chemotherapeutic Agents in Humans

Although retinoids have been applied topically and orally in cancer patients since the 1930s, clinical evaluation has been complicated by the lack of controlled designs. The following section includes the results of clinical trials in the last decade. Phase I (toxicity), II (efficacy), and III (comparison) studies have been performed in a variety of human cancers. Each study will be grouped according to intent of study (phase).

1.5.1. Phase I Trials

Goodman and others (1983) evaluated the toxicity of oral retinol in 13 cancer patients; eight had advanced cancers and five patients received vitamin A as adjuvant therapy. Retinol was given in oral doses of $100,000-300,000$ IU/m^2, with three or more patients at each level. Treatment continued for 1 year or until disease progression was documented. One of three patients receiving 150,000 IU and five of nine patients receiving 300,000 IU developed central nervous system changes. Hepatomegaly or abnormal liver function results also occurred in five of the nine patients receiving the highest dose. Cholesterol and triglyceride abnormalities were noted in subjects receiving 200,000 IU or more. The researchers suggested that future trials use a retinol dose of 200,000 IU/m^2.

Band *et al.* (1982) studied 13-*cis*-retinoic acid in 16 patients with head and neck cancers. The retinoid was given in doses of 20 (two patients), 35 (six subjects), and 90 (one patient) mg/m^2. One patient took 120 mg/m^2 as a single dose in error. Doses of 60 mg/m^2 or higher were associated with grade II toxicity or higher. Headaches and desquamation were noted in the two patients with doses above 60 mg/m^2. The researchers suggest limiting doses of 13-*cis*-retinoic acid to 60 mg/m^2 or lower.

Gold and others (1983) also studied 13-*cis*-retinoic acid, using doses ranging from 40 to 120 mg/m^2, in patients with myelodysplastic syndrome. Two patients were diagnosed with leukemias. Five patients did have improved hematological parameters. Toxicity was noted in 90% of patients at levels above 80 mg/m^2. Transient liver function abnormalities were noted in patients receiving 120 mg/m^2 and hepatotoxicity was the dose-limiting factor. No central nervous system effects or severe skin reactions were described. The researchers suggested starting doses of 100 mg/m^2.

1.5.2. Phase II Studies

Cassidy and others (1981) used 13-*cis*-retinoic acid in 42 patients with advanced cancer of the breast, testes, ovary, skin, or hematopoietic system. Patients were given escalating doses of retinoid, ranging from 0.5 mg/kg to 8 mg/kg for 1 month. Doses were regulated by toxicity. Three patients developed hypercalcemia, two patients complained of earaches, and several patients reported nausea, vomiting, and abdominal cramping. Although some patients with cutaneous disease noted reduction in tumor size and one patient had improved platelet function, there were no objective responses among the patients.

Mickshe and colleagues (1977) used either 13-*cis*-retinoic acid (100 mg/day) or vitamin A palmitate (1.5 million IU/day) in nine male patients with metastatic squamous cell lung cancer. Patients were treated with 3-week courses followed by several weeks of rest; up to seven cycles were given in a period of 60 weeks. Six of the patients had improved responses in at least two of four skin tests and a significant increase in lymphocyte blastogenesis response to phytohemagglutinin. No improvement in overall survival was noted by the researchers, although one patient did achieve a complete response.

Warrell and others (1982) evaluated 13-*cis*-retinoic acid (100 mg/m^2 daily) in the treatment of 13 lymphoma patients. Some improvement in blood counts or cutaneous disease was noted in patients with chronic lymphocytic leukemia and mycosis fungoides, respectively. No benefit has been demonstrated in patients with non-Hodgkin's lymphoma. Toxicity was reported as "mild." Daenen and others (1986) and Fontana *et al.* (1986) presented case reports of individual patients with acute promyelocytic leukemia who achieved responses from 13-*cis*-retinoic acid. Both patients relapsed, at 6 and 12 months, respectively.

Levine and Meyskens (1980) applied a tropical vitamin A solution, 0.05%, to satellite lesions in two patients with melanoma. The vitamin A was covered with an occlusive dressing. One patient had a complete response in 22 lesions.

Thatcher and colleagues (1980) treated 25 patients with advanced head and neck cancers with Adriamycin, bleomycin, 5-fluorouracil, methotrexate, and retinol palmitate (400,000 IU/m^2, intramuscularly). Patients who responded had a significantly longer survival time; however, retinoid therapy was not associated with a higher response rate. The authors did state that the patients receiving vitamin A may have had a reduced incidence of mucositis.

A Phase II trial of 13-*cis*-retinoic acid in 14 patients with advanced germ cell tumors has been conducted by Bosl and others (1983). All patients received 100 mg/m^2 per day orally and all patients had some skin toxicity. No patient had an objective response.

1.5.3. Phase III Studies

Stam and colleagues (1982) reported preliminary data from a randomized trial of placebo versus Tigason, an aromatic retinoid, in 54 patients who have recuperated from curative surgical resection of an epidermoid lung cancer. Data on 27 patients were presented: 11 complete remissions, 13 deaths, three with active disease. The 3-year survival rate was 48%. There was no difference between the placebo and the retinoid groups. Weber and others (1985) compared the results of treatment with bleomycin, CCNU, with or without etretinate in 46 patients with squamous cell lung cancers. No difference in response rates was found. A randomized study of 13-*cis*-retinoic acid with or without busulfan in patients with chronic myelocytic leukemia has not shown a difference between the groups in the time to blast crisis development (Presant and Bearman, 1981). No difference in toxicity levels was noted.

1.6. Summary

Retinoids have been used in a variety of human preneoplastic or early neoplastic conditions. The finding that retinoids might be helpful in the prevention of lung and oral cancers is certainly worth further study, since the cure rate once cancer has developed is poor. Further study of retinoids in the treatment of early mucosal changes in the mouth and cervix has also been supported in clinical trials. Long-term control has not been achieved. Retinoid therapy in skin cancer does not, at this time, offer the control provided by other modalities. Thus far, research into retinoid therapy in esophageal cancer prevention has not been fruitful. There is a need for an expansion of studies with larger patient groups, control of intervening variables, consistent choices of retinoids to be studied, and consistent evaluation criteria. Retinoid therapy in the treatment of human cancers is still being explored in all phases. Thus far, there have been no reports of retinoid studies conducted by cooperative research groups; consequently, the majority of the trials have included only small patient numbers. However, the increased interest in vitamin A, especially in adjuvant settings, may alter the problem of small patient populations in the near future.

2. Vitamin D

2.1. Background

Investigations of associations between vitamin D and cancer have been relatively few (DeLuca and Ostrem, 1986; Manolagas, 1987). This is partly due to the lack of understanding of the biochemical mechanism of action of vitamin D, which is rapidly changing as receptors for 1-alpha, 25-dihydroxyvitamin D_3 are being characterized and their functions elucidated. At this time, the major points of investigation are the relation of vitamin D deficiency and colon cancer incidence and the activity of 1-alpha, 25-dihydroxyvitamin D_3 receptors on cancer cells. There have also been a few reports on vitamin D as a therapeutic agent in cancer patients. These topics will be discussed below, following a general discussion of the pharmacology, biology, and biochemical activity of vitamin D.

Vitamin D, like other fat-soluble vitamins, exists as several related compounds. The two forms important to humans are ergocalciferol (vitamin D_2) and cholecalciferol (vitamin D_3). These two substances are produced from the UV irradiation of ergosterol, found in yeast and molds, and 7-dehydrocholesterol, found in skin. Vitamin D_3 undergoes hydroxylation at position 25 in the liver and at the 1-alpha-position in kidney before becoming biologically active in calcium transport, endochondral calcification, and prevention of tetany. 1-Alpha, 25-dihydroxyvitamin D_3 and other biologically active forms of vitamin D are thought to function in a manner analogous to steroid hormones.

There are relatively few natural dietary sources of vitamin D. Fish oils, sardines, salmon, and herring are rich sources of vitamin D. Vitamin D is now available through the supplementation of milk products which are treated with irradiated yeast. For populations that do not use radiated milk, conversion of 7-dehydrocholesterol by sunlight is the most common source of the vitamin.

2.2. Epidemiologic Evidence Relating Cancer and Vitamin D

Teppo and Saxen (1979) reviewed cases of colon cancer in four Scandanavian countries and noted that milk consumption was inversely related to the incidence of cancer. Age and seasonal adjustments, which could influence milk intake and UV exposure, respectively, were not made by the researchers.

Garland and others (1980, 1985) carried out a 19-year study of vitamin D and calcium intake among workers at a single workplace. Nutritionists obtained 28-day dietary histories at baseline and at 1 year. At the end of the follow-up period, 49 persons had developed colon or rectal cancer. These subjects had a lower dietary calcium and vitamin D intake than healthy participants or participants with other cancers. The difference persisted even when adjustment for body size, fat intake, and age was made. The researchers admitted that it was not possible to determine the relative strength of calcium and vitamin D deficiency in colon cancer incidence and suggested further study in this area. Since calcium intake has been shown to have a protective effect in colon cancer, the need for more study is evident before the relationship between vitamin D deficiency and colon cancer can be evaluated adequately.

2.3. Experimental Evidence Relating Cancer and Vitamin D

Several *in vitro* studies have indicated that some tumor cells have a cytosol protein that specifically binds 1-alpha, 25-dihyroxyvitamin D_3. The mechanism of the effects of 1,25-dihydroxyvitamin D_3 in inhibiting the growth of transformed cells appears to be via the receptor (Haussler *et al.*, 1986) because analogs of this compound have been found to suppress colony formation in soft agar by a number of cultured cancer cell lines in accordance with their binding affinity for the receptor for 1,25-dihydroxyvitamin D_3. The remainder of this section will discuss briefly some of the findings with various cell lines.

2.3.1. Breast Cancer Cells

Both animal and human breast cancer cell lines have been found to have 1-alpha, 25-dihydroxyvitamin D_3 receptors (Colston and Coombes, 1985; Eisman *et al.*, 1980a; Martin *et al.*, 1980). In addition, receptors have been found in surgically removed mastectomy specimens (Eisman *et al.*, 1980b). However, the presence of receptor does not identify a role for the vitamin D_3 compound in breast cancers. Optimal measurement of receptor level and sampling procedures have not been identified, but are being actively studied. Studies *in vivo* have indicated that 1-alpha, 25-dihydroxyvitamin D_3 can either stimulate (Freake *et al.*, 1981) or inhibit (Frampton *et al.*, 1982) cancer cell growth, depending on concentration, growth media, time, and addition of other substances (insulin, calcitonin, etc.) (Eisman, 1980).

2.3.2. Malignant Melanoma

Several human melanoma cell lines have demonstrated the presence of 1-alpha, 25-dihydroxyvitamin D_3 receptors (Frampton *et al.*, 1982; Colston *et al.*, 1981). It is not clear that these receptors are present in normal melanocytes. Colston and colleagues (1981) noted that the inclusion of 1-alpha, 25-dihydroxyvitamin D_3 significantly increased the doubling time of the tumor cells.

2.3.3. Leukemia

Mouse and human myeloid leukemia cells also have 1-alpha, 25-dihydroxyvitamin D_3 receptors (Abe *et al.*, 1981; Miyaura *et al.*, 1981). Studies in M1 (mouse) and HL-60 (human) lines have suggested that cell growth is reduced and differentiation of immature ells is enhanced when 1-alpha, 25-dihydroxyvitamin D_3 is supplied (Miyaura *et al.*, 1981).

2.3.4. Colon Cancer

Receptors for vitamin D_3 have been demonstrated in some, but not all, colon cancer cell lines (Frampton *et al.*, 1982). Wargovich and Lointier (1987) have recently observed a relationship between calcium and vitamin D in the modulation of mouse colon epithelial proliferation and the growth of a human colon tumor cell line.

2.4. Clinical Intervention with Vitamin D

Sato and others (1984) induced hepatoma in rats and then administered 1-alpha, 25-dihydroxyvitamin D_3 or placebo by gastric tube. Although morphological changes in the primary tumor and metastatic lesions were similar in both groups of animals, the weight of tumors formed and the number of metastases beyond the liver were significantly reduced in the group given the vitamin D_3 compound. Kyle and Jowsey (1980) administered fluoride plus calcium or fluoride, calcium, and vitamin D to 15 patients with multiple myeloma. There was no difference in bone formation between the groups, and the authors suggested further study.

3. Vitamin E

Interest in vitamin E as a chemopreventive agent for cancer began with Jaffe's work in 1946, when he reported that rats fed wheat germ oil had a lower incidence of induced tumors. Recent investigations have included epidemiologic surveys as well as chemopreventive and therapeutic trials in both animals and humans (Birt, 1986). The relationship of vitamin E to cancer will be explored following a mention of the biology and biochemistry of vitamin E.

3.1. Background

There are eight compounds referred to as vitamin E. All of the forms are called tocopherols and are distinguished by the position of the methyl groups in the chroman ring. The common forms of vitamin E studied in humans are the alpha, beta, and gamma formulations. Alpha-tocopherol has been the primary vitamin E investigated in cancer trials; it is about four times more active than the beta and gamma formulations.

Vegetable oil, eggs, and whole grains are the major source of vitamin E in the normal diet. Although reproductive problems, myopathy, neurological, and vascular injuries are associated with vitamin E deficiency from investigations with laboratory animals and some human studies, deficiency states in normal populations are uncommon. However, malabsorptive disorders (pancreatic deficiencies, hepatobiliary obstruction) or massive resections can interfere with vitamin E absorption and potentially can produce deficiency.

The activities of vitamin E as an antioxidant and free radical scavenger have been most often suggested as a possible antineoplastic function (Prasad, 1988). Fiddler *et al.* (1978), Mergens (1979), and Mirvish (1986) have reported that vitamin E competes for nitrates, thereby blocking formation of carcinogenic nitrosamines and nitrosamides. Vitamin E may also act as a repressor, regulating coenzyme Q functions and specific enzymes and proteins required for tissue differentiation. Pascoe *et al.* (1987) have shown that vitamin E protects isolated hepatocytes against the toxicity of Adriamycin, a chemotherapeutic agent that undergoes redox cycling, and ethacrynic acid, which depletes cellular glutathione. The prevention of cell injury was associated with maintenance of cellular protein thiols. Alpha-tocopherol ($7\mu M$) has been shown to decrease the transformation of C3H/10T-1/2 cells by both chemical carcinogens (benzo[a]pyrene and tryptophan pyrolysate) and X-rays, and further protection was obtained with selenium in an additive fashion (Borek *et al.*, 1986). Immunostimulatory activity has been suggested as another anticancer mechanism (Carpenter, 1986; Watson, 1986).

3.2. Epidemiologic Evidence Relating Vitamin E and Cancer

Epidemiologic investigations of vitamin E and cancer incidence have been performed only relatively recently, with mixed results. Willett and others (1984) prospectively studied 111 participants in a hypertension project, who subsequently developed cancer. The 111 were compared with 210 healthy participants, who were matched for age, sex, race, and venipuncture date. Although serum vitamin E levels were lower in the cancer patients than the case controls, the differences were not significant. This group has reviewed other human epidemiologic studies of the possible protective effect of vitamin E against cancer and noted that much of the data are sparse and inconclusive (Willett, 1986; Colditz *et al.*, 1987).

Salonen and colleagues (1985) used a similar design with 51 cancer patients, controlling only for age, sex, and smoking. As in the Willett study, vitamin E levels tended to be lower in the cancer patients than the noncancer controls, but not significantly so. Knekt *et al.* (1988) observed that mean levels of serum alpha-tocopherol were similar among controls (8.28 mg/liter) and cancer cases (8.02 mg/liter) in a longitudinal study of 21,172 Finnish men initially aged 15–99 years for whom 453 cancers were diagnosed during the follow-up of 6–10 years. There appeared to be, nonetheless, an association between a high serum alpha-tocopherol level and a reduced risk of cancer. The association was strongest for the cancers unrelated to smoking and persisted when adjusted for cholesterol, serum vitamin A, serum selenium, and various other confounding factors.

Lopez *et al.* (1981, 1982) noted that 45 lung cancer patients had significantly lower serum vitamin E levels than case controls matched for age, sex, and race. Smoking history was not designated as a matching factor, however, and was found to be a risk factor in association with vitamin E. Menkes and Comstock (1984) noted in a prospective study that serum vitamin E levels of 88 persons who developed lung cancer were significantly lower than those of 76 controls matched by age, sex, venipuncture date, and smoking history. Menkes *et al.* (1986) determined the levels of vitamin E using serum that had been collected during a large blood collection study performed in Washington County, Maryland. Sampled were 99 persons who were later found to have lung cancer and who were compared with 196 controls matched for age, sex, race, month of blood donation, and smoking history. Persons with serum levels of vitamin E in the lowest quintile had a 2.5 times higher risk of lung cancer than those in the highest quintile.

Wald and others (1984) found that low levels of vitamin E were associated with higher risk of breast cancer in a prospective study of 39 women who developed breast cancer subsequent to the original sampling. The control group consisted of 78 women. Matching for menopausal history, familial tendency, parity, and other factors was done. However, Russell *et al.* (1988) report that in an 8-year prospective study on breast cancer involving 5086 women, no relationship was found between serum levels of vitamins A and E or retinol-binding protein and subsequent development of breast cancer.

Stahelin and others (1984) noted a relationship between low vitamin E levels in persons with colon and stomach cancers. But a later study of prediagnostic vitamin E status of colon cancer cases compared with matched, population-based controls (Schober *et al.*, 1987) did not support a strong association of low serum levels of vitamin E and an increased risk of subsequent colon cancer. A study in Columbia (Haenszel *et al.*, 1985) found a correlation between significantly lower carotene and (for men only) vitamin E in subjects with gastric dysplasia, but no significant correlation with ascorbic acid. However, in a case-controlled study of factors associated with gastric cancer that was controlled for age, sex, and residence, with calculation of daily nutrient consumption from interview responses, no association with vitamin E was found (Choi *et al.*, 1987).

Kayden *et al.* (1984) noted a markedly reduced tocopherol content in the B cells of patients with chronic lymphocytic leukemia compared to B cells from nonleukemics. The investigators reported no data to indicate when reduced vitamin E levels developed in these patients. Dawson and others (1984) reported a negative finding regarding vitamin E levels and cervical dysplasia. They compared vitamin E levels in 36 women with cervical dysplasia and 36 age-matched controls. No significant difference in serum vitamin E levels was found.

In summary, from the few epidemiologic studies of vitamin E levels that have been done, there is some evidence that lung and breast cancer may be related to vitamin E deficiency, but more research in both site-specific and general surveys is vital to determine the role of vitamin E in cancer incidence.

3.3. Experimental Evidence of the Relationship of Vitamin E and Cancer Incidence

In vitro studies of alpha-tocopherol acid succinate in cultures of mouse melanoma, rat gliomas, and mouse neuroblastomas revealed that vitamin E inhibited the growth of the tumor cells. Interestingly, vitamin E at 5 μg/ml was inhibitory to mouse melanoma and neuroblastomas; at higher doses (10 μg/ml and 8 μg/ml, respectively) the vitamin was lethal (Rama and Prasad, 1983). A study by Tekenaga and colleagues (1981) revealed that alpha-tocopherol could inhibit the differentiation of mouse myeloid leukemia cells; the mechanism of this inhibition was not investigated.

Studies have also evaluated the effect of low vitamin E intake on cancer incidence in intact animals. Cook and McNamara (1980) fed mice either a vitamin E–deficient or a high–vitamin E diet and then induced colonic tumors with dimethylhydrazine (DMH). At the end of the study period, 42 of 65 of the vitamin E–deprived and 51 of 65 of the vitamin E–supplemented mice survived. The researchers noted that, although the number of survivors was not statistically different, the low vitamin E–fed mice had more adenomas and more invasive carcinomas than the mice fed higher levels of vitamin E. In contrast, Toth and Patil (1983) found that vitamin E supplementation increased the incidence of 1,2-DMH-induced intestinal tumors. One possible link between vitamin E and colon cancer, pointed out by Chester *et al.* (1986), is that vitamin E can decrease the occurrence of ulcerative colitis, which predisposes an animal to colonic cancer.

Ip (1982) combined a vitamin E–deficient diet with a high intake of polyunsaturated fats and noted an increased incidence of mouse mammary tumors. Low vitamin E intake had "minimal effect" on mammary tumor development when mice were given a low (5%) polyunsaturated fat diet. Ip also noted that high vitamin E intake did not reverse tumorogenesis associated with a low-selenium diet. Lee and Chen (1979) fed rats 0, ½, 1, 5, or 50 times the minimal level of vitamin E recommended by the National Research Council prior to, during, and following exposure to a carcinogen. The rats with no or low levels of vitamin E intake developed significantly more mammary tumors than the rats fed adequate vitamin E. Chow and colleagues (1984) studied the relationship of vitamin E status to the response of rats to cigarette smoke; higher animal mortality was observed in the vitamin E–deficient group than in the vitamin E–supplemented rats. Thus, there has been some suggestion from animal experimentation that low vitamin E intake increases susceptibility to mammary and lung, but not colon, cancer.

3.4. Experimental Evidence of the Effect of Vitamin E in Cancer Prevention

There have been several studies of vitamin E as a chemopreventive agent in animal models of connective tissue, oral, epidermal, and mammary cancers. The results have been mixed. The information regarding the effect of vitamin E on each of these sites will be discussed briefly.

3.4.1. Connective Tissue Tumors

Vitamin E supplementation has been tested as a preventive agent in sarcomas since 1962, when Haber and Wissler noted some inhibition of sarcoma formation in 3-methylcholanthrene-injected mice. However, Epstein *et al.* (1967) failed to note any suppression of sarcoma growth with the administration of alpha-tocopherol. Constantinides and Harkey (1985) reported that alpha-tocopherol, administered subcutaneously in a soya oil base, produced vigorously growing sarcomas at the site of the injections in 77% of the animals. It was, however, difficult to determine the differential effect of the soya oil, vitamin E, or the combination on tumor promotion.

3.4.2. Oral Tumors

Shklar (1982) divided hamsters into four groups: animals with application of 9,10-dimethyl-1,2-benzanthracene (DMBA) three times weekly, animals with application of DMBA three times weekly and vitamin E supplementation twice weekly, animals fed vitamin E only, and animals acting as controls only. The third and fourth groups developed no tumors; the second group developed fewer, smaller tumors at a slower rate than the first animal group. The researcher also noted that the tumors in the second group were less invasive. Subsequent studies by this laboratory (Trickler and Shklar, 1987) have shown complete suppression of tumors for 28 weeks when lower doses of DMBA were used. Odukoya *et al.* (1984) topically applied a carcinogen with or without vitamin E to hamster buccal mucosa. Animals treated with topical application of vitamin E developed fewer and smaller tumors than animals without vitamin E application. The investigators suggested that both topical and oral routes of vitamin E administration were effective in reducing tumor formation.

3.4.3. Skin

Several researchers have studied the effect of vitamin E supplementation on skin tumor development. Shamberger (1978) demonstrated that alpha-tocopherol did not inhibit mouse skin cancer incidence when the vitamin E preparation was given at the same time as the carcinogen; however, when vitamin E was given with a promoting agent (croton oil), inhibition of skin tumor development was seen. Other groups have also seen evidence for effects on promotion (Perchellet *et al.*, 1987). However, Slaga and Bracken (1977) noted only minimal effect of vitamin E on the assay used to measure epidermal metabolic activity. Pauling and others (1982) noted no effect from vitamin E supplementation on the incidence of squamous cell carcinomas in hairless mice exposed to UV light.

3.4.4. Mammary Tumors

The effect of vitamin E supplementation on mammary tumors has been investigated by several researchers. Wattenberg (1972) found that vitamin E given before cancer induction did not influence the incidence of tumor development. Harmon (1969) found that the incidence of induced tumors was lower (8 of 20) in mice fed 20 mg of vitamin E compared to the incidence (14 of 19) in mice fed 5 mg of vitamin E. King and McCay (1983), in contrast, did not find effective inhibition of mammary tumors in rats fed 0.2% alpha-tocopherol. However, the investigators were also manipulating the amount and type of fat ingested; high polyunsaturated and high saturated fat intakes were related to tumor production regardless of vitamin E supplementation levels.

3.4.5. Liver Tumors

Ura *et al.* (1987) found that dietary vitamin E had an inhibitory effect on the diameter and volume of liver foci induced by dimethylnitrosamine; however, vitamin E did not have an effect on the evolution of the foci into nodules.

3.5. Evidence of the Effect of Vitamin E in Cancer Therapy

Vitamin E has been evaluated in combination with both radiation therapy and chemotherapy, as well as a single modality. This material will be discussed next.

3.5.1. Vitamin E and Radiation Therapy

The function of vitamin E as an antioxidant led to several trials combining radiation with tocopherol in an attempt to improve radiation-induced tumor effect and/or reduce radiation-induced side effects. The findings in these studies have been mixed. Kagerud and others (1980) reported a significantly enhanced effect of radiation given in combination with vitamin E in rat sarcomas and hepatomas. Kagerud also noted that the amount of tumor necrosis was not influenced by tocopherol and suggested that the influence of vitamin E was not based on antioxidant action. Rostock *et al.* (1980), in a study of radiation with and without intraperitoneal vitamin E in cancer-free mice, noted no significant difference in survival in the groups. They concluded that vitamin E offered no mitigation of radiation effects. This contrasts with the results of Malick *et al.* (1978), who found that postirradiation intraperitoneal injection of tocopherol could reduce the death rate in tumor-free mice. In a later study, Kagerud and Peterson (1981) found that tumor growth was significantly enhanced in animals pretreated with tocopherol in doses of 5, 25, and 50 mg/100 g of body weight. However, larger doses of tocopherol did not influence the treatment effect.

3.5.2. Vitamin E and Standard Chemotherapy

Vitamin E has been studied in combination with standard antimetabolite and antibiotic chemotherapy. Waxman and Bruckner (1982) noted that alpha-tocopherol potentiated the antimetabolic activity of 5-fluorouracil (5-FU) in mouse erythroleukemia cell lines. Capel *et al.* (1983) reported that vitamin E provided a protective effect in 5-FU administration of non-tumor-bearing animals. Myers and others (1976) observed similar protective effects of tocopherol administration in mice given doxirubicin. A theoretical advantage of administration of vitamin E is the reduction of free radicals, which are thought to contribute to the cardiotoxicity of doxirubicin. SonneVeld (1978) noted a similar decrease in doxirubicin-induced cardiac effects in leukemic rats pretreated with D-alpha-tocopherol. Van Vleet and Ferrans (1980) and Wang *et al.* (1980) reported similar results in a rabbit model. However, Whittaker and Al-Ismail (1983) failed to find any benefit from vitamin E on cardiac function in a randomized study of 63 acute myeloid leukemia patients treated with doxirubicin. Moreover, Alberts *et al.* (1978) noted that pretreatment with tocopherol in mice treated with doxirubicin was associated with a significant potentiation of bone marrow toxicity.

Vitamin E topical application has been used to reduce the tissue damage associated with the infiltration of vesicant chemotherapeutic agents. Although Svingen *et al.* (1981) reported that alpha-tocopheryl acetate and succinate could reduce the ulceration associated with extravasation of doxirubicin, Dorr and Alberts (1983) and Coleman and others (1983) found no benefit from the administration of vitamin E in doxirubicin-induced skin ulceration.

3.5.3. Vitamin E as a Therapeutic Agent in Cancer

At least two Phase I studies have been reported. Helson (1984) administered escalating doses (from 330 mg/m^2 twice weekly to 2300 mg/m^2 daily) of intravenous vitamin E for 10 days to children with neuroectodermal tumors. Side effects included reduced clotting factor synthesis and prolonged prothrombin times. Short objective responses were reported in 5 of 15 patients. A second Phase I trial is being conducted at the University of Arizona in patients with advanced disease (Loescher and Sauer, 1984). Side effects reported with high doses of vitamin E include the clotting problems noted earlier, thrombophlebitis, pulmonary embolism, hypertension, gynecomastia, and breast tumors (Horwitt, 1980). Interestingly, tocopherol administration has produced clinical response in women with mammary dysplasia (London *et al.*, 1981). Further studies may be warranted since vitamin E has been seen to promote the regression of established epidermoid carcinomas in animal models (i.e., tumors of the Syrian hamster buccal pouch induced by 0.5% 7,12-dimethylbenz[a]anthracene) (Shklar *et al.*, 1987).

3.6. Summary

The effect of vitamin E on standard treatment methods has not yet been consistently identified and the data regarding the use of vitamin E as a single agent in cancer care are too preliminary for evaluation. In view of the uncertain benefits of vitamin E in cancer prevention, it is prudent to employ discretion in the use of supplements considering the limitations of our knowledge about the effects of high doses (Horwitt, 1986). Furthermore, the levels that are effective when combined with other nutrients may be much lower than the amounts that would be indicated by studies in which only vitamin E has been supplemented (Ip, 1988).

4. Vitamin K

Vitamin K analogs have been investigated in cancer patients since 1958. The interest in vitamin K grew in part from its chemical structure, which, though a substituted methyl-1,4-napthoquinone, is similar to the commonly employed anthracyclic chemotherapeutic agents doxirubicin and daunorubicin. Some of the early trials of the vitamin K–based drugs were associated with hematological toxicity in the form of prolonged bleeding times; hence, extensive exploration was suspended. Renewed interest in vitamin K therapy has occurred with better understanding of the biochemical mechanisms of vitamin K activity and different methods of analog production.

4.1. Background

The three compounds considered as vitamin K are: K_1 (phylloquinone), K_2 (menaquinone), and K_3 (menadione). All are lipid-soluble derivatives of 1,4-naphthoquinone and are capable of participating in oxidation–reduction reactions. Vitamin K_1 and K_2 occur naturally; menadione is a synthetic compound. Vitamin K is widely available in plant and animal food sources. Vitamin K deficiency is most often seen in persons with processes that interfere with bile flow or normal bowel absorption, such as cirrhosis, biliary obstruction, or sprue. Certain antibiotics and salicylates act as vitamin K antagonists.

Vitamin K is involved in synthesis of the gamma-carboxyglutamyl residues of proteins that participate in many processes, which include prothombin synthesis, globulin synthesis, reduction of phosphate incorporation, inhibition of benzpyrene metabolism, direct effect on DNA synthesis, radiosynergistic activity, and inhibition of the mixed-function oxidase system. Some proteins with gamma-carboxyl groups have been used as tumor markers (see Fujiyama *et al.*, 1988, for example).

4.2. Experimental Studies of Vitamin K and Cancer

Chlebowski and colleagues have done a great deal of research on the effect of vitamin K_3 on human and animal cell lines. In a study of a variety of human tumor lines, including explants from breast, colon, kidney, ovary, and lung, the vitamin resulted in decreased tumor colony forming units (1983a). Vitamin K_3 was found to be cytotoxic at much lower doses than vitamin K_1. In a related animal study, Chlebowski *et al.* (1983b) used warfarin (a vitamin K antagonist) or vitamin K in conjunction with two standard chemotherapeutic agents (5-FU and methotrexate) in L1210 cells. Both warfarin and vitamin K were noted to inhibit the salvage pathways used by the L1210 cells; the authors suggest that the cytotoxicity of 5-FU and methotrexate could be enhanced with the addition of either vitamin K or warfarin.

Gold (1986) recently observed synergy between menadione and methotrexate in rats bearing Walker 256 carcinosarcoma, and Su *et al.* (1987) have reported interactions between vitamin K_3 and standard chemotherapeutic agents (e.g., mechlorethamine, vincristine, and dexamethasone) in studies of fresh specimens of human lymphatic neoplasms. The combination of vitamins C and K_3 has been found to influence the survival of mice bearing ascitic liver tumors and treated with different cytotoxic drugs (Taper *et al.*, 1987).

Israels and others (1983) studied the effect of vitamin K_1 and vitamin K_3 in ICR/Ha mice. Mice receiving vitamin K_3 developed tumors at a significantly slower rate than control mice or mice receiving vitamin K_1. Indeed, in some animals, vitamin K_1 was associated with accelerated benzo(a)pyrene tumorigenesis. The researchers indicated that vitamin K_1 and K_3 act at different metabolic sites in reference to benzo(a)pyrene activation and detoxification.

4.3. Clinical Trials of Vitamin K in Cancer

4.3.1. Phase I Trials

Vitamin K was given as a therapeutic agent as early as 1968 by Rao and others. The form used was lapachol and work was discontinued because of prolonged bleeding times.

Block and others (1983) reinitiated studies in 19 patients; side effects included prolonged prothrombin time and nausea. Only one minor response was noted among the 19 patients. Chlebowski and others (1983b) extended their previous findings regarding the effects of vitamin K_3 on cells already sensitized by 5-FU adn administered warfarin and vitamin K to patients with advanced colon cancer. Four of the patients responded. Toxicity was reported as mild, without specific details.

4.3.2. Phase II Trials

Activity of a synthetic vitamin K compound (Synkavit) as a radiosensitizer was suggested by work of Mitchell (1960). Krishnamurthi *et al.* (1971) also indicated that Synkavit improved the results of radiotherapy in patients with buccal lesions. However, the Mitchell and Shanta studies used small patient numbers. Mitchell *et al.* (1965) carried out a randomized study comparing combinations of Synkavit, oxygen, and radiation; Synkavite and radiation; oxygen and radiation; and Compound 28 and radiation in 240 patients with lung cancer. Compound 28 was included to examine its effectiveness as a radiosensitizer. No significant differences were noted between the treatment groups, although the authors stated that there was a small increase in mean survival in the group receiving Synkavit, oxygen, and radiation therapy, which was "probably significant at the 5% level." Evans and Todd (1969) carried out a randomized trial of 504 patients with bronchial carcinoma. A total of 273 patients received Synkavit and radiation and 231 patients received radiation only. Although survival at 3 months tended to favor the Synkavit group, the difference was not statistically significant. No differences were found in the groups at 3-year follow-up.

Thus, the experimental evidence that vitamin K_3 may have some inhibitory effect on tumor cell growth in experimental studies bears further exploration. Especially interesting are the indications that vitamin K can be used to improve the cytotoxicity of standard treatment agents. However, the role of vitamin K treatment in cancer therapy is far from clear at this time.

5. Ascorbic Acid (Vitamin C)

Vitamin C (ascorbic acid and dehydroascorbic acid) is both a general antioxidant (e.g., to prevent formation of nitrosamine and of other *N*-nitroso compounds) and a specific redox donor for a limited number of enzyme systems (e.g., those involved in the hydroxylation of proline and lysine) (Englard and Seifter, 1986). There is considerable evidence that ascorbic acid is also involved in inhibition of lipid peroxidation in association with vitamin E (McCay, 1985).

Rich sources of vitamin C include citrus fruits (fresh, canned, and frozen), other fruits, leafy vegetables, tomatoes, and potatoes. Ascorbic acid is interconvertible between the reduced (ascorbic acid) and oxidized (dehydroascorbic acid) forms in tissues. It is excreted in urine unchanged, as the dead-end catabolite oxalic acid, and as the sulfate ester. Block and Sorenson (1987) have noted that orange juice is the leading dietary source of vitamin C in all demographic subgroups, but that the importance of other sources varies among different subgroups. For example, fortified foods are major contributors among the young but not the old, and greens are important sources among blacks but not whites. The

Recommended Daily Allowance for ascorbic acid has undergone considerable debate in recent years; Olson and Hodges (1987) have recently summarized the rationale behind the current recommendations.

A complete presentation of the studies on vitamin C and cancer is beyond the scope of this chapter (there have been over 500 publications on this topic since 1980). The reader is referred to other recent reviews (e.g., Bright-See, 1983; Shamberger, 1984; Newberne and Suphakarn, 1984; Hanck, 1986, 1988; Meyskens and Prasad, 1986; Birt, 1986; Colditz *et al.*, 1987; Bertram *et al.*, 1987). As summarized by Birt (1986): "The most convincing evidence for the involvement of vitamin C in cancer prevention is the ability of ascorbic acid to prevent formation of nitrosamine and of other *N*-nitroso compounds. In addition, vitamin C supplementation was shown to inhibit skin, nose, tracheal, lung, and kidney carcinogenesis, to either not influence or enhance skin, mammary gland, and colon carcinogenesis, and to enhance urinary bladder carcinogenesis, when given as sodium ascorbate, but not when given as ascorbic acid." Additional information, and some updating of this summary, will be given below.

5.1. Epidemiologic Evidence Relating Vitamin C and Cancer

Several indirect lines of evidence initially suggested that vitamin C might lower the risk of cancer, especially of the esophagus and stomach (Committee on Diet, Nutrition, and Cancer, 1982).

Using data collected between 1960 and 1980 on over 4000 men in a study of diet and cardiovascular disease, Stahelin *et al.* (1984) found that plasma vitamin C was consistently lower in cancer cases than in controls. The largest differences were between lung cancer (0.79 ± 0.44 mg/dl, $n = 35$) and matched controls (0.90 ± 0.43, $n = 102$) and stomach cancer (0.72 ± 0.42, $n = 19$) and controls (0.93 ± 0.35, $n = 37$). They also found a strong direct correlation between the consumption of citrus fruits and plasma vitamin C. However, Colditz *et al.* (1987) have recently reviewed the human epidemiologic studies of vitamin C and lung cancer and conclude that "there is little evidence that vitamin C provides protection against human lung cancer. It is likely that cessation of cigarette smoking would have a far greater influence on reducing lung cancer incidence than any known dietary modification."

Boing *et al.* (1985) analyzed regional nutritional data from a national survey on income and consumption in the Federal Republic of Germany to correlate mortality rates due to carcinomas with the consumption data for 15 nutrients. Significant positive correlations were found between vitamin C and breast, prostate, liver, and colon cancer. A prospective follow-up study by Enstrom *et al.* (1986) of noninstitutionalized adult residents of Alameda County, California, did not reveal a relationship between vitamin C intake at levels above and below 25 mg/day and subsequent mortality from cancer.

Another recent study in Columbia (Haenszel *et al.*, 1985) found a correlation between significantly lower carotene and (for males only) vitamin E in subjects with gastric dysplasia, but no significant correlation with ascorbic acid. The Melbourne study of diet and colorectal cancer (Kune *et al.*, 1987) involving 715 cases and 727 age- and sex-matched community controls found that consumption of greater than 230 mg/day of vitamin C appeared to be protective against large-bowel cancer. A study by Potter and McMichael (1966) using cancer cases reported to the South Australian Central Cancer

Registry concluded that the most consistent risk factor for colorectal cancer was dietary protein, but that reduced risk of rectal cancer was also associated with vitamin C. Lyon *et al.* (1987) have cautioned against concluding that vitamin C is protective against colon cancer unless total energy intake has been evaluated.

In a case-controlled study (Wassertheil-Smoller *et al.,* 1981), mean vitamin C intake was lower (80 mg/day, $n = 87$) for women with cervical abnormalities than controls (107 mg/day, $n = 82$) ($p < 0.01$). Analysis of matched pairs showed that a 10-fold higher percentage of the women with cervical dysplasia had vitamin C intakes less than 50% of the recommended dietary allowance. Brock *et al.* (1988) have also suggested that vitamin C and fruit juices show protective effects against cervical cancer. A case–control investigation involving interviews with 564 stomach cancer patients and 1131 population-based controls in Shandong Province, China, found that stomach cancer risk also declined with increasing dietary intake of carotene, vitamin C, and calcium (You *et al.,* 1988).

5.2. Vitamin C Status of Cancer Patients

It is often found that blood from patients with cancer has lower levels of ascorbic acid than blood from healthy subjects (Hoffman, 1985). This is sometimes interpreted as evidence that low vitamin C is a causative factor in the development of cancer, although it is equally plausible that cancer alters the handling of this micronutrient. For example, Ghosh and Das (1985) observed that the serum level of vitamin C was lower than normal for patients with cancer of the uterine cervix or ovary and for leukemia and lymphoma patients. Differences in vitamin C utilization have also been observed on a cellular level. Stahl *et al.* (1985) compared lymphocytes from patients with chronic lymphocytic luekemia and normal subjects and found that the V_{max} for dehydroascorbic acid uptake of the former was only about half that of the latter.

Marcus *et al.* (1987) have reported that vitamin C status may be severely compromised in patients receiving immunotherapy. Plasma ascorbate dropped by 80% during treatment of human cancer by immunotherapy and remained severely depleted throughout the treatment, becoming undetectable in 8 of 11 patients.

5.3. Vitamin C in the Treatment of Cancer

This issue has been debated by Linus Pauling and Charles Moertel (1986). Pauling cites earlier work by E. Cameron and himself (1974, 1976, 1978, 1979a,b) that led him to believe that "high-dose vitamin C, given as an adjunct to appropriate conventional therapy, had value for essentially every cancer patient." He also comments that cancer patients receiving high-dose vitamin C feel better. Moertel describes subsequent investigations in which he and his co-workers (1985) have conducted randomized, double-blind studies of the effect of high-dose ascorbic acid on advanced colorectal cancer patients who had and had not been exposed to cytotoxic drugs. These and other (Creagan *et al.,* 1979) studies found no benefits from vitamin C, and sometimes found that treated patients deteriorated more rapidly. Moertel concludes that "high-dose vitamin C has no discernible value in the treatment of advanced cancer."

Wittes' editorial (1985) cautions that the negative results with colorectal cancer may not be a reliable indicator of the ineffectiveness of a treatment against other neoplasms, but suggests that "additional controlled trials in patients with other types of tumor do not appear warranted" until additional laboratory experiments have been conducted. This view is not universally accepted (Morishige *et al.*, 1986); however, the use of megadoses of ascorbic acid should be assessed in conjunction with evaluation of its possible adverse effects (Sestili, 1983).

Park (1985) has found that L-ascorbic acid has variable effects on the growth of human leukemic colony-forming cells. Analyses of cells from bone marrow aspirates from 163 leukemic patients revealed that L-ascorbic acid suppressed growth in approximately one-sixth of the cases, but enhanced growth in one-third. No growth enhancement was observed in analyses of 34 normal bone marrows.

Ascorbic acid (and dehydroascorbic acid) has also been used in conjunction with hydroxocobalamin to prolong the life of mice bearing the P388 lymphoma (Pierson *et al.*, 1985). The basis behind this combination is that it promotes oxidation of cysteine to cystine, which is taken up poorly by many cancer cells. Taper *et al.* (1987) found that ascorbic acid increased the survival of mice bearing ascitic liver tumors and treated with various cytotoxic drugs.

5.4. Effects of Vitamin C on Carcinogen Metabolism and Action

N-nitroso compounds are among the most potent cancer-promoting agents and are formed through the reaction of nitrites with amines. It is generally thought that ascorbate and other antioxidants may protect against the formation of these species. Wagner *et al.* (1985b) found that healthy adults excrete relatively constant amounts of nitrosoproline and that this is unaffected by daily supplementation with 2 g of ascorbic acid. However, consumption of nitrate and proline caused a significant increase in nitrosoproline excretion, which was prevented to a varying extent by ascorbic acid supplements. Ascorbic acid (and vitamin E) supplementation inhibited the incorporation of [^{15}N]nitrate into nitrosoproline. Vitamin C consumption was also found to decrease the urinary excretion of *N*-nitrosoproline and other nitrosamine acids after a proline load by subjects in an area of Japan associated with a high risk for stomach cancer (Kamiyama *et al.*, 1987).

Lu *et al.* (1986) have studied the effect of ascorbate consumption (100 mg three times daily) on the excretion of *N*-nitrosoamino acids and nitrate in urine from individuals in high- and low-risk areas for esophageal cancer in Northern China. In control groups, it was found that the subjects in high-risk areas excreted more *N*-nitroso compounds than did those in the low-risk areas, and that upon ingestion of L-proline (100 mg 1 hr after each meal) subjects from both areas excreted increased amounts of urinary *N*-nitrosoproline. Ascorbate consumption decreased the levels of *N*-nitrosoamino acids in urine from subjects in the high-risk area to those found in subjects in the low-risk area who had not received additional vitamin C. Hence, if formation of nitroso compounds is a factor in the formation of esophageal cancer, these findings indicate that ascorbic acid may be beneficial.

Werner *et al.* (1985) found that rats given *N*-ethyl-*N*-nitrosoguanidine (ENNG) had no lower incidence of tumors of the small intestine when given ascorbic acid (3 g/100 g of food). Survival time was slightly shorter for the rats receiving both ascorbate and ENNG (207 $\pm$ 45 days) than with ENNG alone (238 $\pm$ 40 days). Ascorbic acid caused a significantly increased numbers of adenomas (and number of colon tumors per rat) when given in the postinitiation phase of colon tumor induction with 1,2-dimethylhydrazine (Shirai *et al.*, 1985a).

Based on the work cited in their review, Newberne and Suphakarn (1984) comment that "certainly one cannot doubt the real or potential value of dietary ascorbic acid to prevent the nitrosation of amines which are in themselves highly carcinogenic to animal species." This is supported by subsequent findings, such as the observation by O'Connor *et al.* (1985) that ascorbic acid significantly reduced the mutagenic activity of fasting gastric juice.

Ascorbic acid has been found to decrease the time of appearance, rate of growth, and multiplicity of spontaneous mammary tumors in RIII mice (Pauling *et al.*, 1985). Douglas *et al.* (1984) have observed a dose-related decline in several lesions usually seen in aged female rats; furthermore, high doses of L-ascorbate (2.5–5% in the diet) had no observable toxic or carcinogenic effects with male or female F344/N rats or B6C3F1 mice.

Using a two-stage gastric carcinogenesis model in F344 rats initiated with *N*-methyl-*N'*-nitro-*N*-guanidine, Shirai *et al.* (1985b) observed that sodium erythrobate was more effective than ascorbate in decreasing the incidence of papilloma of the forestomach. Harada *et al.* (1985) compared the development of tumors in hamsters exposed to cigarette smoke and receiving subcutaneous injections of diethylnitrosamine. Hamsters given a dietary supplementation with vitamin C (1%) had significantly lower incidence of nasal cavity tumors but exhibited a significantly earlier appearance of tracheal tumors. Laryngeal tumors also tended to develop earlier.

Miyata *et al.* (1985) observed that sodium L-ascorbate had significant promoting effects on the incidences and numbers of urinary bladder hyperplasias and papillomas in rats treated with *N*-butyl-*N*-(4-hydroxybutyl)nitrosamine. The sodium salt, but not ascorbic acid, acts as a copromoter in a process that also depends on increased urinary pH and sodium ion concentration (Fukushima *et al.*, 1986). High concentrations of sodium ascorbate potentiate DNA damage in guinea pigs receiving oral 1-methyl-1-nitrosourea; and concentrations greater than 0.5 mM increase the frequency of DNA strand breaks caused by MNU in both L1210 murine leukemia cells and guinea pig pancreatic cells in tissue culture (Woolley *et al.*, 1987). In view of these observations, sodium ascorbate should not be recommended as a "buffered" form of vitamin C, as it recently has been promoted by some health food stores.

Ascorbic acid is thought to influence the formation and/or disposition of reactive electrophiles generated by the microsomal cytochrome P450 system. For example, van Maanen *et al.* (1985) observed that ascorbic acid depressed by 85% covalent binding of VP 16-213 to rat liver microsomal proteins. The inhibition of virus expression by ascorbic acid has been demonstrated in the MT-1 cell line using human T-cell leukemia virus type I induced by *N*-methyl-*N'*-nitro-N-nitrosoguanidine and by 5-iodo-2'-deoxyuridine (Blakeslee *et al.*, 1985). Vitamin C also increases interferon induction, although it does not augment natural killer cell activity (Siegel and Morton, 1984).

5.5. Summary

The evidence to date indicates that consumption of adequate ascorbic acid is important in the prevention of some types of tumors, such as gastric cancer caused by nitrates, nitrites, and nitrosamines. However, the optimal dosage for humans has not yet been proven to be higher than that achievable by consumption of a well-balanced diet containing foods rich in vitamin C, such as fresh vegetables and fruits. The promise of ascorbic acid in benefiting cancer patients has not been fullfilled, and this should undergo additional investigation.

6. Thiamin

Thiamin is utilized as a cofactor by a limited number of enzymes in mammals: pyruvate dehydrogenase, alpha-ketoglutarate dehydrogenase, branched-chain alpha-keto acid dehydrogenase, and transketolase. These enzymes utilize thiamin pyrophosphate (TPP), which is formed directly from thiamin and ATP by thiamin pyrophosphokinase. In addition, periperal nerve membranes contain thiamin triphosphate, which appears to be involved in the transmission of nerve impulses. Good sources of thiamin include meat, milk, fruits, whole grains and rice, nuts, and legumes. In grains, most is located in the germ and refinement removes much of the thiamin from wheat and polished rice.

6.1. Evidence Relating Thiamin and Cancer

Few studies have found associations between thiamin and tumor incidence. Kaul *et al.* (1987) conducted a one-to-one, age- and race-matched case–control study of 55 histologically confirmed black prostate cancer patients and 55 controls. There was a significant negative association between thiamin and iron for the group aged 30–49 years, and for riboflavin in the 50 and older group. These results may indicate that thiamin and iron could be protective against prostate cancer; however, the association is too weak for definitive conclusions at this time.

Since TPP is a cofactor for the transketolase reaction of the pentose phosphate pathway, ribose synthesis for DNA depends on the availability of this coenzyme. The pentose phosphate cycle is required for NADPH formation; hence, the microsomal drug-metabolizing systems would be expected to be affected by deficiencies in thiamin. In fact, thiamin deficiencies are known to enhance the metabolism of some xenobiotics (Wade *et al.*, 1969), perhaps by increasing the ratio of one species of cytochrome P450 (Wade *et al.*, 1973). As is often the case with factors that alter drug metabolism, however, the outcome depends on the compound studied. Whereas thiamin deficiencies increased the metabolism of heptachlor and aniline, the metabolism of hexobarbital was somewhat depressed. Furthermore, high-thiamin diets reduced zoxazolamine metabolism (Grosse and Wade, 1971).

6.2. Thiamin Status of Cancer Patients

Basu *et al.* (1974) noted that although none of 38 patients with advanced cancer exhibited clinical signs of thiamin deficiency, 25% had transketolase activity indices beyond the limit of normal and on this basis could be considered to have some degree of deficiency. They also found that the antitumor drug 5-fluorouracil (5-FU) was a cocarboxylase antagonist *in vitro*. Similar findings were made with breast cancer (Basu and

Dickerson, 1976). Aksoy *et al.* (1980) analyzed patients before and after chemotherapy with 5-FU and reported a significant increase in the transketolase activity index, which was not different, however, for patients treated with other cytotoxic drugs. Furthermore, administration of thiamin during chemotherapy resulted in an index similar to that before administration of 5-FU or for healthy controls.

De Reuck *et al.* (1980) observed Wernicke's encephalopathy in three patients with tumors of the lymphoid–hematopoietic system. Since all the patients had gastrointestinal bleeding, hepatic failure, and sepsis, they concluded that malabsorption was a probable cause of thiamin deficiency. Thiamin levels in adenocarcinoma specimens differ from those in uninvolved adjacent tissue, as occurs with several water-soluble vitamins (Baker *et al.*, 1981).

It appears that cancer patients undergoing irradiation consume lower levels of thiamin. Hulshof *et al.* (1987) examined the dietary intakes of 105 adult Dutch Caucasian patients and found that there was a decrease in thiamin intake for both women treated with abdominal irradiation and men treated with radiotherapy. The authors note that this may be partly due to the observation that many of the patients had chosen a "constipating diet" because of diarrhea.

7. Riboflavin

Riboflavin participates in over 40 biological oxidation/reduction reactions that encompass the metabolism of most nutrients, neurotransmitters, antioxidants (e.g., glutathione), steroid hormones, xenobiotics, and many other compounds (Merrill *et al.*, 1981). Interest in riboflavin and cancer (Rivlin, 1975; Shamberger, 1984) has centered mainly on the effects of dietary deficiencies on the growth of spontaneous or transplanted tumors and on carcinogen metabolism, since cytochrome P450 reductases contain flavin coenzymes; however, other relationships have begun to surface.

7.1. Background

Riboflavin (vitamin B_2) is obtained from various dietary sources, with significant amounts in organ meats (liver, heart, kidney, etc.), milk and milk products, eggs, green leafy vegetables, whole grains, and legumes. After intestinal absorption, riboflavin is transported to tissues via plasma, where it is found free and bound by albumin and immunoglobulins. It is taken up from plasma by diffusion and facilitated transport followed by metabolic trapping involving its conversion to the coenzymatic forms riboflavin 5′-phosphate (FMN), flavin adenine dinucleotide phosphate (FAD), and a number of modified derivatives, such as 8-alpha-peptidyl-FMN and -FAD.

7.2. Evidence Relating Riboflavin and Cancer

7.2.1. Epidemiologic Evidence

The possibility of a relationship between riboflavin deficiency and esophageal cancer dates from the early observations that Plummer–Vinson disease, which is often associated with esophageal cancer, is also linked with riboflavin deficiency (Wynder *et al.*, 1957).

Esophageal cancer has been correlated with diets marginal or deficient in riboflavin, nicotinic acid, magnesium, and zinc (see van Rensburg, 1981; Thurnham *et al.*, 1982). Although these and many other factors (e.g., alcohol consumption) may contribute to the development and progression of esophageal cancer, riboflavin deficiency is well known to cause lesions in the esophageal epithelium of humans (Foy and Mbaya, 1977) that may be precursors of cancer.

In an endoscopic study of 527 people in Linxian, Henan Province, China, Thurnham *et al.* (1982) found that 97% had ariboflavinosis based on the erythrocyte glutathione reductase activation coefficients compared to 66% with esophagitis, 88% with clear-cell acanthosis, and 26% with intermittent dysphagia. Although there was no clear relationship between these factors, the authors comment that the two factors that appear to be common are the consumption of hot beverages and riboflavin deficiency. They cautioned that nutritional deficiencies may not be cancer inducing *per se,* but may render the esophagus more susceptible to other agents. In a later double-blind intervention trial in China, supplementation of apparently healthy individuals with a combination of retinol, riboflavin, and zinc did not lead to a different prevalence of precancerous lesions of the esophagus among those receiving the active treatment compared to a placebo group (Munoz *et al.*, 1988; Wahrendorf *et al.*, 1988). However, individuals who showed large increases in retinol, riboflavin, and zinc blood levels were more likely to have a histologically normal esophagus at the end of the trial.

Foy and Kondi (1984) found that male baboons fed a diet lacking riboflavin developed cutaneous lesions with hyperkeratosis, gross derangement of keratinization with acanthosis, and impressive pseudocarcinomatous hyperplasia. In some animals, the esophageal epithelium was thin and pale and there was esophagitis and large chronic, disorganized lesions. In many, there were numerous mitotic figures that were distinguishable from carcinomas only by the absence of muscular invasion and by the disorganized, highly active epithelial growth. The authors note that this may reflect a "precursor" state that could take years to become invasive; furthermore, chronic esophagitis is common in Iran and China, which also have a relatively high incidence of esophageal cancer. Riboflavin deficiencies and esophageal cancer are widespread in Africa and other areas, as well.

More study is needed to determine the role, if any, that riboflavin deficiency plays in this syndrome. It is interesting that zinc deficiency is also associated with esophageal cancer since riboflavin metabolism may be affected by zinc status because this divalent cation maximally activates flavokinase (Merrill and McCormick, 1980). Munoz *et al.* (1985) have recently obtained results that question the hypothesis that riboflavin deficiencies are associated with precancerous lesions of the esophagus. In a randomized double-blind intervention trial, a high-risk population in China received weekly supplements of retinol, riboflavin, and zinc, or a placebo. The two groups exhibited no differences in the prevalence of esophagitis with or without atrophy or dysplasia.

7.2.2. Therapeutic Trials

Since riboflavin deficiencies reduce tumor growth in experimental animals, Lane (1971) tested riboflavin deficiency along with galactoflavin (an analog that often accelerates the appearance of deficiency symptoms) administration in treating patients with polycythemia vera and lymphoma. Two of four patients with lymphoma showed partial remissions, as did one of two with Hodgkin's disease. Two patients with polycythemia vera had prolonged remissions.

7.2.3. Riboflavin and the Action of Chemical Carcinogens

A relationship between consumption of this vitamin and susceptibility to chemically induced carcinogenesis was reported almost a half-century ago by Kensler *et al.* (1941) in studies of dimethylaminoazobenzene. This observation has been confirmed and elaborated by many subsequent investigations (for reviews, see Miller and Miller, 1953; Rivlin, 1975; Bidlack *et al.,* 1986).

In a fairly detailed study of the effects of riboflavin deficiency on nitrosamine metabolism by rat liver microsomes, Wang *et al.* (1985) found that the relationship can be complex. The NADPH–cytochrome c reductase activity was lower for riboflavin-deficient rats, but cytochrome P450 content was higher. During mild deficiency, *N*-nitrosodimethylamine demethylase activity was elevated but the metabolism of *N*-nitrosomethylbenzylamine and three other nitrosamines was slightly decreased. During more severe deficiency, the metabolism of *N*-nitrosodimethylamine and the oxidation of benzo[a]pyrene were decreased. From these results, they suggest that differences in the response of the monooxygenase enzyme system to riboflavin deficiency result in varying effects on the metabolism of nitrosamines and other carcinogens. Hara and Taniguchi (1985) have reported that the decrease in the NADPH–cytochrome P450 reductase activity is due to a decrease in the FMN content from 9.5 to 4.9 nmole/mg of protein, with a seeming increase in the riboflavin and FAD content.

7.2.4. Riboflavin and Lipid Peroxides

The level of lipid peroxides in serum and the lens has been reported to increase when rats are fed a riboflavin-deficient diet (Hirano *et al.,* 1983). This may be due to a decrease in glutathione reductase activity that developed during the 4 weeks the animals were maintained on this diet. Riboflavin has also been observed to alter the phospholipid metabolism of rat liver impaired with carbon tetrachloride (Horiuchi and Ono, 1984).

7.2.5. Riboflavin and Light-Induced Carcinogenesis

Riboflavin undergoes photoreduction to its dihydro- and seimiquinone forms in the presence of suitable reductants and light. These can react with various electron acceptors, such as oxygen, to yield reactive products (e.g., superoxide). Alvi *et al.* (1984) have reported complexes between riboflavin and DNA that could account for the toxic and mutagenic effects of exposing cultured cells and microorganisms to riboflavin and light in the presence of oxygen.

The importance of this damage is unclear; Pacernick *et al.* (1975) did not observe an effect of massive doses of riboflavin (10,000 times the daily requirement) on the incidence of squamous cell carcinomas in mice exposed to high doses of UV light. Nonetheless, since phototherapy is being used extensively for treatment of neonatal hyperbilirubinemia, this question warrants further investigation. Interestingly, lumichrome, a major photolysis product of riboflavin, has been found to be a ligand for the receptor for the polycyclic hydrocarbon 2,3,7,8-tetrachloro-dibenzo-p-dioxin (TCDD) (Kurl and Villee, 1985).

7.3. Aberrant Utilization of Riboflavin in Cancer

Patients with cancer frequently exhibit signs of aberrant handling of this vitamin. They excrete lower-than-normal amounts of riboflavin in urine (Kagan, 1960) and do not show significant increases in excretion after oral or intravenous doses of this vitamin (Kagan, 1957, 1960). Possible causes of this abnormality include trapping of riboflavin by the tumor or the host. Evidence for the former is the finding by Baker *et al.* (1981) that samples of colon adenocarcinoma obtained at autopsy contained nearly twofold more riboflavin (as well as elevated amounts of other water-soluble vitamins) than neighboring tissue. Liver adenocarcinoma, on the other hand, contained about the same levels as controls (the amounts of several other vitamins were lower, however).

Innis *et al.* (1985) found that the major proteins responsible for riboflavin binding in human plasma are immunoglobulins, and that their levels are higher for patients with breast cancer and melanoma (Innis *et al.*, 1986). Therefore, increased plasma protein binding could contribute to the lower urinary levels and clearance seen in cancer. The best-characterized riboflavin-binding immunoglobulin was first described by Farhangi and Osserman (1976) as the factor responsible for the yellow skin and hair developed by a patient with multiple myeloma. This individual exhibited normal glutathione reductase activities and excreted typical levels of riboflavin, although a major fraction (70–75%) was protein bound (Pinto *et al.*, 1975). Upon riboflavin loading the immediate increase in excretion was only 10% of the controls and the peak was delayed. Subsequent studies have provided detailed information about the properties of this IgG (Chang *et al.*, 1981; Pologe *et al.*, 1982; Kiefer *et al.*, 1983). The possible relationships between this unique immunoglobulin and the types widely found in human circulation have not been determined. Other riboflavin-binding proteins are associated with embryogenesis (White and Merrill, 1988) and might be expressed aberrantly in cancer, but the appearance of these has not been explored for patients.

8. Niacin

The coenzymatic forms of nicotinamide, nicotinamide adenine dinucleotide (NAD) and nicotinamide adenine dinucleotide phosphate (NADP), are utilized at some point in nearly every pathway in cells. The nicotinamide moiety is also used as a leaving group in the synthesis of poly(ADP-ribose), an event that is associated with DNA damage (see below). Nonetheless, deficiency of this vitamin is not generally considered to be a major contributor to the development of cancer (Shamberger, 1984; Bryan, 1986), although nicotinamide analogs are being explored as chemotherapeutic agents.

8.1. Background

Niacin (nicotinic acid) is obtained from various dietary sources, with significant amounts in meats, yeast, grains, and vegetables, although that in some plant sources may not be completely available. Nicotinic acid is also synthesized from tryptophan, and it is estimated that for approximately every 60 mg of tryptophan ingested, 1 mg of niacin is made. Nicotinamide and nicotinic acid are ribosylated using 5'-phosphoribosyl pyrophosphate, then adenylated with ATP to form NAD and the nicotinic acid equivalent, which is converted to NAD using glutamine. NADP is synthesized from NAD by an ATP-dependent kinase. Henderson (1983) has published an excellent review of niacin nutrition, biochemistry, and physiology.

8.2. Evidence Relating Niacin and Cancer

Although epidemiologic data linking niacin and cancer are lacking, Warwick and Harrington (1973) noted that areas where esophageal cancer is becoming more frequent often have a rising incidence of pellagra. In interpreting this, they caution, however, that pellagra may reflect an extreme deficiency of nicotinic acid complicated by other vitamin and mineral deficiencies, and the predisposition to cancer of the esophagus and other possible sites may be due to damaging effects on the organs.

Miller and Burns (1984) found an accelerated rate of tumor incidence in rats administered N-nitrosodimethylamine upon establishment of a significant depression in the coenzymes by feeding diets low in protein (5.5%) (control rats received the same diet supplemented with nicotinamide). Both the oxidized and reduced forms of NAD and NADP were lower than normal in liver, but only NADH and NADPH were below normal in kidney.

8.3. Nicotinamide as a Tumor Promoter

It appears that consumption of very high levels of nicotinamide, instead of protecting against cancer, actually promotes tumor formation in response to some chemical carcinogens. Lanzen *et al.* (1985), following up earlier work by Rakieten *et al.* (1971), reported that nicotinamide enhanced the induction of pancreatic endocrine tumors by streptozotocin. Immunochemical analyses of the tumors identified them as an average of 91% B cells, 8% D cells, and less than 1% of A and PP cells. Insulin release was responsive to glucose, although reduced, and the pattern of enzyme activities was typical for pancreatic endocrine tissue. Shoentel (1977) reported an increased incidence of kidney neoplasias in rats given diethylnitrosamine when nicotinamide (300–500 mg/kg of body weight) was administered before and after each dose. Rosenberg *et al.* (1985) found that administration of nicotinamide in the drinking water (6.7 or 30 mM) of male Fischer 344 rats receiving diethylnitrosamine caused a 28–59% increase in the incidence of kidney tumors. Rats given nicotinamide alone had no kidney tumors. A later study (Rosenberg *et al.*, 1986) found that injection of rats with nicotinamide caused an initial decrease in kidney ornithine decarboxylase activity, which was followed by a substantial increase by 24 hr (administration of nicotinamide in drinking water had a similar effect), but DNA synthesis was unaffected.

8.4. Nicotinamide in Cancer Therapy

Poly(ADP-ribose) polymerase catalyzes the synthesis of poly(ADP-ribose) from NAD in response to DNA damage. Attachment of this polymer to chromosomal proteins is presumed to facilitate the repair of DNA strand breaks. Since a number of NAD analogs inhibit poly(ADP-ribose) polymerase, several laboratories have investigated their effects on DNA repair (Barra *et al.*, 1982) and as potentiators of the cytoxic effects of gamma-irradiation (Nduka *et al.*, 1980; Kjellen *et al.*, 1986; Horsman *et al.*, 1987) and antitumor drugs (Berger *et al.*, 1982). Sulfur-containing analogs of nicotinamide have been shown to be decrease the number of pulmonary metastases in C57BL/6 mice implanted with Lewis lung carcinoma and to inhibit the growth rate of the primary implanted tumors (Grassetti, 1986).

Berger *et al.* (1982) found that treatment of mice bearing tumors from L1210 cells with 6-aminonicotinamide and 1,3-bis(2-chloroethyl)-1-nitrosourea resulted in a synergistic increase in lifespan with, in some cases, production of long-term disease-free survivors. Shapiro *et al.* (1957) reported that 6-aminonicotinamide had antitumor activity against mammary adenocarcinoma in mice. Another analog, 3-aminobenzamide, also inhibited poly(ADP-ribose) polymerase (synthetase) and rat hepatoma (HTC) cell proliferation at a concentration (2 mM) that has been reported to be nontoxic for other cell types (Lea *et al.*, 1984). This compound and a related analog (3-methoxylbenzamide) inhibited the increase in poly(ADP-ribose) in C3H10T1/2 cells following *N*-methyl-*N'*-nitro-*N*-nitrosoguanidine (MNNG) treatment (Jacobson *et al.*, 1984). Lea *et al.* (1984) found that nicotinamide itself had only a small or insignificant effect on hepatoma cells. A single dose of nicotinamide given to hamsters after *N*-nitroso-bis (2-oxopropyl) amine stimulated repair of DNA damage (Lawson, 1983). Nicotinamides have also been observed to potentiate the cytotoxicity of bleomycin in L1210 cultured cells and the antitumor activity of bleomycin in mice bearing Ehrlich ascites tumors (Kato *et al.*, 1988).

In contrast, Schmitt-Graff and Scheulen (1986) have suggested that niacin may be useful in reducing the cardiotoxic side effects of adriamycin. A study by Popov (1987) involving 106 patients with bladder carcinoma suggests that nicotinic acid and aspirin may decrease relapses after radiation therapy.

8.5. Aberrant Metabolism in Cancer

Carcinogens appear to affect niacin metabolism by decreasing the NAD/NADH and NADP/NADPH content of tissues (Schein, 1969; Miller and Burns, 1984). A similar effect has been seen with cells in culture (Jacobson *et al.*, 1980). Treatment of 3T3 cells with 130 µM MNNG for 1 hr caused a rapid lowering of the intracellular levels of NAD by 50%, without altering the NADP pool. MNNG did not affect the synthesis of NAD from nicotinamide or the activity of NAD glycohydrolase, but there was a sevenfold increase in poly(ADP-ribose) polymerase. The lowering of cellular NAD could be reduced by theophylline, an inhibitor of the polymerase. Hence, Jacobson *et al.* conclude that the lowering of NAD is due to an increased synthesis of poly(ADP-ribose) in response to damage to DNA. The excretion of 1-methyl-nicotinamide is increased in rats given alkylating agents (Chu and Lawley, 1975).

A number of other interesting links exist between nicotinamide and cancer. Kull *et al.* (1987) have identified one of the angiogenic factors obtained from an extract of Walker 256 carcinoma as nicotinamide. Another active fraction contained nicotinamide as part of a more complex, unidentified compound. It has also been proposed that some of the effects of nicotinamide may be attributable to its action as a protease inhibitor (Troll *et al.*, 1987).

9. Vitamin B_6

The coenzymatic forms of vitamin B_6 are central to a wide range of biochemical transformations, including racemizations, decarboxylations, transaminations, beta- and gamma-eliminations, and a variety of synthetase reactions. Vitamin B_6-dependent enzymes are most prominent in the many pathways of amino acid and nucleotide anabolism and catabolism, but also figure in the metabolism of carbohydrates (glycogen phosphorylase), lipids (e.g., phosphatidylserine decarboxylase and serine palmitoyltransferase), heme (delta-aminolevulinate synthetase), polyamines (ornithine decarboxylase), and neurotransmitters (e.g., DOPA decarboxylase), to name representative examples. Vitamin B_6 deficiencies are not generally considered to the major contributors to the development of cancer (Shamberger, 1984); however, since this micronutrient is so vital to growth, attempts have been made to limit tumor growth by induction of deficiencies. There have been a number of recent reviews of vitamin B_6 and cancer (Reynolds, 1986; Ladner and Salkeld, 1988) as well as an overview of diseases associated with defects in vitamin B_6 metabolism or utilization (Merrill and Henderson, 1987).

9.1. Background

Vitamin B_6 is obtained from various dietary sources, with significant amounts in organ meats (liver, heart, kidney, etc.), grains (soybean, whole wheat bread, cornmeal), eggs, green leafy vegetables, some fruits, and legumes. The bioavailability can vary considerably (Gregory and Kirk, 1981). Foods contain varying proportions of the three vitaminic forms pyridoxine, pyridoxamine, and pyridoxal.

After intestinal absorption of the unphosphorylated forms, most of the vitamin B_6 is transported to liver, where it is taken up by facilitated diffusion and phosphorylated by pyridoxal kinase (Kozik and McCormick, 1984). The pyridoxine and pyridoxamine 5'-phosphates are converted to pyridoxal 5'-phosphate by an FMN-dependent oxidase (Kazarinoff and McCormick, 1975; Ink and Henderson, 1984). Pyridoxal 5'-phosphate is bound by apoenzymes or released into plasma and carried to tissues as a tight complex with albumin. Upon hydrolysis by alkaline phosphatase, free pyridoxal is taken up by cells and rephosphorylated to the active coenzyme.

9.2. Evidence Relating Vitamin B_6 and Cancer

A recent article titled "Theoretical Involvement of Vitamin B_6 in Tumor Initiation" (Prior, 1985) fairly accurately states current knowledge—there is so little concrete information relating vitamin B_6 to cancer that its association with this disease is mainly "theoretical." Given the major pathways involved in neoplasia that utilize pyridoxal 5'-phosphate (e.g., polyamine biosynthesis, nucleotide formation, lipotrope metabolism, *inter alia*), it is difficult to believe that vitamin B_6 status is not in some way related to susceptibility to cancer. It is also generally felt that there may be a role for vitamin B_6 in the immune system (Robson and Schwartz, 1980). Nonetheless, epidemiologic data to date associates vitamin B_6 and cancer only in the general grouping of B vitamins.

There are some signs that this topic warrants further study. Foy *et al.* (1974) have proposed from studies of the effects of pyridoxine deficiency on baboons that there might be a link with liver cancer. Adjuklewicz and Pollitt (1976), in a letter to the editor, reported that they have seen no association between liver carcinoma and pyridoxine deficiency in their patient population. Bell (1980) reported that women excreting less pyridoxic acid than average, one reflection of vitamin B_6 status, have a higher probability of recurrence of breast cancer than those with more normal excretion. The issue of the vitamin B_6 status of breast cancer patients is complex, however. The studies by Schrijver *et al.* (1987) of postmenopausal women with advanced breast cancer indicate that water-soluble vitamin status is adequate; however, a significantly higher excretion of xanthurenic acid in urine after an oral tryptophan load was observed for women administered the progestin megestrol acetate or the antiestrogen tamoxifen. The authors concluded that hormonal treatment accounted for these differences.

9.3. Therapeutic Trials

Gailani *et al.* (1968) did not observe an effect of treating patients with a pyridoxine-deficient diet for 10–80 days or of administration of a pyridoxine antagonist, 4-deoxypyridoxine. Ladner and Holtz (1979) have claimed, however, that correction of vitamin B_6 deficiency increases the survival of patients with cervix and uterine carcinoma. Vitamin B_6 antagonists have been studied as inhibitors of tumor growth and as chemotherapeutic agents (Rosen *et al.*, 1964a,b; Korytnyk, 1979), but do not appear to be particularly effective except in model systems.

Byar and Blackard (1977) conducted a prospective trial with 121 patients which compared the effects of administering a placebo, pyridoxine, or topical thiothepa on the recurrence of stage 1 bladder cancer. Although the outcome was similar when the groups were compared as a whole, significant differences were obtained when patients having recurrences within the first 10 months or followed up in less than 10 months were excluded.

Since there appears to be an association between tryptophan and bladder cancer, these effects of B_6 may be related through the requirement of this vitamin for tryptophan metabolism. Brown *et al.* (1969) observed such an association between tryptophan and bladder cancer, but it did not appear to be related to vitamin B_6 status.

9.4. Other Studies Relating Vitamin B_6 and Cancer

Studies with experimental animals have found that the growth of some types of tumors is inhibited when the diet is deficient in pyridoxine (Kline *et al.*, 1943; Mihich and Nichol, 1959; Tryfiates and Morris, 1974). Ha *et al.* (1984) have reported that vitamin B_6 deficiencies affect host susceptibility to Maloney sarcoma virus-induced tumor growth in mice. However, the growth of not all tumors is affected by vitamin B_6 status: the growth of spontaneous mammary tumors in strain C3H mice is unaffected by pyridoxine deficiency (Morris, 1947).

Gridley *et al.* (1987) examined the effects of a wide range of vitamin B_6 amounts on the development of herpes simplex virus type 2-transformed (H238) cell-induced tumors and on *in vitro* responses relating to cell-mediated immunity. Mice were fed diets containing 0.2–74.3 mg pyridoxine (PN) per kg diet (0.2 mg PN caused mild deficiency symptoms). The tumor incidence among the groups was similar, except at 13–16 days after tumor cell injection, when mice mice fed the highest dosage of pyridoxine had a lower incidence. Mice fed 0.2 mg pyridoxine had the lowest tumor volume; the 1.2-mg group had the largest primary tumor volume, the highest incidence of lung metastases, and the greatest number of metastatic nodules per animal at 7 weeks, and lower tumor volumes were found in animals fed 7.7 and 74.3 mg pyridoxine. The lymphoproliferative response tended to be higher in the groups with higher pyridoxine; however, all tumor-bearing groups had decreased mitogen-stimulated responsiveness compared to control mice. These findings illustrate that pyridoxine can affect both tumor size and the ability of the host to maintain immune function; however, whether or not these are causally related remains unknown.

DiSorbo *et al.* (1982) reported that pyridoxine at millimolar concentrations is toxic to hepatoma cells in culture, and they have isolated a resistant cell line. They have also reported (DiSorbo *et al.*, 1985) that pyridoxal inhibited the growth of B-16 melanoma cells in culture and after establishment in mice.

Inculet *et al.* (1987) have noted that most cancer patients receiving total parenteral nutrition had normal blood or urine levels of all water-soluble vitamins and there was no clinical evidence of water-soluble vitamin deficiency or toxicity. Since some patients had low vitamin B_6 levels, and intravenous doses of vitamin B_6 appear to be safe and well tolerated, increased daily amounts of these vitamins could be given to cancer patients on parenteral nutrition.

9.5. Aberrant Metabolism of Vitamin B_6 in Cancer

Several groups have reported that cancer patients have signs of unusual metabolism of vitamin B_6, such as lower plasma pyridoxal 5'-phosphate despite normal urinary pyridoxic acid in patients with breast cancer (Potera *et al.*, 1977). Low plasma pyridoxal 5'-phosphate has been found in Hodgkin's disease (Chabner *et al.*, 1970), and abnormalities in tryptophan metabolism have also been reported in Hodgkin's disease (Chabner *et al.*, 1970), hemoblastosis (Crepaldi and Parpajola, 1964), breast cancer (Rose and Sheff, 1967), and bladder cancer (Brown *et al.*, 1969). Thanassi and co-workers (Thanassi *et al.*, 1981, 1985; Nutter *et al.*, 1983; Meisler and Thanassi, 1988) have conducted detailed investigations of vitamin B_6 metabolism by tumors (see these references for earlier citations). They have found that pyridoxine (pyridoxamine) 5'-phosphate oxidase is low or absent from hepatomas, which implies that pyridoxal 5'-phosphate must be obtained from another source. This could lead to a strategy for controlling this type of tumor if a way could be found to prevent it from taking up or utilizing the precursors to pyridoxal. There is also some evidence that tumors may form a novel metabolite of pyridoxine (Tryfiates *et al.*, 1983).

Lander and Salkeld (1988) have observed that the percentage of cancer patients with erythrocyte pyridoxal 5'-phosphate below 3 ng/ml increased from 31 to 83% during radiation therapy for gynecological carcinoma. They also noted that the 5-year survival rate of patients with stage II endometrial carcinoma was increased by administration of pyridoxine.

10. Folate

Folic acid, present mostly in mammalian tissues in various forms of tetrahydrofolate (THF) and as the pentaglutamyl conjugate, is central to one-carbon metabolism. These pathways include purine and pyrimidine biosynthesis (including DNA methylation) and amino acid metabolism. Many of these processes also utilize vitamin B_{12} (Shane and Stokstad, 1985). Plentiful sources of folate include whole grains, yeast, and liver. The form of folate taken up from food and in circulation is primarily the monoglutamate, which is elaborated intracellularly to the polyglutamates. The major serum and tissue form is 5-methylTHF, with lesser amounts of 10-formylTHF in most tissues, and even less 5,10-methyleneTHF, THF, and others (Erbe and Wang, 1984).

10.1. Evidence Relating Folate and Cancer

Much of the early attention on folate and cancer centered on the use of folate antagonists as chemotherapeutic agents (Bleyer, 1978). Methotrexate, for example, is taken up by cells, converted into polyglutamates, and inhibits dihydrofolate reductase (Baugh *et al.*, 1973; Samuels *et al.*, 1985). A number of investigators have concluded that intake of folate obtained by patients on methotrexate therapy does not compromise the effectiveness of chemotherapy (van Eys, 1985), although this point is undergoing reevaluation.

Folate is also involved in the metabolism of methyl groups, which is thought to be associated with cancer through the effects of DNA methylation on gene expression (Hoffman, 1985; Newberne and Rogers, 1986). Folate, together with vitamin B_{12}, methionine, and choline, controls the methyl group pool of cells. Serine, which can be synthesized *de novo* from carbohydrates, is the most abundant source of endogenously formed methyl groups. Other sources available from the diet include methionine, serine, glycine, choline, betaine, dimethylglycine, sarcosine, and histidine. The relationships between folate and vitamin B_{12} and cancer have been reviewed recently (Herbert, 1986; Eto and Krumdieck, 1986), as well as their role with other lipotrophic factors in carcinogenesis (Newberne, 1986).

Wagner *et al.* (1985a) have proposed that glycine *N*-methyltransferase, which is the major folate-binding protein of some tissues and contains the endogenous ligand 5-methyltetrahydropterolylpentaglutamate, controls the ratio of *S*-adenosylmethonine to *S*-adenosylhomocysteine in cells. Human tumor cells have an unusually low ratio of *S*-adenosylmethionine to *S*-adenosylhomocysteine (Steen *et al.*, 1984). Diets deficient in methyl groups lead to increased incidence of tumors (Rogers, 1975; Lombardi and Shinozuka, 1979; Mikol *et al.*, 1983; Ghoshal and Farber, 1984; Hoover *et al.*, 1984).

Hoover *et al.* (1984) found that feeding rats a diet deficient in choline, methionine, folate, and vitamin B_{12} for 15 weeks was sufficient to predispose them to a high incidence of hepatic tumors after a single dose of diethylnitrosamine. The effects of methyl group–deficient diets on hepatocarcinogenesis have been attributed to the severe lipidosis and cell death (Giambarresi *et al.*, 1982; Ghoshal *et al.*, 1983; Shinozuka and Lombardi, 1980).

There appears to be a link between folate and esophageal cancer. Individuals from areas of South Africa known to have a high incidence of esophageal cancer differ significantly from those in low-risk areas with respect to vitamins A, E, and B_{12} in addition to folate (van Helden *et al.*, 1987). Heimburger *et al.* (1988) have recently conducted a randomized, controlled, prospective intervention trial of smokers with bronchial squamous metaplasia given either placebo or 10 mg of folate plus 500 μg of hydroxocobalamin.

Direct cytological comparison of the two groups after 4 months showed significantly greater reduction of atypia in the supplemented group. The authors note that this provides preliminary evidence that atypical bronchial squamous metaplasia may be reduced by folate and vitamin B_{12}, but caution against concluding that supplementation with these vitamins is desirable for the prevention or cure of cancer because of spontaneous variation in the small study population, the short duration of the trial, and the supraphysiological doses used.

10.2. Metabolism of Folate and Other Pterins in Cancer (Nichol *et al.*, 1985)

Serum folate concentrations have been reported to be lower for patients with leukemia and various solid tumors (Hoogstraten *et al.*, 1961; Hellman *et al.*, 1964; Rama Rao *et al.*, 1965). However, Clamon *et al.* (1984) found that serum folate levels were elevated for most patients with small-cell lung cancer. Elevated serum B_{12} levels have been observed (Buamah *et al.*, 1987) in 5 of 11 patients with primary hepatocellular carcinoma and levels rose during chemotherapy; there did not appear to be much necrosis of the tumor or the liver.

Halpern *et al.* (1977) identified pterin-6-aldehyde as a folate degradation product formed by tumor cells in culture, but not normal human epithelial and fibroblastic cells, human amniotic cells, or mouse embryonic fibroblasts. This metabolite was not detected in human urine unless the individual's diet had been supplemented with folic acid. Pterin-6-aldehyde was found, however, in urine from cancer patients and disappeared after successful surgical removal of the tumor. Elevated levels of various pterins (neopterin, biopterin, etc.) have also been reported in blood (Ziegler *et al.*, 1982; Kokolis and Ziegler, 1977) and urine (Rokos *et al.*, 1980; Stea *et al.*, 1981) from patients with different types of neoplastic disease. Biopterin is a cofactor for the enzymes that convert phenylalanine to tyrosine and tryptophan to melatonin and neopterin is one of the intermediates in the biosynthesis of biopterin from GTP. Urinary neopterin levels were found (Hausen *et al.*, 1982; Bichler *et al.*, 1982) to be significantly higher in patients with hematological disease, except for Stage I multiple myeloma or when the disease was benign or in remission.

Perhaps because inhibition of folate utilization is a major chemotherapeutic strategy, relatively little is known about the potential benefits of folate supplementation in cancer. One study noted that supplementation with oral folate gradually decreased cervical dysplasia (Ziegler, 1986).

10.3. Folate-Binding Proteins in Cancer

Folate-binding proteins (for a review see Wagner, 1985) are higher in serum from some patients with cancer (Eichner *et al.*, 1978). This might be due to elevations in folate binders in tumor tissue (Corrocher *et al.*, 1978). Sheppard *et al.* (1984) found that a wide variety of tumor tissues contain increased concentrations of both folate-binding proteins and vitamin B_{12}–binding proteins. No abnormalities in serum folate-binding proteins were observed. These may account for the elevated folate levels in tumors (Baker *et al.*, 1981); however, Samuels *et al.* (1986) have reported that folylpolyglutamate hydrolase activities of normal mouse tissues are 10- to 20-fold higher than from sarcoma 180,

Ehrlich ascites cells, and L1210 cells. This could result in net accumulation of the polyglutamates in most proliferative tissues as well as contributing to the cytotoxicity of folate analogs, such as methotrexate.

11. Vitamin B_{12}

Vitamin B_{12} is involved in two known reactions in humans, the transfer of a methyl group from 5-methyltetrahydrofolate to homocysteine to form methionine (catalyzed by 5-methyltelate-homocysteine methyltransferase) (Shane and Stokstad, 1985), and the rearrangement of L-methylmalonyl-CoA to succinyl-CoA (catalyzed by methylmalonyl-CoA mutase). The former is vital because it removes homocysteine (the converse reaction—methionine synthesis—is minimal), which can be converted to homocysteic acid, a compound with growth-promoting characteristics (Clopath *et al.*, 1975), and because it is the major route for regeneration of tetrahydrofolate (Taheri *et al.*, 1982). Furthermore, *S*-adenosylhomocysteine is a competitive inhibitor of many enzymes that utilize *S*-adenosylmethionine and its relative amount is increased in some tissues of animals consuming lipotrope-deficient diets (Shivapurkar and Poirier, 1983). Hence, vitamin B_{12}, together with folate, methionine, and choline, controls many aspects of the utilization of the methyl group pool of cells, which has already been discussed in relationship to cancer (see preceding section).

Vitamin B_{12} is actually a group of cobalt-containing compounds termed cobalamins. The principal cobalamins in animal products are thought to be methylcobalamin, 5'-deoxyadenosylcobalamin, and hydroxycobalamin, whereas, the predominant form available commercially is cyanocobalamin, which is heat-stable and convertable to active forms by humans. Good food sources are liver, kidney, eggs, and cheese, although most diets (except strict vegetarian) provide reasonable amounts of vitamin B_{12}.

11.1. Evidence Associating Vitamin B_{12} and Cancer

Lipotrope deficiencies have been shown to enhance chemical carcinogenesis in the liver and sometimes other tissues of rats (for example, see Rogers, 1975, and Mikol *et al.*, 1983). Hoover *et al.* (1984) found that feeding rats a diet deficient in choline, methionine, folate, and vitamin B_{12} for 15 weeks was sufficient to predispose them to a high incidence of hepatic tumors after a single dose of diethylnitrosamine. Altered methionine metabolism, from whatever cause, appears to be a general feature of cancer (Stern *et al.*, 1984). Since the observation by Kaplan and Rigler (1945) that patients with pernicious anemia have a higher incidence of gastric carcinoma, this association has been confirmed by several laboratories and expanded to leukemias, erythremic myelosis, polycythemia vera, multiple myeloma, and other cancers (see Arvanitakis *et al.*, 1979). Ruddell *et al.* (1978) have proposed that the mechanism of increased gastric cancer could be the increased formation of carcinogenic *N*-nitroso compounds. Arvanitakis *et al.* (1979) note that an altered immune response in pernicious anemia may be important in the incidence of cancer. Ahmann and Durie (1984) have cautioned that excessive replacement of vitamin B_{12} in patients with leukemia may have the potential to accelerate such disorders.

11.2. Evidence that Vitamin B₁₂ Supplementation Enhances Chemically Induced Cancers

Despite the likely benefits of maintaining normal levels of vitamin B_{12}, the efficacy of vitamin B_{12} supplementation has not been established. In fact, supplementation appears to be contraindicated. Day *et al.* (1960) observed that vitamin B_{12} can have a procarcinogneic effect for rats treated with *p*-dimethylaminoazobenzene. Temcharoen *et al.* (1978) have reported that vitamin B_{12} supplementation significantly enhanced the induction of hyperplastic nodules and hepatomas by aflatoxin in rats fed high-, but not low-, protein diets. Rats on a vitamin B_{12}–deficient diet have also been found to develop fewer tumors of the small intestine and colon upon treatment with azoxymethane than rats on the same diet supplemented with vitamin B_{12} (Yamamoto, 1980). Furthermore, the supplemented diet was more effective in yielding colon tumors than a mixed commercial diet.

11.3. Serum Vitamin B₁₂ and Vitamin B₁₂–Binding Proteins in Cancer

Abnormalities in serum vitamin B_{12}–binding proteins were first reported by Beard *et al.* (1954) in patients with luekemia. Elevations in serum transcobalamin I and serum vitamin B_{12} are now well documented in chronic myelogenous leukemia and other hematopoietic disorders (e.g., Mendelson *et al.*, 1958; Meyer *et al.*, 1961; Hall and Wanko, 1971; Rachmilewitz *et al.*, 1971). Liver tumors are also often associated with higher serum vitamin B_{12} and B_{12}–binding proteins (Waxman and Gilbert, 1973; Nexo *et al.*, 1975). A recent study by van Tonder *et al.* (1985) of serum vitamin B_{12} binders in South African blacks with hepatocellular carcinoma found that over 80% had slightly raised serum vitamin B_{12} and unsaturated vitamin B_{12}–binding capacity. Carmel and Eisenberg (1977) studied 139 patients with other types of malignancies (28 breast, 19 colon, 17 stomach, 12 lung, eight pancreas, eight prostate, eight ovary, and other less prevalent types of cancer) and concluded that they fell in these major subgroups: (1) normal (50% of the total); (2) high transcobalamin I and vitamin B_{12} levels (6%); (3) high vitamin B_{12} but relatively normal transcobalamin levels (11%); (4) high vitamin B_{12}–binding capacity, but normal transcobalamin and vitamin B_{12} levels (23%); and (5) low vitamin B_{12} without obvious cause (10%). Groups 3 and 4 were associated with hepatic (and some other) metastases and early death. They conclude that elevations in serum vitamin B_{12} and B_{12}–binding proteins frequently occur in malignancies involving organs other than granulocytic proliferation or hepatic tumors, as had been indicated by prior studies (e.g., Carmel, 1975). Clamon *et al.* (1984) did not find a correlation between serum vitamin B_{12} and small-cell lung cancer. Sheppard *et al.* (1984) found that brain, heart, and lung tumors had both higher cobalamin binding and unsaturated cobalamin-binding capacity, whereas liver had only an increased unsaturated cobalamin-binding capacity and the total was lower. The results with liver are consistent with the observation by Baker *et al.* (1981) that liver adenocarcinomas had lower vitamin B_{12} content than specimens from adjacent uninvaded liver.

11.4. Vitamin B₁₂ Status of Cancer Patients

From 5 to 20% of the patients who receive radiotherapy for pelvic tumors develop some degree of bowel complication, which can include malabsorption of vitamin B_{12}.

Kinn and Lantz (1984) found that patients given full irradiation because of inoperable bladder cancer had malabsorption of vitamin B_{12} and suggested that serum vitamin B_{12} be evaluated after radiotherapy. Ludgate and Merrick (1985) have proposed that B_{12} absorption be used as an index of bowel damage. Another potential source of vitamin B_{12} deficiencies arises among cancer patients who require total parenteral nutrition (Kirkemo *et al.*, 1982).

12. Biotin

Biotin is utilized as a cofactor by carboxylases for pyruvate, acetyl-CoA, propionyl-CoA, and 3-methylcrotonyl-CoA in mammalian organisms. Biotin is obtained from various dietary sources, with significant amounts in eggs, nuts, and chocolate, and is also synthesized by intestinal microflora.

Evidence Relating Biotin and Cancer

There have been few reports relating biotin to cancer. Since avidin binds biotin with a high affinity and can induce a deficiency (for example, if one eats large amounts of raw egg white), attempts have been made to use avidin to limit tumor growth. Kaplan (1944), in a preliminary study with nine patients, concluded that some benefit might exist, but that high levels must be consumed. Kline *et al.* (1945) found a much greater effect with rats given *p*-dimethylaminoazobenzene and fed a suboptimal level of riboflavin. These observations do not appear to have been followed up with additional human or animal studies. However, avidin has been studied with cells in culture (for example, see Korpela, 1984). If humans have biotin-binding proteins (which has never been convincingly ruled out), they could be involved in cancer since avidin appears to serve as a host defense factor in avian species (Korpela, 1984).

Biotin has proven useful as a tool in cancer research. Biotinylated lectins or antibodies against cell surface proteins or glycolipids can be sensitively detected by avidin conjugated to an easily detected enzyme such as horseradish peroxidase or acid phosphatase (Weber *et al.*, 1985). The recent development of techniques to detect specific regions of DNA using biotinylated nucleotides (Murer-Orlando and Peterson, 1985) may also prove useful in the detection of specific regions of DNA modification and expression in transformed cells.

13. Pantothenic Acid

Pantothenic acid is a precursor of coenzyme A, which is utilized in numerous acyltransferase reactions, and of the phosphopantetheine moiety of fatty acid synthetase. Because pantothenate derivatives are present in significant amounts in most foods, deficiencies are rare. There is little evidence linking pantothenic acid and cancer. Morris (1941) reported that the rate of growth of spontaneous mammary carcinoma was markedly retarded in mice fed a diet deficient in pantothenic acid. However, he concluded that the diet so severely interfered with the host's nutrition that this offered no practical application in cancer therapy. Bulovskaia (1976) found inhibition of tumor growth by sodium omega-methylpantothenate, an antoganist of pantothenic acid, in mice bearing transplanted tumors. As with many other vitamins, the levels of pantothenate in tumors may be higher or lower than in adjacent uninvolved tissues (Baker *et al.*, 1981).

14. Summary

Maintenance of a well-balanced diet with respect to vitamins (and other nutrients) has a role in minimizing the likelihood of developing cancer. Furthermore, ongoing research is identifying several exciting areas in which vitamins may be useful agents in therapy, although these require considerable additional study. Caution is advisable in extrapolating these results; however, because vitamins may not be uniformly beneficial since they act as promoters in some instances. As summarized by Young and Newberne (1981): "On the basis of current evidence, it would be inappropriate to recommend either substantial changes in habitual vitamin intakes, as provided by an adequate, well-balanced diet, or promotion of megavitamin intakes, as a means of reducing risk from cancers in the human population. However, a prudent approach toward diet and food habits, as a means of better optimizing the health consequences of our complex lifestyles, is to be recommended."

ACKNOWLEDGMENTS. The authors thank Mary Miller, Debbie Johnson, Jennifer Saarinen, Winnie Scherer, and Minal Patel for assistance in the preparation of this manuscript, and Dr. Tim Moore and Sharon Landvik of Veris (Henkel Corporation) for providing a bibliography of reports on vitamin E and cancer. The authors' work described in this chapter was supported by grants from the NIH (AM26746) and the Winship Cancer Center of Emory University.

15. References

Abe, E., Miyaura, C., Sakagami, H., Takeda, M., Konno, K., Yamazaki, T., Yoshiki, S., and Suda, T., 1981, Differentiation of mouse myeloid leukemia cells induced by 1-alpha, 25-dihydroxyvitamin D_3, *Proc. Natl. Acad. Sci. USA* **78**:4990–4994.

Ahmann, F. R., and Durie, B. G. M., 1984, Acute myelogenous leukemia modulation by B_{12} deficiency: A case with bone marrow blast cell assay corroboration, *Br. J. Haematol.* **58**:91–94.

Ajdokiewicz, A., and Pollit, N., 1976, Letter to the editor: Liver carcinoma and pyroxidine deficiency, *Am. J. Clin. Nutr.* **29**(8):813.

Aksoy, M., Basu, T. K., Brient, J., and Dickerson, J. W. T., 1980, Thiamin status of patients treated with drug combinations containing 5-flurouracil, *Eur. J. Cancer* **16**:1041–1045.

Alberts, D., Peng, Y., and Moon, T., 1978, Alpha-tocopherol pretreatment increases adriamycin bone marrow toxicity, *Biomedicine* **29**:189–191.

Alvi, N. K., Ahmad, S., and Hadi, S. M., 1984, Effect of riboflavin and light on the secondary structure of DNA, *Chem. Biol. Interact.* **48**:367–376.

Arvanitakis, C., Holmes, F. H., and Hearne, E., III, 1979, A possible association of pernicious anemia with neoplasia, *Oncology* **36**:127–129.

Atukorala, S., Basu, T., Dickerson, J., Donaldson, D., and Sakula, A., 1979, Vitamin A, zinc and lung cancer, *Br. J. Cancer* **40**:927–931.

Baker, H., Frank, O., Chen, T., Feingold, S., DeAngelis, B., and Baker, E. R., 1981, Elevated vitamin levels in colon adenocarcinoma as compared with metastatic liver adenocarcinoma from colon primary and normal adjacent tissue, *Cancer* **47:**2883–2886.

Band, P., Besner, J., Leclaire, R., Girard, C., Diorio, G., Deschamps, M., Gelinas, G., and Larochelle, D., 1982, Phase II study of 13-*cis*-retinoic acid toxicity, *Cancer Treat. Rep.* **66:**1759–1761.

Barra, R., Randolph, V., Sumas, M. E., Lanighan, K., and Lea, M. A., 1982, Effects of nicotinamide, isonicotinamide and bleomycin on DNA synthesis and repair in rat heptaocytes and hepatoma cells, *J. Natl. Cancer Inst.* **69:**1353–1357.

Basu, T. K., and Dickerson, J. W. T., 1976, The thiamin status of early cancer patients with particular reference to those with breast and bronchial carcinomas, *Oncology* **33:**250–252.

Basu, T. K., Dickerson, J. W. T., Raven, R. W., and Williams, D. C., 1974, The thiamin status of patients with cancer as determined by the red cell transketolase activity, *Int. J. Vit. Nutr. Res.* **44:**53–58.

Basu, T., Donaldson, D., Jenner, M., Williams, D., and Sakula, A., 1976, Plasma vitamin A in patients with bronchial carcinoma, *Br. J. Cancer* **33:**119–121.

Baugh, C. M., Krumdieck, C. L., and Nair, M. S., 1973, Polyglutamyl metabolites of methotrexate, *Biochem. Biophys. Res. Commun.* **52:**27–34.

Beard, M. F., Pitney, W. R., and Sanneman, E. H., 1954, Serum concentration of vitamin B_{12} in patients suffering from leukemia, *Blood* **9:**789–794.

Bell, E., 1980, The excretion of a vitamin B_6 metabolite and the probability of recurrence of early breast cancer, *Eur. J. Cancer* **16:**297–298.

Bellog, W., and Ott, F., 1971, Therapy of actinic keratoses and basal cell carcinomas with local application of vitamin A acid, *Cancer Chemother. Rep.* **55:**59–60.

Berger, N. A., Catino, D. M., and Vietti, T. J., 1982, Synergistic antileukemic effect of 6-aminonicotinamide and 1,3-bis(2-chloroethyl)-1-nitrosourea on L1210 cells *in vitro, Cancer Res.* **42:**4382–4386.

Bertram, J. S., Kolonel, L. N., and Meyskens, F. L., Jr., 1987, Rationale and strategies for chemoprevention of cancer in humans, *Cancer Res.* **47:**3012–3031.

Bichler, A., Fuchs, D., Hausen, A., Hetzel, H., Konig, K., and Wachter, H., 1982, Urinary neopterine excretion in patients with genital cancer, *Clin. Biochem.* **15:**38–40.

Bidlack, W. R., Brown, R. C., and Mohan, C., 1986, Nutritional parameters that alter hepatic drug metabolism, conjugation, and toxicity, *Fed. Proc.* **45:**142–148.

Birt, D. F., 1986, Update on the effects of vitamins A, C, and E and selenium on carcinogenesis, *Proc. Soc. Exp. Biol. Med.* **183:**311–320.

Bjelke, E., 1975, Dietary vitamin A and lung cancer, *Int. J. Cancer* **15:**561–565.

Blakeslee, J. R., Yamamoto, N., and Hinuma, Y., 1985, Human T-cell leukemia virus I induction by 5-iodo-2′-deoxyuridine and *N*-methyl-*N*′-nitro-*N*-nitrosoguanidine: Inhibition by retinoids, L-ascorbic acid, and DL-alpha-tocopherol, *Cancer Res.* **45:**3471–3476.

Bleyer, W. A., 1978, The clinical pharmacology of methotrexate, *Cancer* **41:**36–51.

Block, G., and Sorenson, A., 1987, Vitamin C intake and dietary sources by demographic characteristics, *Nutr. Cancer* **10:**53–65.

Block, J., Chlebowski, R., and Dietrich, M., 1983, Potential for iapachol (NSC-11905) clinical trials reassessment with adjuvant quinone therapy, *Med. Pediatr. Oncol.* **11:**492A–493A.

Boing, H., Martinez, L., Frentzel-Beyme, R., and Oltersdorf, U., 1985, Regional nutritional pattern and cancer mortality in the Federal Republic of Germany, *Nutr. Cancer* **7:**121–130.

Bollag, W., 1974, Therapeutic effects of an aromatic retinoic acid analog on chemically induced skin papillomas and carcinomas of mice, *Eur. J. Cancer* **10:**731–737.

Bollag, W., 1975, Prophylaxis of chemically-induced epithelial tumors with an aromatic retinoid acid analog, *Eur. J. Cancer* **11:**721–724.

Bollag, W., and Matter, A., 1981, From vitamin A to retinoids in experimental and clinical oncology, *Ann. NY Acad. Sci.* **27:**9–23.

Bond, G. G., Thompson, F. E., and Cook, R. R., 1987, Dietary vitamin A and lung cancer: Results of a case–control study among chemical workers, *Nutr. Cancer* **9:**109–121.

Borek, C., Ong, A., Mason, H., Donahue, L., and Biaglow, J. E., 1986, Selenium and vitamin E inhibit radiogenic and chemically induced transformation *in vitro* via different mechanisms, *Proc. Natl. Acad. Sci. USA* **83:**1490–1494.

Bosl, G., Whitmore, W., Myers, W., and Goldbey, R., 1983, Phase II trial of 13-*cis*-retinoic acid in the treatment of patients with advanced germ cell tumors, *Proc. Am. Assoc. Cancer Res.* **24:**150.

Brandes, D., Anton, E., Schofield, B., and Barnard, S., 1966, Role of lysosomal labilizers in treatment of mammary gland carcinomas with cyclophosphamide, *Cancer Chemother. Rep.* **50**:47–53.

Bright-See, E., 1983, Vitamin C and cancer prevention, *Semin. Oncol.* **10**:294–298.

Brock, K. E., Berry, G., Mock, P. A., MacLennan, R., Truswell, A. S., and Brinton, L. A., 1988, Nutrients in diet and plasma and risk of *in situ* cervical cancer, *J. Natl. Cancer Inst.* **80**:580–585.

Brown, R. R., Price, J. M., Friedell, G. H., and Burney, S. W., 1969, Tryptophan metabolism in patients with bladder cancer: Geographical differences, *J. Natl. Cancer Inst.* **53**:295–301.

Bryan, G. T., 1986, The influence of niacin and nicotinamide on *in vivo* carcinogenesis, *Adv. Exp. Med. Biol.* **206**:331–338.

Buamah, P. K., James, O. F., Skillen, A. W., and Harris, A. L., 1987, Serum vitamin B_{12} levels in patients with primary hepatocellular carcinoma during treatment with CB3717, *J. Surg. Oncol.* **34**:100–103.

Bulovskaia, L. N., 1976, Acetylation reaction in mice in the normal state and in tumors, *Vopr. Onkol.* **22**:59–63.

Byar, D., and Blackard, C., 1977, Comparisons of placebo, pyridoxine, and topical thiothepa in preventing recurrence of stage 1 bladder cancer, *Urology* **10**:556–561.

Byers, T., Marshall, J., and Graham, S., 1986, Dietary vitamin A and cancer—A multisite case-control study, *Nutr. Cancer* **8**:107–116.

Byers, T. E., Graham, S., Haughey, B. P., Marshall, J. R., and Swanson, M. K., 1987, Diet and lung cancer risk: findings from the Western New York Diet Study, *Am. J. Epidemiol.* **125**:351–363.

Cameron, E., and Campbell, A., 1974, The orthomolecular treatment of cancer. II. Clinical trial of high-dose ascorbic asid supplements in advanced human cancer, *Chem. Biol. Interact.* **9**:285–315.

Cameron, E., and Pauling, L., 1976, Supplemental ascorbate in the supportive treatment of cancer: Prolongation of survival times in terminal human cancer, *Proc. Natl. Acad. Sci. USA* **73**:3685–3689.

Cameron, E., and Pauling, L., 1979a, Supplemental ascorbate in the supportive treatment of cancer: Re-evaluation of prolongation of survival times in terminal human cancer, *Proc. Natl. Acad. Sci. USA* **75**:4538–4542.

Cameron, E., and Pauling, L., 1979b, *Cancer and Vitamin C,* Linus Pauling Institute of Science and Medicine, Menlow Park, CA.

Capel, I., Leach, D., and Dorrell, H., 1983, Vitamin E retards the lipoperoxidation resulting from anticancer drug administration, *Cancer Res.* **43**:59–62.

Carmel, R., 1975, Extreme elevation of serum transcobalamin I in patients with metastatic cancer, *N. Engl. J. Med.* **292**:282–284.

Carmel, R., and Eisenberg, L., 1977, Serum vitamin B_{12} and transcobalamin abnormalities in patients with cancer, *Cancer* **40**:1348–1353.

Carpenter, M. P., 1986, Effects of vitamin E on the immune system, in: *Vitamins and Cancer* (F. L. Meyskens, Jr., and K. N. Prasad, eds.), Humana Press, Clifton, NJ, pp. 199–211.

Cassidy, J., Lippma, M., Lacroix, A., Peck, G., and Ozols, R., 1981, Phase II trial of 13-*cis*-retinoic acid in metastatic breast cancer and other malignancies, *Proc. Am. Soc. Clin. Oncol.* **23**:441.

Chabner, B. A., DeVita, V. T., Livingston, D. M., and Oliverio, V. T., 1970, Abnormalities of tryptophan metabolism and plasma pyridoxal phosphate in Hodgkin's disease, *N. Engl. J. Med.* **282**:838–843.

Chang, M-D., Friedman, F. K., Beychok, S., Shyong, J. S., and Osserman, E. F., 1981, Further studies of the riboflavin-binding immunoglobulin IgG_{gar}. Resolution onto fractions of different riboflavin content and aspects of assembly, *Biochemistry* **20**:2916–2921.

Chester, J. F., Gaissert, H. A., Ross, J. S., Malt, R. A., and Weitzman, S. A., 1986, Augmentation of 1,2-dimethylhydrazine-induced colon cancer by experimental colitis in mice: Role of dietary vitamin E, *J. Natl. Cancer Inst.* **76**:939–942.

Chlebowski, R., Dietrich, M., Akman, S., and Block, J., 1983a, Vitamin K3 (menadione) inhibition of human tumor growth in the soft agar assay system, *Proc. Am. Assoc. Cancer Res.* **24**:563.

Chlebowski, R., Block, J., Dietriich, M., Octay, E., Barth, N., Yanagihara, R., Gota, C., and Ali, I., 1983b, Inhibition of human tumor growth and DNA biosynthetic activity by vitamin K and warfarin *in vitro* and clinical results, *Proc. Am. Assoc. Cancer Res.* **24**:653.

Choi, N. W., Miller, A. B., Fodor, J. G., Jain, M., Howe, G. R., Risch, H. A., and Ruder, A. M., 1987, Consumption of precursors of N-nitroso compounds and human gastric cancer, *IARC Sci. Publ.* **1987**(84):492–496.

Chow, C., Chen, L., Thacker, R., and Griffith, R., 1984, Dietary vitamin E and pulmonary biochemical responses of rats to cigarette smoking, *Environ. Res.* **34**:8–17.

306   *Alfred H. Merrill, Jr. et al.*

Chu, B. C. F., and Lawley, P. D., 1975, Increased urinary excretion of nucleic acid and nicotinamide derivatives by rats after treatment with alkylating reagents, *Chem.–Biol. Interact.* **10**:333–338.

Clamon, G. H., Feld, R., Evans, W. K., Weiner, R. S., Kramer, B. S., Lininger, L. L., Gardner, L. B., Wolfe, E. C., DeWys, W. D., and Hoffman, F. A., 1984, Serum folate and vitamin B$_{12}$ levels in patients with small cell lung cancer, *Cancer* **53**:306–310.

Clopath, P., Smith, V. C., and McCully, K. S., 1975, Growth promotion by homocysteic acid, *Science* **192**:372–374.

Cohen, M., 1972, Enhancement of the antitumor effect of 1,3-bis(2-chloroethyl)-1-nitrosurea by vitamin A and caffeine, *J. Natl. Cancer Inst.* **48**:927–932.

Cohen, M., and Carbone, P. P., 1972, Enhancement of the antitumor effects of 1,3-bis(2-chloroethyl)-1-nitrosourea and cyclophosphamide by Vitamin A, *J. Natl. Cancer Inst.* **48**:921–922.

Cohen, M., Primack, A., Broder, L., and Williams, L., 1977, Vitamin A serum levels and dietary vitamin A intake in lung cancer patients, *Cancer Lett.* **4**:51–54.

Cohen, S., Wattenberg, J., and Bryan, G., 1976, Effect of avitaminosis A and hypervitaminosis A on urinary bladder carciongenicity of N4-5 nitro-2-furyl-2-thiazolyl formamide, *Cancer Res.* **36**:2334–2339.

Colditz, G. A., Stampfer, M. J., and Willett, W. C., 1987, Diet and lung cancer. A review of the epidemiologic evidence in humans, *Arch. Intern. Med.* **147**:157–160.

Coleman, J., III, Walker, A., and Didolkar, M., 1983, Treatment of adriamycin-induced skin ulcers: A prospective controlled study, *J. Surg. Oncol.* **22**:129–135.

Colston, K., and Coombes, R., 1985, Characterization of 1,25 dihydroxyvitamin D$_3$ receptors in rat breast tumor, in: *Vitamin D: Chemical, Biochemical, and Clinical Update, Proceedings of the Sixth Workshop on Vitamin D, Merano, Italy,* (A. W. Norman, K. Schaefer, H.-G. Grigoleit, and D. V. Herrath, eds.), Walter de Gruyter, New York, p. 895.

Colston, K., Colston, M., and Feldman, D., 1981, 1,25-Dihyroxyvitamin D$_3$ and malignant melanoma, *Endocrinology* **108**:1083–86.

Committee on Diet, Nutrition, and Cancer, National Academy of Sciences, 1982, *Diet, Nutrition, and Cancer,* National Academy Press, Washington, DC.

Constantinides, P., and Harkey, M., 1985, Initiation of a transplantable fibrosarcoma by the synergism of two non-initiators, alpha-tocopherol and soya oil, *Virchows Arch.* **405**:285–297.

Cook, M., and McNamara, P., 1980, Effect of dietary vitamin E on dimethylhydrazine-induced colonic tumors in mice, *Cancer Res.* **40**:1329–1331.

Corrocher, R., DeSandre, G., Ambrosetti, A., Pachor, M. L., Bambara, L. M., and Hoffbrand, A. V., 1978, Specific and non-specific folate binding protein in normal and malignant human tissues, *J. Clin. Pathol.* **31**:659–665.

Creagan, E. T., Moertel, C. G., O'Fallon, J. R., Shutt, A. J., O'Connell, M. J., Rubin, J., and Frytak, S., 1979, Failure of high-dose vitamin C (ascorbic acid) therapy to benefit patients with advanced cancer, *N. Engl. J. Med.* **301**:687–690.

Crepaldi, G., and Parpajola, A., 1964, Excretion of tryptophan metabolites in different forms of haemoblastosis, *Clin. Chim. Acta* **9**:106–117.

Daenen, S., Vellenga, E., van Dobbenburgh, O. A., and Halie, M. R., 1986, Retinoic acid as antileukemic therapy in a patient with acute promelocytic leukemia and *Aspergillus pneumonia, Blood* **67**:559–561.

Davies, D., 1967, Effect of vitamin A on 7,12-dimethylbene(a)anthracene-induced papillomas in rhino mouse skin, *Cancer Res.* **27**:237–241.

Dawson, E., Nosovitch, J., and Hannigan, E., 1984, Serum vitamin and selenium changes in cervical dysplasia, *Fed. Proc.* **43**:#1914.

Day, P. L., Payne, L. D., and Dinning, J. S., 1960, Procarcinogenic effect of vitamin B$_{12}$ on *p*-dimethylamino-fed rats, *Proc. Soc. Exp. Biol. Med.* **74**:854–857.

DeLuca, H. F., and Ostrem, V., 1986, The relationship between the vitamin D system and cancer, *Adv. Exp. Med. Biol.* **206**:413–429.

De Reuck, J. L., Sieben, G. J., Sieben-Praet, M. R., Ngendahayo, P., De Coster, J. P., and Vander Eecken, H. M., 1980, Wernicke's encephalopathy in patients with tumors of the lymphoidc systems, *Arch. Neurol.* **37**:338–341.

DiSorbo, D. M., Paavola, L. G., and Litwack, G., 1982, Pyridoxine resistance in a rat hepatoma cell line, *Cancer Res.* **42**:2362–2370.

DiSorbo, D. M., Wagner, R., Jr., and Nathanson, L., 1985, *In vivo* and *in vitro* inhibition of B16 melanoma growth by vitamin B$_6$, *Nutr. Cancer* **7**:43–52.

Dorr, R., and Alberts, D., 1983, Failure of DMSO and vitamin E to prevent doxorubicin skin ulceration in the mouse, *Cancer Treat. Rep.* **67**:499–501.

Douglas, J. F., Huff, J., and Peters, A. C., 1984, No evidence of carcinogenicity of L-ascorbic acid (vitamin C) for rodents, *J. Toxicol. Env. Health* **14**:605–609.

Eichner, E. R., McDonald, C. R., and Dickson, B. A., 1978, Elevated serum levels of unsaturated folate binding protein: Clinical correlates in a general hospital population, *Am. J. Clin. Nutr.* **31**:1988–1992.

Eisman, J., 1985, Regulation of human target cell response to 1,25 dihydroxyvitamin D_3, in: *Vitamin D: Chemical, Biochemical, and Clinical Update*, Proceedings of the Sixth Workshop on Vitamin D, Merano, Italy, (A. W. Norman, K. Schaefer, H.-G. Grigoleit, and D. V. Herrath, eds.), Walter de Gruyter, New York, pp. 879–886.

Eisman, J., MacIntyre, I., Martin, T., and Frampton, R., 1980a, Normal and malignant breast tissue is a target organ for $1,25(OH)_2$ vitamin D_3, *Clin. Endocrinol.* **13**:267–272.

Eisman, J., Martin, T., MacIntyre, I., Frampton, R., Mosley, J., and Whitehead, R., 1980b, 1,25-Dihydroxyvitamin D_3 receptor in a cultured human breast cancer cell line, *Biochem. Biophys. Res. Commun.* **93**:9–15.

England, S., and Seifter, S., 1986, The biochemical functions of ascorbic acid, *Annu. Rev. Nutr.* **6**:365–406.

Enstrom, J. E., Kanim, L. E., and Breslow, L., 1986, The relationship between vitamin C intake, general health practices, and mortality in Alameda County, California, *Am. J. Public Health* **76**:1124–1130.

Epstein, J., 1977, Chemicals and photocarcinogenesis, *Aust. J. Dermatol.* **18**:57–61.

Epstein, J., and Grenkin, D., 1981, Inhibition of ultraviolet-induced carcinogenesis by all-*trans* retinoic acid, *J. Invest. Dermatol.* **76**:178–180.

Epstein, S., Joshi, S., Andrea, J., Forsyth, J., and Mantel, N., 1967, The null effect of antioxidants on the carcinogenecity of 3,4,9,10-dibenzpyrene to mice, *Life Sci.* **6**:225–233.

Erbe, R. W., and Wang, J-C. C., 1984, Folate metabolism in humans, *Am. J. Genet.* **17**:277–287.

Eto, I., and Krumdieck, C. L., 1986, Role of vitamin B_{12} and folate deficiencies in carcinogenesis, *Adv. Exp. Med. Biol.* **206**:313–330.

Evans, C., and Todd, I., 1969, Synkavite and radiotherapy in the treatment of bronchial carcinoma: A randomized trial, *Clin. Radiol.* **20**:228–230.

Farhangi, M., and Osserman, E. F., 1976, Myeloma with xanthoderma due to an IgG monoclonal anti-flavin antibody, *N. Engl. J. Med.* **294**:177–183.

Fiddler, W., Pensabene, J., Piotrowski, E., Philips, J., Keatining, J., Mergens, W., and Newmark, H., 1978, Inhibition of formation of volatile nitrosamines in fried bacon by the use of cure-solubilized alpha-tocopherol, *J. Agric. Food Chem.* **26**:653–56.

Fontana, J. A., Rogers, J. S., and Durham, J. P., 1986, The role of 13 *cis*-retinoic acid in the remission induction of a patient with acute promyelocytic leukemia, *Cancer* **57**:209–217.

Foy, H., and Kondi, A., 1984, The vulnerable esophagus: Riboflavin deficiency and squamous cell dysplasia of the skin and the esophagus, *J. Natl. Cancer Inst.* **72**:941–948.

Foy, H., and Mbaya, V., 1977, Riboflavin, *Prog. Food Nutr. Sci.* **2**:357–394.

Foy, H., Kondi, A., Davies, J. N. P., Anderson, B., Parker, A., Preston, J., and Peers, F. J., 1974, Histologic changes in livers of pyridoxine-deprived baboons—Relation to alpha-fetoprotein and liver cancer in Africa, *J. Natl. Cancer Inst.* **53**:1295–1311.

Frampton, R., Suva, L., Eisman, J., Findley, D., Moore, G., Moseley, J., and Martin, T., 1982, Presence of 1,25-dihydroxyvitamin D_3 receptors in established human cancer cell lines in culture, *Cancer Res.* **42**:1116–1119.

Freake, H., Marocci, C., Iwasaki, J., and MacIntyre, I., 1981, 1,25-Dihydroxyvitamin D_3 specifically binds to a human breast cancer cell line and stimulates growth, *Biochem. Biophys. Res. Commun.* **101**:113–1138.

Fujimaki, I., 1926, Formation of carcinoma in albino rats fed on deficient diets, *J. Cancer Res.* **10**:469–477.

Fujiyama, S., Morishita, T., Hashiguchi, O., and Sato, T., 1988, Plasma abnormal prothrombin (des-gamma-carboxy prothrombin) as a marker of hepatocellular carcinoma, *Cancer* **61**:1621–16288.

Fukushima, S., Shibata, M. A., Shirai, T., Tamano, S., and Ito, N., 1986, Roles of urinary sodium ion concentration and pH in promotion by ascorbic acid of urinary bladder carcinogenesis in rats, *Cancer Res.* **46**:1623–1626.

Gailani, S. D., Holland, N. F., Nussbaum, A., and Olson, K. B., 1968, Chemical and biochemical studies of pyridoxine deficiency in patients with neoplastic diseases, *Cancer* **21**:975–988.

Garland, C., and Garland, F., 1980, Do sunlight and vitamin D reduce the likelihood of colon cancer? *Int. J. Epidemiol.* **9**:227–231.

Garland, C., Shekelle, R., Barrett-Connor, B., Criqui, M., Rossof, A., and Oglesby, P., 1985, Dietary vitamin D and calcium and risk of colorectal cancer, *Lancet* **1**:307–309.

Ghosh, J., and Das, S., 1985, Evaluation of vitamin A and C status in normal and malignant conditions and their possible role in cancer prevention, *Jpn. J. Cancer Res.* **76**:1174–1178.

Ghoshal, A. K., and Farber, E., 1984, The induction of liver cancer by dietary deficiency of choline and methionine without added carcinogens, *Carcinogenesis* **5**:1367–1370.

Ghoshal, A. K., Ahluwalia, M., and Farber, E., 1983, The rapid induction of liver cell death in rats fed a choline-deficient methionine low diet, *Am. J. Pathol.* **113**:309–314.

Giambarresi, L. I., Katyal, S. L., and Lambardi, B., 1982, Promotion of liver carcinogenesis in the rat by a choline-devoid diet: Role of liver cell necrosis and regeneration, *Br. J. Cancer* **46**:825–829.

Gold, E., Mertelsmann, R., Itri, L., Gee, T., Arlen, Z., Kemplin, S., Clarkson, B., and Moore, M., 1983, Phase I clinical trial of 13-*cis*-retinoic acid in myelodysplasitc syndromes, *Cancer Treat. Rep.* **67**:981–986.

Gold, J., 1986, *In vivo* synergy of vitamin K_3 and methotrexate in tumor-bearing animals, *Cancer Treat. Rep.* **70**:1433–1435.

Goodman, G., Alberts, D., Ernst, D., and Meyskens, F., Jr., 1983, Phase I trial of retinol in cancer patients, *J. Clin. Oncol.* **1**:394–399.

Goodwin, T. W., 1986, Metabolism, nutrition, and function of carotenoids, *Annu. Rev. Nutr.* **6**:273–297.

Gouveia, J., Mathew, G., Hergend, T., Gros, F., Lemaigre, G., and Santelli, G., 1982, Degree of bronchial metaplasia in heavy smokers and its regression after treatment with retinoid, *Lancet* **2**:710–712.

Grassetti, D. R., 1986, The antimetastatic and tumor growth retarding effects of sulfur containing analogs of nicotinamide, *Cancer Lett.* **31**:187–195.

Gregor, A., Lee, P., Roe, J., Wilson, M., and Melton, A., 1980, Comparison of dietary histories in lung cancer cases and controls with special reference to Vitamin A, *Nutr. Cancer* **2**:93–97.

Gregory, J. F., III, and Kirk, J. R., 1981, The bioavailability of vitamin B_6 in foods, *Nutr. Rev.* **37**:1–8.

Gridley, D. S., Stickney, D. R., Nutter, R. L., Slater, J. M., and Shultz, T. I., 1987, Suppression of tumor growth and enhancement of immune status with high levels of dietary vitamin B_6 in BALB/c mice, *J. Natl. Cancer Inst.* **78**:951–959.

Grosse, W., III, and Wade, A. E., 1971, The effects of thiamine consumption on liver microsomal drug-metabolizing pathways, *J. Pharmacol. Exp. Ther.* **176**:758–768.

Ha, C., Kerkvilet, N. I., Miller, L. T., 1984, The effect of vitamin B_6 dificiency on host susceptibility to Maloney sarcoma virus-induced tumor growth in mice, *J. Nutr.* **114**:938–945.

Haber, S., and Wissler, R., 1962, Effect of vitamin E on carcinogenicity of methylcholanthrene, *Proc. Soc. Exp. Biol. Med.* **111**:774–775.

Haenszel, W., Correa, P., Lopez, A., Cuello, C., Zarama, G., and Fontham, E., 1985, Serum micronutrient levels in relation to gastric pathology, *Int. J. Cancer* **36**:43–48.

Hall, C. A., and Wanko, M., 1971, Increased transcobalamin I in a leukemoid reaction, *J. Lab. Clin. Med.* **78**:298–301.

Halpern, R., Halpern, B. C., Stea, B., Dunlap, A., Conklin, K., Clark, B., Ashe, H., Sperling, L., Halpern, J. A., Hardy, D., and Smith, R. A., 1977, Pterin-6-aldehyde. A cancer cell catabolite: Identification and application in diagnosis and treatment of human cancer, *Proc. Natl. Acad. Sci. USA* **74**:587–591.

Hanck, A., 1986, Ascorbic acid and cancer, in: *Vitamins and Cancer* (F. L. Meyskens, Jr., and K. N. Prasad, eds.), Humana Press, Clifton, NJ, pp. 365–397.

Hanck, A. B., 1988, Vitamin C and cancer, *Prog. Clin. Biol. Res.* **259**:307–320.

Hara, T., and Taniguchi, M., 1985, Relationship between the changes in properties and contents of riboflavin derivatives of NADPH–cytochrome P450 reductase in liver microsomes of riboflavin-deficient rats, *J. Biochem. (Tokyo)* **97**:473–482.

Harada, T., Kitazawa, T., Maita, K., and Shirasu, Y., 1985, Effects of vitamin C on tumor induction by diethylnitrosamine in the respiratory tract of hamsters exposed to cigarette smoke, *Cancer Lett.* **25**:163–169.

Harmon, D., 1969, Dimethylbenzanthracene induced cancer: Inhibiting effect of dietary vitamin E, *Clin. Res.* **17**:125.

Hausen, A., Fuchs, D., Grunewald, K., Huber, H., Konig, K., and Wachter, H., 1982, Urinary neopterine in the assessment of lymphoid and myeloid neoplasia and neopterine levels in haemolytic anemia and benign monoclonal gammopathy, *Clin. Biochem.* **15**:34–37.

Haussler, C. A., Marion, S. L., Pike, J. W., and Haussler, M. R., 1986, 1,25-Dihydroxyvitamin D_3 inhibits the clonogenic growth of transformed cells via its receptor, *Biochem. Biophys. Res. Commun.* **139**:136–143.

Haydey, R., Reed, M., Dzubow, L., and Shupack, J., 1980, Treatment of keratocanthomas with oral 13-*cis*-retinoic acid, *N. Engl. J. Med.* **303**:560–562.

Heimburger, D. C., Alexander, C. B., Birch, R., Butterworth, C. E., Jr., Bailey, W. C., and Krumdieck, C. L., 1988, Improvement in bronchial squamous metaplasia in smokers treated with folate and vitamin B_{12}. Report of a preliminary randomized, double-blind intervention trial, *JAMA* **259**:1525–1530.

Hellman, S., Ianotti, A. T., and Bertino, J. R., 1964, Determinations of the levels of serum folate in patients with carcinoma of the head and neck treated with methotrexate, *Cancer Res.* **24**:105–113.

Helson, L., 1984, A trial of vitamin E in neuroectodermal tumors, *Proc. Am. Soc. Clin. Oncol.* **3**:80.

Henderson, L. M., 1983, Niacin, *Annu. Rev. Nutr.* **3**:289–307.

Herbert, V., 1986, The role of vitamin B_{12} and folate in carcinogenesis, *Adv. Exp. Med. Biol.* **206**:293–311.

Hill, D. L., and Grubbs, C. J., 1982, Retinoids as chemopreventive and anticancer agents in intact animals, *Anticancer Res.* **2**:111–124.

Hinds, M., Kolonel, L., Hankin, J., and Lee, J., 1984, Dietary vitamin A, carotene, vitamin C, and risk of lung cancer in Hawaii, *Am. J. Epidemiol.* **119**:227–237.

Hirano, H., Hamajima, S., Horiiuchi, S., Niitsu, Y., and Ono, S., 1983, Effects of B_2-deficiency on lipoperoxide and its scavenging system in the rat lens, *Int. J. Vit. Nutr. Res.* **53**:377–382.

Hirayama, T., 1979, Diet and cancer, *Nutr. Cancer* **1**:67–81.

Hoffman, F. A., 1985, Micronutrient requirements of cancer patients, *Cancer* **55**:295–300.

Hoogstraten, B., Baker, H., and Reizenstein, R., 1961, Correlation between serum folic acid activity and response to anti-folate therapy, *Blood* **18**:787.

Hoover, K. L., Lynch, P. H., and Poirier, L. A., 1984, Profound postinitiation enhancement by short-term severe methionine, choline, vitamin B_{12}, and folate deficiency of hepatocarcinogenesis in F344 rats given a single low-dose diethylnitrosamine injection, *J. Natl. Cancer Inst.* **73**:1327–1336.

Horiuchi, S., and Ono, S., 1984, Effects of riboflavin administration on the phospholipid metabolism of rat liver impaired with carbon tetrachloride, *Int. J. Vit. Nutr. Res.* **54**:173–177.

Horsman, M. R., Chaplin, D. J., and Brown, J. M., 1987, Radiosensitization by nicotinamide *in vivo:* A greater enhancement of tumor damage compared to that of normal tissues, *Radiat. Res.* **109**:479–489.

Horwitt, M., 1980, Therapeutic uses of vitamin E in medicine, *Nutr. Rev.* **38**:105–113.

Horwitt, M. K., 1986, The promotion of vitamin E, *J. Nutr.* **116**:1371–1377.

Howard, W. B., and Willhite, C. C., 1986, Toxicity of retinoids in humans and animals, *J. Toxicol.–Toxin Rev.* **5**:55–94.

Hulshof, K. F., Gooskens, A. C., Wedel, M., and Bruning, P. F., 1987, Food intake in three groups of cancer patients. A prospective study during cancer treatment, *Hum. Nutr. Appl. Nutr.* **41**:23–37.

Inculet, R. I., Norton, J. A., Nichoalds, G. E., Maher, M. M., White, D. E., and Brennan, M. F., 1987, Water-soluble vitamins in cancer patients on parenteral nutrition: A prospective study, *J. Parenter. Enter. Nutr.* **11**:243–249.

Ink, S. L., and Henderson, L. M., 1984, Vitamin B_6 metabolism, *Annu. Rev. Nutr.* **4**:455–470.

Innis, W. S. A., McCormick, D. B., and Merrill, A. H., Jr., 1985, Variations in riboflavin binding by human plasma: Identification of immunoglobulins as the major proteins responsible, *Biochem. Med.* **34**:151–165.

Innis, W. S. A., Nixon, D. W., Murray, D. R., McCormick, D. B., and Merrill, A. H., Jr., 1986, Immunoglobulins associated with elevated riboflavin binding by plasma from cancer patients, *Proc. Soc. Exp. Biol. Med.* **181**:237–241.

Ip, C., 1982, Dietary vitamin E and mammary carcinogenesis in rats, *Carcinogenesis* **3**:1453–1456.

Ip, C., 1988, Feasibility of using lower doses of chemopreventive agents in a combination regimen for cancer protection, *Cancer Lett.* **39**:239–246.

Israels, L., Walls, G., Ollmann, D., Friesen, E., and Israels, E., 1983, Vitamin K as a regulator of benzo(a)pyrene metabolism, mutagenesis, and carcinogenesis, *J. Clin. Invest.* **71**:1130–1140.

Ito, Y., 1981, Effect of an aromatic retinoic acid analog on growth of virus-induced papilloma and related neoplasias of rabbits, *Eur. J. Cancer* **17**:35–42.

Jacobson, E. L., Smith, J. Y., Mingmuang, M., Meadows, R., Sims, J. L., and Jacobson, M. K., 1984, Effect of nicotinamide analogues on recovery from DNA damage in C3H10T1/2 cells, *Cancer Res.* **44**:2485–2492.

Jacobson, M. K., Levi, V., Juarez-Salinas, H., Barton, R. A., and Jacobson, E. L., 1980, Effect of carcinogenic *N*-alkyl-*N*-nitroso compounds on nicotinamide adenine dinucleotide metabolism, *Cancer Res.* **40**:1797–1802.

Jaffe, W., 1946, The influence of wheat germ oil on the production of tumors in rats by methylcholanthrene, *Exp. Med. Surg.* **4:**278–282.

Kagan, Y. A., 1957, The effect of internal administration of riboflavine on the content of riboflavine in the urine of cancer patients, *Patol. Fiziol. Eksp. Ter.* **1:**44–48.

Kagan, Y. A., 1960, Riboflavin determination in the urine of patients suffering from malignant neoplasms, *Khirurgiya* **2:**103–108.

Kagerud, A., and Peterson, H., 1981, Tocopherol in tumor irradiation, *Anticancer Res.* **1:**35–38.

Kagerud, A., Klintenberg, C., Lund, N., and Peterson, H., 1980, Influence of tocopherol on tumor cell oxygenation, *Cancer Lett.* **5:**185–9.

Kamiyama, S., Ohshima, H., Shimada, A., Saito, N., Bourgade, M. C., Ziegler, P., and Bartsch, H., 1987, Urinary excretion of *N*-nitrosamino acids and nitrate by inhabitants in high- and low-risk areas for stomach cancer in northern Japan, *IARC Sci. Publ.* **1987**(84):497–502.

Kaplan, H. S., and Rigler, L. G., 1945, Pernicious anemia and carcinoma of the stomach. Autopsy studies concerning their interrelationship, *Am. J. Med. Sci.* **209:**339–348.

Kaplan, I. I., 1944, One year observation of the treatment of cancer with avidin (egg white), *Am. J. Med. Sci.* **207:**733–743.

Kark, J., Smith, A., Sitzer, B., and Hames, C., 1981, Serum vitamin A and cancer incidence in Evans County, Georgia, *J. Natl. Cancer Inst.* **66:**7–16.

Kato, T., Suzumura, Y., and Fukushima, M., 1988, Enhancement of blemoycin activity by 3-aminobenzamide, a poly (ADP-ribose) synthesis inhibitor, *in vitro* and *in vivo*, *Anticancer Res.* **8:**239–243.

Katsouyanni, K., Willett, W., Trichopoulos, D., Boyle, P., Trichopoulou, A., Vasilaros, S., Papadiamantis, J., and MacMahon, B., 1988, Risk of breast cancer among Greek women in relation to nutrient intake, *Cancer* **61:**181–185.

Kaul, L., Heshmat, M. Y., Kovi, J., Jackson, M. A., Jackson, A. G., Jones, G. W., Edson, M., Enterline, J. P., Worrell, R. G., and Perry, S. L., 1987, The role of diet in prostate cancer, *Nutr. Cancer* **9:**123–128.

Kayden, H., Hatam, L., and Traber, M., 1984, Reduced tocopherol content of B cells from patients with chronic lymphocytic leukemia, *Blood* **63:**213–215.

Kazarinoff, M. N., and McCormick, D. B., 1975, Rabbit liver pyridoxamine (pyridoxine) 5'-phosphate oxidase: Purification and properties, *J. Biol. Chem.* **250:**3436–3442.

Kensler, C. J., Sugiura, K., Young, N. F., Halter, C. R., and Rhoads, C. P., 1941, Partial protection of rats by riboflavin with casein against liver cancer caused by dimethylaminobenzene, *Science* **93:**308–310.

Kiefer, C. R., McGuire, B. S., Osserman, E. F., and Garver, F. A., 1983, The modeled structure of the IgG$_{Gar}$ VL region and its implications for anti-flavin and anti-DNP fine specificities, *J. Immunol.* **131:**1871–1875.

King, M., and McCay, P., 1983, Modulation of tumor incidence and possible mechanism of inhibition of mammary carcinogenesis by dietary antioxidants, *Cancer Res.* **43:**2485–2490.

Kinn, A-C., and Lantz, B., 1984, Vitamin B$_{12}$ deficiency after irradiation for bladder carcinoma, *J. Urol.* **131:**888–890.

Kirkemo, A. K., Burt, M. E., and Brennan, M. F., 1982, Serum vitamin level maintenance in cancer patients on total parenteral nutrition, *Am. J. Clin. Nutr.* **35:**1003–1009.

Kjellen, E., Pero, R. W., Cameron, R., and Ranstam, J., 1986, Radiosensitizing effects of nicotinamide on a C3H mouse mammary adenocarcinoma. A study on per os drug administration, *Acta Radiol. (Oncol.)* **25:**281–284.

Kline, B. E., Rusch, H. P., Bauman, C. A., and Lavik, P. S., 1943, The effect of pyridoxine on tumor growth, *Cancer Res.* **3:**825–829.

Kline, B. E., Miller, J. A., and Rusche, H. P., 1945, Certain effects of egg white and biotin on the carcinogenicity of *p*-dimethylaminoazobenzene in rats fed a sub-protective level of riboflavin, *Cancer Res.* **5:**641–643.

Knekt, P., Aromaa, A., Maatela, J., Aaran, R. K., Nikkari, T., Hakama, M., Hakulinen, T., Peto, R., Saxen, E., and Teppo, L., 1988, Serum vitamin E and risk of cancer among Finnish men during a 10-year follow-up, *Am. J. Epidemiol.* **127:**28–41.

Koch, H., 1978, Biochemical treatment of precancerous oral lesions: The effectiveness of various analogs of retinoic acid, *J. Max-Fac. Surg.* **6:**59–63.

Kokolis, N., and Ziegler, I., 1977, On the levels of phenylalanine, tyrosine, and tetrahydrobiopterin in the blood of tumor-bearing organisms, *Cancer Biochem. Biophys.* **2:**79–85.

Kolonel, L. N., Hankin, J. H., and Yoshizawa, C. N., 1987, Vitamin A and prostate cancer in elderly men: Enhancement of risk, *Cancer Res.* **47:**2982–2985.

Korpela, J., 1984, Avidin, a high affinity biotin-binding protein, as a tool and subject of biological research, *Med. Biol.* **62:**5–26.

Korytnyk, W., 1979, Synthesis and biological activity of vitamin B$_6$ analogs, *Meth. Enzymol.* **62:**454–483.

Kozik, A., and McCormick, D. B., 1984, Mechanism of pyridoxine uptake by isolated rat liver cells, *Arch. Biochem. Biophys.* **229:**187–193.

Krishnamurthi, S., Shanta, V., and Sastri, D., 1971, Combined therapy in bucal mucosal cancers, *Radiology* **99:**409–415.

Kull, F. C., Jr., Brent, D. A., Parikh, I., and Cuatrecasas, P., 1987, Chemical identification of a tumor-derived angiogenic factor, *Science* **236:**843–845.

Kune, S., Kune, G. A., and Watson, L. F., 1987, Case–control study of dietary etiological factors: The Melbourne Colorectal Cancer Study, *Nutr. Cancer* **9:**21–42.

Kurl, R. N., and Villee, C. A., 1985, A metabolite of riboflavin binds to the 2,3,7,8-tetrachlorodibenzo-*p*-dioxin (TCDD) receptor, *Pharmacology* **30:**241–244.

Kvale, G., Bjelke, E., and Gart, J., 1983, Dietary habits and lung cancer risk, *Br. J. Cancer* **31:**397–405.

Kyle, R., and Jowsey, J., 1980, Effect of sodium fluoride, calcium carbonate and vitamin D on the skeleton in multiple myeloma, *Cancer* **45:**1669–1674.

Ladner, H. A., and Holtz, F., 1979, Zum verhalten einiger B-vitamine nach strahlen und/oder zytostatikabehandlung gynakolischer karzinome, *Strahlentherapie* **75:**191–195.

Ladner, H. A., and Salkeld, R. M., 1988, Vitamin B$_6$ status in cancer patients: Effect of tumor site, irradiation, hormones and chemotherapy, *Prog. Clin. Biol. Res.* **259:**273–281.

Lane, M., 1971, Induced riboflavin deficiency in treatment of patients with lymphomas and polycythemia vera, *Proc. Am. Assoc. Cancer Res.* **12:**85.

Lawson, T., 1983, Nicotinamide stimulates the repair of carcinogen-induced DNA damage in the hamster pancreas *in vitro*, *Anticancer Res.* **3:**207–210.

Lea, M. A., Barra, R., and Randolph, V., 1984, Effects of nicotinamide and structural analogs on DNA synthesis and cellular replication of rat hepatoma cells, *Cancer Biochem. Biophys.* **7:**195–202.

Lee, C., and Chen, C., 1979, Enhancement of mammary tumorigenesis in rats by vitamin E deficiency, *Proc. Am. Assoc. Cancer Res.* **20:**132.

Lenzen, S., Koppel, G., and Panten, U., 1985, Secretory, enzymatic, and morphological characterization of rat pancreatic endocrine tumours induced by streptozotocin and nicotinamide, *Acta Endocrinol.* **109:**361–368.

Levij, I. S., and Pollack, M. B., 1968, Potentiating effect of vitamin A on 9–10 dimethyl, 1,2-benzathracene-carcinogenesis in the hamster cheek pouch, *Cancer* **22:**300–306.

Levine, N., and Meyskens, F., 1980, Topical vitamin-A-acid therapy for cutaneous metastatic melanoma, *Lancet* **2:**224–226.

Loescher, L., and Sauer, K., 1984, Vitamin therapy for advanced cancers, *Oncol. Nurs. Forum* **11:**38–45.

Lombardi, B., and Shinozuka, H., 1979, Enhancement of 2-AAF liver carcinogenesis in rats fed a choline-deficient diet, *Int. J. Cancer* **23:**565–570.

London, R., Sundaram, G., and Schultz, M., 1981, Endocrine parameters and alpha-tocopherol therapy of patients with mammary dysplasia, *Cancer Res.* **41:**3811–3813.

Lopez, S., and LeGardeur, B., 1982, Vitamin A, C, and E in relation to lung cancer incidence, *Am. J. Clin. Nutr.* **35:**851.

Lopez, S., LeGarrdeur, B., and Johnson, W., 1981, Vitamin A status and lung cancer, *Am. J. Clin. Nutr.* **34:**641.

Lu, S. H., Ohshima, H., Fu, H. M., Tian, Y., Li, F. M., Blettner, M., Wahrendorf, J., and Bartsch, H., 1986, Urinary excretion of *N*-nitrosoamino acids and nitrate by inhabitants of high- and low-risk areas for esophageal cancer in Northern China: Endogenous formation of nitrosoproline and its inhibition by vitamin C, *Cancer Res.* **46:**1485–1491.

Ludgate, S. M., and Merrick, M. V., 1985, The pathogenesis of post-irradiation chronic diarrhea: Measurement of SeHCAT and B$_{12}$ adsorption for differential diagnosis determines treatment, *Clin. Radiol.* **36:**275–278.

Lutzner, M., and Blanchet-Bardon, C., 1980, Oral retinoid treatment of human papillomavirus type 5 induced epidermodysplasia verruciformis, *N. Engl. J. Med.* **302:**1091.

Lyon, J. L., Mahoney, A. W., West, D. W., Gardner, J. W., Smith, K. R., Sorenson, A. W., and Stanish, W., 1987, Energy intake: Its relationship to colon cancer risk, *J. Natl. Cancer Inst.* **78:**853–861.

MacLennon, R., Dacosta, J., Day, N., Law, C., Ng, Y., and Shanmugarartnam, K., 1977, Risk factors for lung cancer in Singapore Chinese, *Int. J. Cancer* **20:**854–860.

Mahmoud, L., and Robinson, W., 1982, Vitamin A levels in human bladder cancer, *Int. J. Cancer* **30:**143–145.

Malick, M., Roy, R., and Sternberg, J., 1978, Effect of vitamin E on post-irradiation death in mice, *Experiential* **34**:1216–1217.

Manolagas, S. C., 1987, Vitamin D and its relevance to cancer, *Anticancer Res.* **7**:625–638.

Marcus, S. L., Dutcher, J. P., Paietta, E., Ciobanu, N., Strauman, J., Wiernik, P. H., Hutner, S. H., Frank, O., and Baker, H., 1987, Severe hypovitaminosis C occurring as the result of adoptive immunotherapy with high-dose interleukin 2 and lymphokine-activated killer cells, *Cancer Res.* **47**:4208–4212.

Marshall, J., Graham, S., and Mettlin, C., 1982, Diet in the epidemiology of oral cancer, *Nutr. Cancer* **3**:145–149.

Martin, T., Findlay, D., MacIntyre, I., Eisamn, J., Michelangeli, V., Moseley, J., and Partridge, N., 1980, Calcitonin receptors in a cloned human breast cancer cell line, *Biochem. Biophys. Res. Commun.* **96**:150–156.

Marubini, E., Decarli, A., Costa, A., Mazzoleni, C., Andreoli, C., Barbieri, A., Capitelli, E., Carlucci, M., Cavallo, F., Monferroni, N., Pastorino, U., and Salvini, S., 1988, The relationship of dietary intake and serum levels of retinol and beta-carotene with breast cancer. Results of a case-control study, *Cancer* **61**:173–180.

McCay, P. B., 1985, Vitamin E: Interaction with free radicals and ascorbate, *Annu. Rev. Nutr.* **5**:323–340.

McCormick, D., Burns, F., and Albert, R., 1980, Inhibition of rat mammary carcinogenesis by short dietary exposure to retinyl acetate, *Cancer Res.* **40**:1140–1143.

McCormick, D. L., May, C. M., Thomas, C. F., and Detrisac, C. J., 1986, Anticarcinogenic and hepatotoxic interactions between retinyl acetate and butylated hydroxytoluene in rats, *Cancer Res.* **46**:5264–5269.

Meisler, N. T., and Thanassi, J. W., 1988, Vitamin B_6 metabolism in McA-RH7777 cells, *Cancer Res.* **48**:1080–1085.

Mendelson, R. W., Watkin, D. M., Horbett, A. P., and Fahey, J. L., 1958, Identification of the vitamin B_{12}-binding protein in the serum of normals and of patients with chronic myelocytic leukemia, *Blood* **13**:740–747.

Menkes, M., and Comstock, J., 1984, Vitamins A and E and lung cancer, *Am. J. Epidemiol.* **120**:491.

Menkes, M. S., Comstock, G. W., Vuilleumier, J. P., Helsing, K. J., Rider, A. A., and Brookmeyer, R., 1986, Serum beta-carotene, vitamins A and E, selenium, and the risk of lung cancer, *N. Engl. J. Med.* **315**:1250–1254.

Mergens, W., Vane, F., Tannenbaum, S., Green, L., and Skipper, P., 1979, *In vitro* nitrosation of methapyrilene, *J. Pharm. Sci.* **68**:827–832.

Merrill, A. H., Jr., and Henderson, J. M., 1987, Diseases associated with defects in vitamin B_6 metabolism or utilization, *Annu. Rev. Nutr.* **7**:137–156.

Merrill, A. H., Jr., and McCormick, D. B., 1980, Affinity chromatographic purification and properties of flavokinase (ATP:riboflavin 5'-phosphotransferase) from rat liver, *J. Biol. Chem.* **255**:1335–1338.

Merrill, A. H., Jr., Lambeth, J. D., Edmondson, D. E., and McCormick, D. B., 1981, Formation and mode of action of flavoproteins, *Annu. Rev. Nutr.* **1**:281–317.

Mettlin, C., 1986, Changing the public's health behaviors by diet and chemopreventive interventions, in: *Vitamins and Cancer* (F. L. Meyskens, Jr., and K. N. Prasad, eds.), Humana Press, Clifton, NJ, pp. 257–266.

Mettlin, C., and Graham, S., 1979, Dietary risk factors in human bladder cancer, *Am. J. Epidemiol.* **110**:255–263.

Mettlin, C., Graham, S., and Swanson, M., 1979, Vitamin A and lung cancer, *J. Natl. Cancer Inst.* **62**:1435–1438.

Meyer, L. M., Bertcher, R. W., Cronkite, E. P., Suarez, R. M., Miller, I. F., Mulzac, I. F., and Olivarreta, S. T., 1961, Co60 vitamin B_{12} binding capacity of serum in persons with hematologic disorders, various medical diseases and neoplasms, *Acta Med. Scand.* **169**:557–575.

Meyskens, F. L., and Prasad, K. N. (eds.), 1986, *Vitamins and Cancer,* Humana Press, Clifton, NJ.

Meyskens, Jr., F., Gilmartin, E., Alberts, D., Levine, N., Brooks, R., Dalmon, S., and Surwit, E., 1982, Activity of isoretinoin against squamous cell cancers and preneoplastic lesions, *Cancer Treat. Rep.* **66**:1315–1319.

Mickshe, M., Cerni, C., Kokron, O., Titscher, R., and Wrba, H., 1977, Stimulation of immune response in lung cancer patients by vitamin A therapy, *Oncology* **34**:234–238.

Mihich, E., and Nichol, C. A., 1959, The effect of pyridoxine deficiency on mouse sarcoma 180, *Cancer Res.* **19**:279–284.

Mikol, Y. B., Hoover, K. L., Creasia, D., and Poirier, L. A., 1983, Hepatocarcinogenesis in rats fed methyl-deficient, amino acid-defined diets, *Carcinogenesis* **4**:1619–1629.

Miller, E. G., and Burns, H., Jr., 1984, *N*-Nitrosodimethylamine carcinogenesis in nicotinamide-deficient rats, *Cancer Res.* **44**:1478–1482.

Miller, J. A., and Miller, E. C., 1953, The carcinogenic aminoazo dyes, *Adv. Cancer Res.* **1**:339–396.

Mills, E., 1983, The role of vitamin A in cancer, *South Afr. Med. J.* **63**:74–77.

Mirvish, S. S., 1986, Effects of vitamins C and E on N-nitroso compound formation, carcinogenesis, and cancer, *Cancer* **58**(Suppl.):1842–1850.

Mitchell, J., 1960, Clinical assessment of tetra-sodium 2-methyl-1,4-napthahydroquinone diphosphate as a radiosensitizer in the radiotherapy of malignant tumors, *Br. J. Cancer* **7**:140.

Mitchell, J., Brinkley, D., and Haybrittle, J., 1965, Clinical trial of radiosensitizers, including synkavit and oxygen inhales at atmospheric pressure, *Acta Radiol. Ther. Physiol. Biol.* **3**:329–341.

Miyata, Y., Fukushima, S., Hirose, M., Masui, T., and Ito, N., 1985, Short-term screening of promoters of bladder carcionogenesis in *N*-butyl-*N*-(4-hydroxybutyl)nitrosamine-initiated, unilaterally ureter-ligated rats, *Jpn. J. Cancer Res.* **76**:828–834.

Miyaura, C., Abe, E., Koribayashi, T., Tanaka, H., Konno, K., Nishii, Y., and Suda, T., 1981, 1α,25-Dihydroxyvitamin D₃ induces differentiation of human myeloid leukemia cells, *Biochem. Biophys. Res. Comm.* **102**:937–943.

Moertel, C. G., Fleming, T. R., Creagan, E. T., Rubin, J., O'Connell, M. J., and Ames, M. M., 1985, High-dose vitamin C versus placebo in the treatment of patients with advanced cancer who have had no prior chemotherapy, *N. Engl. J. Med.* **312**:137–141.

Moon, R., Grubbs, C., Spron, M., and Goodman, D., 1977, Retinyl acetate inhibits mammary carcinogenesis induced by *N*-methyly-*N*-nitrosurea, *Nature* **267**:620–621.

Moon, R. C., McCormick, D. L., and Mehta, R. G., 1986a, Retinoids as chemotherapeutic agents: Alone and in combination, in: *Vitamins and Cancer* (F. L. Meyskens, Jr., and K. N. Prasad, eds.), Humana Press, Clifton, NJ, pp. 161–180.

Moon, T. E., Rodney, S., Peng, Y-M., Alberts, D. S., and Meyskens, F. L., Jr., 1986b, Design and compliance considerations of dietary intervention trials, in: *Vitamins and Cancer* (F. L. Meyskens, Jr., and K. N. Prasad, eds.), Humana Press, Clifton, NJ, pp. 267–282.

Morishige, F., Nakamura, T., Nakamura, N., and Morishige, N., 1986, The role of vitamin C in tumor therapy (human), in: *Vitamins and Cancer* (F. L. Meyskens, Jr., and K. N. Prasad, eds.), Humana Press, Clifton, NJ, pp. 399–427.

Morris, H. P., 1941, Effect of pantothenic acid on growth of the spontaneous mammary carcinoma in female C3H mice, *J. Natl. Cancer Inst.* **2**:47–54.

Morris, H. P., 1947, Effects on the genesis and growth of tumors associated with vitamin intake, *Ann. NY Acad. Sci.* **49**:119–140.

Munoz, N., Wahrendorf, J., Bang, L. J., Crespi, M., Thurnham, D. I., Day, N. E., Ji, Z. H., Grassii, A., Yan, L. W., Lin, L. G., Quan, L. Y., Yun, Z. C., Fang, Z. S., Yao, L. J., Correa, P., O'Conor, G. T., and Bosch, X., 1985, No effect of riboflavine, retinol, and zinc on prevalence of precancerous lesions of oesophagus, *Lancet* **2**:111–114.

Munoz, N., Hayashi, M., Bang, L. J., Wahrendorf, J., Crespi, M., and Bosch, F. X., 1988, Effect of riboflavin, retinol, and zinc on micronuclei of buccal mucosa and of esophagus: A randomized double-blind intervention study in China, *J. Natl. Cancer Inst.* **79**:687–691.

Murer-Orlando, M. L., and Peterson, A. C., 1985, *In situ* nick translation of human and mouse chromosomes detected with a biotinylated nucleotide, *Exp. Cell Res.* **157**:322–334.

Myers, C., McGuire, W., and Young, R., 1976, Adriamycin amelioration of toxicity by alpha tocopherol, *Cancer Treat. Rep.* **60**:961–962.

Narisawa, T., Reddy, B., Wong, Q., and Weisburger, J., 1976, Effect of vitamin A deficiency on rat colon carcinogenesis, *Cancer Res.* **36**:1379–1383.

National Research Council, 1989, *Diet and Health. Implications for reducing chronic disease risk,* Committee on Diet and Health, Food and Nutrition Board, Commission on Life Sciences, National Research Council, National Academy Press, Washington D.C.

Nduka, N., Skidmore, C. J., and Shall, S., 1980, The enhancement of cytotoxicity of *N*-methyl-*N*-nitrosourea and of gamma-radiation by inhibitors of poly(ADP-ribose) polymerase, *Eur. J. Biochem.* **105**:525–530.

Nettlesheim, P., 1980, Inhibition of carcinogenesis by retinoids, *Can. Med. Assoc. J.* **122**:757–765.

Nettlesheim, P., and Williams, M., 1976, The influence of vitamin A on the susceptibility of rat lung to 3-methylcholanthrene, *Int. J. Cancer* **17**:351–357.

Newberne, P. M., 1986, Lipotropic factors and oncogenesis, *Adv. Exp. Med. Biol.* **206**:223–251.

Newberne, P., and Rogers, A., 1973, Rat colon carcinogenesis associated with aflatoxin and marginal vitamin A, *J. Natl. Cancer Inst.* **50**:439–448.

Newberne, P. M., and Rogers, A. E., 1986, Labile methyl groups and the promotion of cancer, *Annu. Rev. Nutr.* **6**:407–432.

Newberne, P. M., and Suphakarn, V., 1984, Influence of the antioxidants vitamins C and E and of selenium on cancer, in: *Vitamins, Nutrition, and Cancer* (K. N. Prasad, ed.), Karger, Basel, pp. 46–67.

Nexo, E., Olesen, H., Norredam, K., and Schwartz, M., 1975, A rare case of megaloblastic anaemia caused by disturbances in the plasma cobalamin binding proteins in a patient with hepatocellular carcinoma, *Scand. J. Haematol.* **14**:320–327.

Nichol, C. A., Smith, G. K., and Duch, D. S., 1985, Biosynthesis and metabolism of tetrahydrobiopterin and molybdopterin, *Annu. Rev. Biochem.* **54**:729–764.

Nomura, A., Stemmermann, G., Heilbrun, L., Salkeld, R., and Vuillemier, J., 1985, Serum vitamin levels and the risk of cancer of specific sites in men of Japanese ancestry in Hawaii, *Cancer Res.* **45**:2369–2372.

Nutrition Policy Board, Department of Health and Human Services, 1988, *The Surgeon General's Report on Nutrition and Health,* U.S. Department of Health and Human Services, U.S. Government Printing Office, Washington, DC, (DHHA(PHS) Publication No. 88-50210.

Nutter, L. M., Meisler, N. T., and Thanassi, J. W., 1983, Absence of pyridoxine-(pyridoxamine-) 5'-phosphate oxidase in Morris hepatoma 7777, *Biochemistry* **22**:1599–1604.

O'Connor, H. J., Habibzedah, N., Schorah, C. J., Axon, A. T., Riley, S. E., and Garner, R. C., 1985, Effect of increased intake of vitamin C on the mutagenic activity of gastric juice and intragastric concentrations of ascorbic acid, *Carcinogenesis* **6**:1675–1676.

Odukoya, O., Hawach, F., and Shklar, G., 1984, Retardation of experimental oral cancer by topical vitamin E, *Nutr. Cancer* **6**:98–104.

Ohno, Y., Yoshida, O., Oishi, K., Okada, K., Yamabe, H., and Schroeder, F. H., 1988, Dietary beta-carotene and cancer of the prostate: A case-control study in Kyoto, Japan, *Cancer Res.* **48**:1331–1336.

Olson, J. A., 1987, Recommended dietary intakes (RDI) of vitamin A in humans, *Am. J. Clin. Nutr.* **45**:704–716.

Olson, J. A., and Hodges, R. E., 1987, Recommended dietary intakes (RDI) of vitamin C in humans, *Am. J. Clin. Nutr.* **45**:693–703.

Ong, D., and Chytil, F., 1983, Vitamin A and cancer, *Vit. Horm.* **40**:105–44.

Pacernick, L. J., Soltani, K., and Lorincz, A. L., 1975, The inefficacy of riboflavin against ultraviolet-induced carcinogenesis, *J. Invest. Dermat.* **65**:547–548.

Paganini-Hill, A., Chao, A., Ross, R. K., and Henderson, B. E., 1987, Vitamin A, beta-carotene, and the risk of cancer: A prospective study, *J. Natl. Cancer Inst.* **79**:443–448.

Park, C. H., 1985, Biological nature of the effect of ascorbic acids on the growth of human leukemic cells, *Cancer Res.* **45**:3969–3973.

Pascoe, G. A., Olafsdottir, K., and Reed, D. J., 1987, Vitamin E protection against chemical-induced cell injury. I. Maintenance of cellular protein thiols as a cytoprotective mechanism. *Arch. Biochem. Biophys.* **256**:150–158.

Pastorino, U., Pisani, P., Berrino, F., Andreoli, C., Barbieri, A., Costa, A., Mazzoleni, C., Gramegna, G., and Marubini, E., 1987, Vitamin A and female lung cancer: A case–control study in plasma and diet, *Nutr. Cancer* **10**:171–179.

Patek, P., Collins, J., Yogeeswaran, G., and Dennert, G., 1979, Antitumor potential of retinoic acid, *Int. J. Cancer* **24**:624–628.

Pauling, L., and Moertel, C., 1986, A proposition: Megadoses of vitamin C are valuable in the treatment of cancer, *Nutr. Rev.* **44**:28–32.

Pauling, L., Willoughby, R., Reynolds, R., Blaisdell, B., and Lawson, S., 1982, Incidence of squamous cell carcinoma in hairless mice irradiated with ultraviolet light in relation to intake of ascorbin acid (vitamin C) and of D,L-alpha-tocopheryl acetate (vitamin E), *Int. Z. vitam. Ernahrungsforsch.* **23**:53–82.

Pauling, L., Nixon, J. C., Stitt, F., Marcuson, R., Dunham, W. B., Barth, R., Bensch, K., Herman, Z. S., Blaisdell, B. E., Tsao, C., Prender, M., Andrews, V., Willoughby, R., and Zuckerkandl, E., 1985, Effect of dietary ascorbic acid on the incidence of spontaneous mammary tumors in RIII mice, *Proc. Natl. Acad. Sci. USA* **82**:5185–5189.

Paveic, Z., Dave, S., Bialkowski, S., Priore, R., and Greco, W., 1980, Antitumor activity of *Cornynebacterium parvum* and retinyl palmitate used in combination on the Lewis lung carcinoma, *Cancer Res.* **40**:4617–4621.

Peck, G., Olsen, T., Butkus, J., Pandya, M., Arnaud-Battandier, J., Yoder, F., and Lewis, W., 1979, Treatment of basal cell carcinomas with 13-*cis*-retinoic acid, *Proc. Am. Assoc. Clin. Res.* **20**:56.

Pelej, I., Heyden, S., Knowles, M., and Hames, O., 1984, Serum retinol and risk of subsequent cancer; extension of the Evans Country, Georgia, study, *J. Natl. Cancer Inst.* **73**:1455–1488.

Percheliet, J. P., Abney, N. L., Thomas, R. M., Guislain, Y. L., and Perchellet, E. M., 1987, Effects of combined treatments with selenium, glutathione, and vitamin E on glutathione peroxidase activity, ornithine decarboxylase induction, and complete and multistage carcinogenesis in mouse skin, *Cancer Res.* **47**:477–485.

Pierson, H. F., Fisher, J. M., and Rabinovitz, M., 1985, Depletion of extracellular cysteine with hydroxocobalamin and ascorbate in experimental murine cancer chemotherapy, *Cancer Res.* **45**:4727–4731.

Pinto, J., Huang, Y. P., Chaudhuri, R., and Rivlin, R. S., 1975, Riboflavin excretion and turnover in an unusual case of multiple myeloma, *Clin. Res.* **23**:426A.

Polliack, A., and Sasson, Z., 1972, Enhancing effect of excess topical vitamin A on Rous sarcomas in chickens, *J. Natl. Cancer Inst.* **48**:407–416.

Pologe, L. G., Goyal, A., and Greer, J., 1982, Nature of the riboflavin interaction with the immunoglobulin IgG$_{gar}$: Analogue binding studies, *Mol. Immunol.* **19**:1499–1507.

Popov, A. I., 1987, Effect of the nonspecific prevention of thrombogenic complications on late results in the combined treatment of bladder cancer, *Med. Radiol. (Mosk.)* **32**:42–45.

Potera, C., Rose, D. P., and Brown, R. R., 1977, Vitamin B$_6$ deficiency in cancer patients, *Am. J. Clin. Nutr.* **30**:1677–1679.

Potter, J. D., and McMichael, A. J., 1986, Diet and cancer of the colon and rectum: A case–control study, *J. Natl. Cancer Inst.* **76**:557–569.

Prasad, K. N., 1984, *Vitamins, Nutrition, and Cancer,* Karger, Basel.

Prasad, K. N., 1988, Mechanisms of action of vitamin E on mammalian tumor cells in culture, *Prog. Clin. Biol. Res.* **259**:363–375.

Presant, C., and Bearman, R., 1981, Randomized study of 13-*cis*-retinoic acid plus busulfan (B) or B alone in chronic phase chronic granulocytic leukemia, *Proc. Am. Soc. Clin. Oncol.* **22**:448.

Prior, F. G. R., 1985, Theoretical involvement of vitamin B$_6$ in tumour initiation, *Med. Hypotheses* **16**:421–428.

Rachmilewitz, B., Rachmilewitz, M., Moshkowitz, B., and Gross, J. 1971, Serum transcobalamin in myeloid leukemia, *J. Lab. Clin. Med.* **78**:275–288.

Rakieten, N., Gordon, B. S., Beaty, A., Cooney, D. A., Davis, R. D., and Schein, P. S., 1971, Pancreatic islet tumors produced by the combined action of streptozotocin and nicotinamide, *Proc. Soc. Exp. Biol. Med.* **137**:280–283.

Rama, B., and Prasad, K., 1983, Study on the specificity of alpha-tocopherol (vitamin E) acid succinate effects on melanoma, glioma, and neuroblastoma cells in culture, *Proc. Soc. Exp. Biol. Med.* **174**:302–307.

Rama Rao, P. B., Lagerlof, B., Einhorn, J., and Reizenstein, P. G., 1965, Folic acid activity in leukemia and cancer, *Cancer Res.* **23**:221–224.

Rao, J., McBride, T., and Oleson, J., 1968, Recognition and evaluation of iapachol as an antitumor agent, *Cancer Res.* **28**:1952–1954.

Reynolds, R. D., 1986 Vitamin B$_6$ deficiency and carcinogenesis, *Adv. Exp. Med. Biol.* **206**:339–347.

Rivlin, R. S., 1975, Riboflavin and cancer, in: *Riboflavin* (R. S. Rivlin, ed.), Plenum Press, New York, pp. 369–391.

Roberts, A., and Sporn, M., 1984, Cellular biology and biochemistry of the retinoids, in: *The Retinoids*, vol. 2 (M. Sporn, A. Roberts, and D. Goodman, eds.), Academic Press, New York, pp. 209–286.

Robson, L. C., and Schwarz, M. R., 1980, The effects of vitamin B$_6$ deficiency on the lymphoid system and immune responses, in: *Vitamin B$_6$ Metabolism and Role in Growth* (G. P. Tryfiates, ed.), Food and Nutrition Press, Westport, CT, pp. 205–222.

Rogers, A. E., 1975, Variable effects of a lipotrope-deficient, high-fat diet on chemical carcinogenesis in rats, *Cancer Res.* **35**:2469–2474.

Rogers, A., Herndon, B., and Newberne, P., 1973, Induction by dimethylhydrazine of intestinal carcinoma in normal rats and rats fed high or low levels of vitamin A, *Cancer Res.* **33**:1003–1009.

Rokos, H., Rokos, K., Frisius, H., and Kirstaeder, H. J., 1980, Altered urinary excretion of pteridines in neoplastic disease. Determination of biopterin, neopterin, xanthipterin, and pterin, *Clin. Chim. Acta* **105**:275–286.

Rose, D. P., and Sheff, M. D., 1967, Tryptophan metabolism in carcinoma of the breast, *Lancet* **1**:239–241.

Rosen, F., Mihich, E., and Nichol, E. E., 1964a, Selective metabolic and chemotherapeutic effects of vitamin B_6 adntimetabolites, *Vit. Horm.* **22**:609–641.

Rosen, F., Satobayashi, H., and Nichol, C. A., 1964b, Different effects of folic acid deficiency and treatment with amethopterin on the growth of several rat tumors, *Proc. Am. Assoc. Cancer Res.* **5**:54.

Rosenberg, M. R., Novicki, D. L., Jirtle, R. L., Novotny, A., and Michalopoulos, G., 1985, Promoting effect of nicotinamide on the development of renal tubular cell tumors in rats initiated with diethylnitrosamine, *Cancer Res.* **45**:809–814.

Rosenberg, M. R., Strom, S. C., Pachman, S., Slotkin, T. A., and Michalopoulos, G., 1986, Induction of rat kidney ornithine decarboxylase by nicotinamide without a concomitant increase in DNA synthesis, *Carcinogenesis* **7**:175–178.

Rostock, R., Stryker, J., and Abt, A., 1980, Evaluation of high dose vitamin E as a radioprotective agent, *Radiology* **136**:763–766.

Ruddell, W. S. J., Bone, E. S., Hill, M. J., and Waters, C. L., 1978, Pathogenesis of gastric cancer in pernicious anemia, *Lancet* **1**:521–523.

Russell, M. J., Thomas, B. S., and Bulbrook, R. D., 1988, A prospective study of the relationship between serum vitamins A and E and risk of breast cancer, *Br. J. Cancer* **57**:213–215.

Saccomanno, G., Moran, P., Schmiidy, R., Hartshorn, D., Brian, D., Dreher, W., and Sowada, B., 1982, Effects of 13-*cis*-retiinoids on premalignant and malignant cells of lung origin, *Acta Cytol.* **26**:78–84.

Saffiotti, U., Montesano, R., Sellakumar, A., and Borg, S., 1967, Experimental cancer of the lung, *Cancer* **20**:857–864.

Salonen, J., Salonen, R., Lappetelainen, R., Maenpaa, P., Alfthan, G., and Puska, P., 1985, Risk of cancer in relation to serum concentrations of selenium and vitamins A and E: Matched case–control analysis of prospective data, *Br. Med. J.* **290**:417–420.

Samuels, L. L., Moccio, D. M., and Sirotnak, F. M., 1985, Similar differential for total polyglutamylation and cytotoxicity among various folate analogues in human and murine tumor cells *in vitro, Cancer Res.* **45**:1488–1485.

Samuels, L. L., Goutas, L. J., Priest, D. G., Piper, J. R., and Sirotnak, F. M., 1986, Hydrolytic cleavage of methotrexate gamma-polyglutamates by folylpolyglutamyl hydrolase derived from various tumors and normal tissues of the mouse, *Cancer Res.* **46**:2230–2235.

Sato, T., Takusagawa, K, and Konno, K., 1984, Effect of 1 alpha-hydroxyvitamin D_3 on metastasis of rat ascites hepatoma K-231, *Br. J. Cancer* **50**:123–125.

Schein, P. S., 1969, 1-Methyl-1-nitrosourea and dialkylnitrosamine depression of nicotinamide adenine dinucleotide, *Cancer Res.* **29**:1226–1232.

Schmaehl, D., and Habs, M., 1978, Experiments on the influence of an aromatic retinoid on the chemical carcinogenesis in rats by butyl-butanol-nitrosamine and 1,2-dimethylhydrazine, *Arzneim. Forsch.* **28**:49–51.

Schmitt-Graff, A., and Scheulen, M. E., 1986, Prevention of adriamycin cardiotoxicity by niacin, isocitrate or *N*-acetyl-cysteine in mice. A morphological study, *Pathol. Res. Pract.* **181**:168–174.

Schober, S. E., Comstock, G. W., Helsing, K. J., Salkeld, R. M., Morris, J. S., Rider, A. A., and Brookmeyer, R., 1987, Serologic precursors of cancer. I. Prediagnostic serum nutrients and colon cancer risk, *Am. J. Epidemiol.* **126**:1033–1041.

Schrijver, J., Alexieva-Figusch, J., van Breederode, N., and van Gilse, H. A., 1987, Investigations on the nutritional status of advanced breast cancer patients. The influence of long-term treatment with megestrol acetate or tamoxifen, *Nutr. Cancer* **10**:231–245.

Schroder, E., and Black, P., 1980, Retinoids: Tumor preventors or tumor enhancers? *J. Natl. Cancer Inst.* **65**:671–674.

Sestili, M. A., 1983, Possible adverse health effects of vitamin C and ascorbic acid, *Semin. Oncol.* **10**:299–304.

Shamberger, R. J., *Nutrition and Cancer,* Plenum Press, New York, 1984, Chapter 4.

Shamberger, R., Beaman, K., Corlett, C., and Kasten, B., 1978, Effect of selenium and other antioxidants on the mutagenicity of malonaldehyde, *Fed. Proc.* **37**:261.

Shane, B., and Stokstad, E. L. R., 1985, Vitamin B_{12}-folate interrelationships, *Annu. Rev. Nutr.* **5**:115–141.

Shapiro, D. M., Dietrich, L. S., and Shies, M. D., 1957, Quantitative biochemical differences between tumor and host as a basis of chemotherapy, *Cancer Res.* **17**:600–604.

Shekelle, R., Lepper, M., Liu, S., Maliza, C., Raynor, W., Rossof, A., Paul, O., Shylock, A., and Stamler, J., 1981, Dietary vitamin A and risk of cancer in the Western Electric study, *Lancet* 2:1186–90.

Sheppard, K., Danbury, D. A., Davies, J. M., and Ryrie, D. R., 1984, Cobalamin and folate binding proteins in human tumour tissue, *J. Clin. Pathol.* 37:1336–1338.

Shinozuka, H., and Lombardi, B., 1980, Synergistic effect of a choline-devoid diet and pheonbarbital in promoting the emergence of foci of gamma-glutamyltranspeptidase-positive hepatocytes in the liver of carcinogen-treated rats, *Cancer Res.* 40:3846–3849.

Shirai, T., Ikawa, E., Hirose, M., Thamavit, W., and Ito, N., 1985a, Modification by five antioxidants of 1,2-dimethylhydrazine-initiated colon carcinogenesis in F344 rats, *Carcinogenesis* 6:637–639.

Shirai, T., Masuda, A., Fukushima, S., Hosoda, K., and Ito, N., 1985b, Effects of L-ascorbate and related compounds on rat stomach carcinogenesis initiated by N-methyl-N'-nitro-N-nitroguanidine, *Cancer Lett.* 29:283–288.

Shivapurkar, N., and Poirier, L. A., 1983, Tissue levels of S-adenosylmethionine and S-adenosylhomocysteine in rats fed methyl-deficient, amino acid-defined diets for one to five weeks, *Carcinogenesis* 4:1051–1057.

Shklar, G., 1982, Oral mucosal carcinogenesis in hamsters: Inhibition by vitamin E, *J. Natl. Cancer Inst.* 68:791–797.

Shklar, G., Flynn, E., Szbo, G., and Marefat, P., 1980, Retinoid inhibition of experimental ligual carcinogenesis, *J. Natl. Cancer Inst.* 65:1307–1316.

Shklar, G., Schwartz, J., Trickler, D. P., and Niukian, K., 1987, Regression by vitamin E of experimental oral cancer, *J. Natl. Cancer Inst.* 78:987–992.

Shoentel, R., 1977, The role of nicotinamide and other modifying factors in diethylnitrosamine carcinogenesis, *Cancer* 40:1833–1840.

Sherman, M. I. (ed.), 1986, *Retinoids and Cell Differentiation*, CRC Press, Boca Raton, FL.

Siegel, B. V., and Morton, J. I., 1984, Vitamin C and immunity: Influence of ascorbate on prostaglandin E_2 synthesis and implications for natural killer cell activity, *Int. J. Vit. Nutr. Res.* 54:339–342.

Silverman, J., Katayama, S., Zelenkas, K., Lauber, J., Musser, T., Reddy, M., Levenstein, M., and Weisburger, J., 1981, Effect of retinoids on the induction of colon cancer in F344 rats by N-methyl-N-nitrosurea or by 1,2 dimethylhydrazine, *Carcinogenesis* 2:1167–1172.

Slaga, T., and Bracken, W., 1977, The effects of antioxidants on skin tumor initiation and aryl hydrocarbon hydroxlase, *Cancer Res.* 37:1631–1635.

Smith, D., Rogers, A., Herndon, B., and Neberne, P., 1975a, Vitamin A and benzo(a)pyrene-induced respiratory tract carcinogenesis in hamsters fed a commercial diet, *Cancer Res.* 35:11–16.

Smith, D., Rogers, A., and Newberne, P., 1975b, Vitamin A and benzo(a)pyrene carcinogenesis in the respiratory tract of hamsters fed a semisynthetic diet, *Cancer Res.* 35:1485–1487.

Sonneveld, P., 1978, Effect of alpha tocopherol on the cardiotoxicity of Adriamycin in the rat, *Cancer Treat. Rep.* 62:1033–36.

Sporn, M., and Newton, D., 1979, Chemoprevention of cancer with retinoids, *Fed. Proc.* 38:2528–2534.

Stahelin, H., Buess, E., Rosel, F., Widmer, L., and Brubacher, G., 1982, Vitamin A, cardiovascular risks, and mortality, *Lancet* 1:394–395.

Stahelin, H. B., Rosel, F., Buess, E., and Brubacher, G., 1984, Cancer, vitamins, and plasma lipids: Prospective Basel study, *J. Natl. Cancer Inst.* 73:1463–1468.

Stahl, R. L., Farber, C. M., Liebes, L. F., and Silber, R., 1985, Relationship of dehydroascorbic acid transport to cell lineage in lymphocytes from normal subjects and patients with chronic lymphocytic leukemia, *Cancer Res.* 45:6507–6512.

Stam, J., Germano, G., and Boorsma, M., 1982, Preliminary results of a 3 year double-blind study of the aromatic retinoid Tigason versus placebo as adjuvant therapy in patients who underwent a curative resection for epidermoid carcinoma of the lung, *Eur. J. Respir. Dis.* 63(Suppl. 125):Abstr. 100.

Stea, B., Halpern, R. M., Halpern, B. C., and Smith, R. A., 1981, Urinary excretion of unconjugated pterins in cancer patients and normal individuals, *Clin. Chim. Acta* 113:231–242.

Steen, P. H., Wallace, C. D., and Hoffman, R. M., 1984, Altered methionine metabolism occurs in all members of a set of diverse human tumor cell lines, *J. Cell. Physiol.* 119:29–34.

Stehr, P., 1983, Vitamin A deficiencies as a predisposing factor in the development of stomach cancer, *Diss. Abstr. Int.* 43:2863-B.

Stern, P. H., Wallace, C. D., and Hoffman, R. M., 1984, Altered methionine metabolism occurs in all members of a set of diverse human tumor cell lines, *J. Cell. Physiol.* 119:29–34.

Stewart, D., Speer, R., Ridgeway, H., and Hill, J., 1979, Combination chemotherapy of leukemia L1210 with platinum compounds and vitamins, *J. Clin. Hematol. Oncol.* **9:**235–239.

Stitch, H., Rosin, M., and Vallejera, M., 1984, Effect of vitamin A and Beta-carotene administration on the frequencies of micronucleated buccal mucosa cells of betel nut and tobacco chewers, *Proc. Am. Assoc. Cancer Res.* **25:**125.

Su, Y. Z., Duarte, T. E., Dill, P. L., and Weisenthal, L. M., 1987, Selective enhancement by menadiol of in vitro drug activity in human lymphatic neoplasms, *Cancer Treat. Rep.* **71:**619–625.

Surwit, E., Graham, V., Doregemueller, W., Alberts, D., Chvapil, M., Dorr, R., Davis, J., and Meyskens, Jr., F., 1982, Evaluation of topically applied trans-retinoic acid in the treatment of cervical intrepithelial lesions, *Am. J. Obstet. Gynecol.* **143:**821–823.

Svingen, B., Powis, G., Appel, P., and Scott, M., 1981, Protection by alpha-tocopherol and dimethylsulfoxide (DMSO) against Adriamycin induced skin ulcers in the rat, *Cancer Res.* **41:**3395–3399.

Taheri, M. R., Wickremasinghe, R. G., Jackson, B. F., and Hoffbrand, A. V., 1982, Effect of folate analogues and vitamin B_{12} on provision of thymine nucleotides for DNA synthesis in megaloblastic anemia, *Blood* **59:**634–640.

Taper, H. S., de Gerlache, J., Lans, M., and Roberfroid, M., 1987, Non-toxic potentiation of cancer chemotherapy by combined C and K_3 vitamin pre-treatment, *Int. J. Cancer* **40:**575–579.

Tekenaga, K., Honma, Y., and Hozumi, M., 1981, Inhibition of differentiation of mouse myeloid leukemia cells by phenolic antioxidants and alpha-tocopherol, *GANN* **72:**104–112.

Temcharoen, P., Anukarahanonta, T., and Bhamarapravati, N., 1978, Influence of dietary protein and vitamin B_{12} on the toxicity and carcinogenicity of aflatoxins in rat liver, *Cancer Res.* **38:**2185–2190.

Teppo, L., and Saxén, E., 1979, Epidemiology of colon cancer in Scandinavia, *Isr. J. Med. Sci.* **15:**322–328.

Thanassi, J. W., Nutter, L. M., Meisler, N. T., Commers, P., and Chiu, J-F., 1981, Vitamin B_6 metabolism by Morris hepatomas, *J. Biol. Chem.* **256:**3370–3375.

Thanassi, J. W., Meisler, N. T., and Kittler, J. M., 1985, Vitamin B_6 metabolism and cancer, in: *Vitamin B_6: Its Role in Health and Disease* (J. E. Leklem, R. D. Reynolds, and E. E. McCoy, eds.), Alan R. Liss, New York, pp. 319–336.

Thatcher, N., Blackledge, G., and Crowther, D., 1980, Advanced recurrent squamous cell carcinoma of the head and neck, *Cancer* **46:**1324–1328.

Thurnham, D. I., Rathakette, P., Hambridge, K. M., Munoz, N., and Crespi, M., 1982, Riboflavin, vitamin A and zinc status in Chinese subjects in a high-risk area for oesophageal cancer in China, *Hum. Nutr. Clin. Nutr.* **36C:**337–349.

Toth, B., and Patil, K., 1983, Enhancing effect of vitamin E on murine intestinal tumorigenesis by 1,2-dimethylhydrazine dihydrochloride, *J. Natl. Cancer Inst.* **70:**1107–1111.

Trickler, D., and Shklar, G., 1987, Prevention by vitamin E of experimental oral carcinogenesis, *J. Natl. Cancer Inst.* **78:**165–169.

Troll, W., Wiesner, R., and Frenkel, K., 1987, Anticarcinogenic action of protease inhibitors, *Adv. Cancer Res.* **49:**265–283.

Trown, P., Byck, M., and Hansen, R., 1976, Inhibition of growth and regression of a transplantable rat chrondrosarcoma by three retinoids, *Cancer Treat. Rep.* **60:**1647–1653.

Tryfiates, G. P., and Morris, H. P., 1974, The effect of pyridoxine deficiency on tyrosine transaminase activity and growth of four mouse hepatomas, *J. Natl. Cancer Inst.* **52:**1259–1262.

Tryfiates, G. P., Bishop, R., and Smith, R. R., 1983, Identification of fatty acids associated with a novel tumor vitamin metabolite by GC-mass spectroscopy, *J. Nutr. Growth Cancer* **1:**1–9.

Ura, H., Denda, A., Yokose, Y., Tsutsumi, M., and Konishi, Y., 1987, Effect of vitamin E on the induction and evolution of enzyme altered foci in the liver of rats treated with diethylnitrosamine, *Carcinogenesis* **8:**1595–1600.

van Eys, J., 1985, Nutrition and cancer, *Annu. Rev. Nutr.* **5:**435–461.

van Helden, P. D., Beyers, A. D., Bester, A. J., and Jaskiewicz, K., 1987, Esophageal cancer: Vitamin and lipotrope deficiencies in an at-risk South African population, *Nutr. Cancer* **10:**247–255.

Van Maanen, J. M., de Ruiter, C., de Vries, J., Koostra, P. R., Gobas, F., and Pinedo, H. M., 1985, The role of metabolic activation by cytochrome P-450 in covalent binding of VP 16-213 to rat liver and He La cell microsomal proteins, *Eur. J. Cancer Clin. Oncol.* **21:**1099–1106.

van Rensburg, S. J., 1981, Epidemiological and dietary evidence for a specific nutritional predisposition to esophageal cancer, *J. Natl. Cancer Inst.* **67:**243–251.

van Tonder, S., Kew, M. C., Hodkinson, J., Metz, J., and Fernandez-Costa, F., 1985, Serum vitamin B_{12} binders in South African blacks with hepatocellular carcinoma, *Cancer* **56:**789–792.

Van Vleet, V., and Ferrans, V., 1980, Evaluation of vitamin E and selenium protection against chronic adriamycin toxicity in rabbits, *Cancer Treat. Rep.* **64:**315–317.

Wade, A. E., Greene, F. E., Ciordia, R. H., Meadows, J. S., and Caster, W. O., 1969, Effect of dietary thiamin intake on hepatic drug metabolism in the rat, *Biochem. Pharmacol.* **18:**2288–2292.

Wade, A. E., Wu, B. C., Holbrooke, C. M., and Caster, W. O., 1973, Effects of thiamin antagonists on drug hydroxylation and properties of cytochrome P-450 in the rat, *Biochem. Pharm.* **22:**1573–1580.

Wagner, C., 1985, Folate-binding proteins, *Nutr. Rev.* **43:**293–299.

Wagner, C., Briggs, W. T., and Cook, R. J., 1985a, Inhibition of glycine *N*-methyltransferase activity by folate derivatives: Implications for regulation of methyl group metabolism, *Biochem. Biophys. Res. Commun.* **127:**746–752.

Wagner, D., Shuker, D. E. G., Blimazes, C., Obiedzinski, M., Baker, I., Young, V. R., and Tannenbaum, S. R., 1985b, Effects of vitamins C and E on endogenous synthesis of *N*-nitrosamino acids in humans: Presursor-product studies with [15N]nitrate, *Cancer Res.* **45:**6519–6522.

Wald, N., Idle, M., and Boreham, J., 1980, Low serum vitamin A and subsequent risk of cancer, *Lancet* **2:**813–815.

Wald, N., Boreham, J., Hayward, J., and Bulbrook, R., 1984, Plasma retinol, beta-carotene, and vitamin E levels in relation to the future risk of breast cancer, *Br. J. Cancer* **49:**321–324.

Wahrendorf, J., Munoz, N., Lu, J. B., Thurnham, D. I., Crespi, M., and Bosch, F. X., 1988, Blood, retinol and zinc riboflavin status in relation to precancerous lesions of the esophagus: Findings from a vitamin intervention trial in the People's Republic of China, *Cancer Res.* **48:**2280–2283.

Wang, Y., Madanat, F., and Kimball, J., 1980, Effect of vitamin E against Adriamycin-induced toxicity in rabbits, *Cancer Res.* **40:**1022–1027.

Wang, T., Miller, K. W., Tu, Y. Y., and Yang, C. S., 1985, Effects of riboflavin deficiency on metabolism of nitrosamines by rat liver microsomes, *J. Natl. Cancer Inst.* **74:**1291–1297.

Ward, J., Sporn, M., Wenk, M., Smith, J., Feeser, D., and Dean, R., 1978, Dose response to intrarectal administration of *N*-methyl-*N*-Nitrosurea and histopatologic evaluation of the effect of two retinoids on colon lesions induced in rats, *J. Natl. Cancer Inst.* **60:**1489–1493.

Wargovich, M. J., and Lointier, P. H., 1987, Calcium and vitamin D modulate mouse colon epithelial proliferation and growth characteristics of a human colon tumor cell line, *Can. J. Physiol. Pharmacol.* **65:**472–477.

Warrell, R., Coonley, C., and Itri, L., 1982, Clinical effects of 13-*cis*-retinoic acid in patients with lymphoid cancer, *Clin. Res.* **30:**692A.

Warwick, G. P., and Harrington, J. S., 1973, Some aspects of the epidemiology and etiology of esophageal cancer with particular emphasis on Transkei, South Africa, *Adv. Cancer Res.* **17:**81–229.

Wassertheil-Smoller, S., Romney, S. L., Wylie-Rosett, J., Slagle, G., Miller, D., Lucido, C., Duttagupta, P., and Palan, R., 1981, Dietary vitamin C and uterine cervical dysplasia, *Am. J. Epiderm.* **114:**714–724.

Watson, R. R., 1986, Retinoids and vitamin E: Modulators of immune functions and cancer resistance, in: *Vitamins and Cancer* (F. L. Meyskens, Jr., and K. N. Prasad, eds.), Humana Press, Clifton, NJ, pp. 439–451.

Wattenberg, L., 1972, Inhibition of carcinogenic and toxic effects of polycyclic hydroxcarbons by phenolic antioxidants and ethoxyquin, *J. Natl. Cancer Inst.* **48:**1425–1430.

Waxman, S., and Bruckner, H., 1982, The enhancement of 5-fluorouracil antimetabolic activity by leucovorin, menadione, and alpha-tocopherol, *Eur. J. Can. Clin. Oncol.* **18:**685–692.

Waxman, S., and Gilbert, H. S., 1973, A tumor-related vitamin B_{12}-binding protein in adolescent hepatoma, *N. Engl. J. Med.* **289:**1053–1056.

Weber, T., Seitz, R. J., Liebert, U. G., Gallasch, E., and Wechsler, W., 1985, Affinity cytochemistry of vascular endothelia in brain tumors by biotinylated Ulex europaeus type I lectin (UEA I), *Acta Neuropathol.* **67:**128–135.

Welsch, C., Goodrich-Smith, M., Brown, C., and Crowe, N., 1981, Enhancement by retinyl acetate of hormone-induced mammary tumorigenesis in female GR/A mice, *J. Natl. Cancer Inst.* **67:**935–938.

Wenk, M., Ward, J., Resnik, G., and Dean, J., 1981, Effects of three retinoids on colon adenocarcinomas, sarcomas, and hyperplastic polyps induced by intrarectal *N*-methyl-*N*-nitrosurea administration in male F344 rats, *Carcinogenesis* **2:**1161–1166.

Werner, B., Hrynyschyn, K., and Schafer, H., 1985, Long-term study on vitamin C: No effect on experimental carcinogenesis, *Langenbecks Arch. Chir.* **363:**185–193.

Whelen, W., Walker, B., and Kelleher, J., 1983, Zinc, vitamin A and prostate cancer, *Br. J. Urol.* **55:**525–528.

White, H. B., III, and Merrill, A. H., Jr., 1988, Riboflavin-binding proteins, *Annu. Rev. Nutr.* **8:**279–299.

Whittaker, J., and Al-Ismail, S., 1983, Effect of digoxin and vitamin E in preventing cardiac damage caused by doxorubicin in acute myeloid leukemia, *Br. J. Med.* **288:**283–284.

Willett, W. C., 1986, Selenium, vitamin E, fiber, and the incidence of human cancer: An epidemiologic perspective, *Adv. Exp. Med. Biol.* **206:**27–34.

Willett, W., Polk, B., Underwood, B., Stampfer, M., Pressel, S., Rosner, B., Taylor, J., Schneider, K., and Hames, C., 1984, Relation of serum vitamins A and E and carotenoids to the risk of cancer, *N. Engl. J. Med.* **310:**430–434.

Wittes, R. E., 1985, Vitamin C and cancer, *N. Engl. J. Med.* **312:**178–179.

Wolbach, S., and Howe, P., 1925, Tissue changes following deprivation of fat-soluble A vitamin, *J. Exp. Med.* **42:**753–777.

Woolley, P. V., Kumar, S., Fitzgerald, P., and Simpson, R. T., 1987, Ascorbate potentiates DNA damage by 1-methyl-nitrosourea *in vivo* and generates DNA strand breaks *in vitro, Carcinogenesis* **8:**1657–1662.

Wynder, E. L., Hultberg, S., Jacobson, F., and Bross, I. J., 1957, Environmental factors in cancer of the upper alimentary tract. A Swedish study with special reference to Plummer–Vinson (Patterson–Kelly) syndrome, *Cancer* **10:**470–479.

Yamamoto, R. S., 1980, Effect of vitamin B_{12}-deficiency in colon carcinogenesis, *Proc. Soc. Exp. Biol. Med.* **163:**350–353.

You, W. C., Blot, W. J., Chang, Y. S., Ershow, A. G., Yang, Z. T., An, Q., Henderson, B., Xu, G. W., Fraumeni, J. F., Jr., and Wang, T. G., 1988, Diet and high risk of stomach cancer in Shandong, China, *Cancer Res.* **48:**3518–3523.

Young, V. R., and Newberne, P. M., 1981, Vitamins and cancer prevention: Issues and dilemmas, *Cancer* **47**(Suppl. 5):1226–1240.

Ziegler, I., Fink, M., and Wimanns, W., 1982, Biopterin levels in peripheral blood cells as a marker for hematopoietic cell proliferation during leukemia and polycythemia vera, *Blut* **44:**231–240.

Ziegler, R. G., 1986, Epidemiologic studies of vitamins and cancer of the lung, esophagus, and cervix, *Adv. Exp. Med. Biol.* **206:**11–26.

Ziegler, R., Mason, T., Stemhagen, A., Hoover, R., Schoenberg, J., Gridley, G., Virgo, P., Altamn, R., and Fraumeni, J., Jr., 1984, Dietary carotene and vitamin A and risk of lung cancer among white men in New Jersey, *J. Natl. Cancer Inst.* **73:**1429–35.

Ziegler, R. G., Mason, T. J., Stemhagen, A., Hoover, R., Schoenberg, J. B., Gridley, G., Virgo, P. W., and Fraumeni, J. F., Jr., 1986, Carotenoid intake, vegetables, and the risk of lung cancer among white men in New Jersey, *Am. J. Epidemiol.* *123:*1080–1093.

13

Interrelationships of Alcohol and Cancer

Adrianne E. Rogers and Michael W. Conner

1. Introduction

Cancers at several sites are associated with ingestion of alcohol. Head and neck cancers (of the mouth, pharynx, esophagus, and larynx) are strongly associated with use of both alcohol and tobacco; other tobacco-related cancers, of the lung and perhaps pancreas, have been found to be associated with alcohol consumption in some studies. Liver cancer is related to alcohol consumption; epidemiologic studies have reported additive or synergistic interactions between alcohol, HBV and AFB_1 in the etiology of liver cancer. Risk for head and neck and liver cancers, all of which occur in much higher incidence in men than in women in the United States, is significantly increased at high alcohol intake (>80 g/day) and may show a dose response to lower alcohol intakes. Epidemiologic and experimental data suggest that malnutrition in alcoholic patients contributes to their increased cancer risk. Influences of alcohol consumption on nutritional status have been known and studied for many years. Understanding of nutritional influences on cancer induction and development is increasing and may contribute to clarification of relationships between alcohol intake and cancer risk.

Risk for colorectal and breast cancer also appears to be related to alcohol ingestion, but the patterns of and evidence for a relationship and dose responses are variable and inconsistent, and there are significant negative results. Colon cancer incidence is similar in men and women; it is a disease that, like breast cancer, occurs in well- or overnourished population groups and appears not to be associated with tobacco smoking. Rectal cancers occur in somewhat higher incidence in men than women; an association with alcohol consumption, while not consistently found, has been reported at relatively low alcohol (particularly beer) intake.

Abbreviations used in this chapter: AFB_1, Aflatoxin B_1; HCC, hepatocellular carcinoma; HBsAg, hepatitis B surface antigen; HBV, hepatitis B virus; MBN, methylbenzylnitrosamine; DMH, symmetrical dimethylhydrazine.

Adrianne E. Rogers and Michael W. Conner • Department of Pathology, Boston University School of Medicine, Boston, Massachusetts 02118.   *Present address for M.W.C.:* Merck, Sharp and Dohme, West Point, Pennsylvania, 19486.

Doll and Peto (1981) attributed 3% of cancer deaths in the United States to alcohol alone. Since heavy drinking is almost always associated with tobacco smoking, and many studies show that the two factors contribute additively or synergistically to cancer incidence, the total contribution of alcohol is significantly greater than 3%. The NIAAA Report to Congress on Alcohol and Health (1984) summarized certain conclusions on alcohol and cancer:

1. Cancers of the oropharynx, larynx, and esophagus are strongly associated with chronic consumption of alcohol. Effects of alcohol and tobacco smoking are synergistic.
2. Heavy alcohol intake is a risk factor for liver, gastric, pancreatic, and colorectal cancer.
3. Alcoholic beverages may contain carcinogenic nitrosamines, polycyclic aromatic hydrocarbons, fusel oils, and asbestos fibers, but there are no animal data showing carcinogenesis by ethanol itself.

2. Alcoholism and Alcohol-Related Diseases

Approximately 7% of the adult (18 years and older) population of the United States and many other countries is alcoholic (Van Thiel *et al.*, 1981) Alcoholic cirrhosis and related diseases of the gastrointestinal tract and other organ systems are a major cause of death in men 30 and older and contribute significantly to morbidity and mortality. Cirrhosis causes 11,000–29,000 deaths per year in the United States, and alcohol-related esophagitis, gastritis, pancreatitis, neurological disease, cardiomyopathy, anemia, renal failure, and malnutrition are major causes of morbidity and mortality.

The difficulties of gathering accurate data on alcohol consumption make demonstration of dose responses highly variable. Risk for cirrhosis, which is much more clearly related to alcohol consumption than is cancer, becomes significant at ethanol intakes of 80–100 g/day for several years. The pattern of increased risk with greater intakes is not clear. Attempts to implicate specific alcoholic beverages in the etiology of cirrhosis or other diseases have generally not succeeded because patterns of consumption vary within and between populations and in individual patients' histories.

In 1981 the average U.S. ethanol consumption per capita (14 years and older) was 2.77 gallons; 51% of intake was in beer, 36% in distilled spirits, and 13% in wine. The average intake by alcohol consumers is about 4.5 gallons of alcoholic beverages per capita based on the estimate that about 60% of women and 77% of men drink some alcohol (Broitman 1984; NIAAA, 1984; Van Thiel *et al.*, 1981). The amount of intake, of course, varies widely. A large survey of intake in 10 areas of the United States in 1978–1979 showed a high percent of abstainers (59% of women, 38% of men) (Thomas *et al.*, 1983). A summary of intake patterns in that study is shown in Table I. About ¼ of the population surveyed had one or fewer drinks per day; ⅓ of men and ⅙ of women consumed one to four drinks per day; and 10% of men and 1% of women had four or more drinks per day. People who drank primarily wine drank less heavily than people who drank distilled spirits or beer. Another large survey reported in 1985, based on intake in the 24 hr (nonweekend) prior to interview only, showed alcohol consumption by 43% of men and

Table I. Patterns of Alcoholic Beverage Consumption in the United States[a]

Alcoholic drinks/week[b]	Men (%)	Women (%)
1–6	21	23
7–27	31	16
≥28	10	1.3

[a]Summarized from Thomas *et al.*, 1983.
[b]Thirty-eight percent of men and 59% of women reported that they drank no alcohol.

25% of women, with age and geographical variations ranging from 13 to 66% of men and 6 to 67% of women interviewed. Percent of calories taken as alcohol showed means of 6–15% for men and 8–18% for women (Dennis *et al.*, 1985). The authors made the interesting observation that the study populations with the lowest relative fat intakes were the populations with the highest consumers of alcohol, and populations with high carbohydrate intakes were low consumers of alcohol. Using the overall average per capita ethanol and caloric consumption figures in the United States, one can calculate that ethanol contributes about 7% of daily caloric intake. Consumption of 30% or more of calories as ethanol, which corresponds to an annual intake of 264,000 kcal or 12.6 gallons, can be considered an alternative to >80 g daily to define heavy intake. Ethanol content in alcoholic beverages is approximately 1.1 g/fl oz of beer, 3 g/fl oz of wine, and 9–10 g/fl oz of distilled spirits. The caloric equivalents are 13 kcal/fl oz beer, 25 kcal/fl oz wine, and 65 kcal/fl oz of hard liquor (Ziegler *et al.*, 1981). Consumption of 30–50% of calories as ethanol by people and laboratory animals leads to reduced nutrient intake and absorption and abnormal nutrient utilization (Broitman, 1984; Rogers *et al.*, 1981; Tamura and Halsted, 1983; Van Thiel *et al.*, 1981).

3. Alcohol Consumption and Cancer at Specific Sites

Alcohol consumption, nutritional status, liver disease, and other factors that modulate the response to alcohol probably interact to induce or enhance the development of cancer and other diseases related to alcoholism. Cirrhosis, alcoholic psychoses, and neuropathies are clearly associated with heavy consumption of alcohol. This appears to be true for cancer of the upper gastrointestinal (GI) and respiratory tracts as well. Since malnutrition alone is a risk factor for these same cancers, it may link or add to their association with alcoholism. Recent epidemiologic studies (Pickle *et al.*, 1984; Pollack *et al.*, 1984; Willett *et al.*, 1987) suggest an effect of alcohol at lower intakes on colorectal, breast, and possibly lung cancer. Nutritional mechanisms may be related to alcohol effects on metabolism of fat, vitamin A, folate, trace minerals, or other nutrients influential in carcinogenesis.

3.1. Hepatocellular Carcinoma

Alcoholism is a risk factor for HCC, a cancer that occurs primarily in cirrhotic patients in all parts of the world. The etiology of the associated cirrhosis varies and can be alcoholism, viral hepatitis, or possibly malnutrition or toxin exposure. Epidemiologic evidence supports the conclusion that the alcohol, viral, and carcinogenic toxin associations with HCC show interactions with each other and with other environmental factors in the etiology of HCC (Austin *et al.*, 1986; Brechot *et al.*, 1982; Bulatao-Jayme *et al.*, 1982; Edmondson and Peters, 1985; Melbye *et al.*, 1984; Ohnishi *et al.*, 1982; Paterson *et al.*, 1985). The association of markers for HBV with alcoholism is well known (Brechot *et al.*, 1982; Gondeau *et al.*, 1981; Yu *et al.*, 1983) and separation of the two factors is often difficult. Demonstration of HBV DNA in malignant hepatocytes and hepatocytes in tumor-bearing liver or in liver of alcoholic patients without evidence of HCC strengthens the evidence for an association of factors in the development of HCC (Brechot *et al.*, 1982).

Hepatocellular carcinoma incidence was studied in 1 to 15-year follow-up of a group of 652 cirrhotic patients in Austria (Ferenci *et al.*, 1984). Of the 416 deaths, 169 (40.6%) were from cancer; primary liver cancer made up 64% of all cancers and occurred in 30% of the men and 15% of the women. Earlier studies in Europe and the United States had shown that HCC occurs in 7–30% of alcoholic cirrhotics and up to 38% of posthepatitic cirrhotics. In the Austrian study total deaths from cancer were approximately twice the expected number, but no single site was increased as prominently as liver cancer. HBsAg was detected in the blood of 19% of male and 6% of female cirrhotics; the prevalence was 0.5% in the general population. The percent of HBsAg positivity was the same in patients with or without HCC. The etiology of cirrhosis was judged to be alcoholism in 56% of the men and 27% of the women; the others were diagnosed as posthepatitic or cryptogenic (unknown) etiology.

Yu *et al.* (1983) interviewed patients with HCC and controls in California and concluded that heavy alcohol consumption (>80 g/day) increased the relative risk for HCC to about 4, that heavy smoking further raised the risk to about 14, and that a history of hepatitis alone gave a risk of about 13. They estimated that alcoholism accounted for about 15% of cases, smoking for 20%, and hepatitis for 43%. Austin *et al.* (1986) interviewed HCC cases and controls at several locations in the United States and examined their blood for HBsAg. Measures of alcohol use and cumulative alcohol consumption both gave evidence of a dose–response effect on relative risk for HCC (Table II). There was no evidence of an effect of tobacco use on HCC risk. The authors concluded that there is a strong association between alcohol use and HCC and that even moderate consumption may increase risk, although the possibility of underreporting of consumption must be considered. HBsAg was positive in 27% of male cases and in no female cases or controls. The average age of HCC cases who were HBsAg positive was 48 years, significantly younger than the 64-year average age of the antigen-negative cases. Interactive effects with alcohol were not discussed.

Evidence for positive interaction between alcohol and HBV in development of HCC was reported in Japanese cases. Ohnishi *et al.* (1982) studied 79 patients with HCC for evidence of alcohol intake and HBV infection. Age at diagnosis of HCC was significantly lower if the patients drank alcohol than if they did not, regardless of evidence of HBV

Table II. Alcohol Use, Cumulative Intake,
and Risk for HCC[a]

Alcohol use	Relative risk for HCC[b]
Frequency	
Infrequent	1.4
1–6 servings/week	2.3
≥7 servings/week	2.6
Cumulative[c]	
<18	1.4
18–65	2.5
>65	3.3

[a]Summarized from Austin *et al.*, 1986.
[b]Compared to nonusers.
[c]Drinks per day × years consumed.

infection (Table III). HBsAg positivity alone was not associated with lower age at diagnosis. This is in contrast to the results of Austin *et al.* (1986) and other studies reviewed by them.

A role of AFB$_1$ and other mycotoxins in HCC etiology has been indicated by many epidemiologic studies and is strongly supported by studies in animals (WHO, 1979). Bulatao-Jayme *et al.* (1982) evaluated diet and alcohol intake by 90 primary liver cancer cases and matched controls and measured aflatoxin content of major staple foods and alcoholic beverages. They found heavy contamination in cassava and other major carbohydrate sources as well as in peanut products. They concluded that alcohol intake above the mean (>24 g/day) or heavy aflatoxin intake (≥4 μg/day) gave a relative risk for HCC of about 18; the two combined gave an additive relative risk of 35. The mean daily alcohol intake of cases was 38.4 g and of controls was 9.8 g. HBV infection was not evaluated.

The data from these and other case follow-up or case–control studies indicate that consumption of alcohol increases the risk for HCC and decreases the latent period for its development. The roles of alcohol, hepatitis or related viruses, other toxins or car-

Table III. Ethanol Consumption, HBV, and Age at Diagnosis
of HCC in Men

HbsAg	Alcohol use	Age at diagnosis of HCC (years)	Reference
+	−	61	Ohnishi *et al.*, 1982
+	+	49[a]	
−	−	61	
−	+	51[b]	
+	Not stated	48[a]	Austin *et al.*, 1986
−	Not stated	64	

[a]Significantly reduced, $p < 0.01$, compared to abstainers (Ohnishi *et al.*), or to HBV-negative patients (Austin *et al.*).
[b]Significantly reduced, $p < 0.05$, compared to abstainers.

cinogens, and malnutrition secondary to alcoholism are not clear. Histopathological evaluation of HCC and surrounding liver in black patients in South Africa and correlation of results with historical evidence of alcohol intake and serological or tissue markers of HBV infection gave evidence of the multifactorial etiology of HCC and of a changing pattern over the past 20–25 years (Paterson *et al.*, 1985). The authors concluded that liver damage associated with alcohol consumption had become more prominent in HCC patients over the period studied and that the contribution of HBV infection, although still highly prevalent, appeared to have decreased. They postulated that reduced mycotoxin exposure in the progressively urbanized population also might play a role in the changing liver histology and demographic characteristics of HCC.

A recent population-based study was negative, however. Data from a 1973 regional food consumption survey in Germany were compared to cancer mortality rates in 1976–1980 in the same regions and showed no association between HCC and alcohol consumption. The average baseline daily alcohol intake was relatively high, 41 g for men and 21 g for women, supplying 9 and 6% of daily caloric intake, respectively (Boing *et al.*, 1985).

3.2. Head and Neck Cancers

3.2.1. Laryngeal Carcinoma

Laryngeal cancer, like other head and neck cancers, is strongly related to tobacco smoking; alcohol consumption increases the risk 1.5–4.4 times and is synergistic with smoking. Ethanol ingestion alone is only weakly associated with laryngeal cancer (Flanders and Rothman, 1982). There are about 11,000 new cases of laryngeal cancer in the United States (about 1.5% of U.S. cancer incidence) annually and 3700 deaths (Cowles, 1983). Herity *et al.* (1982) studied alcohol consumption and tobacco smoking in laryngeal cancer patients in Ireland. The study population (cases and controls) had a median alcohol consumption of 90 g of alcohol per day (4.5 pints of beer or ⅓ pint of spirits) for 10 years and a median tobacco exposure of 20 cigarettes per day for 43 years. Only 12–20% of the population studied did not drink alcohol and 0–16% did not smoke. The relative risk for laryngeal cancer in heavy drinkers (>90 g/day for 10 years) compared to all others, irrespective of smoking, was 6. In heavy smokers, heavy alcohol intake increased the relative risk from 3 to 14 (Table IV).

Table IV. Alcohol and Tobacco Use by Laryngeal and Lung Cancer Patients[a]

Daily alcohol consumption	Laryngeal cancer patients (%)	Lung cancer patients (%)	Other (control) patients (%)
None	14	12	20
≤90 g × 10 years	17	42	51
≥90 g × 10 years	69[b]	46[c]	29

[a]Summarized from Herity *et al.*, 1982.
[b]Significant increase in risk associated with heavy alcohol intake.
[c]No significant effect of alcohol on risk.

3.2.2. Carcinoma of the Oral Cavity and Esophagus

Risk for cancer of the oral cavity is increased by heavy alcohol intake and smoking (Mashberg *et al.*, 1981). Of all patients with oral cancer seen in a VA hospital, 82% drank the equivalent of 6 or more oz of whiskey per day, compared to 37% of controls. Only 5% of patients were considered minimal drinkers, compared to 41% of controls.

Esophageal carcinoma occurs in the poor and malnourished of both sexes in many parts of the world and in the predominantly male, heavy consumers of tobacco and alcohol (who may also be poor and malnourished) in the United States and other Western countries. Esophageal cancer accounts for about 4% of cancer deaths in the United States (Rogers *et al.*, 1982). The black population in the United States is at about 3 times the risk of the white population for esophageal cancer; men have about 3 times the risk of women (Schottenfeld, 1984). Mortality has doubled over the last 25 years in black men. Heavy alcohol intake, tobacco smoking, and poor nutrition have been identified as risk factors (Correa, 1982; Pottern *et al.*, 1984; Rogers *et al.*, 1982; Schottenfeld, 1984; Ziegler *et al.*, 1981).

Risk for esophageal cancer is increased proportionally to the amount of alcohol consumed and may be related particularly to consumption of distilled spirits. Schottenfeld (1984) concluded from his review that total ethanol intake probably was the most important factor. Tuyns *et al.* (1979) gathered data on alcoholic beverage consumption and esophageal cancer in France. They found that the major risk factor was the amount of the daily intake of alcohol, but there was a somewhat higher risk if the alcohol was consumed in fermented or fermented and distilled apple cider than in beer or wine (Table V).

Correa (1982) reviewed studies on risk factors for esophageal carcinoma and concluded that, in international studies, the single most important risk factor is poor nutritional status. Ziegler *et al.*, (1981) collected dietary information from families of esophageal cancer patients and compared the data to information on patients who died of other causes. Relative risk for esophageal cancer was inversely related to consumption of fresh meat, chicken, and fish, dairy products, fruits, and vegetables. The inverse correlation with good nutritional history persisted after adjustment for alcohol intake. Relative risk of esophageal cancer was 8 in patients with poor nutritional history and alcohol intake >56 g/day (about 6 oz distilled spirits), compared to a relative risk of 3 with only one of the two risk factors.

Table V. Alcohol Consumption and Esophageal Cancer Risk[a]

Beverage	Daily ethanol consumption (g)		
	1–40	41–80	≥81
Cider	0.9–1.5	2.9–3.1	13.8–16.4
Beer	1.0	1.8	10.5
Wine	0.7	2.3	10.4

[a]Summarized from Tuyns *et al.*, 1979.

3.3. Colorectal Carcinoma

Colorectal carcinoma occurs characteristically in a patient population that differs greatly from the populations at risk for hepatocellular and head and neck cancers. Over-rather than undernutrition and other correlates of Western lifestyle are risk factors for colorectal cancer; several studies have reported associations with alcohol intake. Beer consumption has been found correlated to colon and rectal cancer (Breslow and Enstrom, 1974; Pickle *et al.*, 1984) or only to colon cancer (Kono and Ikeda, 1979) or only to rectal cancer (Miller *et al.*, 1983; Pollack *et al.*, 1984). Other studies have reported no association (Hinds *et al.*, 1980; Jensen, 1983).

In a case–control study of patients with colorectal cancer, Miller *et al.* (1983) found a significantly increased risk for rectal cancer in women who drank 47.6 g/day or more of ethanol in beer (about 1.5 liters); men who drank 143 g/day or more (more than 4 liters of beer) had a nonsignificantly increased risk. There was no evidence of increased risk for colon cancer in either group. Pickle *et al.* (1984) reported a significant positive association between colon cancer and consumption of seven or more servings of beer per week; there was an association also between beer consumption and rectal cancer, but it was not significant.

In a prospective study of alcohol intake and cancer in Japanese men in Hawaii, rectal cancer was associated with beer consumption (Pollack *et al.*, 1984). Alcohol intake data were collected from approximately 7800 men, 45–65+ years old. Average alcohol consumption was about 10 g/day in men aged 45–54 and 8 g/day in men aged 55–65. Average wine consumption was 3 oz/mo in younger men, 45–49, and 30 oz/mo in older men. Beer consumption in the same age groups was 308 and 169 oz/mo, respectively. Spirits intake was 7.8 and 6.4 oz/mo in the two groups, respectively. Cancers diagnosed in five organs in an average follow-up of 14 years were recorded. The incidence of rectal cancer correlated significantly with amount of alcohol consumed; the incidence of colon cancer did not show a correlation. The relative risk for rectal cancer was significantly increased in men whose beer intake was ≥500 oz (15 liters) per month (about 20 g ethanol per day).

In a second study of five ethnic groups in Hawaii, Hinds *et al.* (1980) reported a correlation between cancer incidences at several sites and mean group intake of alcoholic beverages, calculated from data derived from interviews. They found a statistically significant relationship between alcohol consumption and head and neck cancers; a weak association with lung, gastric, pancreatic, and renal cancers; and no association with colorectal cancer. The different results with respect to colorectal cancer in the two studies from Hawaii are of interest. Pollack *et al.* (1984) reviewed several recent studies of associations of rectal cancer and beer consumption that yielded highly variable results. They emphasized the importance of taking individual consumption data that permit separate assessment of effects of high intake on risk.

Important negative results for an association between colorectal cancer and beer consumption were reported by Jensen (1983). He found no increased risk for colorectal cancer in brewery workers, who consumed 2.1–2.5 l of beer per day, compared to controls, who drank little or no alcohol. The brewery workers did have the expected increased incidence of cancers of the oropharynx, larynx, esophagus, and liver. Reexamination of data for colorectal and other cancers from a large prospective study in men, designed to study cardiovascular disease, has given negative results for an association between alcohol and colorectal cancer (Garland *et al.*, 1985). In a 20-year follow-up of men initially aged 40–55 years, 14.8/1000 had a diagnosis of colon cancer, 10.2/1000 a diagnosis of rectal cancer, and 95.1/1000 a diagnosis of other cancer. Alcohol intake history, obtained at initiation of the study, was not different in the colorectal cancer cases than in other cancer cases or in subjects who did not have a diagnosis of cancer.

In an attempt to study the question of alcohol and colon cancer in an animal model, rats given DMH, a colon carcinogen, were fed 5% ethanol or beer in place of drinking water. Colon tumor induction apparently was not increased by ethanol, but since tumor incidence was 100%, only tumor number was analyzed. In rats fed beer, tumor induction was reported to be decreased rather than increased. However food, ethanol, and beer intake were not measured, and body weights were not reported, so the experiments are not definitive (Nelson and Samelson, 1985). Seitz *et al.* (1985) reported increased rectal tumor number but not incidence in rats given intermittent feeding of 36% of calories as ethanol.

3.4. Breast Cancer

There are several case–control studies of the association, if any, between history of alcohol intake and development of breast cancer. A relative risk of 1.4–2.0 has been reported associated with moderate alcohol intake, in studies from several countries (Rosenberg *et al.*, 1982; Le *et al.*, 1984; La Vecchia *et al.*, 1985). Others have found no association (Webster *et al.*, 1983). The inconsistent results do not appear to be due to interference by known genetic or reproductive risk factors for breast cancer; dietary influences were not studied in any detail. Two prospective studies have demonstrated increased risk. Hiatt and Bawol (1984) reported a 40% increase in risk associated with consumption of three or more alcoholic drinks per day compared to nondrinkers. Willett *et al.* (1982) have found an association in a 4-year follow-up of almost 90,000 female registered nurses, aged 34–59, examined by mailed questionnaire about dietary practices and history. For consumers of up to 5 g ethanol per day (less than one drink), there was no increase in breast cancer risk compared to abstainers. For consumers of 5–14.9 g (less than 1 to 1½ drinks per day) the relative risk was 1.3 and for heavier consumers the relative risk was 1.6. The population was approximately equally divided into the three intake groups. The data did not indicate strong associations with particular beverages, smoking, or reproductive, familial, dietary, or anthropomorhophic factors known or thought to be related to breast cancer. The reliability of the history of alcohol intake was established by highly correlated results on repeat questionnaires and by measurement of high-density lipoprotein (HDL) cholesterol in the blood. Several of the authors cited have reviewed their own and others' results without identifying compelling reasons for the differences. Inclusion of data on diet and possibly on indicators of lipid metabolism and examination of effects of ethanol on mammary tumorigenesis in animal models may resolve the current questions.

In summary, the head and neck cancers consistently associated with ingestion of alcohol are associated also with tobacco use and arise from epithelia that are in direct contact with both agents. Tobacco smoking–related cancers at sites not directly in contact with the alcoholic beverages, the lung, bladder, and pancreas, do not consistently show a relationship to alcohol consumption, although lung and pancreatic tumors have been associated with alcohol in some studies. Pollack *et al.* (1984) found an association of lung cancer with alcohol intake and reviewed related studies. A significant increase in relative risk for lung cancer was seen in men whose wine or spirits intake was ≥50 oz (1.5 liters) per month (7–15 g ethanol per day). They found that reported associations often disappear when correction is made for tobacco smoking, although the association persisted in their study after adjustment for smoking. They raised the question of a contribution to lung cancer risk of low vitamin A intake in moderate to heavy drinkers, as suggested by Kvale *et al.* (1983). Hinds *et al.* (1980) also reported a 2–3 times increase in risk for lung cancer with alcohol ingestion.

Colorectal cancers form a different category. They occur about equally in men and women in well-nourished populations and are not associated with tobacco smoking. The association with alcohol consumption is not consistent, occurs apparently at relatively low alcohol intakes, and is often stronger for consumption of beer than of other alcoholic beverages. The recent data on breast cancer–alcohol associations have some of the same characteristics.

Most of the studies cited are of cancers in men, and many of the cancers of interest in alcohol studies (mouth, upper gastrointestinal (GI) tract, respiratory tract, and liver) occur in much lower incidence in women than in men. Hinds *et al.* (1980) found similar results in men and women in their studies in Hawaii in which head and neck, lung, gastric, renal, and pancreatic cancer showed some association with alcohol intake and colorectal cancer did not. Two reports of an association of colorectal cancer with beer consumption gave similar results in men and women (Miller *et al.*, 1983; Pickle *et al.*, 1984). Gastric cancer was associated with alcohol intake in both men and women in the Federal Republic of Germany (Boing *et al.*, 1985).

4. Mechanisms by Which Alcohol Consumption May Influence Cancer Risk

Mechanisms by which alcoholic consumption can influence carcinogenesis are summarized in Table VI. Studies in laboratory animals have not yielded evidence of carcinogenesis by ethanol itself, but there is some evidence of cocarcinogenesis in esophagus (Gabrial *et al.*, 1982), nasopharynx (Castonguay *et al.*, 1984), liver (Porta *et al.*, 1985; Schwartz *et al.*, 1983), and colon (Seitz *et al.*, 1985; Nelson and Samelson, 1985). In most studies of chronic ethanol administration to rats, weight gain is reduced and interpretation of results, therefore, complicated by caloric and other considerations. Studies are needed in which nutrient and alcohol intake and weight gain are carefully controlled, different carcinogens for the important target organs are tested, and timing of ethanol administration is well defined. The powerful effect of lipotrope deficiency on hepatocarcinogenesis in rats suggests that the metabolic effects of ethanol on the liver, for which lipotrope deficiency provides a partial model, probably are of major importance at that site (Rogers and Newberne, 1982; Rogers *et al.*, 1987).

Involvement of ethanol in carcinogenesis has been proposed to occur through effects on carcinogen metabolism. Castonguay *et al.* (1984) proposed a metabolic hypothesis for variations in effects of ethanol reported on nitrosamine tumorigenesis in laboratory ani-

Table VI. *Summary of Mechanisms Which Consumption of Alcoholic*
Beverages May Influence Cancer Risk

1. Direct effects on target tissues:
   Cell damage leading to increased turnover or permeability to carcinogens
   Altered carcinogen metabolism
   Altered nutrient requirements for maintenance of normal structure and
       function
2. Presence of carcinogens, promoters, enzyme inducers or inhibitors, other
       toxins in beverages
3. Systemic effects:
   Hepatic metabolic, physiological, and structural alternations
   Pancreatic and GI tract injury and malfunction
   Malnutrition

mals. They found that ethanol induced carcinogen-activating enzymes and increased nitrosamine carcinogenesis in the nasal, but not the esophageal mucosa. However, in other studies rats fed ethanol for 3 weeks and then injected with a different nitrosamine, MBN, methylation of esophageal DNA was increased (Kouros *et al.*, 1983), a result that indicated increased activation and was consistent with the enhancement of MBN esophageal tumorigenesis reported by Gabrial *et al.* (1982).

Inhibition by acute exposure to ethanol of xenobiotic metabolism in the hepatic cytochrome P450 system has been demonstrated; the pathways by which xenobiotic metabolism is or may be altered have been reviewed (Lieber, 1983; Muhoberac *et al.*, 1984; Sellers and Holloway, 1978). The end result of changes in metabolism is not easily predictable because of the additional influence of hepatic glutathione stores, other aspects of Phase II metabolism, and changes in the characteristics of tissue oxidation–reduction potential attendant on ethanol catabolism. In rats, hepatic glutathione was decreased by a single large (6 g/kg) dose of ethanol, an effect that was blocked by administration of *S*-adenosylmethionine (Feo *et al.*, 1986). Potentiation of acetaminophen, cocaine, and CCl_4 toxicity by prior ethanol exposure is one of the clinically significant effects of alcohol on drug metabolism (Muhoberac *et al.*, 1984).

It is likely that malnutrition has a role in excessive cancer risk in the alcoholic. Byers and Graham (1984) reviewed methods and results of a large number of epidemiologic investigations of diet and cancer. They cited one or more case–control studies in each of which alcohol had been found to be a statistically significant risk factor for cancers of colon and rectum, mouth, esophagus, all GI sites, larynx, or liver. In discussion of the data they emphasized potential interactions of alcohol and dietary or nutritional status. Specific nutrient deficiencies or marginal general nutritional status has been demonstrated in alcoholic patients by clinical and laboratory examinations in many studies (reviewed in Rogers and Conner, 1986) and probably contributes to the cancers associated with heavy alcohol intake. Causes of malnutrition in alcoholics include poor dietary intake and dysfunction of the salivary glands, GI tract, liver, and pancreas leading to malabsorption or excessive loss of nutrients. Liver damage causes malabsorption, as well as reduced synthesis and secretion of nutrient transport proteins and excessive nutrient demands resulting from abnormal energy and other metabolism. Chronic ingestion of alcohol induces a hypermetabolic state in which calories are inefficiently utilized and requirements for cofactors, as well as for calories, are increased (Van Thiel *et al.*, 1981). Failure of ethanol-fed rodents (Misslbeck *et al.*, 1984; Seitz *et al.*, 1985) and primates (Rogers *et al.*, 1981) to gain weight normally is evidence for the poor utilization of calories supplied by ethanol.

Alcohol–folate–one-carbon interactions may be particularly important in carinogenesis. Folate deficiency is well documented and clinically significant in alcoholics (Russell *et al.*, 1983). The folate coenzymes are central to one-carbon metabolism, and the storage form, 5-methyl-tetrahydrofolate, is proposed as a major regulator of methyl metabolism (Wagner *et al.*, 1985). This is, of course, the biochemical site of interest in the lipotrope-deficient model for alcoholic liver disease. Ethanol-fed rats have increased hepatic folate polyglutamate stores and decreased utilization and enterohepatic circulation of folate (McMartin, 1984). Ethanol-fed monkeys have abnormal folate metabolism (Tamura and Halsted, 1983). This is an area of active and fruitful investigation at present.

Mineral deficiencies induced by alcoholism may be important in cancer risk. Epidemiologic and experimental evidence suggests that deficiencies of zinc and selenium, in particular, may increase cancer risk at GI tract and other sites (Committee on Diet, Nutrition, and Cancer, 1982). Decreased blood selenium has been reported in alcoholics, particularly if cirrhosis is present (Dworkin *et al.*, 1984; Valimaki *et al.*, 1983). Ethanol ingestion by humans results in increased urinary and fecal excretion of zinc; alcoholic patients may have reduced serum zinc content (Mellow *et al.*, 1983). In rats fed 30–36% of calories as alcohol, zinc absorption and serum and liver zinc were decreased (Antonson and Vanderhoof, 1983; Bogden *et al.*, 1984; Yeh and Cerklewski, 1984). Long-term ingestion of a lower ethanol dose, 4% in drinking water, had no detectable effect on zinc status (Gabrial *et al.*, 1982).

Hepatic stores of vitamin A are reduced in ethanol-fed rats, a reduction that is increased if a high-fat diet is fed (Misslbeck *et al.*, 1984; Grummer and Erdman, 1986). Vitamin A absorption or β-carotene absorption, which is much lower, appeared not to be reduced by ethanol feeding in one study in rats, but hepatic storage of the administered dose was reduced (Grummer and Erdman, 1986).

A recent study of diet intake and nutritional and health status in men classified as middle-class alcoholics, alcohol consumers, or abstainers is of interest (Hillers and Massey, 1985). Subjects were 179 men in Washington State drawn in equivalent numbers from four groups: university students, nonfaculty university employees, men arrested for driving while intoxicated, and men in an alcoholism treatment center. Nutritional histories, blood chemistries, hematological indices, and height and weight were evaluated. The subjects were divided into tertiles on the basis of alcohol intake: ≤0.28 oz/day, 0.28–1.25 oz/day, ≥1.25 oz/day. They showed alcohol–dose-related decreases in intake of several nutrients (Table VII). The results were similar to those of other studies reviewed by the authors, who concluded that excessive alcohol intake is associated with decreased diet quality. However, in the socioeconomic group studied, nutrient intake still remained above the Recommended Daily Allowance (RDA), with a few exceptions. Even in the exceptional cases, nutrient intake was at about 75% of the RDA. Hematological and clinical chemistry studies showed evidence of liver damage, borderline abnormalities of red blood count, and elevated HDL cholesterol in subjects in the highest tertile for alcohol intake.

Table VII. Changes in Dietary Intake
with Alcohol Consumption[a]

Nutrient	Changes in consumption per day per ounce of alcohol consumed
Energy	+93 kcal
Protein	−4 g
Fat	−6 g
Calcium	−81 mg
Vitamin A[b]	−550 IU
Vitamin C[b]	−10 mg
Thiamin[b]	−0.1 mg
Iron	−0.5 mg
Fiber	−0.2 g

[a]Adapted from Hillers and Massey, 1985.
[b]Intake 73–79% of RDA in highest tertile of alcohol consumption; intake of other nutrients was above RDA.

In summary, nutritional and metabolic mechanisms proposed for the influence of heavy alcohol intake on carcinogenesis are supported by studies in human subjects and laboratory animals. There is a need for animal models in which effects of ethanol on carcinogenesis can be consistently demonstrated and which can then be used to examine mechanisms. The relationships between moderate alcohol intake and carcinogenesis are less well established but have been found in many studies. Availability of animal models would permit significant advances in determining the significance of the relationships, if any, and demonstrating the mechanisms that explain them.

ACKNOWLEDGMENTS. This work was supported in part by USPHS Grants CA39222 and ES02429.

5. References

Antonson, D. L., and Vanderhoof, J. A., 1983, Effect of chronic ethanol ingestion on zinc absorption in rat small intestine, *Dig. Dis. Sci.* **28:**604–608.

Austin, H., Delzell, E., Grufferman, S., Levine, R., Morrison, A., Stolley, P. D., and Cole, P., 1986, A case control study of hepatocellular carcinoma and the hepatitis B virus, cigarette smoking, and alcohol consumption, *Cancer Res.* **46:**962–966.

Bogden, J. D., Al-Rabiai, S., and Gilani, S. H., 1984, Effect of chronic ethanol ingestion on the metabolism of copper, iron, manganese, selenium, and zinc in an animal model of alcoholic cardiomyopathy, *J. Toxicol. Environ. Health* **14:**407–417.

Boing, H., Martinez, L., Frentzel-Beyme, R., and Oltersdorf, U., 1985, Regional nutritional pattern and cancer mortality in the Federal Republic of Germany, *Nutr. Cancer* **7:**121–130.

Brechot, C., Nalpas, B., Courouce, A., Duhamel, G., Callard, P., Carnot, F., Tiollais, P., and Berthelot, P., 1982, Evidence that hepatitis B virus has a role in liver-cell carcinoma in alcoholic liver disease, *N. Engl. J. Med.* **306:**1384–1387.

Breslow, N. E., and Enstrom, J. E., 1974, Geographic correlations between cancer mortality rates and alcohol-tobacco consumption in the U.S., *J. Natl. Cancer Inst.* **53:**639, 1974.

Broitman, S. A., 1984, Relationship of ethanolic beverages and ethanol to cancers of the digestive tract, in: *Vitamins, Nutrition, and Cancer* (A. Prasad, ed.), S. Karger, Basel.

Bulatao-Jayme, J., Almero, E. M., Castro, M. C. A., Jardeleza, M. R., and Salamat, L. A., 1982, A case-control dietary study of primary liver cancer risk from aflatoxin exposure, *Int. J. Epidemiol.* **11:**112–119.

Byers, T., and Graham, S., 1984, The epidemiology of diet and cancer, *Adv. Cancer Res.* **41:**1–61.

Castonguay, A., Rivenson, A., Trushin, N., Reinhardt, J., Spathopoulos, S., Weiss, C., Reiss, B., and Hecht, S., 1984, Effects of chronic ethanol consumption on the metabolism and carcinogenicity of N'-nitrosonornicotine in F344 rats, *Cancer Res.* **44:**2285–2290.

Committee on Diet, Nutrition, and Cancer, Assembly of Life Sciences, National Research Council, *Diet, Nutrition, and Cancer,* National Academy Press, Washington, DC.

Correa, P., 1982, Precursors of gastric and esophageal cancer, *Cancer* **50:**2554–2565.

Cowles, S. R., 1983, Cancer of the larynx: Occupational and environmental associations, *South. Med. J.* **76:**894–898.

Dennis, B. H., Haynes, S. G., Anderson, J. J. B., Liu-Chi, S., Hosking, J. D., and Rifkind, B. M., 1985, Nutrient intakes among selected North American populations in the Lipid Research Clinics Prevalence Study: Composition of energy intake, *Am. J. Clin. Nutr.* **41:**312–329.

Doll, R., and Peto, R., 1981, The causes of cancer: Quantitative estimates of avoidable risks of cancer in the U.S. today, *J. Natl. Cancer Inst.* **66:**1191–1308.

Dworkin, B. M., Rosenthal, W. S., Gordon, G. G., and Jankowski, R. H., 1984, Diminished blood selenium levels in alcoholics. *Alcoholism Clin. Exp. Res.* **8:**535–538.

Edmondson, H. A., and Peters, R. L., 1985, Liver, in: *Anderson's Pathology* (J. M. Kissane, ed.), C. V. Mosby, St. Louis, pp. 1096–1212.

Feo, F., Pascale, R., Garcea, R., Daino, L., Pirisi, L., Frassetto, S., Ruggiu, M. E., Di Padova, C., and Stramentinoli, G., 1986, Effect of the variations of S-adenosyl-L-methionine liver content on fat accumulation and ethanol metabolism in ethanol-intoxicated rats, *Toxicol. Appl. Pharmacol.* **83:**331–341.

Ferenci, P., Dragosics, B., Marosi, L., and Kiss, F., 1984, Relative incidence of primary liver cancer in cirrhosis in Austria. Etiological considerations, *Liver* **4:**7–14.

Flanders, W. D., and Rothman, K. J., 1982, Occupational risk for laryngeal cancer, *Am. J. Public Health* **72:**369–372.

Gabrial, G. N., Schrager, T. F., and Newberne, P. M., 1982, Zinc deficiency, alcohol, and a retinoid: Association with esophageal cancer in rats, *J. Natl. Cancer Inst.* **68:**785–789.

Garland, C., Barrett-Connor, E., Rossof, A. H., Shekelle, R. B., Criqui, M. H., and Paul, O., 1985, Dietary vitamin D and calcium and risk of colorectal cancer: A 19-year prospective study in men, *Lancet* **1:**307–309.

Gondeau, A., Maupas, P., Dubois, F., Coursaget, P., and Boughoux, P., 1981, Hepatitis B infection in alcoholic liver disease and primary hepatocellular carcinoma in France, *Prog. Med. Virol.* **27:**26–34.

Grummer, M. A., and Erdman, J. W., 1986, Effect of chronic ethanol consumption and moderate or high fat diet upon tissue distribution of vitamin A in rats fed either vitamin A or B-carotene, *Nutr. Res.* **6:**61–73.

Herity, B., Moriarty, M., Daly, L., Dunn, J., and Bourke, G. J., 1982, The role of tobacco and alcohol in the aetiology of lung and larynx cancer, *Br. J. Cancer* **46:**961–1964.

Hiatt, R. A., and Bawol, R. D., 1984, Alcoholic beverage consumption and breast cancer incidence, *Am. J. Epidemiol.* **120:**676–683.

Hillers, V. N., and Massey, L. K., 1985, Interrelationships of moderate and high alcohol consumption with diet and health status, *Am. J. Clin. Nutr.* **41:**356–362.

Hinds, M. W., Kolonel, L. N., Lee, J., and Hirohata, T., 1980, Associations between cancer incidence and alcohol/cigarette consumption among five ethnic groups in Hawaii, *Br. J. Cancer* **41:**929–940.

Jensen, O. M., 1983, Cancer risk among Danish male Seventh Day Adventists and other temperance society members, *J. Natl. Cancer Inst.* **70:**1011–1014.

Kono, S., and Ikeda, S., 1979, Correlation between cancer mortality and alcoholic beverages in Japan, *Br. J. Cancer* **40:**449–455.

Kouros, M., Monch, W., Reiffer, F. J., and Dehnen, W., 1983, The influence of various factors on the methylation of DNA by the oesophageal carcinogen N-nitrosomethylbenzylamine. I. The importance of alcohol, *Carcinogenesis* **4:**1081–1084.

Kvale, G., Bjelke, E., and Gart, J. J., 1983, Dietary habits and lung cancer risk, *Int. J. Cancer* **31:**397–405.

La Vecchia, Decaril A., Franceshci, S., Pampallona, S., and Tognon, G., 1985, Alcohol consumption and the risk of breast cancer in women, *J. Natl. Cancer Inst.* **75:**61–65.

Le, M. G., Hill, C., Kramar, A., and Flamani, R., 1984, Alcoholic beverage consumption and breast cancer incidence, *Am. J. Epidemiol.* **120**:350–357.

Lieber, C. S., 1983, Microsomal ethanol oxidizing system (MEOS). Interaction with ethanol, drugs and carcinogens, *Pharm. Biochem. Behav.* **18**:181–187.

Mashberg, A., Garfinkel, L., and Harris, S., 1981, Alcohol as a primary risk factor in oral squamous carcinoma, *CA— Cancer J. for Clinicians* **31**:146–156.

McMartin, K. E., 1984, Increased urinary folate excretion and decreased plasma folate levels in the rat after acute ethanol treatment, *Alcoholism Clin. Exp. Res.* **8**:172–178.

Melbye, M., Skinhoj, P., Nielsen, N. H., Vestergaard, B. F., Ebbesen, P., Hansen, J. P. H., and Biggar, R. J., 1984, Virus-associated cancers in Greenland: Frequent hepatitis B virus infection but low primary hepatocellular carcinoma incidence, *J. Natl. Cancer Inst.* **73**:1267–1272.

Mellow, M. H., Layne, E. A., Lipman, T. O., Kaushik, M., Hostetler, C., and Smith, J. C., 1983, Plasma zinc and vitamin A in human squamous carcinoma of the esophagus, *Cancer* **51**:1615–1620.

Miller, A. B., Howe, G. R., Jain, M., Craib, K. J., and Harrison, L., 1983, Food items and food groups as risk factors in a case-control study of diet and colorectal cancer, *Int. J. Cancer* **32**:155–161.

Misslbeck, N. G., Campbell, T. C., and Roe, D. A., 1984, Effect of ethanol consumed in combination with high or low fat diets on the postinitiation phase of hepatocarcinogenesis in the rat, *J. Nutr.* **114**:2311–2323.

Muhoberac, B. B., Roberts, R. K., Hoyumpa, A. M., and Schenker, S., 1984, Mechanism(s) of ethanol-drug interaction, *Alcoholism Clin. Exp. Res.* **8**:583–593.

National Inst. on Alcohol Abuse and Alcoholism, 1984, Alcohol Health and Research World: Summary of Fifth Special Report to the U.S. Congress on Alcohol and Health, Vol. 9, NIAAA, pp. 4–67.

Nelson, R. L., and Samelson, S. L., 1985, Neither dietary ethanol nor beer augments experimental colon carcinogenesis in rats, *Dis. Colon Rectum* **28**:460–462.

Ohnishi, K., Iida, S., Iwama, S., Goto, N., Nomura, F., Takashi, M., Mishima, A., Knon, K., Kimura, K., Musha, H., Kotota, K., and Okuda, K., 1982, The effect of chronic habitual alcohol intake on the development of liver cirrhosis and hepatocellular carcinoma: Relation to hepatitis B surface antigen carriage, *Cancer* **49**:672–677.

Paterson, A. C., Kew, M. C., Herman, A. A. B., Becker, P. J., Hodkinson, J., and Isaacson, C., 1985, Liver morphology in Southern Africa blacks with hepatocellular carcinoma: A study within the urban environment, *Hepatology* **5**:72–78.

Pickle, L. W., Greene, M. H., Ziegler, R. G., Toledo, A., Hoover, R., Lynch, H. T., and Fraumeni, J. F., 1984, Colorectal cancer in rural Nebraska, *Cancer Res.* **44**:363–369.

Pollack, E. S., Nomura, A. M. Y., Heilbrun, L. K., Stemmermann, G. N., and Green, S. B., 1984, Prospective study of alcohol consumption and cancer, *N. Engl. J. Med.* **310**:617–621.

Porta, E. A., Markell, N., and Dorato, R. D., 1985, Chronic alcoholism enhances hepatocarcinogenicity of diethylnitrosamine in rats fed a marginally methyl-deficient diet, *Hepatology* **5**:1120–1125.

Pottern, L. M., Morris, L. E., Blot, W. J., Ziegler, R. G., and Fraumeni, J. F., 1984, Esophageal cancer among black men in Washington, D.C. I. Alcohol, tobacco and other risk factors, *J. Natl. Cancer Inst.* **67**:777–783.

Rogers, A. E., and Conner, M. W., 1986, Alcohol and cancer, in: *Essential Nutrients in Carcinogenesis* (L. Poirier, P. M. Newberne, and M. W. Pariza, eds.) Plenum Press, New York, pp. 473–496.

Rogers, A. E., and Newberne, P. M., 1982, Lipotrope deficiency in experimental carcinogenesis, *Nutri. Cancer* **2**:104–112.

Rogers, A. E., Fox, J. G., and Murphy, J. C., 1981, Ethanol and diet interactions in male rhesus monkeys, *Drug-Nutrient Interact.* **1**:3–14.

Rogers, A. E., Nields, H. M., and Newberne, P. M., 1986, Nutritional and dietary influences on liver tumorigenesis in mice and rats, *Arch. Toxicol. Suppl.* **10**:231–243.

Rogers, E. L., Goldkind, L., and Golkind, S. F., 1982, Increasing frequency of esophageal cancer among black male veterans, *Cancer* **49**:610–617.

Rosenberg, L., Slone, D., and Shapiro, S., 1982, Breast cancer and alcoholic beverage consumption, *Lancet* **1**:267–271.

Russell, R. M., Rosenberg, I. H., Wilson, P. D., Iber, F. L., Oaks, E., Giovetti, A., Atradovic, C., Karwaski, P., and Press, A., 1983, Increased urinary excretion and prolonged turnover time of folic acid during ethanol ingestion, *Am. J. Clin. Nutr.* **38**:64–70.

Schottenfeld, D., 1984, Epidemiology of cancer of the esophagus, *Semin. Oncol.* **11**:92–100.

Schwartz, M., Buchmann, A., Wiesbeck, G., and Kunz, W., 1983, Effect of ethanol on early stages in nitrosamine carcinogenesis in rat liver, *Cancer Lett.* **20:**305–312.

Seitz, H. K., Czygan, P., Waldherr, R., Veith, S., and Kommerell, B., 1985, Ethanol and intestinal carcinogenesis in the rat, *Alcohol* **2:**491–494.

Sellers, E. M., and Holloway, M. R., 1978, Drug kinetics and alcohol ingestion, *Clin. Pharmacokinet.* **3:**440–452.

Tamura, T., and Halsted, C. H., 1983, Folate turnover in chronically alcoholic monkeys, *J. Lab. Clin. Med.* **101:**623–628.

Thomas, D. B., Uhl, C. N., and Hartge, P., 1983, Bladder cancer and alcoholic beverage consumption, *Am. J. Epidemiol.* **118:**720–727.

Tuyns, A. J., Pequignot, G., and Abbatucci, J. S., 1979, Oesophageal cancer and alcohol consumption: Importance of type of beverage, *Int. J. Cancer* **23:**443–447.

Valimaki, M. J., Harju, K. J., and Ylikahri, R. H., 1983, Decreased serum selenium in alcoholics—A consequence of liver dysfunction, *Clin. Chim. Acta* **130:**291–296.

Van Thiel, D. H., Lipsitz, H. D., Porter, L. E., Schade, R. R., Gottlieb, G. P., and Graham T. O., 1981, Gastrointestinal and hepatic manifestations of chronic alcoholism, *Gastroenterology* **81:**594–615.

Wagner, C., Briggs, W. T., and Cook, R. J. 1985, Inhibition of glycine *n*-methyltransferase activity by folate derivatives: implications for regulation of methyl group metabolism, *Biochem. Biophys. Res. Commun.* **127:**746–752.

Webster, L. A., Wingo, P. A., Layde, P. M., and Ory, H. W., 1983, Alcohol consumption and risk of breast cancer, *Lancet* **2:**724–726.

Willett, W. C., Stampfer, M. J., Colditz, G. A., Rosner, B. A., Hennekens, C. H., and Speizer, F. E., 1987, Moderate Alcohol consumption and risk of breast cancer *N. Engl. J. Med.* **316:**1174–1180.

World Health Organization, 1979, *Environmental Health Criteria 11. Mycotoxins,* WHO, Geneva.

Yeh, L-C. C., and Cerklewski, F. L., 1984, Interaction between ethanol and low dietary zinc curing gestation and lactation in the rat, *J. Nutr.* **114:**2027–2033.

Yu, M. C., Mack, T., Hanisch, R., Peters, R. L., Henderson, B. E., and Pike, M. C., 1983, Hepatisis, alcohol consumption, cigarette smoking, and hepatocellular carcinoma in Los Angeles, *Cancer Res.* **43:**6077–6079.

Ziegler, R. G., Morris, L. E., Blot, W. J., Pottern, L. M., Hoover, R., and Fraumeni, J. F., 1981, Esophageal cancer among black men in Washington, D.C. II. Role of nutrition, *J. Natl. Cancer Inst.* **67:**1199–1206.

Appendix

Effects of Dietary Constituents on Carcinogenesis in Different Tumor Models
An Overview from 1975 to 1988

Gabriele Angres and Maren Beth

1. Preface

What people eat is known to have a great influence on their risk of developing cancer, yet there has been little systematic analysis of the influence of diet on cancer in laboratory animals, despite the fact that results in animals are widely used to make estimates of carcinogenic risks for humans. ICPEMC felt that a comprehensive survey of the literature on the influence of dietary factors on carcinogenesis (both spontaneous and induced) in animals would be useful and would encourage a wider awareness of the effects of diet. Through the good offices of a member of the Commission, Professor D. Schmähl, the following survey was commissioned from Drs. Angres and Beth.

B. A. Bridges, Chairman
International Commission for Protection against Environmental Mutagens and Carcinogens

Abbreviations

AFB$_1$	Aflatoxin B$_1$
AFB	Aflatoxin
AOM	Azoxymethane

Gabriele Angres and Maren Beth • Institute of Toxicology and Chemotherapy, German Cancer Research Center, D-6900 Heidelberg, Federal Republic of Germany. This chapter was originally published by the International Commission for Protection against Environmental Mutagens and Carcinogens as ICPEMC Working Paper No. 8. ICPEMC is affiliated with the International Association of Environmental Mutagen Societies (IAEMS) and is sponsored by the Institut de la Vie. All correspondence and reprint requests should be addressed to the secretary of ICPEMC: Dr. J. D. Jansen, Medical Biological Laboratory TNO, P. O. Box 45, 2280 AA Rijswijk (The Netherlands).

BBN	*N*-butyl-*N*(4-hydroxybutyl)nitrosamine
BMA	Benzylmethylamine
BOP	Bis(2-oxopropyl)nitrosamine
B(a)p	Benzo(a)pyrene
DMAB	3,2′-Dimethyl-4-aminobiphenyl
DMBA	7,12-Dimethylbenzanthracene
DMH	Dimethylhydrazine
2,7-FAA	*N*,*N*′-2,7-fluorenylene
FANFT	Nitrofurylthiazolylformamide
MAM	Methylazomethanol
MCA	3-Methylcholanthrene
3′-MeDAB	3′-Methyl-4-dimethylaminoazobenzene
MonN-Pip	Mononitrosopiperazine
NAMM	*N*-nitroso-acetoxymethylmethylamine
NDEA	Nitrosodiethylamine
NMBA	*N*-nitrosomethylbenzylamine
NMNG	Nitrosomethylnitroguanidine
NMOR	Nitrosomorpholine
NMU	Nitrosomethylurea
NPip	*N*-nitrosopiperidine
NQO	4-Nitroquinoline-1-oxide
N-SAR-ethylester	*N*-nitrososarcosine-ethylester
Pb	Phenobarbital
SD	Sprague–Dawley
TPA	12-*O*-tetradecanoylphorbol-13-acetate
ad lib	*Ad libitum*
dw	Drinking water
hr	Hour
ig	Intragastral
im	Intramuscular
inj	Injection
ip	Intraperitoneal
ir	Intrarectal
it	Intratracheal
iv	Intravenous
po	Peroral
sc	Subcutane
wk	Week
*	Number of tumors/animal
b	Diet given before carcinogen administration
d	Diet given during carcinogen administration
a	Diet given after carcinogen administration
↑	Significant increase
↓	Significant decrease
Ø	No significant effect, significance not noted
→	Increasing tumor manifestation time
←	Decreasing tumor manifestation time

The first column reflects the nutrition factor in the diet when no other gavage is noted.

2. Introduction

For many years, diet has been discussed as a major factor in several types of carcinogenesis. Particular attention has been focused on the "fat hypothesis" according to which breast cancer in women, prostate cancer in men, and colonic cancer in both sexes are said to be caused alone or in part by high dietary fat content. On the other hand, a high dietary fiber content is said to especially inhibit colonic carcinogenesis. Furthermore, it has been discussed whether overweight and the total amount of energy ingested might cause some types of cancer, such as endometrium or colonic carcinoma.

Since Doll and Peto published their paper in 1981, it has been public opinion that 35% (10–70%) of all carcinomas are diet-related. This is, however, a global number that does not apply to all geographic sites. In some Asian countries, for instance, chewing of betel nuts wrapped in raw tobacco leaves and glued together is responsible for the exceedingly high number of oral carcinomas observed in these countries (incidence of 30% compared to 1% in Germany). This, indeed, is a dietary component with a high carcinogenic potential. Another example is the extremely high incidence of esophageal cancer in some areas of China and India, which wholly or in part might be due to the intake of very hot food and beverages. For this specific type of cancer, too, a dietary habit would thus be causal.

With regard to our own diet and the incidence of certain tumor types, a general statement is not possible. In numerous studies the etiology of colonic carcinoma is related to high meat and fat, but low fiber consumption (Reddy *et al.*, 1980; Rose *et al.*, 1986). In other studies a correlation between these dietary habits and the incidence of colonic cancer was not established (Berry *et al.*, 1986; Carr, 1985; Philips and Snowdon, 1985; Shimizu *et al.*, 1987; Zaridse, 1983). Some authors even found an inverse relationship between fat consumption and colonic cancer (Stemmermann *et al.*, 1984). The same applies to gastric and mammary carcinoma, for which the causality of high dietary fat consumption has also been postulated (Willett *et al.*, 1984).

In addition to these widely discussed dietary problems, there are studies in which, for instance, the consumption of black tea is claimed to cause colonic cancer (Heilbrun, 1986). However, the results have not been reproduced and have to be interpreted with special caution.

Evidence has been supplied that in Western countries overweight may play a role in the development of some tumor types (Garfinkel, 1986). This applies in particular to endometrium carcinoma in women, to a certain degree to postmenopausal mammary carcinoma, and to colonic carcinoma. The finding coincides with experimental results according to which a certain "carcinogenic potential" is inherent in hypercaloric nutrition as opposed to hypocaloric diets. The composition of the diets, however, is of no relevance (Albaner, 1987; Beth *et al.*, 1987a; Kritchevsky *et al.*, 1984); the surplus of energy is the decisive factor.

Thus, the relationships between diet and cancer are by no means clear, but warrant further studies (Carr, 1985; Preussmann, 1985). In critically reviewing the available literature on this topic Byers and Graham (1984) stated: "This entire effort has not led to a single unequivocal conclusion regarding the relationship between dietary factors and cancer risk." The English epidemiologist Sir Richard Doll, coauthor of the study cited in the first paragraph (Doll and Peto, 1981), now obviously has a more critical opinion, because in a lecture given July 4, 1986, in Heidelberg he stated: "Epidemiological enquiry alone has been frustratingly inconclusive in explaining the correlation between diet and cancers of the breast and large bowel."

Therefore, it does not seem justified to disconcert the public by statements on diet-induced cancer, particularly in the lack of "hard data." If at all, recommendations should be of very general, aiming at the intake of high-vitamin, high-protein, and high-fiber diets and avoiding overweight.

It is therefore highly estimable that my co-workers, G. Angres and M. Beth, set out to compile and give a detailed presentation of the essential experimental data published on diet and cancer in recent years. G. Angres is responsible for colon, urinary bladder, liver, skin, esophagus, forestomach, glandular stomach, and respiratory tract investigations whereas M. Beth dealt with the papers on mammary gland and pancreas. This survey, too, shows the controversial nature of results obtained in different experimental designs. The experimental data do not contain any clear scientific evidence on which recommendations for certain cancer risk–reducing diets might be based. Thus, the topic of diet and cancer will doubtless be of major relevance in future clinical and experimental studies.

D. Schmähl

3. Materials and Methods

The results of animal experiments concerning dietary influences on chemical carcinogenesis, as well as on the incidence of spontaneous tumors, published from 1975 to August 1988 have been obtained by online search. Cancerlit and Medline system identified and analyzed approximately 300 articles describing dietary effects on the following organs: colon, urinary bladder, liver, esophagus, forestomach, glandular stomach, skin, respiratory tract, mammary gland, and pancreas. Influences on transplanted tumors were not considered. In evaluating the tumor incidence in the mammary gland and pancreas, only carcinomas were counted, whereas at all other tumor sites carcinomas as well as adenomas were included in the study. The effects of dietary factors on liver carcinogenesis were described when the investigators induced liver tumors, while reports on γ-glutamyl-transferase–positive foci were not considered.

If no differentiation was made by the respective authors, the influence on overall tumor development was evaluated. The effects on carcinogenesis are described in the tables as follows: ↑ = significant increase, ↓ = significant decrease of either cancer incidence or number of tumors per tumor-bearing animals. If the parameter "number of tumors" was only given per rat, it is marked by an * in the respective column. ← or → means that the manifestation time of carcinomas was significantly shortened or prolonged. Effects that were not significant or not clearly designated as significant are marked by an ø in the respective column, whereas effects that were not observed or described by the authors are marked —.

Differences in the statistical test systems, evaluation modes, and levels of significance between the various studies were not worked out. The designation as significant effect was based on a significant influence described in comparison to the respective control group. The disparity between control groups, especially the difference in dietary compositions, was not taken into consideration. When there was no clearly designated control group, the group that logically functioned as control group was selected. Neither differences in animal numbers nor differences in experimental periods between the various studies were taken into account. Only those effects significant at the respective end of the study were discussed, but not effects observed during the experimental period. The carcinogen and the dose used as well as the mode of administration were mentioned without giving the precise time schedule of tumor initiation. The feeding schedule of the respective diets was described in relation to carcinogen administration as b = before and/or d = during and/or a = after tumor initiation. No further differentiation was made. The nutritional constituents described in this review are shown in the tables. The dose of the nutrient factors refers to the diet, unless otherwise provided. It was not taken into consideration whether the respective diets were fed *ad libitum* or isocalorically. Our aim was to show the influence of dietary factors on carcinogenesis most comprehensively. We therefore mentioned the different experimental designs. This was necessary because many authors described the influence of several different types of diets on carcinogenesis.

A total of 84 tables were compiled, which show details of the experimental designs. The most important trends are summarized in the result tables. These summary tables describe enhancing or inhibiting effects with regard to either tumor incidences or the number of tumors per tumor-bearing animal or both. The influence of diet on tumor manifestation time was not taken into account, because in most papers, except those dealing with mammary gland tumors, this information was not given.

The difficulties and shortcomings that inevitably arose in an overview designated to be comprehensive become apparent from the methods described and are discussed below.

4. Results

Owing to the abundance of data compiled in this study, the results deal only with major trends. It is striking that for nearly every dietary factor and every organ site all three influences were seen: i.e., enhancing, reducing, and no effects. In summary, the overall picture was very heterogeneous.

4.1. Colon

For the induction of colon tumors many different carcinogens were used (DMH, AOM, NMU, MAM, DMAB, NAMM, AFB_1, NMNG, and BOP). In the experiments carried out with fiber diets the results were controversial. Comparison of the experimental designs is problematic, because the fibers used in experiments belong to a very heterogeneous group of foodstuffs. There are studies which show enhancing as well as inhibiting effects of fibers on colon carcinogenesis. In some experiments wheat bran exerted inhibitory activity, whereas no trend could be seen for corn bran, soybean bran, oat bran, or rice bran. For alfalfa, lignin, guar gum, carrageenan, and pectin a clear trend could not be observed either; in most cases no effects were seen (20 of 33, Table 1.1). The same applies to the effect of fiber-free diets on colon carcinogenesis (4 of 5; Table 1.1).

Cellulose and hemicellulose diminished the effects of carcinogens, as usually expressed in a significant reduction of the number of tumors per tumor-bearing animal, whereas the tumor incidence was not influenced significantly (Table 1.1).

The influence of a diet consisting of different types of fat on colon carcinogenesis resulted in heterogeneous findings. In more than half of the experimental designs (23 of 40) increased tumor incidences were obtained. The fat types involved were beef fat and lard, representing mainly saturated fats (increasing effects in 10 of 17). Various other oils (coconut oil, menhaden oil, olive oil, soybean oil, safflower oil, and corn oil) enhanced the carcinogenic effect in 13 of 23 experiments (Table 1.3). The oils used consisted of fatty acids with different saturation. It was not possible to detect a trend proving that more unsaturated fatty acids increase carcinogenesis whereas more saturated fatty acids do not.

In studies of the combination of fat and fibers, a trend toward higher tumor incidence and more tumors per tumor-bearing animal was seen for decreasing percentage of fibers and increasing percentage of fat (Table 1.2). Vitamin A and synthetic retinoids had basically no influence on colon tumor induction in the cited animal experiments, which is the only clear effect seen in colon investigations. Vitamin A deficiency showed heterogeneous results, too. One author found a lower tumor incidence for vitamin A–deficient diets when a high dose of the respective carcinogen was given, while another report described a decreasing effect of vitamin A deficiency on carcinogenesis by AFB_1 (Table 1.4).

In summary, vitamin C had almost no effect on colon carcinogenesis (9 of 11). One investigator found a reduction in tumor incidence only when a high dose of DMH was administered (Table 1.6). In three experiments vitamin E caused either an enhancing, an inhibiting, or no effect (Table 1.7).

Table I. Effect of Dietary Factors
on Colon Carcinogenesis

Dietary factor	Effect		
	∅	↑	↓
Fiber free	4		1
Bran	18	1	11
Cellulose and hemicellulose	4	1	8
Other fibers	20	7	6
High fiber and low fat	2		8
low fiber and high fat	4	3	4
Saturated fat	7	10	
Oils	10	13	
Vitamin A and synthetic retinoids	22		
Vitamin A deficiency	2	2	1
Vitamin C	9		2
Vitamin E		1	1
Vitamin E deficiency	2		
Selenium	7		10
Selenium in combination	2		5
Protein	2	2	1
Carbohydrates	2	2	
Caloric restriction	4		5

Selenium, usually given as sodium selenite in the drinking water, lowered the incidence of colon tumors (in 10 of 17 investigations). In a few experimental designs no effect of selenium on colon carcinogenesis was observed (Table 1.8), whereas selenium in combination with other dietary factors usually diminished the effect of the carcinogen (Table 1.9). No influence of carbohydrates on chemical carcinogenesis in the colon was seen. One author found more tumors after administration of glucose and DMH than in the DMH control group. However, the observation period lasted only 22 weeks (Table 1.11). Caloric restriction led to a significant decrease of tumor incidence or tumors per tumor-bearing animal in five of nine experimental designs (Table 1.13).

4.2. Urinary Bladder

The induction of urinary bladder tumors was effected by BBN, FANFT, and NMU. Vitamin A mainly caused a diminished bladder tumor incidence. This effect was observed in 30 of 70 experiments. The results include experiments on synthetic retinoids (Table 2.1). Vitamin C, given as sodium ascorbate (5% in diet), enhanced tumor incidence only when a dose of 0.05% BBN in the drinking water was administered for at least 4 weeks. This effect, however, was observed only in male rats. Lower doses of BBN or gavage to female rats showed no influence on bladder carcinogenesis (Table 2.2). The results with tryptophan were heterogeneous. There were increasing trends (one of four), as well as no effects. Leucin and isoleucin enhanced the carcinogenic activity of BBN in two experiments (Table 2.4). No influence of sodium chloride or other salts on urinary bladder tumorigenesis was found (Table 2.5).

4.3. Liver

Liver carcinogenesis was induced by AOM, 2,7-FAA, 3'-MeDAB, AFB_1, NDEA + Pb + partial hepatectomy, and DMH. In general, no effect of fat on liver tumorigenesis was found, although one experimental group showed an increase in liver tumors when corn oil was added to the

Table II. Effect of Dietary Factors
on Urinary Bladder Carcinogenesis

Dietary factor	Effect		
	$\varnothing$	↑	↓
Vitamin A and synthetic retinoids	30	1	39
Vitamin C	8	4	
Tryptophan	3	1	
Leucin and isoleucin		4	
Different salts	4	1	

diet. Another investigator used mice in the experiments and fed fats with different saturation, but no influence was seen (Table 3.1). Vitamin A and protein had no influence on tumor incidence or number of tumors of the liver per tumor-bearing animals (Table 3.2, 3.7). Selenium compounds had an inhibiting effect on liver carcinogenesis in three of eight experimental designs (Table 3.5). Trypthophan decreased the tumor incidence in all three experiments (Table 3.6). Carbohydrates were given as sucrose, but in summary no clear trend was seen (Table 3.8). Restricted diets were examined in mice with spontaneous tumors. A diminishing effect of the restricted diet was seen only in male mice (Table 3.11).

4.4. Esophagus

Vitamin A and synthetic retinoids had no effect on tumor incidence and number of tumors of the esophagus per tumor-bearing animal (Table 4.1). Feeding of the trace element selenium caused a decreasing effect in two of four investigations (Table 4.3). Three of four experimental designs showed decreasing effects of the metal molybdenum (Table 4.5).

Feeding of the metal zinc caused inhibition in two of three investigations. Zinc deficiency, on the other hand, enhanced tumor incidence in 3 of 10 experiments (Table 4.6). Sodium chloride, when given during and after administration of the carcinogen, enhanced esophageal tumorigenesis (one of three, Table 4.4). One study dealt with the influence of cereals in different preparations on NMBA-induced esophageal carcinogenesis in 26 different experimental designs. In 16 of these 26 investigations the cereals (white and yellow corn, white and brown wheat, polished and brown rice, sorghum, millet) reduced the tumor incidence (Table 4.7).

Table III. Effect of Dietary Factors
on Liver Carcinogenesis

Dietary factor	Effect		
	$\varnothing$	↑	↓
Fat	23	6	
Vitamin A and synthetic retinoids	5		
Selenium	5		3
Tryptophan			3
Protein	7		2
Carbohydrates	5	1	
Restricted diet	2		2

Table IV. Effect of Dietary Factors
on Esophagus Carcinogenesis

	Effect		
Dietary factor	∅	↑	↓
Vitamin A and synthetic retinoids	5		
Selenium	2		2
Sodium chloride	2	1	
Molybdenum	1		3
Zinc	1		2
Zinc deficiency	7	3	
Cereals	10	16	

4.5. Forestomach

The influence of diet on forestomach carcinogenesis was not investigated very often. One report dealt with the influence of different sorts of fat on spontaneous tumor incidence in mice; no effect was seen (Table 5.1). No clear trend was found when the effect of vitamin A and synthetic retinoids and selenium on forestomach carcinogenesis was investigated (Table 5.3, Table 5.4) whereas sodium chloride had either enhancing (three of seven) or no effect (Table 5.5).

4.6. Glandular Stomach

Glandular stomach carcinogenesis was seldom used as a model for the investigation of dietary influences. One important dietary factor affected glandular stomach carcinogenesis by enhancing tumor incidence—i.e., sodium chloride, when given in high concentration and during administration of the carcinogen NMNG (Table 6.3).

4.7. Skin

Only a limited number of reports dealing with skin carcinogenesis and diet were found. In many experiments vitamin A and synthetic retinoids were administered topically, but not in the diet.

Table V. Effect of Dietary Factors
on Forestomach Carcinogenesis

	Effect		
Dietary factor	∅	↑	↓
Fat	6		
Synthetic retinoids	5		1
Selenium	3		2
Sodium chloride	4	3	

Table VI. Effect of Dietary Factors
on Glandular Stomach Carcinogenesis

	Effect		
Dietary factor	∅	↑	↓
Sodium chloride	12	5	

Table VII. Effect of Dietary Factors
on Skin Carcinogenesis

Dietary factor	Effect		
	$\varnothing$	$\uparrow$	$\downarrow$
Fat	3		1
Vitamin A and synthetic retinoids	5		6
Vitamin C			3
Selenium	1		2

Therefore, these papers could not be included in our review. Administration as retinylpalmitate and as retinylacetate or as a synthetic analog resulted in a decreased tumor incidence or number of tumors per tumor-bearing animal in 6 of 11 cases of chemical skin carcinogenesis (Table 7.2). Fat, vitamin C, and selenium decreased UV-induced carcinogenesis of the skin in one of four, three of three, and two of three experiments, respectively (Table 7.1, Table 7.3, Table 7.4).

4.8. Respiratory Tract

It was difficult to compare the experiments on effects of dietary factors on chemical carcinogenesis in the respiratory tract. This was due to the fact that some authors evaluated the carcinogenic potential of respective diets on the complete respiratory system whereas others related only to the lung or trachea. Another aspect concerned the different histological evaluation; sometimes preneoplastic lesions were included, sometimes only adenomas and carcinomas were counted. Fats as dietary constituents generally caused no effect on respiratory carcinogenesis (Table 8.1). One result which can be substantiated was that vitamin A as well as vitamin A deficiency usually had no influence on the carcinogenic effect of B(a)p, MCA, or NMU in the respiratory tract (Table 8.3, Table 8.2). Vitamin C had an increasing influence on tumor incidences or tumors per tumor-bearing animal. When endogenous nitrosation was practiced, vitamin C diminished the parameters in six (i.e., in all) experimental designs examined (Table 8.4). With sodium selenite, protein, and restricted diets almost no enhancement or inhibition was detected (Table 8.5–8.7).

4.9. Mammary Gland

To summarize the effects of saturated animal fats, no significant effect on mammary carcinogenesis was observed for beef tallow and lard fed to different strains of rats, as described 8 to 26 times, respectively (Table 9.1, Table 9.2). Coconut oil, a phytogenic saturated fat, was analyzed 12

Table VIII. Effect of Dietary Factors
on Respiratory Tract Carcinogenesis

Dietary factor	Effect		
	$\varnothing$	$\uparrow$	$\downarrow$
Fat	3	1	
Vitamin A deficiency	6		
Vitamin A and synthetic retinoids	17	3	1
Vitamin C	4	6	
Vitamin C endogen nitrosation			6
Selenium	5		1
Protein	4		
Restricted diet	2		2

Table IX. Effect of Dietary Factors
on Mammary Gland Carcinogenesis

Dietary factor	Effect		
	∅	↑	↓
Saturated fat	28	5	1
Low oil	6		4
Oils	49	15	15
Different fatty acids	8	1	1
Vitamin A	14		35
Synthetic retinoids	3		7
Selenium	10		5
Oils in combination with selenium	16	2	15
Protein in combination	23		2
Dextrose in combination	4		7
Caloric restriction	1		14
Calories	1		3
Coffee and caffeine	22	7	11

times and showed no significant effect either (Table 9.4). Regarding the studies dealing with the influence of unsaturated phytogenic sunflower seed oil, rapeseed oil, palm oil, olive oil, and corn oil, described 10, 2, 4, 2, and 43 times, respectively, most of the results were not significant, as depicted in Tables 9.6 and 9.4. When corn oil was fed in combination with the carbohydrate dextrose, as investigated in seven studies (Table 9.14), and when different combinations of fats were fed, most of the effects observed were not significant. Menhaden oil, a marine fat, did not have any significant effects in most of the six experiments (Table 9.5).

The effect of vitamin A administered at different forms and doses was described 49 times. To summarize the results, a significant decrease of tumor incidence was observed in 35 of the 49 experiments. A more marked effect was observed when retinyl methyl ether was fed. In three of four experiments, the tumor incidence was significantly reduced and in four investigations the manifestation time of DMBA-induced mammary carcinomas was prolonged (Table 9.8). When retinyl acetate was given to NMU-induced female SD rats after carcinogen administration at the high dose of 328 ppm (= 328 mg/kg diet, = 1 mM), tumor incidence was significantly decreased in 12 of the 15 experimental designs, and even the development of tumor numbers per tumor-bearing rats was significantly inhibited in all analyses. When the high dose of 656 ppm (= 2 mM) was given, all three evaluated parameters of tumorigenesis were significantly changed in both studies (Table 9.10). 4–hydroxyphenylretinamide (4-HPR), a synthetic vitamin A analog, decreased the tumor incidence in four of six and the number of tumors per tumor-bearing animal in four of five experiments when fed to DMBA- and NMU-induced rats and mice (Table 9.11). Vitamin E in combination with other dietary factors showed no significant effects on mammary carcinogenesis (Table 9.12). The same applies to vitamin C (five analyses, Table 9.12).

The influence of sodium selenite on spontaneous and chemically induced mammary carcinogenesis was investigated 15 times and selenium in combination with different oils in 33 experimental designs (Table 9.10, Table 9.11). To sum up the results, irrespective of the great variety of experimental designs, no unequivocal effect of sodium selenite was observed. Only in 5 of 15 analyses, the authors described a significant reduction of mammary cancer incidence. In four of five experiments, however, sodium selenite given to mice significantly reduced the number of spontaneous mammary carcinomas (Table 9.10). Administration together with corn oil diets decreased the tumor incidence in 15 of 33 investigations (Table 9.11). When protein was administered as casein together with different fatty diets, as described in 25 experimental designs (Table 9.13), no significant effect on mammary carcinoma development was observed in most of the experiments.

Table X. Effect of Dietary Factors
on Pancreas Carcinogenesis

Dietary factor	Effect		
	∅	↑	↓
Corn oil	9	4	
Other oils	3	1	
Vitamin A and synthetic retinoids	25	12	
Selenium	7		
Casein	10	2	2
Soya flour	14	8	
Caloric restriction	1		2

Only the effect of caloric restriction on mammary carcinogenesis was unequivocal and uniform, as described 15 times: in 14 of 15 experiments, the tumor incidence was significantly decreased (Table 9.15). On the other hand, when high-calorie diets were fed, the incidence of mammary cancer was increased in three of four experiments (Table 9.15). Caffeine and coffee, investigated 24 and 16 times, respectively, exerted no clear effect on mammary cancer development. The number of tumors per tumor-bearing animal decreased, however, in 4 of 16 experiments when different doses were given before, during, and shortly after DMBA administration to female SD rats, whereas gavage only after DMBA initiation produced no significant effects (Table 9.17). When mice received caffeine, the number of tumors per mouse was decreased in four of four investigations (Table 9.17).

4.10. Pancreas

When corn oil, an unsaturated plant fat, was fed, no significant effect on carcinoma development in the pancreas was observed in most of the 13 studies evaluated (Table 10.1). The same applies to coconut oil, a saturated vegetarian fat (Table 10.1). The dietary supplementation of vitamin A and analogs resulted in increased pancreatic cancer incidence and number of tumors per animal in rats and hamsters in 12 of 37 investigations (Table 10.2). The influence of sodium selenite on BOP-induced pancreatic carcinogenesis was investigated seven times. It did not exert any significant effect (Table 10.3). The effect of casein, a protein, was heterogeneous. In 4 of 14 investigations a significant enhancement or decrease in pancreatic cancer incidence was found, whereas casein deficiency had no effect in all experiments (Table 10.4). Combination of casein with a corn oil diet enhanced the cancer incidence of BOP-initiated hamsters in two experiments (Table 10.5). Soya flour, given either raw or heated, enhanced the pancreatic cancer incidence in 8 of 22 investigations (Table 10.6). Caloric restriction decreased the pancreatic cancer incidence as well as the number of tumors per tumor-bearing rat in two of three investigations in azaserine-induced rats (Table 10.7).

5. Comments

It is impossible to review all the papers published in recent years on this topic, but we strove to select the most important and respective investigations.

The animal study is used as a model of the human situation, implying that the results of animal studies can be extrapolated to a great extent to the human situation.

But on the other hand, many problems arise when comparing the results of different animal experiments with one another and even more when extrapolating to the human situation.

Comparison of animal experiments with the human situation is difficult, because of differences in metabolism, caloric composition, and dietary habits. In summary, we can conclude that in nearly all cases included in this review a definite effect of the different dietary factors on carcinogenesis could not be established. Owing to different conditions and consequently different effects of dietary factors on carcinogenesis in different organs, it is advisable to avoid the general term "diet" when speaking about dietary factors and cancer. On the whole, it is difficult to precisely evaluate the influence of dietary factors on carcinogenesis, because the experimental designs differ to a great extent.

1. The influence of a specific dietary factor on chemical carcinogenesis is extremely difficult to describe exactly. One major problem concerns the different groups referred to as controls to assess the influences of the diet. The different fat diets used in colon carcinogenesis studies, for example, include a 5% fat content diet, a normal fat diet, and diets with different fatty acids. Often a positive control fed the carcinogen and a normal diet was not included.
2. Moreover, differences in the amount of carcinogen used and duration of administration are found in different experimental designs. An influence on the tumor incidence, diminishing or increasing, was found after administration of the high dose as well as the low dose of the carcinogen.
3. The experimental animals were not always observed until their natural end, but were sacrificed at varying intervals in different studies. We found studies that describe significant effects of dietary factors on carcinogenesis in comparison to the control group after a short observation period. However, if the observation period was prolonged, these effects disappeared.
4. At present, the effect of caloric restriction in diet on carcinogenesis is discussed. Therefore, the diets fed in this type of investigation should by all means be isocaloric. This prerequisite has seldom been met.
5. Another interesting factor is the difference in housing conditions of the animals when specific pathogen-free and conventional housing are compared. While under conventional settings a significant increasing effect of the diet on carcinogenesis was observed by combined administration of the two high doses of retinylacetate, the same diet failed in a germ-free surrounding (Smith *et al.,* 1975b).
6. Some investigators did not use statistical tests for the evaluation of their data and others did not mention the level of significance they chose.
7. Very deviating effects of the carcinogen used and the diet fed were found in different species of laboratory animals. There are also sex differences in the influence of dietary constituents on cancer, mostly seen in mice.

In spite of these restrictions, the animal experiment seems to be an appropriate tool to investigate dietary influences on carcinogenesis, because common basic principles do exist. Interindividual variations in metabolism are found in humans, too, e.g., different tolerances to alcoholic beverages. Everyone must be aware of the fact that dietary habits influence human life and the quality of life to a great extent. On the basis of this complex situation, great caution should be exercised in giving recommendations concerning diets to the public. In 1982, the Committee on Diet, Nutrition, and Cancer (1983) of the National Cancer Institute drafted interim guidelines on diet and cancer. We think such recommendations to the general public should be given in a more general nature in view of the heterogeneity of the results and the lack of a fundamental scientific basis. Under the present circumstances the public who generally believes in published scientific results should not be confused by unwarranted recommendations. Instead, further investigations on the basis of the general recommendations mentioned here should be pursued to obtain more relevant data.

Table 1.1. The Effect of Fibers on Colon Carcinogenesis

The Effect of Different Fiber-Free Diets on Colon Carcinogenesis

Diet	Feeding schedule	Carcinogen	Dose/duration	Species, strain/sex	Tumor incidence	No. of tumors/tumor-bearing animal	Reference
Low fiber + vitamin A palmitate (500 IU/rat/day)	b + d + a	DMH	20 mg/kg/wk sc 20 weeks	Chester Beatty male rats	∅	∅	Fleiszer et al. (1980)
Fiber free	d + a	DMH	20 mg/kg/wk sc 20 weeks	Chester Beatty male rats	∅	∅	Fleiszer et al. (1980)
Flexical diet (fiber free)	d + a	DMH	20 mg/kg/wk sc 20 weeks	Chester Beatty male rats	∅	—	Fleiszer et al. (1978)
Fiber free, then wheat bran (20%)[a]	d + a	DMH	20 mg/kg/wk sc 20 weeks	SD male rats	∅	∅	L. R. Jacobs (1983)
Wheat bran (20%), then fiber free[a]	b + d	DMH	20 mg/kg/wk sc 20 weeks	SD male rats	→	∅	L. R. Jacobs (1983)
Fibers (15%)	d + a	DMH	20 mg/kg/wk sc 20 weeks	Chester Beatty male rats	∅	—	Fleiszer et al. (1980)
Bran (20%)	b + d + a	DMH	40 mg/kg/wk sc 13 weeks	Wistar male rats	∅	—	Cruse et al. (1978)
Bran cereal (28%)	d + a	DMH	20 mg/kg/wk sc 20 weeks	Chester Beatty male rats	→	∅	Fleiszer et al. (1980)
Bran (28%)	d + a	DMH	20 mg/kg/wk sc 20 weeks	Chester Beatty male rats	→	—	Fleiszer et al. (1978)
Wheat bran (10%)	a	DMH	30 mg/kg/wk sc 5 weeks	F344 male rats	→	→	Calvert et al. (1987)
Wheat bran (15%)	b + d + a	AOM	8 mg/kg/wk sc 10 weeks	F344 male rats	→	→	Reddy et al. (1981)
Wheat bran (15%)	b + d + a	AOM	8 mg/kg/wk sc 10 weeks	F344 female rats	→	∅	Watanabe et al. (1979)
Wheat bran (15%)	b + d + a	NMU	2×2 mg/rat/wk ir 3 weeks	F344 female rats	∅	∅	Watanabe et al. (1979)
Wheat bran (15%)	b + d + a	DMAB	50 mg/kg/wk sc 20 weeks	F344 male rats	→	→	Reddy and Mori (1981)

(continued)

Table 1.1. (Continued)

Diet	Feeding schedule	Carcinogen	Dose/duration	Species, strain/sex	Tumor incidence	No. of tumors/ tumor-bearing animal	Reference
Wheat bran (20%)	b + d + a	DMH	30 mg/kg/wk ig 10 weeks	SD male rats	∅	→	Barbolt and Abraham (1980)
Wheat bran (20%)	b + d + a	DMH	15 mg/kg/wk ig 10 weeks	SD male rats	∅	→	Barbolt and Abraham (1980)
Wheat bran (20%)	b + d + a	DMH	30 mg/kg/wk ig 10 weeks	SD female rats	∅	∅	Barbolt and Abraham (1980)
Wheat bran (20%)	b + d + a	DMH	15 mg/kg/wk ig 10 weeks	SD female rats	∅	→	Barbolt and Abraham (1980)
Wheat bran (20%)	b + d + a	DMH	30 mg/kg/wk ig 10 weeks	SD male rats	∅	→	Barbolt and Abraham (1978)
Wheat bran (20%)	b + d + a	DMH	15 mg/kg/wk sc 12 weeks	SD male rats	∅	∅*	Bauer et al. (1979)
Wheat bran (20%)	b + d + a	DMH	135 mg/kg sc 2 weeks later 150 mg/kg sc	F344 rats male rats	∅	∅	Barnes et al. (1983)
Wheat bran (20%) (soft winter)	b + d + a	DMH	20 mg/kg/wk sc 10 weeks	Balb/C male mice	∅	∅	Clapp et al. (1984)
Wheat bran (20%) (hard spring)	b + d + a	DMH	20 mg/kg/wk sc 10 weeks	Balb/C male mice	∅	∅	Clapp et al. (1984)
Wheat bran (20%)	d + a	DMH	20 mg/kg/wk ig 13 weeks	SD male rats	←	∅	L. R. Jacobs (1983)
Wheat bran (20%)	a	DMH	20 mg/kg/wk ig 13 weeks	SD male rats	∅	∅	L. R. Jacobs (1983)
Wheat bran (20%)	a	DMH	135 mg/kg sc 2 weeks later 150 mg/kg sc	F344 rats male rats	→	∅	Barnes et al. (1983)
Wheat bran (40%)	b + d + a	DMH	20 mg/kg/wk sc 26 weeks	CF-1 female mice	→	∅	Chen et al. (1978)
Corn bran (15%)	b + d + a	DMAB	50 mg/kg sc 20 times	F344 male rats	∅	∅	Reddy et al. (1983)
Corn bran (20%)	b + d + a	DMH	135 mg/kg sc 2 weeks later 150 mg/kg	F344 male rats	∅	∅	Barnes et al. (1983)
Corn bran (20%)	b + d + a	DMH	20 mg/kg/wk sc 10 weeks	Balb/C male mice	∅	∅	Clapp et al. (1984)

Substance	Treatment	Carcinogen	Dose	Animal	Effect	Effect	Reference
Soy bean bran (20%)	b + d + a	DMH	135 mg/kg sc 2 weeks later 150 mg/kg	F344 male rats	∅	∅	Barnes et al. (1983)
Soy bean bran (20%)	b + d + a	DMH	20 mg/kg/wk sc 10 weeks	Balb/C male mice	∅	∅	Clapp et al. (1984)
Oat bran (20%)	b + d + a	DMH	20 mg/kg/wk sc 12 weeks	SD male rats	∅[b]	∅	Jacobs and Lupton (1986)
Rice bran (20%)	b + d + a	DMH	135 mg/kg sc 2 weeks later: 150 mg/kg	F344 male rats	∅	∅	Barnes et al. (1983)
The Effect of Cellulose on Colon Carcinogenesis							
Cellulose (0.37%) (Metamucil)	d	DMH	10 mg/kg/wk sc	Wistar male rats	∅	—	Castleden (1977)
Cellulose (0.37%) (Metamucil)	d	DMH	20 mg/kg/wk sc up to 20 weeks	Wistar male rats	∅	—	Castleden (1977)
Cellulose (4.5%)	b + d + a	DMH	25 mg/kg/wk sc 16 weeks	Wistar male rats	∅	→ *	Freeman et al. (1980)
Cellulose (4.5%)	b + d + a	DMH	25 mg/kg/wk sc 14 weeks	Wistar male rats	∅	→ *	Freeman (1986)
Cellulose (4.5%)	d + a	DMH	25 mg/kg/wk sc 16 weeks	Wistar male rats	∅	→ *	Freeman et al. (1980)
Cellulose (9.0%)	b + d + a	DMH	25 mg/kg/wk sc 16 weeks	Wistar male rats	∅	→ *	Freeman et al. (1980)
Cellulose (9.0%)	b + d + a	DMH	25 mg/kg/wk sc 16 weeks	Wistar male rats	∅	→ *	Freeman (1986)
Cellulose (9.0%)	d + a	DMH	25 mg/kg/wk sc 14 weeks	Wistar male rats	∅	→ *	Freeman et al. (1980)
Cellulose (10%)	b + d + a	DMH	20 mg/kg/wk sc 12 weeks	SD male rats	∅	—	Jacobs and Lupton (1986)
Cellulose (20%) (Metamucil)	b + d + a	DMH	20 mg/kg/wk sc 10 weeks	Swiss Albino male mice	↑	—	Toth (1984)
Cellulose (20%) (Metamucil)	b + d + a	DMH	20 mg/kg/wk sc 10 weeks	Swiss Albino female mice	∅	—	Toth (1984)
Hemicellulose (4.5%)	b + d + a	DMH	25 mg/kg/wk sc 14 weeks	Wistar male rats	∅	→ *	Freeman (1986)
Hemicellulose (9.0%)	b + d + a	DMH1	25 mg/kg/wk sc 14 weeks	Wistar male rats	∅	→ *	Freeman (1986)

(continued)

Table 1.1. (Continued)

Diet	Feeding schedule	Carcinogen	Dose/duration	Species, strain/sex	Tumor incidence	No. of tumors/ tumor-bearing animal	Reference
The Effect of Pectin on Colon Carcinogenesis							
Pectin (0.87%)	d	DMH	10 mg/kg/wk sc up to 20 weeks	Wistar male rats	∅	—	Castleden (1977)
Pectin (0.87%)	d	DMH	20 mg/kg/wk sc up to 20 weeks	Wistar male rats	∅	—	Castleden (1977)
Pectin (4%)	b + d + a	DMH	25 mg/kg/wk sc 16 weeks	Wistar male rats	∅	∅*	Freeman et al. (1980)
Pectin (4%)	d + a	DMH	25 mg/kg/wk sc 16 weeks	Wistar male rats	∅	∅*	Freeman et al. (1980)
Pectin (4.5%)	b + d + a	DMH	25 mg/kg/wk sc 14 weeks	Wistar male rats	∅	∅*	Freeman (1986)
Pectin (5%) (low methoxylated and high methoxylated.)	b + d + a	DMH	10 mg/kg/wk sc 12 weeks	SD male rats	∅	↑	Bauer et al. (1981)
Citrus pectin (6.5%)	b + d + a	DMH	15 mg/kg/wk sc 12 weeks	SD male rats	↑	↑	Bauer et al. (1979)
Pectin (9%)	b + d + a	DMH	25 mg/kg/wk sc 16 weeks	Wistar male rats	∅	∅*	Freeman et al. (1980)
Pectin (9%)	b + d + a	DMH	25 mg/kg/wk sc 14 weeks	Wistar male rats	∅	∅*	Freeman (1986)
Pectin (9%)	d + a)	DMH	25 mg/kg/wk sc 16 weeks	Wistar male rats	∅	∅*	Freeman et al. (1980)
Pectin (10%)	b + d + a	DMH	20 mg/kg/wk sc 12 weeks	SD male rats	∅	—	Jacobs and Lupton (1986)
Pectin (15%)	b + d + a	AOM	8 mg/kg/wk sc 10 weeks	F344 female rats	→	∅	Watanabe et al. (1979)
Pectin (15%)	b + d + a	NMU	2 × 2 mg/kg/wk ir 3 weeks	F344 female rats	∅	∅	Watanabe et al. (1979)

The Effect of Other Fibers on Colon Carcinogenesis

Fiber		Carcinogen	Dose	Animal			Reference
Citrus fiber (15%)	b + d + a	AOM	8 mg/kg/wk sc 10 weeks	F344 male rats	→	→	Reddy et al. (1981)
Citrus fiber (15%)	b + d + a	DMAB	50 mg/kg/wk sc 20 weeks	F344 male rats	∅	∅	Reddy and Mori (1981)
Carrot fiber (20%)	b + d + a	DMH	15 mg/kg/wk sc 12 weeks	SD male rats	∅	∅*	Bauer et al. (1979)
Lignin (7.5%)	b + d + a	DMAB	50 mg/kg/wk sc 20 weeks	F344 male rats	→	→	Reddy et al. (1983)
Alfalfa (15%)	b + d + a	AOM	8 mg/kg/wk sc 10 weeks	F344 male rats	∅	∅	Watanabe et al. (1979)
Alfalfa (15%)	b + d + a	NMU	2 × 2 mg/kg/wk ir 3 weeks	F344 female rats	↑	∅	Watanabe et al. (1979)
Guargum (0.87%)	d	DMH	10 mg/kg/wk sc up to 20 weeks	Wistar male rats	∅	—	Castleden (1977)
Guargum (0.87%)	d	DMH	20 mg/kg/wk sc up to 20 weeks	Wistar male rats	∅	—	Castleden (1977)
Guargum (5%)	b + d + a	DMH	10 mg/kg/wk sc 12 weeks	SD male rats	∅	∅	Bauer et al. (1981)
Guargum (10%)	b + d + a	DMH	20 mg/kg/wk sc 12 weeks	SD male rats	↑	—	Jacobs and Lupton (1986)
Carrageenan (1%)	—	—	—	SD male and female rats	∅	—	Wakabayashi et al. (1978)
Carrageenan (5% ig)	—	—	—	SD male and female rats	∅	—	Wakabayashi et al. (1978)
Carrageenan (6%)	d + a	DMH	20 mg/kg/wk 16 weeks	F344 male rats	∅	↑	Arakawa et al. (1986)
Carrageenan (10% ig)	—	—	—	SD male and female rats	∅	—	Wakabaysahi et al. (1978)

(continued)

Table 1.1. (*Continued*)

Diet	Feeding schedule	Carcinogen	Dose/duration	Species, strain/sex	Tumor incidence	No. of tumors/tumor-bearing animal	Reference
Carrageenan (15%)	b + d + a	AOM	8 mg/kg/wk sc 10 weeks	F344 female rats	↑	∅	Watanabe et al. (1978)
Carrageenan (15%)	b + d + a	NMU	2 × 2 mg/rat/wk ir 3 weeks	F344 female rats	↑	∅	Watanabe et al. (1978)
Konjacmannan (5%)	—	DMH	20 mg/kg/wk ip	F344 male rats	→	→	Mizutani and Mitsuoka (1983)
Normacol (0.37%)	d	DMH	10 mg/kg/wk sc or 20 mg/kg/wk sc up to 20 weeks	Wistar male rats	∅	—	Castleden (1977)
Elemental diet Vivonex (chemically defined)	d	DMH	20 mg/kg/wk sc up to 20 weeks	Wistar male rats	→	—	Castleden (1977)
Elemental diet Vivonex (chemically defined)	d	DMH	10 mg/kg/wk sc up to 20 weeks	Wistar male rats	→	—	Castleden (1977)

[a]Change: 13 after initiation.
[b]Significant reduction of tumors in the proximal colon.

Table 1.2. The Effect of a Combination of Fat and Fibers on Colon Carcinogenesis

Diet	Feeding schedule	Carcinogen	Dose/duration	Species, strain/sex	Tumor incidence	No. of tumors/ tumor-bearing animal	Reference
Wheat bran (30%) + beef fat (4.9%)	b + d	AOM	8 mg/kg/wk sc 23 weeks	SD male rats	—	→*	Nigro et al. (1979)
Alfalfa (30%) + beef fat (4.9%)	b + d	AOM	8 mg/kg/wk sc 23 weeks	SD male rats	—	→*	Nigro et al. (1979)
Cellulose (30%) + beef fat (4.9%)	b + d + a	AOM	8 mg/kg/wk sc 24 weeks	SD male rats	—	→*	Nigro et al. (1979)
Cellulose (26.9%) + beef tallow (2.1%)	b + d + a	AOM	10 mg/kg/wk sc 12 weeks	Albino Swiss male rats	∅	→	Galloway et al. (1987)
Cellulose (26.9%) + beef tallow (2.1%)	b + d + a	AOM	10 mg/kg/wk sc 12 weeks	Albino Swiss male rats	∅	→	Galloway et al. (1986)
Wheat bran (20%) + beef fat (5.6%)	b + d	AOM	8 mg/kg/wk sc 23 weeks	SD male rats	∅	∅*	Nigro et al. (1979)
Alfalfa (20%) + beef fat (6%)	b + d	AOM	8 mg/kg/wk sc 23 weeks	SD male rats	—	∅	Nigro et al. (1979)
Cellulose (20%) + beef fat (4.9%)	b + d + a	AOM	8 mg/kg/wk sc 24 weeks	SD male rats	—	→*	Nigro et al. (1979)
Cellulose (15%) + fat[a] (5%)	b + d + a	DMH	30 mg/kg/wk sc 15 weeks	Wistar male rats	∅	→	Wilpart and Roberfroid (1987)
Fybogel (15%) + fat[a] (5%)	b + d + a	DMH	30 mg/kg/wk sc 15 weeks	Wistar male rats	→	→	Wilpart and Roberfroid (1987)
Fybogel (15%) + fat[a] (20%)	b + d + a	DMH	30 mg/kg/wk sc 15 weeks	Wistar male rats	→	→	Wilpart and Roberfroid (1987)
Wheat bran (20%) + beef fat (20%)	b + d + a	DMH	30 mg/kg/wk ig 4 weeks or 8 weeks	SD male rats	→	∅	Wilson et al. (1977)
Wheat bran (20%) + corn oil (20%)	b + d + a	DMH	30 mg/kg/wk ig 4 weeks or 8 weeks	SD male rats	→	∅	Wilson et al. (1977)
Cellulose (26.6%) + beef tallow (25.1%)	b + d + a	AOM	10 mg/kg/wk sc 12 weeks	Albino Swiss male rats	∅	→	Galloway et al. (1986)

(continued)

Table 1.2. (*Continued*)

Diet	Feeding schedule	Carcinogen	Dose/duration	Species, strain/sex	Tumor incidence	No. of tumors/ tumor-bearing animal	Reference
Cellulose (26.6%) + beef tallow (25.1%)	b + d + a	AOM	10 mg/kg/wk sc 12 weeks	Albino Swiss male rats	∅	→	Galloway et al. (1986)
Cellulose (26.6%) + beef tallow (25.1%)	b + d + a	AOM	10 mg/kg/wk sc 12 weeks	Albino Swiss male rats	∅	→	Galloway et al. (1987)
Wheat bran (10%) + beef fat (35%)	b + d + a	AOM	8 mg/kg/wk sc 24 weeks	SD male rats	∅	∅*	Nigro et al. (1979)
Alfalfa (10%) + beef fat (36%)	b + d + a	AOM	8 mg/kg/wk sc 24 weeks	SD male rats	—	∅*	Nigro et al. (1979)
Cellulose (10%) + beef fat (35%)	b + d + a	AOM	8 mg/kg/wk sc 24 weeks	SD male rats	—	∅*	Nigro et al. (1979)
Cellulose + safflower oil (20%)	b + d + a	DMH	20 mg/kg/wk sc 20 weeks	SD male rats	→	→	Trudel et al. (1983)
Cellulose + lard (20%)	b + d + a	DMH	20 mg/kg/wk sc 20 weeks	SD male rats	→	→	Trudel et al. (1983)
Cellulose (15%) + fat[a] (20%)	b + d + a	DMH	30 mg/kg/wk sc 15 weeks	Wistar male rats	∅	→	Wilpart and Roberfroid (1987)
Agar (9.2%) + tallow (18.2%)	b + d + a	DMH	20 mg/kg/wk sc 20 weeks	CF-1 male mice	←	∅	Glauert and Bennink (1981)
Fybogel (5%) + fat[a] (20%)	b + d + a	DMH	30 mg/kg/wk sc 15 weeks	Wistar male rats	∅	→	Wilpart and Roberfroid (1987)
Cellulose (5%) + fat[a] (20%)	b + d + a	DMH	30 mg/kg/wk sc 15 weeks	Wistar male rats	∅	∅	Wilpart and Roberfroid (1987)
Cellulose (2.1%) + beef tallow (25.2%)	b + d + a	AOM	10 mg/kg/wk sc 12 weeks	Albino Swiss male rats	∅	←	Galloway et al. (1987)
Cellulose (2.1%) + beef tallow (25.1%)	b + d + a	AOM	10 mg/kg/wk ig 12 weeks	Albino Swiss male rats	∅	←	Galloway et al. (1986)

[a]Fat is a mixture of corn oil and palm oil.

Table 1.3. The Effect of Fat on Colon Carcinogenesis

Diet	Feeding schedule	Carcinogen	Dose/duration	Species, strain/sex	Tumor incidence	No. of tumors/tumor-bearing animal	Reference
			The Effect of Beef Fat on Colon Carcinogenesis				
Beef fat (20%)	b + d + a	DMH	150 mg/kg sc	F344 male rats	↑	∅	Reddy et al. (1977)
Beef fat (20%) (tallow)	b + d + a	DMH	20 mg/kg/wk sc 20 weeks	CF-1 male mice	∅	∅	Glauert and Bennink (1981)
Beef fat (20%) (tallow)	b + d + a	NMU	2.5 mg/kg/wk ir 2 weeks	F344 male rats	↑	↑	Reddy et al. (1977)
Beef fat (20%) (tallow)	b + d + a	MAM	35 mg/kg ip	F344 male rats	↑	↑	Reddy et al. (1977)
Beef fat (23.3%) (tallow)	b + d + a	DMAB	50 mg/kg/wk sc 20 weeks	F344 male rats convention-al	↑	↑	Reddy and Ohmori (1981)
Beef fat (23.3%) (tallow)	b + d + a	DMAB	50 mg/kg/wk sc 20 weeks	F344 male rats germ free	∅	∅	Reddy and Ohmori (1981)
Beef fat (24%)	b + d + a	DMH	10 mg/kg/wk sc 20 weeks	F344 male rats	∅	∅	Nauss et al. (1983)
Beef fat (24%)	b + d + a	NMU	2 × 1.5 mg/rat ir 2 weeks	SD male rats	∅	∅	Nauss et al. (1984)
Beef fat (30%)	b + d	AOM	8 mg/kg/wk sc 8 weeks	SD male rats	—	∅	Bull et al. (1979)
Beef fat (30%)	a	AOM	8 mg/kg/wk sc 8 weeks	SD male rats	—	↑	Bull et al. (1979)
Beef fat (35%)	b + d	AOM	8 mg/kg/wk sc until death	SD male rats	∅	↑*	Nigro et al. (1975)

(continued)

Table 1.3. (Continued)

Diet	Feeding schedule	Carcinogen	Dose/duration	Species, strain/sex	Tumor incidence	No. of tumors/ tumor-bearing animal	Reference
The Effect of Lard on Colon Carcinogenesis							
Lard (13.5%)	b + d	AOM	15 mg/kg	F344 male and female rats	∅	↑	Reddy and Maruyama (1986b)
Lard (20%)	b + d + a	DMH	20 mg/kg/wk sc 20 weeks	SD male rats	↑	∅	Trudel et al. (1983)
Lard (20%)	b + d + a	DMH	10 mg/kg/wk sc 20 weeks	F344[a] male and female rats	∅	∅*	Reddy et al. (1976a)
Lard (23.5%)	b + d	AOM	15 mg/kg	F344 male rats	↑	∅	Reddy and Maruyama (1986b)
Lard (23.5%)	a	AOM	15 mg/kg	F344 male rats	↑	↑	Reddy and Maruyama (1986b)
Lard (30%)	b + d + a	DMH	15 mg/kg/wk sc 2 weeks	W/FU male rats	∅↓	—	Bansal et al. (1978)
The Effect of Corn Oil on Colon Carcinogenisis							
Corn oil (13.6%)	b + d	AOM	15 mg/kg/wk sc 2 weeks	F344 male rats	∅	∅	Reddy and Maruyama (1986b)
Corn oil (13.6%)	a	AOM	15 mg/kg/wk sc 2 weeks	F344 male rats	↑	↑	Reddy and Maruyama (1986b)
Corn oil (20%)	b + d + a	DMH	10 mg/kg/wk sc 20 weeks	F344[a] male and femal rats	∅	∅*	Reddy et al. (1976a)
Corn oil (23%)	b + d	DMH	19,24,29,26,45 mg/kg/wk/sc 5 weeks	Swiss Webster mice	↑	↑	Temple and El-Khatib (1987)
Corn oil (23%)	b + d + a	DMH	19,24,29,26,45 mg/kg/sc 5 weeks	Swiss Webster mice	↑	∅	Temple and El-Khatib (1987)

							Reference
Corn oil (23.5%)	b + d	AOM	15 mg/kg/wk sc 2 weeks	F344 male rats	∅	∅	Reddy and Maruyama (1986b)
Corn oil (23.5%)	a	AOM	20 mg/kg sc	F344 female rats	↑	∅	Reddy and Maeura (1984)
Corn oil (23.5%)	a	AOM	15 mg/kg/wk sc 2 weeks	F344 male rats	↑	↑	Reddy and Maruyama (1986b)
Corn oil (23.5%)	a	AOM	15 mg/kg/wk sc 2 weeks	F344 male rats	↑	↑	Reddy and Maruyama (1986a)
Corn oil (24%)	b + d + a	DMH	15 mg/kg/wk ig	SD male rats	∅	∅	Nauss et al. (1983)
Corn oil (24%)	b + d + a	NMU	2 × 15 mg/kg/ wk ir 2 weeks	SD male rats	∅	∅	Nauss et al. (1984)
Corn oil (30%)	b + d + a	DMH	15 mg/kg/wk sc 2 weeks	W/FU male rats	∅	—	Bansal et al. (1978)

The Effect of Different Other Oils on Colon Carcinogenesis

Coconut oil (20%)	b + d + a	DMH	10 mg/kg/wk im 20 weeks	SD male rats	↑	↑	Broitman et al. (1977)
Coconut oil (20%)	b + d + a	DMH	10 mg/kg/wk im 20 weeks	Lewis male rats	↑	∅	Vitale et al. (1977)
Coconut oil (23.52%)	a	AOM	20 mg/kg/sc	F344 female rats	∅	∅*	Reddy and Maeura (1984)
Olive oil (23.52%)	a	AOM	20 mg/kg sc	F344 female rats	∅	∅*	Reddy and Maeura (1984)
Menhaden oil (4%)	b + d + a	AOM	15 mg/kg/wk sc 2 weeks	F344 male rats	∅	∅*	Reddy and Maruyama (1986a)
Menhaden oil (22.5%)	b + d + a	AOM	15 mg/kg/wk sc 2 weeks	F344 male rats	∅	∅*	Reddy and Maruyama (1986a)
Soy bean oil in beef fat (1 : 1) (30%)	d	DMH	20 mg/kg/wk sc 20 weeks	D/A male rats	↑	—	Howarth and Pihl (1985)
Safflower oil (20%)	b + d + a	DMH	20 mg/kg/wk sc 20 weeks	SD male rats	↑	∅	Trudel et al. (1983)
Safflower oil (20%)	b + d + a	DMH	10 mg/kg/wk im 20 weeks	SD male rats	↑	↑	Broitman et al. (1977)

(continued)

Table 1.3. (Continued)

Diet	Feeding schedule	Carcinogen	Dose/duration	Species, strain/sex	Tumor incidence	No. of tumors/ tumor-bearing animal	Reference
Safflower oil (20%)	b + d + a	DMH	10 mg/kg/wk im 20 weeks	Lewis male rats	↑	∅	Vitale et al. (1977)
Safflower oil (23.52%)	a	AOM	20 mg/kg sc	F344 female rats	↑	∅*	Reddy and Maeura (1984)
Crisco[b] (24%)	b + d + a	DMH	10 mg/kg/wk sc 20 weeks	F344 male rats	∅	∅	Nauss et al. (1983)
Crisco[b] (24%)	b + d + a	NMU	2 × 15 mg/kg/ wk ir 2 weeks	SD male rats	∅	∅	Nauss et al. (1984)
Unsaturated fat diet (5% linoleic acid ethyl ester + 40 IU vitamin E)	b + d + a	AOM	7.4 mg/kg/wk sc 11 weeks	Donryu male rats	↑	↑	Sakaguchi et al. (1984)
High fat (10 g)	d	DMH	30 mg/kg/month sc 7 months	SD male and female rats	∅	—	Schmähl et al. (1979)
High cholesterol (fat, 17 g)	d	DMH	30 mg/kg/month sc 7 months	SD male and female rats	∅	—	Schmähl et al. (1979)
High fat (10 g)	b + d	NAMM	0.1 mg/rat/14 days ir 24 times	SD[c] male and female rats	∅	—	Schmähl et al. (1983)
High fat (pork, butter, egg powder)	d + a	DMH	30 mg/kg/month sc 10 months	SD male and female rats	∅	—	Schmähl et al. (1976)

[a]Mothers were fed special diets since mating.
[b]Crisco = partially hydrogenated fat.
[c]Parental and F_1 generations were fed the diets.

Table 1.4. The Effect of Vitamin A and Synthetic Retinoids on Colon Carcinogenesis

Diet	Feeding schedule	Carcinogen	Dose/duration	Species, strain/sex	Tumor incidence	No. of tumors/ tumor-bearing animal	Reference
Vitamin A deficient (retinyl acetate, 0.3 μmole/g)	d	AFB₁	25 μg/rat/day ig 15 days	SD male and female rats	↑	—	Newberne and Suphakarn (1977)
Vitamin A deficient (retinyl acetate, 0.3 μmole/g)	d	AFB₁	1 ppm in diet	SD male and female rats	↑	—	Newberne and Suphakarn (1977)
Vitamin A deficient (Vitamin A palmitate at end of study, 10 IU/rat/wk)	b + d + a	NMMG	3 × 1.25 mg/ rat/wk ir 30 weeks	F344 female rats	→	—	Narisawa et al. (1976)
Vitamin A deficient (Vitamin A palmitate at end of study, 10 IU/rat/wk)	b + d + a	NMMG	3 × 0.63 mg/ rat/wk ir 30 weeks	F344 female rats	∅	—	Narisawa et al. (1976)
Vitamin A deficient (Vitamin A palmitate at end of study, 10 IU/rat/wk)	b + d + a	NMMG	3 × 0.31 mg/ rat/wk ir 30 weeks	F344 female rats	∅	—	Narisawa et al. (1976)
Retinyl acetate (0.8 mmole/kg)	a	DMH	150 mg/kg sc	F344 male rats	∅	∅	Silverman et al. (1981)
Retinyl acetate (0.8 mmole/kg)	a	NMU	2.5 mg/rat/wk ir 2 weeks	F344 male rats	∅	∅	Silverman et al. (1981)
Retinyl acetate (30 μmole/g)	d	AFB₁	25 μg/rat/day ig 15 days	SD male and female rats	∅	—	Newberne and Suphakarn (1977)
Retinyl acetate (30 μmole/g)	d	AFB₁	1 ppm in diet	SD male and female rats	∅	—	Newberne and Suphakarn (1977)

(continued)

Table 1.4. (Continued)

Diet	Feeding schedule	Carcinogen	Dose/duration	Species, strain/sex	Tumor incidence	No. of tumors/ tumor-bearing animal	Reference
Vitamin A palmitate (500 IU/rat/day)	d + a	DMH	20 mg/kg/wk sc 20 weeks	Chester Beatty male rats	∅	—	Fleiszer et al. (1980)
13-Cis-retinoic acid (50 mg/kg)	d + a	AOM	8 mg/kg/wk sc 8 weeks	SD male rats	∅	∅*	Nigro et al. (1982)
13-Cis-retinoic acid (240 mg/kg)	a	NMU	2 × 2 mg/kg/wk ir 8 weeks	F344 male rats	∅	∅*	Ward et al. (1978)
13-Cis-retinoic acid (240 mg/kg)	a	NMU	2 × 1 mg/kg/wk 8 weeks	F344 male rats	∅	∅*	Ward et al. (1978)
13-Cis-retinoic acid (240 mg/kg)	a	NMU	2 × 0.5 mg/ kg/wk 8 weeks	F344 male rats	∅	∅*	Ward et al. (1978)
N-ethylretinamide (654 mg/kg)	a	NMU	2 × 0.5 mg/ rat/wk ir 4, 6, or 8 weeks	F344 male rats	∅	∅	Wenk et al. (1981)
N-ethylretinamide (2.0 mmole/kg)	a	DMH	15 mg/kg sc	F344 male rats	∅	—	Silverman et al. (1981)
N-ethylretinamide (2.0 mmole/kg)	a	NMU	2.5 mg/rat/wk ir 2 weeks	F344 male rats	∅	—	Silverman et al. (1981)
N-2-hydroxyethylretin-amide (686 mg/kg)	a	NMU	2 × 0.5 mg/ rat/wk ir 4, 6, or 8 weeks	F344 male rats	∅	∅	Wenk et al. (1981)
N-2-hydroxyethylretin-amide (2.0 mmole/kg)	a	DMH	150 mg/kg sc	F344 male rats	∅	—	Silverman et al. (1981)

Compound		Carcinogen	Dose/route	Strain			Reference
N-2-hydroxyethylretin-amide (2.0 mmole/kg)	a	NMU	2.5 mg/rat/wk ir 2 weeks	F344 male rats	∅	—	Silverman et al. (1981)
N-(4-hydroxyphenyl)-all-trans-retinamide (2.0 mmole/liter)	a	DMH	150 mg/kg sc	F344 male rats	∅	∅	Silverman et al. (1981)
N-(4-hydroxyphenyl)-all-trans-retinamide (2.0 mmole/liter)	a	NMU	2.5 mg/rat/wk ir 2 weeks	F344 male rats	∅	∅	Silverman et al. (1981)
Retinylidene dimedone (406 mg/kg)	a	NMU	2 × 0.5 mg/rat/wk ir 4, 6, or 8 weeks	F344 male rats	∅	∅	Wenk et al. (1981)
Trimethylmethoxy-phenyl analog of retinoic acid ethyl-amide (60 mg/kg)	a	NMU	2 × 2 mg/kg/wk ir	F344 male rats	∅	∅*	Ward et al. (1978)
Trimethylmethoxy-phenyl analog of retinoic acid ethyl-amide (60 mg/kg)	a	NMU	2 × 1 mg/kg/wk ir	F344 male rats	∅	∅*	Ward et al. (1978)
Trimethylmethoxy-phenyl analog of retinoic acid ethyl-amide (60 mg/kg)	a	NMU	2 × 0.5 mg/kg/wk ir	F344 male rats	∅	∅*	Ward et al. (1978)
Ethyl-allyl-trans-9-(4-methoxy-2,3,6-tri-methylphenyl)-3,7-dimethyl-2,4,6,8-nonatetraenoate (8, 16, or 32 mg/kg bw ig 3 times/wk)	d + a	DMH	10 mg/kg/wk sc 10 weeks	SD male rats	∅	—	Schmähl and Habs (1978)

Table 1.5. The Effect of Vitamin B_{12} on Colon Carcinogenesis

Diet	Feeding schedule	Carcinogen	Dose/duration	Species, strain/sex	Tumor incidence	No. of tumors/ tumor-bearing animal	Reference
Vitamin B_{12} deficient	b + d + a	AOM	14, 8 mg/kg/wk sc 10 weeks	F344/cr male rats	$\emptyset$	$\emptyset$	Yamamoto (1980)

Table 1.6. The Effect of Vitamin C on Colon Carcinogenesis

Diet	Feeding schedule	Carcinogen	Dose/duration	Species, strain/sex	Tumor incidence	No. of tumors/ tumor-bearing animal	Reference
Sodium ascorbate (0.25%)	b + d + a	DMH	150 mg/kg sc 10 weeks	F344 female rats	→	∅	Reddy *et al.* (1982)
Sodium ascorbate (0.25%)	b + d + a	DMH	20 mg/kg sc 10 weeks	F344 female rats	∅	∅	Reddy *et al.* (1982)
Sodium ascorbate (1%)	b + d + a	DMH	150 mg/kg sc 10 weeks	F344 female rats	→	∅	Reddy *et al.* (1982)
Sodium ascorbate (1%)	b + d + a	DMH	20 mg/kg sc 10 weeks	F344 female rats	∅	∅	Reddy *et al.* (1982)
Sodium ascorbate (1%)	b + d + a	NMU	2 × 2 mg/rat/wk ir 2 weeks	F344 female rats	∅	∅	Reddy *et al.* (1982)
Sodium ascorbate (5%)	a	DMH	20 mg/kg/wk sc 4 weeks	F344 male rats	∅	—	Shirai *et al.* (1985)
L-Ascorbic acid (25 mg/kg/day)	b + d + a	DMH	20 mg/kg/wk sc 24 weeks	CF-1 male mice	∅	—	Jones *et al.* (1984)
L-Ascorbic acid (50 mg/kg/day)	b + d + a	DMH	20 mg/kg/wk sc 24 weeks	CF-1 male mice	∅	—	Jones *et al.* (1984)
L-Ascorbic acid (100 mg/kg/day)	b + d + a	DMH	20 mg/kg/wk sc 24 weeks	CF-1 male mice	∅	—	Jones *et al.* (1984)
L-Ascorbic acid (200 mg/kg/day)	b + d + a	DMH	20 mg/kg/wk sc 24 weeks	CF-1 male mice	∅	—	Jones *et al.* (1984)
L-Ascorbic acid (500 mg/kg/day)	b + d + a	DMH	20 mg/kg/wk sc 24 weeks	CF-1 male mice	∅	—	Jones *et al.* (1984)

Table 1.7. The Effect of Vitamin E on Colon Carcinogenesis

Diet	Feeding schedule	Carcinogen	Dose/duration	Species, strain/sex	Tumor incidence	No. of tumors/ tumor-bearing animal	Reference
Vitamin E deficient (<0.5 mg/100 g)	b + d + a	DMH[a]	20 mg/kg/wk sc 20 weeks	Wistar male rats	∅[b] →	∅[b]	Sumiyoshi (1985)
Vitamin E deficient (<0.5 mg/100 g)	d + a	DMH[a]	20 mg/kg/wk sc 20 weeks	Wistar male rats	∅[b] →	∅[b]	Sumiyoshi (1985)
Vitamin E (1750 IU/kg)	b + d + a	DMH	15 mg/kg/wk sc 20 weeks	CD-1 male mice	∅	—	Chester *et al.* (1986)
Vitamin E (600 mg/kg)	b + d	DMH	10 mg/kg/wk sc 28 weeks	LACA male mice	→	—	Cook and McNamara (1980)
Vitamin E (4%)	d + a	DMH	20 µg/g/wk sc 10 weeks	Swiss albino male and female mice	↑	—	Toth and Patil (1983)

[a]Additional induction of colitis.
[b]Intestinal tumors.

Table 1.8. The Effect of Selenium on Colon Carcinogenesis

Diet	Feeding schedule	Carcinogen	Dose/duration	Species, strain/sex	Tumor incidence	No. of tumors/ tumor-bearing animal	Reference
Selenium deficient	b + d	DMH	20 mg/kg/wk ip 20 weeks	SD male rats	∅	∅	Pence and Buddingh (1985)
Sodium selenite (0.5 ppm dw)	b + d	AOM	15 mg/kg/wk ig 2 weeks	F344 male rats	∅	∅*	Reddy *et al.* (1988)
Sodium selenite (0.5 ppm dw)	a	AOM	15 mg/kg/wk sc 2 weeks	F344 male rats	∅	∅*	Reddy *et al.* (1988)
Sodium selenite (2 ppm dw)	d + a	AOM	8 mg/kg/wk sc 8 weeks	SD male rats	∅	∅*	Nigro *et al.* (1982)
Sodium selenite (2 ppm dw)	b + d	BOP	5 mg/kg/wk sc 50 weeks	Wistar male and female rats	∅	→*	Birt *et al.* (1982)
Sodium selenite (2.5 ppm dw)	b + d	AOM	15 mg/kg/wk sc 2 weeks	F344 male rats	∅	→*	Reddy *et al.* (1988)
Sodium selenite (2.5 ppm dw)	a	AOM	15 mg/kg/wk sc 2 weeks	F344 male rats	→	→*	Reddy *et al.* (1988)
Sodium selenite (4 ppm dw)	b + d + a	DMH	20 mg/kg/wk inj 18 weeks	SD male rats	→	∅*	Jacobs *et al.* (1977)
Sodium selenite (4 ppm dw)	b + d + a	DMH	10 mg/kg/wk sc 18 weeks	SD male rats	→	∅*	M. M. Jacobs (1983)

(continued)

Table 1.8. (Continued)

Diet	Feeding schedule	Carcinogen	Dose/duration	Species, strain/sex	Tumor incidence	No. of tumors/ tumor-bearing animal	Reference
Sodium selenite (4 ppm dw)	b + d + a	DMH	10 mg/kg/wk sc 10 weeks	SD male rats	→	∅*	M. M. Jacobs (1983)
Sodium selenite (4 ppm dw)	b	DMH	20 mg/kg/wk sc 20 weeks	SD male rats	→	∅	Jacobs et al. (1981)
Sodium selenite (4 ppm dw)	b + d	DMH	20 mg/kg/wk sc 20 weeks	SD male rats	→	∅	Jacobs et al. (1981)
Sodium selenite (4 ppm dw)	d + a	DMH	20 mg/kg/wk sc 20 weeks	SD male rats	→	∅	Jacobs et al. (1981)
Sodium selenite (4 ppm dw)	a	DMH	20 mg/kg/wk sc 20 weeks	SD male rats	∅	∅	Jacobs et al. (1981)
Sodium selenite (4 ppm dw)	b + d + a	MAM	20 mg/kg/wk inj 18 weeks	SD male rats	∅	∅*	Jacobs et al. (1977)
Sodium selenite (8 ppm dw)	b + d + a	AOM	8 mg/kg/wk sc 8 weeks	SD male rats	∅	∅[b]	Soullier et al. (1981)
Sodium selenite (4 µg/ml dw)	d + a	DMH	15 mg/kg/wk sc 15 weeks	Wistar Furth[a] rats	∅ →	∅*	Ankerst and Sjögren (1982)
p-Methoxybenzeneselenol (50 ppm dw)	b + d + a	AOM	15 mg/kg/wk sc 30 weeks	F344 female rats	→	↓*	Reddy et al. (1985)

[a]Mothers were given sodium selenite since mating.
[b]Significant reduction of distal colon tumor only.

Table 1.9. The Effect of Selenium in Combination with Other Dietary Factors on Colon Carcinogenesis

Diet	Feeding schedule	Carcinogen	Dose/duration	Species, strain/sex	Tumor incidence	No. of tumors/ tumor-bearing animal	Reference
Selenium deficient + vitamin E (50 mg/kg) + lard (20%)	b + d + a	AOM	15 mg/kg/wk sc 2 weeks	F344 male rats	∅	∅*	Reddy and Tanaka (1986)
Selenium deficient + vitamin E (750 mg/kg) + lard (20%)	b + d + a	AOM	15 mg/kg/wk sc 2 weeks	F344 male rats	→	→ *	Reddy and Tanaka (1986)
Selenium deficient + vitamin E (50 mg/kg) + corn oil (20%)	b + d + a	AOM	15 mg/kg/wk sc 2 weeks	F344 male rats	→	→ *	Reddy and Tanaka (1986)
Selenium deficient + vitamin E (750 mg/kg) + corn oil (20%)	b + d + a	AOM	15 mg/kg/wk sc 2 weeks	F344 male rats	→	→ *	Reddy and Tanaka (1986)
Sodium selenite (2 ppm) + 13-*cis*-retinoic acid (50 mg/kg)	d + a	AOM	8 mg/kg/wk sc 8 weeks	SD male rats	∅	→ *	Nigro *et al.* (1982)
Sodium selenite (2 ppm) + 13-*cis*-retinoic acid (50 mg/kg) + β-sitosterol (2 g/kg)	d + a	AOM	8 mg/kg/wk sc 8 weeks	SD male rats	∅	→ *	Nigro *et al.* (1982)
13-*Cis*-retinoic acid (50 mg/kg) + β-sitosterol (2 g/kg)	d + a	AOM	8 mg/kg/wk sc 8 weeks	SD male rats	∅	∅	Nigro *et al.* (1982)

Table 1.10. *The Effect of Protein in Combination with Other Dietary Factors on Colon Carcinogenesis*

Diet	Feeding schedule	Carcinogen	Dose/duration	Species, strain/sex	Tumor incidence	No. of tumors/ tumor-bearing animal	Reference
Low casein (7.5%)	d + a	DMH	15 mg/kg/wk ip 24 weeks	SD male rats	→	—	Topping and Visek (1976)
High casein (22.5%)	d + a	DMH	15 mg/kg/wk ip 24 weeks	SD male rats	∅	—	Topping and Visek (1976)
High casein (22.5%) + urea	d + a	DMH	15 mg/kg/wk ip 24 weeks	SD male rats	∅	—	Topping and Visek (1976)
Soybean protein (40%) + corn oil (25%)	b + d	DMH	10 mg/kg/wk/sc 20 weeks	F344 male rats	∅	←	Reddy *et al.* (1976b)
Beef protein (60%) + corn oil (5%)	b + d	DMH	10 mg/kg/wk sc 20 weeks	F344 male rats	∅	←	Reddy *et al.* (1976b)

Table 1.11. The Effect of Carbohydrates on Colon Carcinogenesis

Diet	Feeding schedule	Carcinogen	Dose/duration	Species, strain/sex	Tumor incidence	No. of tumors/ tumor-bearing animal	Reference
Carbohydrate (72%)	b + d + a	DMH	15 mg/kg/wk sc 2 weeks	W/FU male rats	∅	—	Bansal *et al.* (1978)
Carbohydrate (12 g)	d	DMH	30 mg/kg/month sc 7 months	SD male and female rats	∅	—	Schmähl *et al.* (1979)
Protein-bound poly-saccharide prepa-ration (2%)	d	DMH	15 mg/kg/wk sc 16 weeks	Wistar male rats	↑ [a]	∅	Sakita *et al.* (1983)
Glucose (1.6% dw ad lib)	d	DMH	10 mg/kg/wk sc 22 weeks	Wistar male rats	↑	—	Ingram and Castleden (1981)

[a]Well-differentiated carcinomas.

Table 1.12. The Effect of a Vegetarian Diet on Colon Carcinogenesis

Diet	Feeding schedule	Carcinogen	Dose/duration	Species, strain/sex	Tumor incidence	No. of tumors/ tumor-bearing animal	Reference
Vegetarian diet (lettuce, carrots, apples, oatflakes)	d	DMH	30 mg/kg/month sc 7 months	SD male and female rats	$\emptyset$	—	Schmähl et al. (1979)
Vetarian diet (salad, carrots, apples, kohlrabi, oatflakes)	d + a	DMH	30 mg/kg/month sc 10 months	SD male and female rats	$\emptyset \rightarrow$	—	Schmähl et al. (1976)

Table 1.13. The Effect of a Calorie-Restricted Diet on Colon Carcinogenesis

Diet	Feeding schedule	Carcinogen	Dose/duration	Species, strain/sex	Tumor incidence	No. of tumors/ tumor-bearing animal	Reference
Calorie restricted (25%)	b + d + a	NMU	0.8% 3 × 0.5 ml ir on alternate days	SD male rats	∅	→	Pollard and Luckert (1985)
Calorie restricted (25%)	b + d + a	MAM	30 mg/kg sc	SD male rats	∅	∅	Pollard and Luckert (1985)
Calorie restricted (25%)	b + d + a	MAM + NMU 2 weeks later	30 mg/kg sc + 0.8% 3 × 0.5 ml ir on alternate days	SD male rats	∅	→	Pollard and Luckert (1985)
Calorie restricted (25%)	a	MAM	30 mg/kg sc	SD male rats	→	→*	Pollard et al. (1984)
Calorie restricted (25%)	a^a	MAM	30 mg/kg sc	SD male rats	∅	∅*	Pollard et al. (1984)
Calorie restricted, high-fat diet 30% (23% corn oil)	a	AOM	15 mg/kg/wk sc 2 weeks	F344 male rats	→	→	Reddy et al. (1987)
Calorie restricted (40%)	b + d + a	DMH	30 mg/kg/wk 6 weeks	F344 male rats	→	→	Kritchevsky et al. (1986)
Calorie restricted ad lib but alternate days	a	MAM	30 mg/kg sc	SD male rats	∅	∅*	Pollard et al. (1984)
Calorie restricted ad lib but alternate days	a^a	MAM	30 mg/kg sc	SD male rats	∅	∅*	Pollard et al. (1984)

^a Diet was fed 53 days later as in the other group.

Table 2.1. The Effect of Vitamin A and Retinoids on Urinary Bladder Carcinogenesis

Diet	Feeding schedule	Carcinogen	Dose/duration	Species, strain/sex	Tumor incidence	No. of tumors/ tumor-bearing animal	Reference
The Effect of Vitamin A on Urinary Bladder Carcinogenesis							
Vitamin A deficient	b + d + a	FANFT	0.188% in diet 12 weeks 0.1% in diet following 8 weeks	SD male rats	∅	—	Cohen et al. (1976)
Retinyl palmitate (5 IU/g)	b + d + a	FANFT	0.188% in diet 12 weeks + 0.1% in diet following 8 weeks	SD female rats	∅	—	Cohen et al. (1976)
Retinyl palmitate (250 IU/g 4 weeks, then 500 IU/g)	b + d + a	FANFT	0.188% in diet 12 weeks + 0.1% in diet following 8 weeks	SD female rats	∅	—	Cohen et al. (1976)
Vitamin A acetate (100 IU/g)	d	BBN	0.025% dw 20 weeks	Wistar male rats	→	—	Miyata et al. (1978)
Vitamin A acetate (100 IU/g)	d	BBN	0.01% dw 20 weeks	Wistar male rats	∅	—	Miyata et al. (1978)
Vitamin A acetate (200 IU/g)	d	BBN	0.025% dw 20 weeks	Wistar male rats	→	—	Miyata et al. (1978)
Vitamin A acetate (200 IU/g)	d	BBN	0.01% dw 20 weeks	Wistar male rats	∅	—	Miyata et al. (1978)
13-Cis-retinoic acid (120 mg/kg)	d + a	NMU	1.5 mg/rat/2 wk intravesical 3 times	Lewis female rats	→	—	Sporn et al. (1977)
13-Cis-retinoic acid (120 mg/kg)	a	NMU	1.5 mg/rat/2 wk intravesical 3 times	Lewis female rats	→	—	Sporn et al. (1977)
13-Cis-retinoic acid (120 mg/kg)	d + a	NMU	1.5 mg/rat/2 wk intravesical 3 times	Wistar or Lewis female rats	→	—	Squire et al. (1977)
13-Cis-retinoic acid (120 mg/kg)	a	NMU	1.5 mg/rat/2 wk intravesical 3 times	Wistar or Lewis female rats	→	—	Squire et al. (1977)
13-Cis-retinoic acid (150 mg/kg)	a	BBN	2 × 10 mg/wk ig 9 weeks	B6D2F1 male mice	∅	—	Becci et al. (1981)
13-Cis-retinoic acid (150 mg/kg)	a	BBN	2 × 5 mg/wk ig 9 weeks	B6D2F1 male mice	∅	—	Becci et al. (1981)
13-Cis-retinoic acid (200 mg/kg)	a	BBN	2 × 10 mg/kg ig 9 weeks	B6D2F1 male mice	→	—	Becci et al. (1981)
13-Cis-retinoic acid (200 mg/kg)	a	BBN	2 × 5 mg/kg ig 9 weeks	B6D2F1 male mice	→	—	Becci et al. (1981)
13-Cis-retinoic acid (240 mg/kg)	a	BBN	2 × 100 mg/rat/wk ig 6 weeks	F344 male rats	→	—	Becci et al. (1979)

13-*Cis*-retinoic acid (240 mg/kg)	a	BBN	2 × 150 mg/rat/wk ig 6 weeks	F344 male rats	→	—	Becci *et al.* (1979)
13-*Cis*-retinoic acid (240 mg/kg)	a	BBN	2 × 200 mg/rat wk ig 6 weeks	F344 male rats	→	—	Becci *et al.* (1979)
13-*Cis*-retinoic acid (240 mg/kg)	a	BBN	2 × 0.5 ml/wk ig 6 weeks total dose: 1200 mg/rat	F344 female rats	∅[a]	∅	Hicks *et al.* (1982)
13-*Cis*-retinoic (240 mg/kg)	a	BBN	2 × 200 mg/rat/wk ig 8 weeks	F344 male rats	∅	→	Thompson *et al.* (1981a)
13-*Cis*-retinoic (240 mg/kg)	a	BBN	2 × 150 mg/rat/wk ig 6 weeks	F344 female rats	→	→	Thompson *et al.* (1981a)
13-*Cis*-retinoic acid (300 mg/kg)	d + a	NMU	1.5 mg/rat/2 wk intravesical 3 times	Wistar female rats	→	—	Sporn *et al.* (1977)
13-*Cis*-retinoic acid (300 mg/kg)	a	NMU	1.5 mg/rat/2 wk intravesical 3 times	Wistar female rats	→	—	Sporn *et al.* (1977)
13-*Cis*-retinoic acid (300 mg/kg)	d + a	NMU	1.5 mg/rat/2 wk intravesical 3 times	Wistar or Lewis female rats	→	—	Squire *et al.* (1977)
13-*Cis*-retinoic acid (300 mg/kg)	a	NMU	1.5 mg/rat/2 wk intravesical 3 times	Wistar or Lewis female rats	→	—	Squire *et al.* (1977)
The Effect of Different Synthetic Retinoids on Urinary Bladder Carcinogenesis							
N-(ethyl)-all-*trans*-retinamide (164 mg/kg)	a	BBN	2 × 10 mg/mouse/wk ig 9 weeks	B6D2F1 male mice	∅	—	Thompson *et al.* (1981b)
N-(ethyl)-all-*trans*-retinamide (164 mg/kg)	a	BBN	2 × 5 mg/mouse/wk ig 9 weeks	B6D2F1 male mice	∅	—	Thompson *et al.* (1981b)
N-(ethyl)-all-*trans*-retinamide (327 mg/kg)	a	BBN	2 × 0.5 ml/rat/wk ig 6 weeks total dose: 1200 mg/rat	F344 female rats	∅ →	∅	Hicks *et al.* (1982)
N-(ethyl)-all-*trans*-retinamide (327 mg/kg)	a	BBN	2 × 10 mg/mouse/wk ig 5 weeks	B6D2F1 male mice	→	—	Thompson *et al.* (1981b)
N-(ethyl)-all-*trans*-retinamide (327 mg/kg)	a	BBN	2 × 5 mg/mouse/wk ig 3 weeks	B6D2F1 male mice	→	—	Thompson *et al.* (1981b)
N-(ethyl)-all-*trans*-retinamide (654 mg/kg)	a	BBN	2 × 200 mg/rat/wk ig 8 weeks	F344 male rats	∅	∅*	Thompson *et al.* (1981b)
N-(ethyl)-all-*trans*-retinamide (654 mg/kg)	a	BBN	2 × 150 mg/rat/wk ig 6 weeks	F344 male rats	→	→*	Thompson *et al.* (1981b)
N-(ethyl)-all-*trans*-retinamide (654 mg/kg)	a	BBN	2 × 0.5 ml/rat/wk ig 6 weeks total dose: 1200 mg/rat	F344 female rats	∅[a]	∅	Hicks *et al.* (1982)

(*continued*)

Table 2.1. (*Continued*)

Diet	Feeding schedule	Carcinogen	Dose/duration	Species, strain/sex	Tumor incidence	No. of tumors/ tumor-bearing animal	Reference
(654 mg/kg)		BBN	weeks total dose: 600 mg/rat	female rats	⊘[a]	⊘	Hicks et al. (1982)
N-(ethyl)-all-*trans*-retinamide (654 mg/kg)	a	BBN	2 × 0.5 ml/rat/wk ig 6 weeks total dose: 300 mg/rat	F344 female rats	→	—	Moon et al. (1982)
13-*Cis*-ethyl-retinamide (1.5 mmol/kg)	a	BBN	7.5 mg/mouse/wk ig 8 weeks	BDF male mice	→	—	Moon et al. (1982)
All-*trans*-ethyl-retinamide (1.5 mmol/kg)	a	BBN	7.5 mg/mouse/wk ig 8 weeks	BDF male mice	→	→	Moon et al. (1982)
N-(2-hydroxyethyl-all-*trans*-retinamide (686 mg/kg)	a	BBN	2 × 200 mg/rat/wk ig 6 weeks	F344 male rats	→	→	Thompson et al. (1981b)
N-(2-hydroxyethyl-all-*trans*-retinamide (686 mg/kg)	a	BBN	2 × 200 mg/rat/wk ig 6 weeks	F344 female rats	⊘	—	Thompson et al. (1981b)
N-(2-hydroxyethyl-all-*trans*-retinamide (172 mg/kg)	a	BBN	2 × 10 mg/mouse/wk ig 9 weeks	B6D2F1 male mice	⊘	—	Thompson et al. (1981b)
N-(2-hydroxyethyl-all-*trans*-retinamide (172 mg/kg)	a	BBN	2 × 5 mg/mouse/wk ig 9 weeks	B6D2F1 male mice	→	—	Thompson et al. (1981b)
N-2-hydroxyethyl-all-*trans*-retinamide (343 mg/kg)	a	BBN	2 × 10 mg/mouse/wk ig 9 weeks	B6D2F1 male mice	→	—	Thompson et al. (1981b)
N-2-hydroxyethyl-all-*trans*-retinamide (343 mg/kg)	a	BBN	2 × 5 mg/mouse/wk ig 9 weeks	B6D2F1 male mice	⊘	—	Thompson et al. (1981b)
2-Hydroxyethylretinamide (515 mg/kg)	b + d	BBN	2 × 50 mg/rat/wk ig 6 weeks	F344 female rats	⊘	—	Quander et al. (1985)
2-hydroxyethylretinamide (515 mg/kg)	a	BBN	2 × 50 mg/rat/wk ig 6 weeks	F344 female rats	↑	—	Quander et al. (1985)
All-*trans*-2-hydroxyethyl-retinamide (1.0 mmol/kg)	a	BBN	2 × 5 mg/kg/wk ig 9 weeks	BDF male mice	→	—	Moon et al. (1982)
All-*trans*-2-hydroxyethyl-retinamide (1.0 mmol/kg)	a	BBN	7.5 mg/mouse/wk ig 8 weeks	BDF male mice	→	—	Moon et al. (1982)
13-*Cis*-2-hydroxyethyl-retinamide (1.5 mmol/kg)	a	BBN	7.5 mg/mouse/wk ig 8 weeks	BDF male mice	→	—	Moon et al. (1982)
N-4-hydroxyphenylretinamide (391 mg/kg)	a	BBN	7.5 mg/mouse/wk inj 8 weeks	C57BL/6 × DBA2F1 male mice	→	—	McCormick et al. (1982a)

Compound		Carcinogen	Dose	Animal			Reference
All-*trans*-4-hydroxyphenyl-retinamide (1.5 mmol/kg)	a	BBN	7.5 mg/mouse/wk ig 8 weeks	BDF male mice	→	—	Moon *et al.* (1982)
13-*Cis*-4-hydroxyphenyl-retinamide (1.5 mmol/kg)	a	BBN	7.5 mg/mouse/wk ig 8 weeks	BDF male mice	→	—	Moon *et al.* (1982)
2-Hydroxypropylretinamide (1.5 mmol/kg)	a	BBN	2 × 5 mg/kg/wk ig 9 weeks	BDF male mice	→	—	Moon *et al.* (1982)
3-Hydroxypropylretinamide (1.5 mmol/kg)	a	BBN	2 × 5 mg/kg/wk ig 9 weeks	BDF male mice	∅	—	Moon *et al.* (1982)
2.3-Dihydroxypropylretinamide (1.5 mmol/kg)	a	BBN	2 × 5 mg/kg/wk ig 9 weeks	BDF male mice	∅	—	Moon *et al.* (1982)
All-*trans*-5-tetrazolylretinamide (1.5 mmol/kg)	a	BBN	7.5 mg/kg/wk ig 8 weeks	BDF male mice	→	—	Moon *et al.* (1982)
13-*Cis*-5-tetrazolylretinamide (1.5 mmol/kg)	a	BBN	7.5 mg/kg/wk ig 8 weeks	BDF male mice	∅	—	Moon *et al.* (1982)
All-*trans*-butylretinamide (1.5 mmol/kg)	a	BBN	7.5 mg/mouse/wk ig 8 weeks	BDF male mice	∅	—	Moon *et al.* (1982)
13-*Cis*-butylretinamide (1.5 mmol/kg)	a	BBN	7.5 mg/mouse/wk ig 8 weeks	BDF male mice	∅	—	Moon *et al.* (1982)
All-*trans*-4-hydroxybutyl-retinamide (1.5 mmol/kg)	a	BBN	7.5 mg/mouse/wk ig 8 weeks	BDF male mice	∅	—	Moon *et al.* (1982)
Bis-4-hydroxybutyl-retinamide (1.5 mmol/kg)	a	BBN	7.5 mg/mouse/wk ig 8 weeks	BDF male mice	∅	—	Moon *et al.* (1982)
Ethyl-all-*trans*-9-(4-methoxy-2,3,6-trimethylphenyl)-3,7-dimethyl-2,4,6,8-nonatetraenoate (50 ppm)	b	BBN	0.025% dw 8 weeks	F344 male rats	→	∅	Murasaki *et al.* (1980)
Ethyl-all-*trans*-9-(4-methoxy-2,3,6-trimethylphenyl)-3,7-diemthyl-2,4,6,8-nonatetraenoate (50 ppm)	d	BBN	0.025% dw 8 weeks	F344 male rats	∅	∅	Murasaki *et al.* (1980)
Ethyl-all-*trans*-9-(4-methoxy-2,3,6-trimethylphenyl)-3,7-dimethyl-2,4,6,8-nonatetraenoate (50 ppm)	b + d + a	BBN	0.025% dw 8 weeks	F344 male rats	∅	∅	Murasaki *et al.* (1980)
Ethyl-all-*trans*-9-(4-methoxy-2,3,6-trimethylphenyl)-3,7-dimethyl-2,4,6,8-nonatetraenoate (50 ppm)	a	BBN	0.025% dw 8 weeks	F344 male rats	∅	∅	Murasaki *et al.* (1980)

(continued)

Table 2.1. (Continued)

Diet	Feeding schedule	Carcinogen	Dose/duration	Species, strain/sex	Tumor incidence	No. of tumors/ tumor-bearing animal	Reference
Ethyl-all-*trans*-9-(4-methoxy-2,3,6-trimethylphenyl)-3,7-dimethyl-2,4,6,8-nonatetraenoate (100 ppm)	b	BBN	0.025% dw 8 weeks	F344 male rats	→	→	Murasaki *et al.* (1980)
Ethyl-all-*trans*-9-(4-methoxy-2,3,6-trimethylphenyl)-3,7-dimethyl-2,4,6,8-nonatetraenoate (100 ppm)	d	BBN	0.025% dw 8 weeks	F344 male rats	→	→	Murasaki *et al.* (1980)
Ethyl-all-*trans*-9-(4-methoxy-2,3,6-trimethylphenyl)-3,7-dimethyl-2,4,6,8-nonatetraenoate (100 ppm)	b + a + d	BBN	0.025% dw 8 weeks	F344 male rats	→	→	Murasaki *et al.* (1980)
Ethyl-all-*trans*-9-(4-methoxy-2,3,6-trimethylphenyl)-3,7-dimethyl-2,4,6,8-nonatetraenoate (100 ppm)	a	BBN	0.025% dw 8 weeks	F344 male rats	→	→	Murasaki *et al.* (1980)
Ethyl-all-*trans*-9-(4-methoxy-2,3,6-trimethylphenyl)-3,7-dimethyl-2,4,6,8-nonatetraenoate (3 × 8 mg/kg/wk ig)	d + a	BBN	10 mg/kg/day dw until death	SD male rats	∅	—	Schmähl and Habs (1978)
Ethyl-all-*trans*-9-(4-methoxy-2,3,6-trimethylphenyl)-3,7-dimethyl-2,4,6,8-nonatetraenoate (3 × 16 mg/kg/wk ig)	d + a	BBN	10 mg/kg/day dw until death	SD male rats	∅	—	Schmähl and Habs (1978)
Ethyl-all-*trans*-9-(4-methoxy-2,3,6-trimethylphenyl)-3,7-dimethyl-2,4,6,8-nonatetraenoate (3 × 32 mg/kg/wk ig)	d + a	BBN	10 mg/kg/day dw until death	SD male rats	∅	—	Schmähl and Habs (1978)

[a] But effects concerning the tumor volume were seen.

Table 2.2. *The Effect of Vitamin C on Urinary Bladder Carcinogenesis*

Diet	Feeding schedule	Carcinogen	Dose/duration	Species, strain/sex	Tumor incidence	No. of tumors/ tumor-bearing animal	Reference
Ascorbic acid (250 mg/100 cc dw)	a	FANFT	0.01% in diet	C3/He female mice	∅	—	Soloway et al. (1975)
Ascorbic acid (1%)	a	BBN	0.05% 4 weeks dw	F344 male rats	∅	∅[a]	Fukushima et al. (1983b)
Ascorbic acid (1%)	a	BBN	0.01% 4 weeks dw	F344 female rats	∅	∅[a]	Fukushima et al. (1983b)
Ascorbic acid (5%)	a	BBN	0.05% 4 weeks dw	F344 male rats	↑	↑[a]	Fukushima et al. (1983b)
Ascorbic acid (5%)	a	BBN	0.01% 4 weeks dw	F344 female rats	∅	∅[a]	Fukushima et al. (1983b)
Ascorbic acid (5%)	a	BBN	0.05% 4 weeks dw	F344 male rats	∅	∅[a]	Fukushima et al. (1984)
Ascorbic acid (5%)	a	BBN	0.05% 4 week dw	F344 male rats	∅	∅[a]	Fukushima et al. (1986)
Sodium ascorbate (5%)	a	BBN	0.05% 4 weeks dw	F344 male rats	↑	↑[a]	Mori et al. (1987)
Sodium ascorbate (5%)	a	BBN	0.05% 4 weeks dw	Lewis male rats	↑	↑[a]	Mori et al. (1987)
Sodium ascorbate (5%)	a	BBN	0.05% 4 weeks dw	F344 male rats	↑	↑[a]	Fukushima et al. (1986)
Sodium ascorbate (5%)	a	BBN	0.01% 4 weeks dw	F344 male rats	∅	∅[a]	Fukushima et al. (1983a)
Sodium ascorbate (5%)	a	NMU	20 mg/kg/wk ip 4 weeks	F344 male rats	∅	∅[a]	Imaida et al. (1984)

[a]No. of tumors/10 cm of basal membrane.

Table 2.3. The Effect of Vitamin B₆ and Vitamin D Deficiency on Urinary Bladder Carcinogenesis

Diet	Feeding schedule	Carcinogen	Dose/duration	Species, strain/sex	Tumor incidence	No. of tumors/ tumor-bearing animal	Reference
Vitamin D deficient (<0.002%)	a	BBN	0.01% 4 weeks dw	F344 male rats	Ø	Øᵃ	Fukushima et al. (1983a)
Vitamin B₆ deficient (10 mg/kg)	a	FANFT	0.2% 4 weeks dw	F344 male rats	→	—	Birt et al. (1987)

ᵃNo. of tumors/10 cm of basal membrane.

Table 2.4. *The Effect of Tryptophan and Leucine on Urinary Bladder Carcinogenesis*

Diet	Feeding schedule	Carcinogen	Dose/duration	Species, strain/sex	Tumor incidence	No. of tumors/ tumor-bearing animal	Reference
L-Tryptophan (2%)	a	FANFT	0.2% in diet 4 weeks	F344 male rats	∅	—	Birt et al. (1987)
L-Tryptophan (2%)	a	FANFT	0.2% in diet 6 weeks	F344 male rats	↑	—	Cohen et al. (1979)
L-Tryptophan (2%)	a	FANFT	0.2% in diet 4 weeks	F344 male rats	∅	—	Fukushima et al. (1981)
DL-Tryptophan (5%)	a	BBN	0.01% 4 weeks dw	F344 male rats	∅	∅[a]	Fukushima et al. (1983a)
L-Isoleucine (2%)	a	BBN	0.05% 4 weeks dw	F344 rats	∅	↑[a]	Nishio et al. (1986)
L-Isoleucine (4%)	a	BBN	0.05% 4 weeks dw	F344 rats	↑	↑[a]	Nishio et al. (1986)
L-Leucine (2%)	a	BBN	0.05% 4 weeks dw	F344 rats	↑	↑[a]	Nishio et al. (1986)
L-Leucine (4%)	a	BBN	0.05% 4 weeks dw	F344 rats	↑	↑[a]	Nishio et al. (1986)

[a]No. of tumors/10 cm of basal membrane.

Table 2.5. *The Effect of NaHCo₃, NH₄Cl, CaCo₂, and NaCl on Urinary Bladder Carcinogenesis*

Diet	Feeding schedule	Carcinogen	Dose/duration	Species, strain/sex	Tumor incidence	No. of tumors/ tumor-bearing animal	Reference
NaHCO₃ (3%)	a	BBN	0.05% 4 weeks dw	F344 male rats	↑	↑	Fukushima et al. (1986)
NH₄Cl (1%)	a	BBN	0.05% 4 weeks dw	F344 female rats	∅	∅	Fukushima et al. (1986)
CaCO₃ (5%)	a	BBN	0.1% 4 weeks dw	F344 male rats	∅	∅[a]	Fukushima et al. (1983a)
NaCl (5%)	a	BBN	0.01% or 0.05% dw	F344 male rats	∅	∅	Shibata et al. (1986)
NaCl (10%)	a	BBN	0.01% or 0.05% dw	F344 male rats	∅	∅	Shibata et al. (1986)

[a]No. of tumors/10 cm basal membrane.

Table 3.1. The Effect of Different Fats on Liver Carcinogenesis

Diet	Feeding schedule	Carcinogen	Dose/duration	Species, strain/sex	Tumor incidence	No. of tumors/ tumor-bearing animal	Reference
High fat (10 g)	d	DMH	30 mg/kg/month sc 7 months	SD male and female rats	∅	—	Schmähl et al. (1979)
High cholesterol fat (17 g)	d	DMH	30 mg/kg/month sc 7 months	SD male and female rats	∅	—	Schmähl et al. (1979)
High fat (pork bellies, butter, egg powder)	d + a	DMH	30 mg/kg/month sc 10 months	SD male and female rats	∅	—	Schmähl et al. (1976)
Beef fat (28%) + corn oil (2%)	d + a	AFB$_1$	7 mg/kg ig	SD male rats	∅	—	Newberne et al. (1979)
Beef fat (28%) + corn oil (2%)	d + a	AFB$_1$	15 × 25 µg/day ig	SD male rats	∅	—	Newberne et al. (1979)
Beef fat (28%) + corn oil (2%)	d + a	AFB$_1$	5 × 25 µg/day ig	SD male rats	∅	—	Newberne et al. (1979)
Beef fat (28%) + corn oil (2%)	a	AFB$_1$	7 mg/kg ig	SD male rats	∅	—	Newberne et al. (1979)
Beef fat (28%) + corn oil (2%)	a	AFB$_1$	15 × 25 µg/day ig	SD male rats	∅	—	Newberne et al. (1979)
Beef fat (28%) + corn oil (2%)	a	AFB$_1$	5 × 25 µg/day ig	SD male rats	∅	—	Newberne et al. (1979)
Palm oil (25.8%)	a	70% partial hepatectomy + NDEA + PB	20 hours later 10 mg/kg ig + 0.05% in diet	CD female rats	∅	—	Glauert and Pitot (1986)

(continued)

Table 3.1. (Continued)

Diet	Feeding schedule	Carcinogen	Dose/duration	Species, strain/sex	Tumor incidence	No. of tumors/ tumor-bearing animal	Reference
Safflower margarine (30%)	d + a	2,7-FAA	0.03% in diet 7 months	CD-1 male mice	∅	—	Yanagi *et al.* (1984)
Safflower oil (25.8%)	d + a	70% partial hepatectomy + NDEA + Pb	20 hours later: 10 mg/kg ig + 0.05% in diet	CD female rats	∅	—	Glauert and Pitot (1986)
Safflower oil (30%)	d + a	2,7-FAA	0.03% in diet 7 months	CD-1 male mice	∅	—	Yanagi *et al.* (1984)
Corn oil (30%)	d + a	AFB_1	7 mg/kg ig	SD male rats	↑	—	Newberne *et al.* (1986)
Corn oil (30%)	d + a	AFB_1	15 × 25 µg/day ig	SD male rats	↑	—	Newberne *et al.* (1986)
Corn oil (30%)	d + a	AFB_1	5 × 25 µg/day ig	SD male rats	↑	—	Newberne *et al.* (1986)
Corn oil (30%)	a	AFB_1	7 mg/kg ig	SD male rats	↑	—	Newberne *et al.* (1986)
Corn oil (30%)	a	AFB_1	15 × 25 µg/day ig	SD male rats	↑	—	Newberne *et al.* (1986)
Corn oil (30%)	a	AFB_1	5 × 25 µg/day ig	SD male rats	↑	—	Newberne *et al.* (1986)
Saturated fat (17%) (palm oil, palm stearin, safflower oil)	b + d	DMH	0.25 mg/wk sc 10 weeks	CD-1 male and female mice	∅	—	Brown (1981)
Saturated fat (17%) (palm	During	—	—	CH3	∅	—	Brown (1981)

Diet	Timing	Carcinogen	Dose	Animal	Effect	Reference
oil, palm stearin, saf-flower oil)	the whole experiment			female mice	∅	Brown (1981)
Monounsaturated fat (17%) (safflower oil, high oleic palm oil)	b + d	DMH	0.25 mg/wk sc 10 weeks	CD-1 male and female mice	∅	Brown (1981)
Monounsaturated fat (17%) (safflower oil, high oleic palm oil)	During the who experiment	—	—	CH3 female mice	∅	Brown (1981)
Diunsaturated fat (17%) (safflower oil, high oleic palm oil)	b + d	DMH	0.25 mg/wk sc 10 weeks	CD-1 male and female mice	∅	Brown (1981)
Diunsaturated fat (17%) (safflower oil, high oleic palm oil)	During the whole experiment	—	—	CD-1 female mice	∅	Brown (1981)
Transmonounsaturated fat (17%) (transstock, palm stearin, safflower oil)	b + d	DMH	0.25 mg/wk sc 10 weeks	CD-1 male and female mice	∅	Brown (1981)
Transmonounsaturated fat (17%) (transstock, palm stearin, safflower oil)	During the whole experiment	—	—	CH3 female mice	∅	Brown (1981)
Triunsaturated fat (17%) (soy bean oil, safflower oil, high oleic palm oil)	b + d	DMH	0.25 mg/wk sc 10 weeks	CD-1 male and female mice	∅	Brown (1981)
Triunsaturated fat (17%) (soy bean oil, safflower oil, high oleic palm oil)	During the whole experiment	—	—	CH3 female mice	∅	Brown (1981)

Table 3.2. The Effect of Vitamin A on Liver Carcinogenesis

Diet	Feeding schedule	Carcinogen	Dose/duration	Species, strain/sex	Tumor incidence	No. of tumors/tumor-bearing animal	Reference
Vitamin A deficient (retinyl acetate, 0.3 μ/g)	d	AFB$_1$	25 μg/rat/day ig 15 days	SD male and female rats	∅	—	Newberne and Suphakarn (1977)
Vitamin A deficient (retinyl acetate, 0.3 μg/g)	d	AFB$_1$	1 ppm in diet	SD male and female rats	∅	—	Newberne and Suphakarn (1977)
Retinoic acid (0.002% 4 weeks)	d	3'-MeDAB	0.05% in diet 9 weeks	SD male rats	∅	—	Daoud and Griffin (1980)
Retinyl acetate (0.02%)	During the whole experiment	—	—	C3H/He(+) male and female mice	∅	—	Stenbäck et al. (1987)
Ethyl-allyl-*trans*-9(-4-methoxy-2,3,6 trimethylphenyl)-3,7-dimethyl-2,4,6,8 non-atetrenoate (3 × 8 mg/kg/wk ig)	d + a	DMH	10 mg/kg/wk sc 10 weeks	SD male rats	∅	—	Schmähl and Habs (1978)
Ethyl-allyl-*trans*-9(-4-methoxy-2,3,6 trimethylphenyl)-3,7-dimethyl-2,4,6,8 non-atetrenoate (3 × 16 mg/kg/wk ig)	d + a	DMH	10 mg/kg/wk sc 10 weeks	SD male rats	∅	—	Schmähl and Habs (1978)
Ethyl-allyl-*trans*-9(-4-methoxy-2,3,6 trimethylphenyl)-3,7-dimethyl-2,4,6,8 non-atetrenoate (3 × 32 mg/kg/wk ig)	d + a	DMH	10 mg/kg/wk sc 10 weeks	SD male rats	∅	—	Schmähl and Habs (1978)

Table 3.3. The Effect of Vitamin C on Liver Carcinogenesis

Diet	Feeding schedule	Carcinogen	Dose/duration	Species, strain/sex	Tumor incidence	No. of tumors/ tumor-bearing animal	Reference
L-Ascorbic acid (22.7 g/kg)	d	Morpholine + NaO_2	10 g/kg in diet + 3 g/l dw	MRC–Wistar male rats	$\varnothing \rightarrow$	—	Mirvish *et al.* (1976)
L-Ascorbic acid (22.7 g/kg)	d	NMOR	0.15 g/l dw	MRC–Wistar male rats	$\varnothing$	—	Mirvish *et al.* (1976)

Table 3.4. The Effect of Riboflavin on Liver Carcinogenesis

Diet	Feeding schedule	Carcinogen	Dose/duration	Species, strain/sex	Tumor incidence	No. of tumors/ tumor-bearing animal	Reference
Riboflavin (25 ppm dw)	d	AFB$_1$	7 mg/kg ig	Wistar female rats	$\varnothing$	—	Scotto *et al.* (1975)

Table 3.5. The Effect of Selenium on Liver Carcinogenesis

Diet	Feeding schedule	Carcinogen	Dose/duration	Species, strain/sex	Tumor incidence	No. of tumors/ tumor-bearing animal	Reference
Sodium selenite (2 ppm dw)	d	3'-MeDAB	0.05% in diet 9 weeks	SD male rats	∅	—	Daoud and Griffin (1980)
Sodium selenite (3 ppm in 4 cycles) (cycle: 4 weeks selenium + 1 week control diet)	a	2.7 FAA	0.02% in diet	F344 male rats	∅	∅	LeBoeuf et al. (1985)
Sodium selenite (4 ppm dw)	b + d + a	2.7 FAA	0.03% in diet 4 weeks	SD male rats	∅	—	Marshall et al. (1979)
Sodium selenite (4 ppm dw)	d	3'-MeDAB	0.05% in diet 9 weeks	SD male rats	∅	—	Daoud and Griffin (1980)
Sodium selenite (6 ppm dw)	b + d	3'-MeDAB	0.05% in diet 8 weeks	SD male rats	→	—	Griffin and Jacobs (1977)
Sodium selenite (6 ppm)	b + d	3'-MeDAB	0.05% in diet 8 weeks	SD male rats	→	—	Griffin and Jacobs (1977)
Sodium selenite (6 ppm in 4 cycles) (cycle: 4 weeks selenium + 1 week control diet)	a	2.7 FAA	0.02% in diet	F344 male rats	∅	∅	LeBoeuf et al. (1985)
p-Methoxybenzene-selenol (50 ppm)	b + d + a	AOM	15 mg/kg/wk sc 3 weeks	F344 female rats	→	→	Tanaka et al. (1985)

Table 3.6. The Effect of Tryphophan on Liver Carcinogenesis

Diet	Feeding schedule	Carcinogen	Dose/duration	Species, strain/sex	Tumor incidence	No. of tumors/ tumor-bearing animal	Reference
L-Tryphophan (1%)	d + a	3'-MeDAB	0.05% in diet 96 days	Wistar male rats	→	—	Evarts and Brown (1977)
L-Tryphophan (1%)	d + a	NDEA	0.002% dw 128 days	Wistar male rats	→	—	Evarts and Brown (1977)
DL-Tryphophan (2%)	d	Benzidine	0.02% in diet 20 weeks	ICR female rats	→	—	Miyakawa and Yoshida (1980)

Table 3.7. The Effect of Protein in Combination with Other Dietary Factors on Liver Carcinogenesis

Diet	Feeding schedule	Carcinogen	Dose/duration	Species, strain/sex	Tumor incidence	No. of tumors/ tumor-bearing animal	Reference
Casein (8%)	d	AFB_1	1.7 ppm in diet 3 months	USC male rats	∅	—	Wells et al. (1975)
Casein (8%) + cystein (0.6%)	d	AFB_1	1.7 ppm in diet 3 months	USC male rats	∅	—	Wells et al. (1975)
Casein (20%)	d	AFB (mixture)	1 ppm in diet 3 months	F344 male rats	∅[a]	—	Temcharoen et al. (1978)
Casein (20%) + vitmain B_{12}	d	AFB (mixture)	1ppm in diet 3 months	F344 male rats	↓[a]	—	Temcharoen et al. (1978)
Casein (30%)	d	AFB_1	1.7 ppm diet 3 months	USC male rats	∅	—	Wells et al. (1975)
Casein (30%) + cystein (0.6%)	d	AFB_1	1.7 ppm diet	USC male rats	∅	—	Wells et al. (1975)
Casein (49.5%)	d	AFB_1	2,6,18 or 54 ppb in diet	Rainbrow trout	∅	∅	Lee et al. (1978)
Fish protein (32% concentrate)	d	AFB_1	2,6,18 or 54 ppm in diet	Rainbrow trout	→	∅	Lee et al. (1978)
Fish protein (49% concentrate)	d	AFB_1	2 or 6 ppm in diet	Rainbrow trout	∅	∅	Lee et al. (1978)

[a]Hyperplastic nodules and hepatomas.

Table 3.8. The Effect of Carbohydrates on Liver Carcinogenesis

Diet	Feeding schedule	Carcinogen	Dose/duration	Species, strain/sex	Tumor incidence	No. of tumors/ tumor-bearing animal	Reference
Cornstarch (68%)	a	70% partial hepatectomy + NDEA + Pb	20 hr later 10 mg/kg ig + 0.05% in diet	CD female rats	∅	—	Glauert and Pitot (1986)
Cornstarch (68%) + safflower oil (2%)	a	70% partial hepatectomy + DEN + Pb	20 hr later 10 mg/kg + 0.05% in diet	CD female rats	∅	—	Glauert and Pitot (1986)
Sucrose (53.3%) + safflower oil (2%)	a	70% partial hepatectomy + DEN + Pb	20 hr later 10 mg/kg + 0.05% in diet	CD female rats	∅	—	Glauert and Pitot (1986)
Low sucrose (3.64 g/day)	d	3'-MeDAB	10 mg/rat/day 20 weeks	Wistar male rats	↑	↑[a]	Sato et al. (1984)
High sucrose (14.04 g/day)	d	3'-MeDAB	10 mg/rat/day 20 weeks	Wistar male rats	∅	∅[a]	Sato et al. (1984)
High carbohydrate (12 g)	d	DMH	30 mg/kg/month sc 7 months	SD male and female rats	∅	—	Schmähl et al. (1979)

[a]No. of liver tumors per mm².

Table 3.9. The Effect of Orot Acid on Liver Carcinogenesis

Diet	Feeding schedule	Carcinogen	Dose/duration	Species, strain/sex	Tumor incidence	No. of tumors/ tumor-bearing animal	Reference
Orot acid (1%)	b + d + a	2/3 partial hepatectomy + DMH + CCl$_4$	100 mg/kg ip + 2 ml/kg	F344 male rats	↑	—	Laurier *et al.* (1984)
Orot acid (1%)	b + d + a	2/3 partial hepatectomy + DMH	100 mg/kg/ip	F344 male rats	↑	—	Laurier *et al.* (1984)

Table 3.10. The Effect of a Vegetarian Diet on Liver Carcinogenesis

Diet	Feeding schedule	Carcinogen	Dose/duration	Species, strain/sex	Tumor incidence	No. of tumors/ tumor-bearing animal	Reference
Vegetarian diet (lettuce, carrots, apples, oat flakes)	d	DMH	30 mg/kg/month sc 7 months	SD male and female rats	∅	—	Schmähl et al. (1979)
Vegetarian diet (salad, carrots, apples, kohlrabi, oat flakes)	d + a	DMH	30 mg/kg/month sc 10 months	SD male and female rats	→	—	Schmähl et al. (1976)
Cabbage (25%) (freeze dried)	d	AFB₁	1 ppm in diet	F344 male rats	—	→	Boyd et al. (1982)
Table beets (25%)	d	AFB₁	1 ppm in diet	F344 male rats	—	←	Boyd et al. (1982)
Konjac Mannan (10%)	During the whole experiment	—	—	C3H/He mice	∅	↓*	Mizutani and Mitsuoka (1982)

Table 3.11. The Effect of a Restricted Diet on Liver Carcinogenesis

Diet	Feeding schedule	Carcinogen	Dose/duration	Species, strain/sex	Tumor incidence	No. of tumors/ tumor-bearing animal	Reference
PRD diet (75% restricted) (crude oil, 2.78%; crude protein, 19.79%)	During the whole experiment	—	—	Swiss male mice	→	—	Conybeare (1980)
PRD diet (75% restricted) (crude oil, 2.78%; crude protein, 19.79%)	During the whole experiment	—	—	Swiss female mice	∅	—	Conybeare (1980)
41B diet (75% restricted) (crude oil, 2.87%; crude protein, 16.61%)	During the whole experiment	—	—	Swiss male mice	→	—	Conybeare (1980)
41B diet (75% restricted) (crude oil, 2.87%; crude protein, 16.61%)	During the whole experiment	—	—	Swiss female mice	∅	—	Conybeare (1980)

Table 4.1. *The Effect of Vitamin A on Esophagus Carcinogenesis*

Diet	Feeding schedule	Carcinogen	Dose/duration	Species, strain/sex	Tumor incidence	No. of tumors/tumor-bearing animal	Reference
Vitamin A deficient (0.3 mg/kg) (870 IU)	b + d + a	NMBA	2 × 2.5 mg/kg/wk 5 weeks	SD male rats	∅	∅	Nauss *et al.* (1987)
Retinyl acetate (27 mg/kg)	a	NMBA	5 × 3 mg/kg sc 2.5 weeks	BD IX rats	∅	∅	van Rensburg *et al.* (1986)
Vitamin A acetate (29.9 mg/kg) (87,000 IU)	b + d + a	NMBA	2 × 2.5 mg/kg/wk 5 weeks	SD male rats	∅	∅	Nauss *et al.* (1987)
Vitamin A acetate (29.9 mg/kg) (87,000 IU)	a	NMBA	2 × 2.5 mg/kg/wk 5 weeks	SD male rats	∅	∅	Nauss *et al.* (1987)
Ethyl-all-*trans* 9-4-methoxy-2,3,6-trimethylphenyl-3,7-dimethyl-2,4,6,8-nonatetraenoate (30 mg/kg)	d + a	NMBA	25 mg/kg/wk sc 15 times	SD male and female rats	∅ →	—	Schmähl and Habs (1981)
Ethyl-all-*trans* 9-4-methoxy-2,3,6-trimethylphenyl-3,7-dimethyl-2,4,6,8-nonatetraenoate (60 mg/kg)	d + a	NMBA	25 mg/kg/wk sc 15 times	SD male and female rats	∅ →	—	Schmähl and Habs (1981)

Table 4.2. *The Effect of Riboflavin and Nictonic Acid on Esophagus Carcinogenesis*

Diet	Feeding schedule	Carcinogen	Dose/duration	Species, strain/sex	Tumor incidence	No. of tumors/ tumor-bearing animal	Reference
Riboflavin (5 mg/kg)	b + d + a	NMBA	5 × 3 mg/kg sc 2.5 weeks	BD IX rats	→	→	van Rensburg *et al.* (1986)
Riboflavin (5 mg/kg)	a	NMBA	5 × 3 mg/kg sc 2.5 weeks	BD IX rats	→	→	van Rensburg *et al.* (1986)
Nicotinic acid (10 mg/kg)	b + d + a	NMBA	5 × 3 mg/kg sc 2.5 weeks	BD IX rats	→	→	van Rensburg *et al.* (1986)
Nictonic acid (10 mg/kg)	a	NMBA	5 × 3 mg/kg sc 2.5 weeks	BD IX rats	→	→	van Rensburg *et al.* (1986)

Table 4.3. The Effect of Selenium on Esophagus Carcinogenesis

Diet	Feeding schedule	Carcinogen	Dose/duration	Species, strain/sex	Tumor incidence	No. of tumors/ tumor-bearing animal	Reference
Selenium deficient	b + d + a	NMBA	2 × 2.5 mg/kg/wk 3 weeks + 21 weeks later 2 × 2.5 mg/kg/wk 5 weeks	SD male rats	∅	—	Nauss et al. (1986)
Sodium selenite (4 ppm dw)	b + d	NMBA	2 × 2.5 mg/kg/wk 7 weeks	SD male rats	→	—	Nauss et al. (1986)
Sodium selenite (4 ppm dw)	b + d + a	NMBA	2 × 2.5 mg/kg/wk 7 weeks	SD male rats	∅	—	Nauss et al. (1986)
Sodium selenite (4 ppm dw)	a	NMBA	2 × 2.5 mg/kg/wk 7 weeks	SD male rats	∅	—	Nauss et al. (1986)
Sodium selenite (0.45 mg/kg)	b + d	NMBA	5 × 3 mg/kg sc 2.5 weeks	BD IV inbred rats	→	→*	van Rensburg et al. (1986)

Table 4.4. The Effect of Sodium Chloride on Esophagus Carcinogenesis

Diet	Feeding schedule	Carcinogen	Dose/duration	Species, strain/sex	Tumor incidence	No. of tumors/ tumor-bearing animal	Reference
NaCl (10%)	d + a	NPip	0.06% in diet 8 weeks	F344 male rats	↑	—	Konishi *et al.* (1986)
NaCl (10%)	d	NPip	0.06% in diet 8 weeks	F344 male rats	∅	—	Konishi *et al.* (1986)
NaCl (10%)	a	NPip	0.06% in diet 8 weeks	F344 male rats	∅	—	Konishi *et al.* (1986)

Table 4.5. The Effect of Tungsten, Molybdenum, and Magnesium on Esophagus Carcinogenesis

Diet	Feeding schedule	Carcinogen	Dose/duration	Species, strain/sex	Tumor incidence	No. of tumors/ tumor-bearing animal	Reference
Na_2WO_4 (100 ppm dw)	b + d + a	N-SAR-ethylester	2 × 10 ml/kg/wk ig 8 weeks	SD male rats	∅	—	Luo et al. (1983)
Na_2MoO_4 (2 ppm dw)	b + d + a	N-SAR-ethylester	2 × 10 ml/kg/wk ig 8 weeks	SD male rats	→	—	Luo et al. (1983)
Na_2MoO_4 (20 ppm dw)	b + d + a	N-SAR-ethylester	2 × 10 ml/kg/wk ig 8 weeks	SD male rats	→	—	Luo et al. (1983)
Mo (0.5 mg/kg)	b + d + a	NMBA	5 × 3 ml/kg/wk sc 2.5 weeks	BD IX rats	→	→	van Rensburg et al. (1986)
Mo (0.5 mg/kg)	a	NMBA	5 × 3 ml/kg/wk sc 2.5 weeks	BD IX rats	∅	∅	van Rensburg et al. (1986)
Mg (250 mg/kg)	b + d + a	NMBA	5 × 3 mg/kg sc 2.5 weeks	BD IX rats	→	→	van Rensburg et al. (1986)
Mg (250 mg/kg)	a	NMBA	5 × 3 mg/kg sc 2.5 weeks	BD IX rats	∅	∅	van Rensburg et al. (1986)

Table 4.6. The Effect of Zinc on Esophagus Carcinogenesis

Diet	Feeding schedule	Carcinogen	Dose/duration	Species, strain/sex	Tumor incidence	No. of tumors/tumor-bearing animal	Reference
Zinc deficient (2.3 ppm)	b + d + a	NMBA	2 × 2 mg/kg/wk ig 8.5 weeks	SD male rats	↑	↑	Barch et al. (1984)
Zinc deficient (7 ppm)	b + d	NMBA	2 × 2 mg/kg/wk ig 4 weeks	SD male rats	↑	∅	Gabrial et al. (1982)
Zinc deficient (7 ppm)	b + d + a	NMBA	2 × 2 mg/kg/wk 4 weeks	SD male rats	∅	∅	Gabriel et al. (1982)
Zinc deficient (7 ppm)	b + d	BMA + NaNO$_2$	0.25% dw + 0.5% dw	SD male rats	∅	∅	Fong et al. (1984)
Zinc deficient (7 ppm)	b + d	BMA + NaNO$_2$	0.05% dw + 0.5% dw	SD male rats	∅	∅	Fong et al. (1984)
Zinc deficient (7 ppm)	b + d + a	NMBA	2 × 2 mg/kg/wk ig 12 weeks	CD male rats	∅	∅	Fong et al. (1978)
Zinc deficient (7 ppm)	b + d + a	NMBA	2 × mg/kg/wk ig 9 weeks	CD male rats	∅	∅	Fong et al. (1978)
Zinc deficient (7 ppm)	b + d + a	NMBA	2 × 2 mg/kg/wk ig 4 weeks	CD male rats	∅	∅	Fong et al. (1978)
Zinc deficient (7 ppm)	b + d + a	NMBA	2 × 2 mg/kg/wk ig 2 weeks	CD male rats	∅	∅	Fong et al. (1978)
Zinc carbonate (15 mg/kg) + sodium phytate (0.3%)	b + d	NMBA	2 × 2 mg/kg/wk ig	BD IX male rats	↑	—	van Rensburg et al. (1980)
Zinc carbonate (15 mg/kg) + sodium phytate (0.3%) + zinc carbonate without phytate	a	NMBA	2 × 2 mg/kg/wk ig	BD IX male rats	∅	—	van Rensburg et al. (1980)
Zinc carbonate (30 mg/kg)	b + d + a	NMBA	5 × 3 mg/kg/sc 2.5 weeks	BD IX rats	→	→	van Rensburg et al. (1986)
Zinc carbonate (30 mg/kg)	a	NMBA	5 × 3 mg/kg/sc 2.5 weeks	BD IX rats	→	→	van Rensburg et al. (1986)

Table 4.7. The Effect of Cereals in Different Preparations on Esophagus Carcinogenesis

Diet	Feeding schedule	Carcinogen	Dose/duration	Species, strain/sex	Tumor incidence	No. of tumors/ tumor-bearing animal	Reference
Whole white cornmeal (75%)	b + d + a	NMBA	3 mg/kg/wk sc 6 weeks	BD IX male rats	∅	—	van Rensburg et al. (1985)
Whole yellow corn- meal (75%)	b + d + a	NMBA	3 mg/kg/wk sc 6 weeks	BD IX male rats	∅	—	van Rensburg et al. (1985)
White cornmeal (75%) + suppl.[a]	b + d + a	NMBA	3 mg/kg/wk sc 6 weeks	BD IX male rats	→	—	van Rensburg et al. (1985)
White wheat bread flour (75%)	b + d + a	NMBA	3 mg/kg/wk sc 6 weeks	BD IX male rats	∅	—	van Rensburg et al. (1985)
Brown wheat bread flour (75%)	b + d + a	NMBA	3 mg/kg/wk sc 6 weeks	BD IX male rats	∅	—	van Rensburg et al. (1985)
Polished rice (75%)	b + d + a	NMBA	3 mg/kg/wk sc 6 weeks	BD IX male rats	∅	—	van Rensburg et al. (1985)
Brown rice (75%)	b + d + a	NMBA	3 mg/kg/wk sc 6 weeks	BD IX male rats	→	—	van Rensburg et al. (1985)
Polished rice (75%) + bananas	b + d + a	NMBA	3 mg/kg/wk sc 6 weeks	BD IX male rats	∅	—	van Rensburg et al. (1985)
Commercial malt sorghum (75%)	b + d + a	NMBA	3 mg/kg/wk sc 6 weeks	BD IX male rats	∅	—	van Rensburg et al. (1985)
Bird-resistant sorghum (75%)	b + d + a	NMBA	3 mg/kg/wk sc 6 weeks	BD IX male rats	∅	—	van Rensburg et al. (1985)
Traditional, red sor- ghum (75%)	b + d + a	NMBA	3 mg/kg/wk sc 6 weeks	BD IX male rats	→	—	van Rensburg et al. (1985)
Dehusked millet (75%)	b + d + a	NMBA	3 mg/kg/wk sc 6 weeks	BD IX male rats	→	—	van Rensburg et al. (1985)
Whole millet (75%)	b + d + a	NMBA	3 mg/kg/wk sc 6 weeks	BD IX male rats	→	—	van Rensburg et al. (1985)
Whole millet (75%) + suppl.[a]	b + d + a	NMBA	3 mg/kg/wk sc 6 weeks	BD IX male rats	→	—	van Rensburg et al. (1985)

Table 4.7. (Continued)

Diet	Feeding schedule	Carcinogen	Dose/duration	Species, strain/sex	Tumor incidence	No. of tumors/ tumor-bearing animal	Reference
Dried potatoes (75%)	b + d + a	NMBA	3 mg/kg/wk sc 6 weeks	BD IX male rats	∅	—	van Rensburg et al. (1985)
White bread flour (75%)	b + d + a	NMBA	3 mg/kg/wk sc 5 weeks	BD IX male rats	∅	∅*	van Rensburg et al. (1985)
Millet flour (75%)	b + d + a	NMBA	3 mg/kg/wk sc 5 weeks	BD IX male rats	→	→*	van Rensburg et al. (1985)
Brown rice (75%)	b + d + a	NMBA	3 mg/kg/wk sc 5 weeks	BD IX male rats	→	→*	van Rensburg et al. (1985)
Cornmeal (75%) + minerals[b]	b + d + a	NMBA	3 mg/kg/wk sc 5 weeks	BD IX male rats	→	→*	van Rensburg et al. (1985)
Cornmeal (75%) + vitamins[c]	b + d + a	NMBA	3 mg/kg/wk sc 5 weeks	BD IX male rats	→	→*	van Rensburg et al. (1985)
Cornmeal (75%) + vitamins[a] + minerals[b]	b + d + a	NMBA	3 mg/kg/wk sc 5 weeks	BD IX male rats	→	→*	van Rensburg et al. (1985)
Cornmeal (75%) + minerals[b]	a	NMBA	3 mg/kg/wk sc 5 weeks	BD IX male rats	→	→	van Rensburg et al. (1985)
Cornmeal 75% + vitamins[c]	a	NMBA	3 mg/kg/wk sc 5 weeks	BD IX male rats	→	→	van Rensburg et al. (1985)
Cornmeal 75% + minerals[b] + vitamins[c]	a	NMBA	3 mg/kg/wk sc 5 weeks	BD IX male rats	→	→	van Rensburg et al. (1985)
Brown rice–millet (75%)	a	NMBA	3 mg/kg/wk sc 5 weeks	BD IX male rats	→	∅	van Rensburg et al. (1985)
Cornmeal (75%) + suppl.[d]	a	NMBA	3 mg/kg/wk sc 5 weeks	BD IX male rats	→	∅	van Rensburg et al. (1985)

[a]Suppl. = 5 mg riboflavin, 10 mg nicotinic acid, and 50 mg ZnCO₃ per kg diet.
[b]250 mg Mg, 30 mg Zn, 0.5 mg Mo, and 0.45 mg Se per kg diet.
[c]5 mg riboflavin and 20 mg nicotinic acid per kg diet.
[d]Suppl. = 5 mg riboflavin, 10 mg nicotinic acid, 0.45 mg Se per kg diet.

Table 5.1. The Effect of Fat on Forestomach Carcinogenesis

Diet	Feeding schedule	Carcinogen	Dose/duration	Species, strain/sex	Tumor incidence	No. of tumors/ tumor-bearing animal	Reference
Refined corn oil (no free fatty acids) (200 mg/mouse/day)	During the whole experiment	—	—	T.M. female mice	$\emptyset$	—	Szepsenwol (1978)
Refined corn oil (1.5% free fatty acids) (200 mg/mouse/day)	During the whole experiment	—	—	T.M. female mice	$\emptyset$	—	Szepsenwol (1978)
Refined corn oil (+ free fatty acids) (200 mg/mouse/day)	During the whole experiment	—	—	T.M. female mice	$\emptyset$	—	Szepsenwol (1978)
Monolein (200 mg/mouse/day)	During the whole experiment	—	—	T.M. female mice	$\emptyset$	—	Szepsenwol (1978)
Monostearin (200 mg/mouse/day)	During the whole experiment	—	—	T.M. female mice	$\emptyset$	—	Szepsenwol (1978)
Raw egg yolk (1/50 mice/day, 4 months, then: 1/30 mice/day)	During the whole experiment	—	—	Balb/c or C57 male and female mice	$\emptyset$	—	Szepsenwol (1978)

Table 5.2. The Effect of Synthetic Retinoids on Forestomach Carcinogenesis

Diet	Feeding schedule	Carcinogen	Dose/duration	Species, strain/sex	Tumor incidence	No. of tumors/ tumor-bearing animal	Reference
Ethyl-allyl-*trans* 9-(4-methoxy-2,3,6 trimethylphenyl-3,7-dimethyl-2,4,6,8 non-atetrenoate (3 × 8 mg/kg/wk ig)	d + a	DMH	10 mg/kg/wk sc 10 weeks	SD male rats	∅	—	Schmähl and Habs (1978)
Ethyl-allyl-*trans* 9-(4-methoxy-2,3,6 trimethylphenyl-3,7-dimethyl-2,4,6,8 non-atetrenoate (41.82 mg/kg/wk ig)	d + a	DMBA + TPA	25 mg/kg ig + 10 mg/kg/wk po until death	C57BL6 female mice	∅	—	Wagner *et al.* (1983)
Ethyl-allyl-*trans* 9-(4-methoxy-2,3,6 trimethylphenyl-3,7-dimethyl-2,4,6,8 non-atetrenoate (3 × 16 mg/kg/wk ig)	d + a	DMH	10 mg/kg/wk sc 10 weeks	SD male rats	∅	—	Schmähl and Habs (1978)

(continued)

Table 5.2. (Continued)

Diet	Feeding schedule	Carcinogen	Dose/duration	Species, strain/sex	Tumor incidence	No. of tumors/ tumor-bearing animal	Reference
Ethyl-allyl-*trans* 9-(4-methoxy-2,3,6 trimethylphenyl-3,7-dimethyl-2,4,6,8 non-atetrenoate (3 × 32 mg/kg/wk ig)	d + a	DMH	10 mg/kg/wk sc 10 weeks	SD male rats	∅	—	Schmähl and Habs (1978)
Ethyl-allyl-*trans* 9-(4-methoxy-2,3,6 trimethylphenyl-3,7-dimethyl-2,4,6,8 non-atetrenoate (125.46 mg/kg/wk ig)	d + a	DMBA + TPA	25 mg/kg ig + 10 mg/kg/wk po until death	C57BL6 female mice	∅	—	Wagner *et al.* (1983)
Ethyl-allyl-*trans* 9-(4-methoxy-2,3,6 trimethylphenyl-3,7-dimethyl-2,4,6,8 non-atetrenoate (376.38 mg/kg/wk ig)	d + a	DMBA + TPA	25 mg/kg ig + 10 mg/kg/wk po until death	C57BL6 female mice	↑	—	Wagner *et al.* (1983)

Table 5.3. The Effect of Vitamin C on Forestomach Carcinogenesis

Diet	Feeding schedule	Carcinogen	Dose/duration	Species, strain/sex	Tumor incidence	No. of tumors/ tumor-bearing animal	Reference
Ascorbat (5%)	a	NMU	2 × 20 mg/kg/wk ip 4 weeks	F344 male rats	↑	—	Imaida *et al.* (1984)
L-Ascorbic acid (22.7 g/kg)	d	NMOR	0.15 g/liter dw	MRC–Wistar male rats	∅	—	Mirvish *et al.* (1976)

Table 5.4. The Effect of Selenium on Forestomach Carcinogenesis

Diet	Feeding schedule	Carcinogen	Dose/duration	Species, strain/sex	Tumor incidence	No. of tumors/ tumor-bearing animal	Reference
Sodiumselenite (4 ppm dw)	d	NMNG	75 mg/liter dw 3 months	SD male rats	$\emptyset$	—	Newberne et al. (1986)
Sodiumselenite (4 ppm dw)	d	NMU	20 mg/kg/wk ip 10 times	WE female and male rats	$\emptyset$	—	Warzok et al. (1981)
p-Methoxybenzeneselenol (3.3 μmole/g)	b + d + a	B(a)p	2 × 1 mg/wk/mouse ig 4 weeks	CD-1 female mice	$\emptyset$	↓*	El-Bayoumy (1985)
Phenoselenazine (3.8 μmole/g)	b + d + a	B(a)p	2 × 1 mg/wk/mouse ig 4 weeks	CD-1 female mice	$\emptyset$	$\emptyset$*	El-Bayoumy (1985)
Benzylselenocyanate (0.45 μmole/g)	b + d + a	B(a)p	2 × 1 mg/wk/mouse ig 4 weeks	CD-1 female mice	$\emptyset$	↓*	El-Bayoumy (1985)

Table 5.5. The Effect of Sodium Chloride on Forestomach Carcinogenesis

Diet	Feeding schedule	Carcinogen	Dose/duration	Species, strain/sex	Tumor incidence	No. of tumors/ tumor-bearing animal	Reference
NaCl (5%)	a	NMNG	150 mg/kg ig	F344 male rats	Ø	—	Shirai et al. (1984)
NaCl (10%)	d + a	NQO	1 mg/wk ig 20 weeks	Wistar male rats	↑	—	Tatematsu et al. (1975)
NaCl (10%)	a	NMNG	250 mg/kg ig 20 weeks	Wistar male rats	Ø	—	Shirai et al. (1982)
NaCl (18%) 1 ml/wk ig	d + a	NQO	1 mg/wk ig 20 weeks	Wistar male rats	↑	—	Tatematsu et al. (1975)
NaCl (29%) 1 ml/wk ig	d	NMNG	75 mg/liter dw 3 months	SD male rats	↑	—	Newberne et al. (1986)
NaCl (29%) 2 × 1 mg/wk ig	a	NMNG	250 mg/kg ig	Wistar male rats	Ø	—	Shirai et al. (1982)
DL-Tocopherol (1%) + NaCl (10%) first 8 weeks	a	NMNG	100 mg/liter 8 weeks dw	Wistar male rats	Ø	—	Takahashi et al. (1986a)

Table 5.6. The Effect of Tungsten and Molybdenum on Forestomach Carcinogenesis

Diet	Feeding schedule	Carcinogen	Dose/duration	Species, strain/sex	Tumor incidence	No. of tumors/ tumor-bearing animal	Reference
Na$_2$WO$_4$ (100 ppm dw)	b + d + a	N-SAR- ethyl-ester	2 × 10 ml/kg/wk ig 8 weeks	SD male rats	∅	—	Luo et al. (1983)
Na$_2$MoO$_4$ (20 ppm dw)	b + d + a	N-SAR- ethyl-ester	2 × 10 ml/kg/wk ig 8 weeks	SD male rats	→	—	Luo et al. (1983)
Na$_2$MoO$_4$ (2 ppm dw)	b + d + a	N-SAR- ethyl-ester	2 × 10 ml/kg/wk ig 8 weeks	SD male rats	→	—	Luo et al. (1983)

Table 5.7. The Effect of Zinc on Forestomach Carcinogenesis

Diet	Feeding schedule	Carcinogen	Dose/duration	Species, strain/sex	Tumor incidence	No. of tumors/ tumor-bearing animal	Reference
Zinc deficient (7 ppm)	b + d	BMA + NaNO$_2$	0.05% + 0.05% dw	SD male rats	∅	—	Fong *et al.* (1984)
Zinc deficient (7 ppm)	b + d	BMA + NaNO$_2$	0.25% + 0.05% dw	SD male rats	↑	—	Fong *et al.* (1984)

Table 6.1. *The Effect of Vitamin C on Glandular Stomach Carcinogenesis*

Diet	Feeding schedule	Carcinogen	Dose/duration	Species, strain/sex	Tumor incidence	No. of tumors/ tumor-bearing animal	Reference
Sodium ascorbate (2 g/100 g)	d + a	NMNG	167 μg/ml dw	Wistar male rats	∅	—	Kawasaki *et al.* (1982)
Ascorbate (5%)	a	NMU	2 × 20 mg/kg/wk ip 4 weeks	F344 male rats	∅	—	Imaida *et al.* (1984)

Table 6.2. The Effect of Selenium on Glandular Stomach Carcinogenesis

Diet	Feeding schedule	Carcinogen	Dose/duration	Species, strain/sex	Tumor incidence	No. of tumors/ tumor-bearing animal	Reference
Sodium selenite (4 ppm dw)	d	NMNG	75 mg/liter dw 3 months	SD male rats	→	—	Newberne *et al.* (1987)

Table 6.3. The Effect of Sodium Chloride on Glandular Stomach Carcinogenesis

Diet	Feeding schedule	Carcinogen	Dose/duration	Species, strain/sex	Tumor incidence	No. of tumors/tumor-bearing animal	Reference
NaCl (5%)	a	NMNG	150 mg/kg ig	F344 male rats	∅	—	Shirai et al. (1984)
NaCl (10%)	d + a	NMNG	100 mg/liter dw 8 weeks	Wistar male rats	∅	—	Takashi and Hasegawa (1986)
NaCl (10%)	d + a	NMNG	100 mg/liter dw 20 weeks	Wistar male rats	↑	—	Takahashi and Hasegawa (1986)
NaCl (10%)	d + a	NMNG	100 mg/liter dw 8 weeks	Wistar male rats	∅	—	Takahashi et al. (1984)
NaCl (10%)	a	NMNG	100 mg/liter dw 8 weeks	Wistar male rats	∅	—	Takahashi et al. (1984)
NaCl (10%)	d	NMNG	150 mg/liter dw 20 weeks	Wistar male rats	↑	—	Takahashi et al. (1983)
NaCl (10%)	d	NMNG	100 mg/liter dw 20 weeks	Wistar male rats	↑	—	Takahashi et al. (1983)
NaCl (10%)	a	NMNG	100 mg/liter dw 20 weeks	Wistar male rats	∅	—	Takahashi and Hasegawa (1986)
NaCl (10%)	a	NMNG	150 mg/liter dw 20 weeks	Wistar male rats	∅	—	Takahashi et al. (1983)
NaCl (10%)	a	NMNG	100 mg/liter dw 20 weeks	Wistar male rats	∅	—	Takahashi et al. (1983)
NaCl (10%)	a	NMNG	250 mg/kg ig	Wistar male rats	∅	—	Shirai et al. (1982)
NaCl (10% + 6 g/liter dw)	d + a	NMNG	50 mg/liter dw 20 weeks	Wistar male rats	∅	—	Tatematsu et al. (1975)
NaCl (saturated solution) (1 ml/wk ig)	d	NMNG	75 mg/liter dw 3 months	SD rats	∅	—	Charnley and Tannenbaum (1985)
NaCl (29% 1 ml/wk ig)	d	NMNG	75 mg/liter dw 3 months	SD male rats	↑	—	Newberne et al. (1987)
NaCl (29% 1 ml/wk ig)	d + a	NMNG	50 mg/liter dw 20 weeks	Wistar male rats	↑	—	Tatematsu et al. (1975)
NaCl (29% 2 × 1 ml/wk ig)	a	NMNG	250 mg/kg ig	Wistar male rats	∅	—	Shirai et al. (1982)
DL-Tocopherol + NaCl (10%)	a	NMNG	100 mg/liter dw 8 weeks	Wistar male rats	∅	—	Takahashi et al. (1986)

Table 6.4. The Effect of a Defined Diet on Glandular Stomach Carcinogenesis

Diet	Feeding schedule	Carcinogen	Dose/duration	Species, strain/sex	Tumor incidence	No. of tumors/ tumor-bearing animal	Reference
Defined diet in liquid form (iso-caloric, 14.0 g protein, 70.1 g carbohydrates, 9.3 g fat)	b + d + a	NMNG	50 μg/ml dw 24 weeks	Wistar male rats	↓	↓*	Tatsuta *et al.* (1988)

Table 7.1. The Effect of Fat on Skin Carcinogenesis

Diet	Feeding schedule	Carcinogen	Dose/duration	Species, strain/sex	Tumor incidence	No. of tumors/ tumor-bearing animal	Reference
Orange oil (1%)	a	DMBA	0.2 μmole topical	CD-1 mice	$\emptyset$	$\emptyset$	Elegbede et al. (1986)
d-Limonene (1%)	a	DMBA	0.2 μmole topical	CD-1 mice	$\emptyset$	$\emptyset$	Elegbede et al. (1986)
Corn oil (12%)	b + d	UV light	0.87 J/cm²/day −2.18 J/cm²/day 5 days/wk	Hairless female mice	—	$\emptyset$	Black et al. (1984)
Corn oil (12%) (hydrogenated 60%)	b + d	UV light	0.87 J/cm²/day −2.18 J/cm²/day 5 days/wk	Hairless female mice	$\emptyset$	$\rightarrow$	Black et al. (1984)

Table 7.2. The Effect of Vitamin A and Synthetic Retinoids on Skin Carcinogenesis

Diet	Feeding schedule	Carcinogen	Dose/duration	Species, strain/sex	Tumor incidence	No. of tumors/ tumor-bearing animal	Reference
13-*Cis*-retinoic acid (200 000 IU/kg)	d	DMBA + TPA	150 nmoles topical + 3 weeks later 2 × 8 nmoles/wk during the entire experiment	CD-1 female mice	∅	∅	Gensler et al. (1987)
13-*Cis*-retinoic acid (700 000 IU/kg)	d	DMBA + TPA	150 nmoles topical + 3 weeks later 2 × 8 nmoles/wk during the entire experiment	CD-1 female mice	∅	∅	Gensler et al. (1987)
Retinylacetate (0.75 μg/g)	b + d + a	DMBA + croton oil	2 × 150 μg + 2 × 500 μg/wk topical	CD-1 female mice	∅	→	Muto and Moriwaki (1984)
Retinylacetate (5.2 μg/g)	b + d + a	DMBA + croton oil	2 × 150 μg + 2 × 500 μg/wk topical	CD-1 female mice	∅	→	Muto and Moriwaki (1984)
Retinyl palmitate (60 IU/g)	d	DMBA + TPA	150 nmoles + 3 weeks later 2 × 8 nmoles/wk topical during the entire experiment	CD-1 female mice	∅	∅	Gensler et al. (1987)
Retinyl palmitate (200 IU/g)	d	DMBA + TPA	150 nmoles + 3 weeks later 2 × 8 nmoles/wk topical during the entire experiment	CD-1 female mice	∅	→	Gensler et al. (1987)
Retinyl palmitate (350 IU/g)	d	DMBA + TPA	150 nmoles + 3 weeks later 2 × 8 nmoles/wk topical during the entire experiment	CD-1 female mice	→	→	Gensler et al. (1987)
All-*trans*-N-4-N-2-(hydroxylethyl)retinamide (687 mg/kg)	During the whole experiment	—	—	ACI/segHapBr male rats	∅	—	Ohshima et al. (1985)
All-*trans*-N-4 (4-hydroxyphenyl) retinamide (783 mg/kg)	During the whole experiment	—	—	ACI/segHapBr male rats	→	—	Ohshima et al. (1985)
All-*trans*-N-4 (4-pivaloyloxy) phenyl)retinamide (951 mg/kg)	During the whole experiment	—	—	ACI/segHapBr male rats	∅	—	Ohshima et al. (1985)
Ethyl-all-*trans*-9-(4-methoxy-2,3,6-timethylphenyl)-3,7-dimethyl-2,4,6,8-nonatetraenoate (5 × 30 mg/kg/wk ig)	d	DMBA + croton oil	2 × 150 μg + 2.05 mg/wk topical from day 42	Swiss albino female mice	∅	→	Bollag et al. (1975)

Table 7.3. The Effect of Vitamin C on Skin Carcinogenesis

Diet	Feeding schedule	Carcinogen	Dose/duration	Species, strain/sex	Tumor incidence	No. of tumors/ tumor-bearing animal	Reference
Ascorbic acid (0.3%)	d	UV light	Total 135 J/cm^3 5 days/wk 15 weeks	Hairless female mice (Skh-hr strain)	↓	—	Dunham *et al.* (1982)
Ascorbic acid (0.5%)	d	UV light	Total 135 J/cm^3 5 days/wk 15 weeks	Hairless female mice (Skh-hr strain)	↓	—	Dunham *et al.* (1982)
Ascorbic acid (10%)	d	UV light	Total 135 J/cm^3 5 days/wk 15 weeks	Hairless female mice (Skh-hr strain)	↓ →	—	Dunham *et al.* (1982)

Table 7.4. The Effect of Selenium on Skin Carcinogenesis

Diet	Feeding schedule	Carcinogen	Dose/duration	Species, strain/sex	Tumor incidence	No. of tumors/ tumor-bearing animal	Reference
Sodium selenite (2 mg/liter dw)	b + d + a	UV light	Increasing doses from 0.04 to 0.4 J/cm^2 over 2 weeks 5 days/wk + 0.4 J/cm^2 20 weeks	Nude female mice	∅	—	Overvad *et al.* (1985)
Sodium selenite (4 mg/liter dw)	b + d + a	UV light	Increasing doses from 0.04 to 0.4 J/cm^2 over 2 weeks 5 days/wk + 0.4 J/cm^2 20 weeks	Hairless female mice	→	—	Overvad *et al.* (1985)
Sodium selenite (8 mg/liter dw)	b + d + a	UV light	Increasing doses from 0.04 to 0.4 J/cm^2 over 2 weeks 5 days/wk + 0.4 J/cm^2 20 weeks	Hairless female mice	→	—	Overvad *et al.* (1985)

Table 8.1. The Effect of Fat on Respiratory Tract Carcinogenesis

Diet	Feeding schedule	Carcinogen	Dose/duration	Species, strain/sex	Tumor incidence	No. of tumors/ tumor-bearing animal	Reference
Beef tallow (20%)	b + d + a	B(a)p	4 mg/wk it 15 weeks	Syrian Golden male and female hamsters	$\emptyset^a$	—	Beems and van Beck (1984)
Sunflower seed oil (20%)	b + d + a	B(a)p	4 mg/wk it 15 weeks	Syrian Golden male hamsters	↑ ^{a}	—	Beems and van Beck (1984)
Sunflower seed oil (20%)	b + d + a	B(a)p	4 mg/wk it 15 weeks	Syrian Golden female hamsters	$\emptyset^a$	—	Beems and van Beck (1984)
Sunflower oi (20%)	b + d + a	B(a)p	8 mg/rat/2 wk it 16 weeks	Syrian Golden male and female hamsters	$\emptyset^a$	—	Beems (1986)

^{a}Respiratory tract tumors.

Table 8.2. *The Effect of Vitamin A Deficiency on Respiratory Tract Carcinogenesis*

Diet	Feeding schedule	Carcinogen	Dose/duration	Species, strain/sex	Tumor incidence	No. of tumors/ tumor-bearing animal	Reference
Vitamin A deficient	a	MCA	1 × 10 mg it 10 weeks	F344 female rats	∅[a]	∅[a]	Nettesheim and Williams (1976)
Vitamin A deficient (17.4 µg/wk ig)	b + d + a	MCA	2 × 5 mg/rat it	F344 male and female rat	∅[a]	—	Nettesheim et al. (1979)
Vitamin A deficient (17.4 µg/wk ig)	b + d + a	MCA	2 × 2.5 mg/rat it	F344 male and female rat	∅[a]	—	Nettesheim et al. (1979)
Vitamin A deficient (17.4 µg/wk ig)	b + d + a	MCA	2 × 1.25 mg/rat it	F344 male and female rats	∅[a]	—	Nettesheim et al. (1979)
Vitamin A deficient (17.4 µg/wk ig)	b + d + a	MCA	2 × 0.625 mg/rat it	F344 male and female rats	∅[a]	—	Nettesheim et al. (1979)
Vitamin A deficient (1000 IU/kg)	b + d + a	B(a)P	10 mg/rat/wk it	Wistar male rats	∅[a]	∅[a]	Dogra et al. (1985)

[a] Lung.

Table 8.3. The Effect of Vitamin A on Respiratory Tract Carcinogenesis

Diet	Feeding schedule	Carcinogen	Dose/duration	Species, strain/sex	Tumor incidence	No. of tumors/tumor-bearing animal	Reference
13-Cis-retinoic acid (120 mg/kg)	a	NMU	0.5% 1 × 1 ml/wk it 12 weeks	Syrian Golden male hamsters	↑[a]	—	Stinson et al. (1981)
13-Cis-retinoic acid (128 mg/kg)	a	NMU	1% 2 ×/wk it for 7 seconds total; 18,20,23 exposures 9–11.5 weeks	Syrian Golden male hamsters	Ø[a]	Ø[a]	Yarita et al. (1980)
13-Cis-retinoic acid (172 mg/kg)	a	NMU	1% 2 ×/wk it for 7 seconds total; 18,20,23 exposures 9–11.5 weeks	Syrian Golden male hamsters	Ø[a]	Ø[a]	Yarita et al. (1980)
13-Cis-retinoic acid (3.3 × 10³ nmole/day)	a	MCA	1 × 10 mg/rat it	F344 female rats	Ø[b]	Ø[b]	Nettesheim and Williams (1976)
13-Cis-retinoic acid ethylamide (150 mg/kg) (4-methoxy-2,3,6-trimethylphenyl analog)	a	NMU	1% 2 ×/wi it for 7 seconds total; 18,20,23 exposures 9–11.5 weeks	Syrian Golden male hamsters	Ø[a]	Ø[a]	Yarita et al. (1980)
Retinyl acetate (1744 µg/wk ig)	b + d + a	MCA	2 × 1.25 mg/rat it	F344 male and female rats	Ø[b]	—	Nettesheim et al. (1979)
Retinyl acetate (1744 µg/wk ig)	b + d + a	MCA	2 × 0.625 mg/rat it	F344 male and female rats	Ø[b]	—	Nettesheim et al. (1979)

Retinyl acetate (2 × 5 μg/wk it, then: 2 × 5000 μg/wk ig)	b + d + a	MCA	2 × 2 mg/rat it	F344 female rats	∅[b]	—	Nettesheim et al. (1976)
Retinyl acetate (2 × 800 μ/wk ig)	a	B(a)P	3 mg/rat/wk it 12 weeks	Syrian Golden male hamsters	∅[c]	—	Smith et al. (1975a)
Retinyl acetate (2 × 800 μg/wk ig)	a	B(a)P	3 mg/rat/wk it 12 weeks	Syrian Golden male hamsters convention housing	∅[c]	—	Smith et al. (1975b)
Retinyl acetate (2 × 800 μg/wk ig)	a	B(a)P	3 mg/rat/wk it 12 weeks	Syrian Golden male hamsters laminar flow housing	∅[c]	—	Smith et al. (1975b)
Retinyl acetate (2 × 1650 μg/wk ig, reduction: 2 × 1200 μg/wk ig)	a	B(a)P	3 mg/rat/wk it 12 weeks	Syrian Golden male hamsters conventional housing	∅[c,d]	—	Smith et al. (1975b)
Retinyl acetate (2 × 1650 μg/wk ig, reduction: 2 × 1200 μg/wk ig)	a	B(a)P	3 mg/rat/wk it 12 weeks	Syrian Golden male hamsters laminar flow housing	∅[c]	—	Smith et al. (1975b)
Retinyl acetate (2 × 1650 μg/wk ig after 24 weeks, reduction: 2 × 1200 μg/wk ig)	a	B(a)P	3 mg/rat/wk it 12 weeks	Syrian Golden male hamsters	↑[c]	—	Smith et al. (1975a)
Retinyl acetate (1744 μg/wk ig)	b + d + a	MCA	2 × 5 mg/rat it	F344 male and female rats	∅[b]	—	Nettesheim et al. (1979)
Retinyl acetate (2 × 1650 μg/wk ig, reduction: 2 × 1200 μg/wk ig)	a	B(a)P	3 mg/rat/wk it 12 weeks	Syrian Golden male hamsters conventional housing	∅[c,d]	—	Smith et al. (1975b)

(continued)

Table 8.3. (Continued)

Diet	Feeding schedule	Carcinogen	Dose/duration	Species, strain/sex	Tumor incidence	No. of tumors/ tumor-bearing animal	Reference
Retinyl acetate (2 × 1650 μg/wk ig, reduction: 2 × 1200 μg/wk ig)	a	B(a)P	3 mg/rat/wk it 12 weeks	Syrian Golden male hamsters laminar flow housing	Ø[c]	—	Smith et al. (1975b)
Retinyl acetate (2 × 1650 μg/wk ig after 24 weeks, reduction: 2 × 1200 μg/wk ig)	a	B(a)P	3 mg/rat/wk it 12 weeks	Syrian Golden male hamsters	↑[c]	—	Smith et al. (1975a)
Retinyl acetate (1744 μg/wk ig)	b + d + a	MCA	2 × 5 mg/rat it	F344 male and female rats	Ø[b]	—	Nettesheim et al. (1979)
Retinyl acetate (1744 μg/wk ig)	b + d + a	MCA	2 × 2.5 mg/rat it	F344 male and female rats	Ø[b]	—	Nettesheim et al. (1979)
All-*trans*-retinyl acetate (4.6 × 10³ nmoles/day ig)	a	MCA	1 × 10 mg/rat it	F344 female rats	Ø[b]	Ø[b]	Nettesheim and Williams (1976)
Retinyl acetate (0.02%)	During the whole experiment	—	—	C3H/He(+) male mice	↓[b]	—	Stenbäck et al. (1987)
Retinyl acetate (0.02%)	During the whole experiment	—	—	C3H/He(+) female mice	Ø[b]	—	Stenbäck et al. (1987)
Ethyl retinamide (327 mg/kg)	a	NMU	0.5% 1 × 1 ml/wk it 12 weeks	Syrian Golden male hamsters	↑[a]	—	Stinson et al. (1981)
N-(2-hydroxyethyl) reti-namide (343 mg/kg)	a	NMU	0.5% 1 × 1 ml/wk it 12 weeks	Syrian Golden male hamsters	Ø[a]	—	Stinson et al. (1981)

[a]Trachea.
[b]Lung.
[c]Respiratory tract.
[d]Significant increasing effect of rethinylacetate when two high doses are combined.

Table 8.4. The Effect of Vitamin C on Respiratory Tract Carcinogenesis

Diet	Feeding schedule	Carcinogen	Dose/duration	Species, strain/sex	Tumor incidence	No. of tumors/ tumor-bearing animal	Reference
Ascorbic acid (1%)	d	Cigarette smoke + NDEA	2 × 6 min/day 5 days/wk + 10 mg/hamster sc	Syrian Golden male hamsters	$\emptyset^a$	—	Harada et al. (1985)
Sodium ascorbate (5.75 g/kg)	d	Mon N-pip	69 mg/liter dw 5×/wk 20 weeks	Strain A male mice	$\uparrow^b$	$\uparrow^b$	Mirvish et al. (1975)
Sodium ascorbate (5.75 g/kg)	d	Mon N-pip	50 mg/liter dw 5×/wk 20 weeks	Strain A male mice	$\uparrow^b$	$\uparrow^b$	Mirvish et al. (1975)
Sodium ascorbate (5.75 g/kg)	d	NMOR	20 mg/liter dw 5×/wk 20 weeks	Strain A male mice	$\uparrow^b$	$\uparrow^b$	Mirvish et al. (1975)
Sodium ascorbate (11.5 g/kg)	d	Mon N-pip	69 mg/liter dw 5×/wk 20 weeks	Strain A male mice	$\emptyset^b$	$\emptyset^b$	Mirvish et al. (1975)
Sodium ascorbate (11.5 g/kg)	d	Mon N-pip	50 mg/liter dw 5×/wk 20 weeks	Stain A male mice	$\emptyset^b$	$\emptyset^b$	Mirvish et al. (1975)
Sodium ascorbate (11.5 g/kg)	d	NMOR	20 mg/liter dw 5×/wk 20 weeks	Stain A male mice	$\uparrow^b$	$\uparrow^b$	Mirvish et al. (1975)
Sodium ascorbate (11.5 g/kg)	d	Piperazine + NaNo₂	6.25 g/kg + 1.0 g/liter	Strain A male mice	$\downarrow^b$	$\downarrow$ *	Mirvish et al. (1975)
Sodium ascorbate (11.5 g/kg)	d	Morpholine + NaNO₂	6.33 g/kg + 2.09 g/liter	Strain A male mice	$\downarrow^b$	$\downarrow$ *	Mirvish et al. (1975)

(continued)

Table 8.4. (Continued)

Diet	Feeding schedule	Carcinogen	Dose/duration	Species, strain/sex	Tumor incidence	No. of tumors/ tumor-bearing animal	Reference
Sodium ascorbate (11.5 g/kg)	—	Methylurea + NaNO₂	2.68 g/kg + 1.09 g/liter	Strain A male mice	↓[b]	↓*	Mirvish et al. (1975)
Sodium ascorbate (23.0 g/kg)	d	Mon N-pip	69 mg/iter dw 5×/wk 20 weeks	Strain A male mice	↑[b]	↑[b]	Mirvish et al. (1975)
Sodium ascorbate (23.0 g/kg)	d	Mon N-pip	50 mg/liter dw 5×/wk 20 weeks	Strain A male mice	∅[b]	∅[b]	Mirvish et al. (1975)
Sodium ascorbate (23.0 g/kg)	d	NMOR	20 mg/liter dw 5×/wk 20 weeks	Strain A male mice	∅[b]	∅[b]	Mirvish et al. (1975)
Sodium ascorbate (23 g/kg)	d	Piperazine + NaNO₂	6.25 g/kg + 1.0 g/liter 5×/wk/20 weeks	Strain A male mice	↓[b]	↓[b]	Mirvish et al. (1975)
Sodium ascorbate (23 g/kg)	d	Morpholine + NaNO₂	6.33 g/kg + 2.09 g/liter 5×/wk/20 weeks	Strain A male mice	↓[b]	↓*[b]	Mirvish et al. (1975)
Sodium ascorbate (23 g/kg)	d	Methylurea + NaNO₂	2.68 g/kg + 1.09 g/liter 5×/wk/20 weeks	Strain A male mice	↓[b]	↓*[b]	Mirvish et al. (1975)

[a]Trachea.
[b]Lung.

Table 8.5. The Effect of Selenium on Respiratory Tract Carcinogenesis

Diet	Feeding schedule	Carcinogen	Dose/duration	Species, strain/sex	Tumor incidence	No. of tumors/ tumor-bearing animal	Reference
Selenium (1 mg/kg)	b + d	NMU	1 ×/wk/rat it 12 weeks	Syrian Golden hamsters	∅[a]	—	Thompson and Becci (1979)
Selenium (5 mg/kg)	b + d	NMU	1 ×/wk/rat it 12 weeks	Syrian Golden hamsters	∅[a]	—	Thompson and Becci (1979)
Sodium selenite (2 ppm)	b + d	BOP	5 mg/kg/wk sc 50 weeks	Wistar male rats	↓[b]	—	Birt et al. (1982)
Sodium selenite (2 ppm)	b + d	BOP	5 mg/kg/wk sc 50 weeks	Wistar female rats	∅[b]	—	Birt et al. (1982)
Sodium selenite (5 ppm)	b + d + a	B(a)P	8 mg/rat 2wk it 16 weeks	Syrian Golden male and female hamsters	∅[c]	—	Beems (1986)
Sodium selenite (5 ppm + sunflower oil 20%)	b + d + a	B(a)P	8 mg/rat/2 wk it 16 weeks	Syrian Golden male and female hamsters	∅[c]	—	Beems (1986)

[a]Trachea.
[b]Lung.
[c]Respiratory tract.

Table 8.6. The Effect of Protein on Respiratory Tract Carcinogenesis

Diet	Feeding schedule	Carcinogen	Dose/duration	Species, strain/sex	Tumor incidence	No. of tumors/ tumor-bearing animal	Reference
Casein (9%)	b	BOP	10 mg/kg sc	Syrian Golden male and female hamsters	$\varnothing^a$	—	Pour and Birt (1986)
Casein (9%)	a	BOP	10 mg/kg sc	Syrian Golden male and female hamsters	$\varnothing^a$	—	Pour and Birt (1986)
Casein (36%)	b	BOP	10 mg/kg sc	Syrian Golden male and female hamsters	$\varnothing^a$	—	Pour and Birt (1986)
Casein (36%)	a	BOP	10 mg/kg sc	Syrian Golden male and female hamsters	$\varnothing^a$	—	Pour and Birt (1986)

[a]Lung.

Table 8.7. The Effect of a Calorie-Restricted Diet on Respiratory Tract Carcinogenesis

Diet	Feeding schedule	Carcinogen	Dose/duration	Species, strain/sex	Tumor incidence	No. of tumors/ tumor-bearing animal	Reference
PRD diet (75% restr.) (crude oil 2.78%, crude protein 19.79%)	During the whole experiment	—	—	Swiss male mice	$\varnothing^a$	—	Conybeare (1980)
PRD diet (75% restr.) (crude oil 2.78%, crude protein 19.79%)	During the whole experiment	—	—	Swiss female mice	$\downarrow^a$	—	Conybeare (1980)
41B diet (75% restr.) (crude oil 2.87%, crude protein 16.61%)	During the whole experiment	—	—	Swiss male mice	$\varnothing^a$	—	Conybeare (1980)
41B diet (75% restr.) (crude oil 2.87%, crude protein 16.61%)	During the whole experiment	—	—	Swiss female mice	$\downarrow^a$	—	Conybeare (1980)

[a]Lung.

Table 9.1. The Effect of Beef Tallow on Mammary Gland Carcinogenesis

Diet	Feeding schedule	Carcinogen	Dose/duration	Species, strain/sex	Tumor incidence	No. of tumors/ tumor-bearing animal	Reference
Beef tallow (20%)	b + a	DMBA	2.5 mg ig	SD female rats	∅	—	Lee and Rogers (1983)
Beef tallow (20%)	a	DMBA	5 mg ig	SD female rats	∅	∅	Hopkins and Carroll (1979)
Beef tallow (20%)	b + d + a[a]	DMBA	7.5 mg po	SD female rats	∅	∅	Sylvester *et al.* (1986b)
Beef tallow (20%)	b + d	DMBA	7.5 mg/kg po	SD female rats	∅	—	Sylvester *et al.* (1985)
Beef tallow (20%)	b + a	DMBA	17.5 mg/kg po	SD female rats	→	∅	Clinton *et al.* (1984b)
Beef tallow (24.3 g)	b + d + a	NMU	50 mg/kg iv	Fischer female rats	∅	∅	Chan *et al.* (1983)
Beef tallow (17%) + sunflower seed oil (3%)	a	DMBA	5 mg/rat ig	SD female rats	∅	∅	Hopkins and Carroll (1979)
Beef tallow (5%) + beef tallow (20%)	b a	DMBA	2.5 mg ig	SD female rats	∅	—	Lee and Rogers (1983)

[a]For 1 week only.

Table 9.2. The Effect of Lard on Mammary Gland Carcinogenesis

Diet	Feeding schedule	Carcinogen	Dose/duration	Species, strain/sex	Tumor incidence	No. of tumors/ tumor-bearing animal	Reference
Lard (20%)	b + a	DMBA	2.5 mg ig	SD female rats	∅	—	Wetsel et al. (1981)
Lard (20%)	a	DMBA	2.5 mg ig	SD female rats	∅	—	Wetsel et al. (1981)
Lard (20%)	a	DMBA	5 mg ig	SD female rats	∅	∅	Hopkins and Carroll (1979)
Lard (20%)	b + d	DMBA	7.5 mg/kg po	SD female rats	↑	—	Sylvester et al. (1985)
Lard (20%)	b + d + aᵃ	DMBA	7.5 mg po	SD female rats	↑	↑	Sylvester et al. (1986b)
Lard (20%)	d + a	NMU	50 mg/kg iv	SD female rats	∅	—	Silverman et al. (1980)
Lard (20%)	a	NMU	50 mg/kg iv	SD female rats	∅	—	Chan et al. (1977)
Lard (20%)	a	NMU	50 mg/kg iv	F344 female rats	↑	↑ *	Cohen and Chan (1982)
Lard (20%)	a	NMU	50 mg/kg iv	F344 female rats	↑	—	Chan et al. (1977)
Lard (20%)	d + a	NMU	50 mg/kg iv in 2 doses at days 50 and 80	F344 female rats	∅	—	Chan et al. (1977)
Lard (20%)	d + a	NMU	50 mg/kg iv in 2 doses at days 50 and 80	SD female rats	∅	—	Chan et al. (1977)
Lard (20%)	d + a	NMU	25 mg/kg iv in 2 doses at days 50 and 80	F344 female rats	∅	—	Chan et al. (1977)
Lard (20%)	d + a	NMU	25 mg/kg iv in 2 doses at days 50 and 80	SD female rats	∅	—	Chan et al. (1977)

(continued)

Table 9.2. (Continued)

Diet	Feeding schedule	Carcinogen	Dose/duration	Species, strain/sex	Tumor incidence	No. of tumors/ tumor-bearing animal	Reference
Lard (20%)	d + a	—	Total body X-irradiation	SD female rats	∅	—	Silverman *et al.* (1980)
Lard (23.3%)	b	DMBA	0.25 mg sc	SD female rats	∅	—	Rogers *et al.* (1986)
Lard (23.3%)	b	DMBA	0.5 mg sc	SD female rats	∅	—	Rogers *et al.* (1986)
Lard (23.3%)	b	DMBA	1 mg sc	SD female rats	∅	—	Rogers *et al.* (1986)
Lard (23.3%)	b	DMBA	2.5 mg sc	SD female rats	∅	—	Rogers *et al.* (1986)
Lard (23.3%)	b + a	DMBA	0.25 mg sc	SD female rats	∅	—	Rogers *et al.* (1986)
Lard (23.3%)	b + a	DMBA	0.5 mg sc	SD female rats	∅	—	Rogers *et al.* (1986)
Lard (23.3%)	b + a	DMBA	1 mg sc	SD female rats	∅	—	Rogers *et al.* (1986)
Lard (23.3%)	b + a	DMBA	2.5 mg iv	SD female rats	∅	—	Rogers *et al.* (1986)
Lard (23.3%)	a	DMBA	0.25 mg sc	SD female rats	∅	—	Rogers *et al.* (1986)
Lard (4%) + cholesterol (2%)	a	NMU	50 mg/kg iv	F344 female rats	∅	∅	Cohen and Chan (1982)
Lard (20%) + cholesterol (2%)	a	NMU	50 mg/kg iv	F344 female rats	↑	↑*	Cohen and Chan (1982)
Lard (24.3 g)	b + d + a	NMU	50 mg/kg iv	Fischer female rats	∅	∅	Chan *et al.* (1983)

*a*For 1 week only.

Table 9.3. The Effect of Corn Oil on Mammary Gland Carcinogenesis

Diet	Feeding schedule	Carcinogen	Dose/duration	Species, strain/sex	Tumor incidence	No. of tumors/tumor-bearing animal	Reference
Corn oil (0.5%)	b + a	DMBA	5 mg po at 50 days of age	SD female rats	→	—	Ip (1980)
Corn oil (0.5%)	b + a	DMBA	5 mg po at 150 days of age	SD female rats	∅	—	Ip (1980)
Corn oil (0.5%)	b + d + a	DMBA	5 mg po at 50 days of age	SD female rats	→	∅	Ip and Ip (1980)
Corn oil (0.5%)	b + d + a	DMBA	15 mg po at 150 days of age	SD female rats	→	∅	Ip and Ip (1980)
Corn oil (0.5%)	b + d + a	DMBA	5 mg/rat ig	SD female rats	→	∅	Ip and Ip (1981)
Corn oil (0.5%)	b + d + a	NMU	3 × 50 mg/kg iv	BUF female rats	∅	—	Jurkowski and Cave (1985)
Corn oil (1%)	b + d + a	DMBA	5 mg ig	SD female rats	∅	∅	Ip and Sinha (1981b)
Corn oil (1%)	b + d + a	DMBA	10 mg ig	SD female rats	∅	∅	Ip and Sinha (1981b)
Corn oil (1%)	b + d + a	DMBA	15 mg ig	SD female rats	∅	∅	Ip and Sinha (1981b)
Corn oil (3%)	a	DMBA	5 mg ig	SD female rats	∅	∅	Braden and Carroll (1986)
Corn oil (18%)	a	DMBA	5 mg ig	SD female rats	∅ ↓	∅	Carter et al. (1983)
Corn oil (20%)	b + a	DMBA	2.5 mg ig	SD female rats	↑	—	Wetzel et al. (1981)
Corn oil (20%)	a	DMBA	2.5 mg ig	SD female rats	↑	—	Wetzel et al. (1981)
Corn oil (20%)	b + d + a	DMBA	5 mg ig	SD female rats	↑	∅	Ip and Ip (1981)

(continued)

Table 9.3. (Continued)

Diet	Feeding schedule	Carcinogen	Dose/duration	Species, strain/sex	Tumor incidence	No. of tumors/ tumor-bearing animal	Reference
Corn oil (20%)	b + d + a	DMBA	5 mg ig	SD female rats	↓	—	Ip and White (1986)
Corn oil (20%)	a	DMBA	5 mg ig	SD female rats	∅ ↓	↑*	Aylsworth et al. (1986)
Corn oil (20%)	a	DMBA	5 mg ig	SD female rats	↑	∅	Selenskas et al. (1984)
Corn oil (20%)	a	DMBA	5 mg/kg iv	SD female rats	∅	↑*	Welsch and DeHoog (1988)
Corn oil (20%)	a	DMBA	5 mg/kg iv	SD female rats	∅	∅	Braden and Carroll (1986)
Corn oil (20%)	b + d + a[a]	DMBA	7.5 mg po	SD female rats	∅	∅	Sylvester et al. (1986b)
Corn oil (20%)	b + d	DMBA	7.5 mg/kg po	SD female rats	∅	—	Sylvester et al. (1985)
Corn oil (20%)	a	DMBA	7.5 mg/kg ig	SD female rats	∅	—	Sylvester et al. (1986a)
Corn oil (20%)	b + d + a	DMBA	10 mg ig	SD female rats	↑	—	McCay et al. (1981)
Corn oil (20%)	b + a	DMBA	10 mg ig	SD female rats	↑	—	King and McCay (1983)
Corn oil (20%)	b + a	DMBA	10 mg ig	SD female rats	∅ ↓	—	King et al. (1979)
Corn oil (20%)	b + d + a[b]	DMBA	20 mg/kg iv	SD female rats	∅	∅	Welsch and DeHoog (1988)
Corn oil (20%)	b + d + a	Estrone	implantation of 9 mg pellets	Nb female rats	∅	—	Carroll and Noble (1987)
Corn oil (20%)	b + d + a	NMU	3 × 50 mg/kg iv	BUF female rats	∅	—	Jurkowski and Cave (1985)
Corn oil (23%)	a	NMU	50 mg/kg iv	F344 female rats	∅ ↓	∅	Cohen et al. (1986)
Corn oil (24.6%)	a	DMBA	5 mg ig	SD female rats	∅	↑*	Thompson et al. (1988)

Dietary constituent	Feeding schedule	Carcinogen	Dose	Strain			Reference
Corn oil (24.3%)	b + d + a	NMU	50 mg/kg iv	Fischer female rats	↑	⊘	Chan et al. (1983)
Corn oil (25%)	b + d + a	DMBA	5 mg ig	SD female rats	⊘	⊘	Ip and Sinha (1981b)
Corn oil (25%)	b + d + a	DMBA	5 mg ig	SD female rats	⊘	⊘	Ip (1982)
Corn oil (25%)	b + d + a	DMBA	5 mg ig	SD female rats	↑	⊘	Ip and Sinha (1981a)
Corn oil (25%)	b + d + a	DMBA	20 mg ig	SD female rats	↑	⊘	Clinton et al. (1984b)
Corn oil (30%)	a	DMBA	65 mg/kg	F344 female rats	⊘	—	Boissonneault et al. (1986)
Corn oil (40%)	a	DMBA	2 × 10 mg ig	SD female rats	↑	—	Oyaizu et al. (1985)
Corn oil (48%)	b + d + a	DMBA	2 × 20 mg/kg ig	SD female rats	↑	↑	Clinton et al. (1984b)
Corn oil (20%) + linoleic acid (2%)	b a	DMBA	10 mg ig	SD female rats	→	—	Kollmorgen et al. (1981)
Corn oil (20%) and corn oil (0.5%)	b and d	DMBA	5 mg ig at 50 days of age	SD female rats	→	⊘	Ip and Ip (1980)
Corn oil (20%) and corn oil (0.5%)	b[c] and 2 wks a, 4 wks a, 6 wks a, d	DMBA	5 mg ig	SD female rats	→ ⊘ ⊘	⊘ ⊘	Ip and Ip (1980)
Corn oil (20%) and corn oil (0.5%)	b and d	DMBA	15 mg ig ig at 150 days of age	SD female rats	→	⊘	Ip and Ip (1980)
Corn oil (20%) and corn oil (0.5%)	b[c] and 2 wks a, 4 wks a, 6 wks a, d	DMBA	15 mg ig	SD female rats	→ → →	⊘ ⊘ ⊘	Ip and Ip (1980)

[a] For 1 week only.
[b] Only 3 days after.
[c] Because of different effects, feeding schedule is differentiated.

Table 9.4. The Effect of Coconut Oil on Mammary Gland Carcinogenesis

Diet	Feeding schedule	Carcinogen	Dose/duration	Species, strain/sex	Tumor incidence	No. of tumors/ tumor-bearing animal	Reference
Coconut oil (18%)	b + a	DMBA	10 mg ig	SD female rats	∅	—	King and McCay (1983)
Coconut oil (18.4%)	b + a	DMBA	5 mg ig	SD female rats	∅	∅	Kritchevsky et al. (1984)
Coconut oil (18.4%)	a	DMBA	5 mg ig	SD female rats	∅	∅	Kritchevsky et al. (1984)
Coconut oil (18.4%)	b	DMBA	5 mg ig	SD female rats	∅	∅	Kritchevsky et al. (1984)
Coconut oil (20%)	a	DMBA	5 mg ig	SD female rats	∅	∅	Hopkins and Carroll (1979)
Coconut oil (20%)	a	DMBA	5 mg ig	SD female rats	∅	∅	Hopkins et al. (1981)
Coconut oil (20%)	b + d + a	DMBA	10 mg ig	SD female rats	∅	—	McCay et al. (1981)
Coconut oil (23%)	a	NMU	50 mg/kg iv	F344 female rats	$\downarrow \rightarrow$	∅	Cohen et al. (1986)

Dietary fat		Carcinogen	Dose	Animal			Reference
Coconut oil (20%)	b + a	DMBA	10 mg ig	SD female rats	∅ ↓	—	King et al. (1979)
Coconut oil (24%)	b + d + a	DMBA	5 mg ig	SD female rats	∅	—	Ip and Sinha (1981a)
Coconut oil (24%)	b + d + a	DMBA	5 mg ig	SD female rats	∅	∅	Ip and Sinha (1981b)
Coconut oil (24.3 g)	b + d + a	NMU	50 mg/kg iv	Fischer female rats	∅	∅	Chan et al. (1983)
The Effect of Coconut Oil in Combination with Other Dietary Fats on Mammary Gland Carcinogenesis							
Coconut oil (7%) + sunflower seed oil (3%)	a	DMBA	5 mg ig	SD female rats	∅	∅	Braden and Carroll (1986)
Coconut oil (17%) + sunflower seed oil (3%)	a	DMBA	5 mg ig	SD female rats	∅	∅	Braden and Carroll (1986)
Coconut oil (17%) + sunflower seed oil (3%)	a	DMBA	5 mg ig	SD female rats	∅	∅	Hopkins and Carroll (1979)
Coconut oil (17%) + ethyloleate (3%)	a	DMBA	5 mg ig	SD female rats	∅	∅	Hopkins et al. (1981)
Coconut oil (17%) + ethyl linoleate (3%)	a	DMBA	5 mg/rat ig	SD female rats	↑	∅	Hopkins et al. (1981)

Table 9.5. The Effect of Menhaden Oil on Mammary Gland Carcinogenesis

Diet	Feeding schedule	Carcinogen	Dose/duration	Species, strain/sex	Tumor incidence	No. of tumors/ tumor-bearing animal	Reference
Menhaden oil (0.5%)	b + d + a	NMU	3 × 50 mg/kg	BUF female rats	∅	—	Jurkowski and Cave (1985)
Menhaden oil (3%)	a	DMBA	5 mg ig	SD female rats	∅	∅	Braden and Carroll (1986)
Menhaden oil (3%) + coconut oil (17%)	a	DMBA	5 mg ig	SD female rats	∅	∅	Hopkins et al. (1981)
Menhaden oil (10%)	a	DMBA	5 mg ig	SD female rats	→	→	Braden and Carroll (1986)
Menhaden oil (20%)	a	DMBA	5 mg ig	SD female rats	∅	∅	Braden and Carroll (1986)
Menhaden oil (20%)	b + d + a	NMU	3 × 50 mg/kg	BUF female rats	→	—	Jurkowski and Cave (1985)

Table 9.6. *The Effect of Sunflower Seed Oil, Rapeseed Oil, Palm Oil, Olive Oil, and Soybean Oil on Mammary Gland Carcinogenesis*

Diet	Feeding schedule	Carcinogen	Dose/duration	Species, strain/sex	Tumor incidence	No. of tumors/ tumor-bearing animal	Reference
Sunflower seed oil (3%)	a	DMBA	5 mg ig	SD female rats	∅	∅	Braden and Carroll (1986)
Sunflower seed oil (20%)	a	DMBA	5 mg ig	SD female rats	∅	∅	Hopkins *et al.* (1981)
Sunflower seed oil (20%)	a	DMBA	5 mg ig	SD female rats	∅	∅	Hopkins and Carroll (1979)
Sunflower seed oil (20%)	a	DMBA	5 mg ig	SD female rats	∅	∅	Braden and Carroll (1986)
Sunflower seed oil (20%)	a[a]	DMBA	5 mg ig	SD female rats	—	→	Kalamegham and Carroll (1984)
Sunflower seed oil (20%)	a[b]	DMBA	5 mg ig	SD female rats	—	→	Kalamegham and Carroll (1984)
Sunflower seed oil (20%)	a[c]	DMBA	5 mg ig	SD female rats	—	→	Kalamegham and Carroll (1984)
Sunflower seed oil (20%)	a[d]	DMBA	5 mg ig	SD female rats	∅	→	Kalamegham and Carroll (1984)
Sunflower seed oil (23%)	a	NMU	50 mg/kg iv	F344 female rats	∅↓	∅	Cohen *et al.* (1986)
Sunflower seed oil (15 g/1000 kcal)	a	NMU	25 mg/kg iv	SD female rats	∅	∅	Beth *et al.* (1987a)
Rapeseed oil (20%)	b + a	DMBA	2.5 mg ig	SD female rats	∅	—	Lee and Rogers (1983)
Rapeseed oil (5%) + rapeseed oil (20%)	b a	DMBA	2.5 mg ig	SD female rats	∅	—	Lee and Rogers (1983)

(continued)

Table 9.6. (Continued)

Diet	Feeding schedule	Carcinogen	Dose/duration	Species, strain/sex	Tumor incidence	No. of tumors/ tumor-bearing animal	Reference
Palm oil (20%)	b + d	DMBA	7.5 mg/kg po	SD female rats	∅	—	Sylvester et al. (1985)
Palm oil (20%)	b + d + a[e]	DMBA	7.5 mg/kg po	SD female rats	∅	∅	Sylvester et al. (1986b)
Palm oil (15 g/1000 kcal)	a	NMU	25 mg/kg iv	SD female rats	∅	∅	Beth et al. (1987a)
Palm oil (38 g/1000 kcal)	f	—	—	Brown Norway female rats	∅	—	Kort et al. (1985)
Olive oil (23%)	a	NMU	50 mg/kg iv	F344 female rats	∅	∅	Cohen et al. (1986)
Olive oil (23%)	a	NMU	50 mg/kg iv	F344 female rats	∅ →	∅	Cohen et al. (1986)
Olive oil (11.6%) + cocoa butter (8%) + coconut oil (0.4%) (= cis fat 20%)	a	DMBA	5 mg ig	SD female rats	∅	∅	Selenskas et al. (1984)
Soybean oil (10%) + cotton seed oil (10%) (= trans fat 20%)	a	DMBA	5 mg ig	SD female rats	∅	∅	Selenskas et al. (1984)

[a]After 7 week, from week 8 to 43 a fat-free diet was given.
[b]After 7 week, from week 8 to 43 a coconut oil 10% diet was given.
[c]After 7 week, from week 8 to 43 a lard 10% diet was given.
[d]After 7 week, from week 8 to 43 a butter 10% diet was given.
[e]For 1 week only.
[f]The entire experimental period.

Table 9.7. The Effect of Different Fatty Acids on Mammary Gland Carcinogenesis

Diet	Feeding schedule	Carcinogen	Dose/duration	Species, strain/sex	Tumor incidence	No. of tumors/ tumor-bearing animal	Reference
Saturated fatty acids (18.6%)	b + a	DMBA	10 mg ig	Wistar female rats	∅	∅	Hopkins et al. (1976)
Saturated fatty acids (18.6%) + polyunsaturated fatty acids	b / a	DMBA	10 mg ig	Wistar female rats	↑ ↓	—	Hopkins et al. (1976)
Polyunsaturated fatty acids (18.6%)	b + a	DMBA	10 mg ig	Wistar female rats	∅	∅	Hopkins et al. (1976)
Polyunsaturated fatty acids (18.6%) + saturated fatty acids (18.6%)	b / a	DMBA	10 mg ig	Wistar female rats	→	—	Hopkins et al. (1976)
Corn oil (10%) + beef tallow (10%)	b + a	DMBA	17.5 mg/kg po	SD female rats	∅	∅	Clinton et al. (1984a)
Laboratory chow + fat (10%) (Wesson oil)	a	—	—	C3H/HeJ female mice	∅	—	Waxler et al. (1979)
Laboratory chow + fat (10%) (Wesson oil)	a	—	—	C3H/HeJ[b] female mice	∅ ↓	—	Waxler et al. (1979)
Fat (20%) (unsaturated vegetable fat)	b + d + a	DMBA	20 mg ig	SD female rats	∅	∅	Minton et al. (1983)
Fat (35en%) (palm oil 75%, lard 14%, sunflower seed oil 11%)	a	NMU	25 mg/kg iv	SD female rats	∅	∅	Beth et al. (1987a)
Fat (45en%) (palm oil 75%, lard 14%, sunflower seed oil 11%)	a	NMU	25 mg/kg iv	SD female rats	∅	∅	Beth et al. (1987a)

[a]The entire experimental period.
[b]Obese mice.

Table 9.8. *The Effect of Vitamin A on Mammary Gland Carcinogenesis*

Diet	Feeding schedule	Carcinogen	Dose/duration	Species, strain/sex	Tumor incidence	No. of tumors/tumor-bearing animal	Reference
Retinyl acetate (68 ppm)[a]	a	DMBA	20 mg/rat ig	SD female rats	∅	—	Welsch and DeHoog (1983)
Retinyl acetate (82 ppm)[a]	a	DMBA	1 mg/wk 6 weeks	BD2F1 female mice	∅	—	Welsch et al. (1984)
Retinyl acetate (200 ppm)	b	—	—	C3H/HeJ(+) male and female mice	∅	—	Stenbäck et al. (1987)
Retinyl acetate (204 ppm)[c]	a	DMBA	10 mg/rat ig	SD female rats	→	—	Welsch and DeHoog (1983)
Retinyl acetate (250 ppm)[d]	b + d + a	DMBA	20 mg/rat ig	Lewis female rats	∅	→	McCormick et al. (1980)
Retinyl acetate (250 ppm)	a	DMBA	20 mg/rat ig	Lewis female rats	∅	→	McCormick et al. (1980)
Retinyl acetate (250 ppm)[d]	a	NMU	50 mg/kg iv	SD female rats	→↑	—	Moon et al. (1977)
			25 mg/kg iv		→↑	—	
			12.5 mg/kg iv 2 ×/wk		→↑	—	
Retinyl acetate (250 ppm)[d]	b + d + a[e] −2 − +2 wk or a +1 − +20 wk +1 − +90 wk +20 − +90 wk	B(a)P	50 mg/rat ig single dose or 8 wkly fractions	LEW/Mai female rats	→ ↑ ↑ ↑ ∅	→* →* →* ∅* →* ∅	McCormick et al. (1981)
Retinyl acetate (300 ppm)	a	NMU	50 mg/kg iv	SD female rats	→	∅	Thompson et al. (1981a)
Retinyl acetate (323 ppm)	a	NMU	50 mg/kg iv 2 ×/wk	SD female rats	→	→*	Thompson et al. (1979)
Retinyl acetate (323 ppm)	a[f]	NMU	50 mg/kg iv 2 ×/wk	SD female rats	∅	∅*	Thompson et al. (1979)
Retinyl acetate (323 ppm)	a[g]	NMU	50 mg/kg iv 2 ×/wk	SD female rats	↓→	→*	Thompson et al. (1979)

Compound (ppm)	Treatment	Carcinogen	Dose	Animal	Effect	Reference
Retinyl acetate (328 ppm)[h]	a	NMU	50 mg/kg iv 2 ×/wk	SD female rats	→ ↑ →*	Thompson et al. (1980)
Retinyl acetate (328 ppm)[h]	a +4 wk +8 wk	NMU	50 mg/kg iv	SD female rats	→→↑ ↑∅→ — — — —	McCormick and Moon (1982)
Retinyl acetate (328 ppm)[h]	a	NMU	12.5 mg/kg iv 2 ×/wk	SD female rats	↑ —	Welsch et al. (1980)
Retinyl acetate (328 ppm)[h]	a	NMU	15 mg/kg iv 2 ×/wk and 57	SD female rats	↑ →*	Thompson et al. (1980)
Retinyl acetate (328 ppm)[h]	a	NMU	25 mg/kg iv 2 ×/wk	SD female rats	→ —	Welsch et al. (1980)
Retinyl acetate (328 ppm)[h]	a	DMBA	5 mg/rat ig	SD female rats	→ —	Welsch and DeHoog (1983)
Retinyl acetate (328 ppm)[h]	a	DMBA	5 mg ig	SD female rats	∅ →*	Aylsworth et al. (1986)
Retinyl acetate (328 ppm)	a	DMBA	15 mg ig	SD female rats	∅→ ∅↑ — — —	Thompson et al. (1982b)
Retinyl acetate (328 ppm)	a	DMBA	20 mg ig	SD female rats	∅↑ → — — —	Thompson et al. (1982b)
Retinyl acetate (328 ppm)	a	DMBA	20 mg ig	SD female rats		Thompson et al. (1982b)
Retinyl acetate (328 ppm)	a[e] +1 wk +4 wk +8 wk +12 wk +16 wk +20 wk	NMU	25 mg/kg iv	SD female rats	↑↑↑↑↑ →∅∅ —	McCormick and Moon (1982)
Retinyl acetate (328 ppm)	a[i]	NMU	35 mg/kg iv	SD female rats	→ →*	McCormick et al. (1983)
Retinyl acetate (328 ppm)	a[j]	NMU	35 mg/kg iv	SD female rats	→*	McCormick et al. (1983)
Retinyl acetate (656 ppm)[k]	a	NMU	15 mg/kg iv 2 ×/wk	SD female rats	↑ →*	Thompson et al. (1980)
Retinyl acetate (656 ppm)[k]	a	NMU	50 mg/kg iv 2 ×/wk	SD female rats	↑ →*	Thompson et al. (1980)

(continued)

Table 9.8. (Continued)

Diet	Feeding schedule	Carcinogen	Dose/duration	Species, strain/sex	Tumor incidence	No. of tumors/ tumor-bearing animal	Reference
Retinyl acetate (380 μmoles/kg diet)	a	DMBA	5 mg ig	SD female rats	∅	—	Grubbs et al. (1977)
Retinyl acetate (380 μmoles/kg diet)	a	DMBA	15 mg ig	SD female rats	∅	—	Grubbs et al. (1977)
Retinyl acetate (760 μmoles/kg diet)	a	DMBA	5 mg ig	SD female rats	∅	—	Grubbs et al. (1977)
Retinyl acetate (760 μmoles/kg diet)	a	DMBA	15 mg ig	SD female rats	→	—	Grubbs et al. (1977)
Retinyl methylether (380 μmoles/kg diet)	a	DMBA	5 mg ig	SD female rats	→	—	Grubbs et al. (1977)
Retinyl methylether (380 μmoles/kg diet)	a	DMBA	15 mg ig	SD female rats	∅ →	—	Grubbs et al. (1977)
Retinyl methylether (760 μmoles/kg diet)	a	DMBA	5 mg ig	SD female rats	→	—	Grubbs et al. (1977)
Retinyl methylether (760 μmoles/kg diet)	a	DMBA	15 mg ig	SD female rats	→	—	Grubbs et al. (1977)
Retinyl acetate (328 ppm)[h] + corn oil (20%)	a	DMBA	5 mg ig	SD female rats	∅	—	Aylsworth et al. (1986)

[a] = 0.2 mM.
[b] The entire experimental period.
[c] = 0.6 mM.
[d] = 3 mg/rat per day.
[e] Because of potentially different effects feeding schedule is differentiated.
[f] Only to tumor-bearing rats.
[g] Only to non-tumor-bearing rats.
[h] = 1 mM.
[i] After removal of animals first mammary tumor.
[j] After ovariectomy.
[k] = 2 mM.

Table 9.9. The Effect of Synthetic Retinoids on Mammary Gland Carcinogenesis

Diet	Feeding schedule	Carcinogen	Dose/duration	Species, strain/sex	Tumor incidence	No. of tumors/ tumor-bearing animal	Reference
Axerophthene (270 ppm)[a]	a	NMU	15 mg/kg iv 2×/wk	SD female rats	∅	→*	Thompson *et al.* (1980)
Axerophthene (270 ppm)[a]	a	NMU	50 mg/kg iv 2×/wk	SD female rats	∅	∅	Thompson *et al.* (1980)
Axerophthene (540 ppm)[b]	a	NMU	15 mg/kg iv 2×/wk	SD female rats	∅	→*	Thompson *et al.* (1980)
Axerophthene (540 ppm)[b]	a	NMU	50 mg/kg iv 2×/wk	SD female rats	∅→	∅	Thompson *et al.* (1980)
4-HPR (1.0 mM)	a	DMBA	1 mg/wk ig 6 weeks	BD2F1 female mice	∅	—	Welsch *et al.* (1984)
4-HPR (587 ppm)[c,d]	a	NMU	20 mg/kg iv	SD female rats	∅→	→	McCormick *et al.* (1982b)
4-HPR (782 ppm)[b]	a	DMBA	20 mg ig	SD female rats	→	∅	McCormick *et al.* (1982b)
4-HPR (782 ppm)[b]	a	DMBA	20 mg ig	SD female rats[e]	→	→*	McCormick *et al.* (1982b)
4-HPR (782 ppm)[b]	a	NMU	50 mg/kg iv	SD female rats	→↑	→*	McCormick *et al.* (1982b)
4-HPR (782 ppm)[b]	a	NMU	50 mg/kg iv	SD female rats[b]	→	→*	McCormick *et al.* (1982b)

[a] = 1 mM.
[b] = 2 mM.
[c] = 1.5 mM.
[d] Decreased to 391 ppm from day 20 after NMU administration because of toxic side effects.
[e] Ovariectomized rats.

Table 9.10. The Effect of Selenium on Mammary Gland Carcinogenesis

Diet	Feeding schedule	Carcinogen	Dose/duration	Species, strain/sex	Tumor incidence	No. of tumors/tumor-bearing animal	Reference
Sodium selenite deficiency	b + d + a	DMBA	5 mg/ig	SD female rats	∅	∅	Ip and Sinha (1981b)
Sodium selenite (0.1 ppm)	a	—	—	C3H/St. female mice	∅	—	Schrauzer et al. (1978)
Sodium selenite (0.15 ppm)	b + d + a	DMBA	7.5 mg po	SD female rats	∅	∅	Thompson et al. (1982a)
Sodium selenite (0.15 ppm)	b + d + a	DMBA	15 mg po	SD female rats	∅	∅	Thompson et al. (1982a)
Sodium selenite (0.15 ppm)	a	—	—	C3H/St. female rats	↑	—	Schrauzer et al. (1978)
Sodium selenite (0.5 ppm)	a	—	—	C3H female mice	→	—	Whanger et al. (1982)
Sodium selenite (0.7 ppm)	a	—	—	C3H/St. female mice	↑	—	Schrauzer et al. (1978)
Sodium selenite (1 ppm)	a	—	—	C3H/St. female mice	∅	∅	Thompson et al. (1982a)
Sodium selenite (1.05 ppm)	b + d + a	DMBA	7.5 mg po	SD female rats	∅	∅	Thompson et al. (1982a)
Sodium selenite (1.05 ppm)	b + d + a	DMBA	15 mg po	SD female rats	∅	∅	Thompson et al. (1982a)
Sodium selenite (2.06 ppm)	b + d + a	DMBA	7.5 mg po	SD female rats	∅	∅	Thompson et al. (1982a)
Sodium selenite (2.06 ppm)	b + d + a	DMBA	15 mg po	SD female rats	∅→	→	Thompson et al. (1982a)
Sodium selenite (2.2 ppm)	a	—	—	C3H female mice	→	—	Whanger et al. (1982)
Sodium selenite (2.5 ppm)	b + d + a	DMBA	5 mg ig	SD female rats	∅	∅	Ip and Sinha (1981a)
Sodium selenite (4 ppm)	a	MNU	50 mg/kg iv	SD female rats	∅	∅	Thompson et al. (1981a)
Sodium selenite (4 ppm)	a	MNU	20 mg/kg ip 10 × in 4 wks	WE male and female rats	∅	—	Warzok et al. (1981)

a The entire experimental period.

Table 9.11. The Effect of Oils in Combination with Selenium on Mammary Gland Carcinogenesis

Diet	Feeding schedule	Carcinogen	Dose/duration	Species, strain/sex	Tumor incidence	No. of tumors/tumor-bearing animal	Reference
Corn oil (1%) + sodium selenite deficiency	b + d + a	DMBA	5 mg ig	SD female rats	⊘	⊘	Ip and Sinha (1981b)
Corn oil (1%) + sodium selenite deficiency	b + d + a	DMBA	10 mg ig	SD female rats	⊘	⊘	Ip and Sinha (1981b)
Corn oil (1%) + sodium selenite deficiency	b + d + a	DMBA	15 mg ig	SD female rats	←	⊘	Ip and Sinha (1981b)
Corn oil (25%) + sodium selenite deficiency	b + d + a	DMBA	5 mg ig	SD female rats	⊘	→	Ip (1982)
Corn oil (25%) + sodium selenite deficiency	b + d + a	DMBA	5 mg ig	SD female rats	←	⊘	Ip and Sinha (1981b)
Corn oil (5%) + sodium selenite (2 ppm)	a	DMBA	7.5 mg ig	SD female rats	⊘	—	Ip (1986)
Corn oil (5%) + sodium selenite (3 ppm)	a	DMBA	7.5 mg ig	SD female rats	→	—	Ip (1986)
Corn oil (5%) + sodium selenite (4 ppm)	a	DMBA	7.5 mg ig	SD female rats	→	—	Ip (1986)
Corn oil (10%) + sodium selenite (2.5 ppm)	a	—	—	C3H female mice	⊘	—	Whanger et al. (1982)
Corn oil (20%) + sodium selenite (2.5 ppm)	b + d + a	DMBA	5 mg ig	SD female rats	→	⊘	Ip (1985)
Corn oil (20%) + sodium selenite (4 ppm)	a	NMU	50 mg/kg sc	SD female rats	⊘	⊘	Thompson et al. (1984)

(continued)

Table 9.11. (Continued)

Diet	Feeding schedule	Carcinogen	Dose/duration	Species, strain/sex	Tumor incidence	No. of tumors/ tumor-bearing animal	Reference
Corn oil (20%) + sodium selenite (5 ppm)	a	NMU	50 mg/kg sc	SD female rats	⊘ →	→	Thompson et al. (1984)
Corn oil (20%) + sodium selenite (6 ppm)	a	NMU	50 mg/kg sc	SD female rats	⊘ →	⊘	Thompson et al. (1984)
Corn oil (20%) + sodium selenite (3.4 ppm dw)	a	DMBA	5 mg ig	SD female rats	→	→	Thompson et al. (1984)
Corn oil (25%) + sodium selenite (2.5 ppm)	b + d + a	DMBA	5 mg ig	SD female rats	→	⊘	Ip and Sinha (1981a)
Corn oil (25%) + sodium selenite (5 ppm)	b + d + a[b] -2 − +24 -2 − +2 -2 − +12 or a +2 − +24 +2 − +12 +12 − +24	DMBA	10 mg ig	SD female rats	→↑ →↑ →↑ ⊘↑ ⊘	→⊘ ⊘ ⊘⊘⊘ ⊘	Ip (1981)
Corn oil (5%) + selenoDL-methionine (2 ppm)	a	DMBA	7.5 mg ig	SD female rats	⊘	—	Ip (1986)
Corn oil (5%) + selenoDL-methionine (3 ppm)	a	DMBA	7.5 mg ig	SD female rats	→	—	Ip (1986)

Corn oil (5%) + seleno-DL-methionine (4 ppm)	a	DMBA	7.5 mg ig	SD female rats	→	—	Ip (1986)
Corn oil (20%) + seleno-DL-methionine (3.4 ppm)	a	DMBA	5 mg ig	SD female rats	∅	→	Thompson et al. (1984)
Corn oil (20%) + seleno-DL-methionine (5 ppm)	a	NMU	50 mg/kg sc	SD female rats	∅	∅	Thompson et al. (1984)
Corn oil (20%) + seleno-DL-methionine (6 ppm)	a	NMU	50 mg/kg sc	SD female rats	∅→	∅	Thompson et al. (1984)
Coconut oil (24%) + sodium selenite deficiency	b + d + a	DMBA	5 mg ig	SD female rats	∅	∅	Ip and Sinha (1981b)
Coconut oil (24%) + sodium selenite (2.5 ppm)	b + d + a	DMBA	5 mg ig	SD female rats	∅	—	Ip and Sinha (1981a)
Coconut oil (24%) + sodium selenite (2.5 ppm)	b + d + a	DMBA	10 mg ig	SD female rats	→	—	Ip and Sinha (1981a)
Rapseed oil (10%) + sodium selenite (2 ppm)	[a]	—	—	C3H female mice	∅	—	Whanger et al. (1982)
Lard (10%) + sodium selenite (2 ppm)	[a]	—	—	C3H female mice	∅	—	Whanger et al. (1982)
Butter (10%) + sodium selenite (2 ppm)	[a]	—	—	C3H female mice	∅	—	Whanger et al. (1982)

[a] The entire experimental period.
[b] Because of different effects, feeding schedule is differentiated.

Table 9.12. Different Combination Effects on Mammary Gland Carcinogenesis

Diet	Feeding schedule	Carcinogen	Dose/duration	Species, strain/sex	Tumor incidence	No. of tumors/tumor-bearing animal	Reference
Corn oil (25%) + DL-α-tocopheryl-acetate deficiency (7.5 ppm)	b + d + a	DMBA	5 mg ig	SD female rats	↑	∅	Ip (1982)
Corn oil (20%) + vitamin E deficiency	b + d + a	DMBA	5 mg ig	SD female rats	∅	—	Ip (1985)
Corn oil (20%) + sodium selenite (2.5 ppm) + vitamin E deficiency	b + d + a	DMBA	5 mg ig	SD female rats	∅	—	Ip (1985)
Corn oil (25%) + DL-α-tocopheryl-acetate (1000 ppm) sodium selenite deficiency	b + d + a	DMBA	5 mg ig	SD female rats	∅	∅	Ip (1982)
Corn oil (20%) + α-tocopherol (0.2%)	b + d + a	DMBA	10 mg ig	SD female rats	∅	—	McCay et al. (1981)
Corn oil (20%) + α-tocopherol (0.2%)	b + a	DMBA	10 mg ig	SD female rats	∅	—	King and McCay (1983)
Corn oil (25%) + DL-α-tocopheryl-acetate (1000 mg/kg) (excess)	b + d + a	DMBA	5 mg ig	SD female rats	∅	∅	Ip (1982)
Retinyl acetate (300 ppm) + sodium selenite (4 ppm)	a	NMU	50 mg/kg iv	SD female rats	→	∅	Thompson et al. (1981a)
Safflower oil[a] (20%) + α-tocopherol (387 μg/g)	a	DMBA	5 mg ig	SD female rats	∅	∅	Dayton et al. (1987)
Safflower oil[b] (20%) + α-tocopherol (330 μg/g)	a	DMBA	5 mg ig	SD female rats	↑	←	Dayton et al. (1987)
Coconut oil (18%) + α-tocopherol (0.2%)	b + d + a	DMBA	10 mg ig	SD female rats	∅	—	McCay et al. (1981)
Coconut oil (18%) + α-tocopherol (0.2%)	b + a	DMBA	10 mg ig	SD female rats	∅	—	King and McCay (1983)
Coconut oil (20%) + α-tocopherol (34 μg/g)	a	DMBA	5 mg ig	SD female rats	∅	∅	Dayton et al. (1987)

Treatment	Modifier	Carcinogen	Dose	Strain			Reference
Corn oil (5%) + sodium selenite (3 ppm) + vitamin C (0.5%)	a	DMBA	7.5 mg ig	SD female rats	∅	—	Ip (1986)
Corn oil (5%) + seleno DL-methionine (3 ppm) + vitamin C (0.5%)	a	DMBA	7.5 mg ig	SD female rats	→	—	Ip (1986)
Corn oil (5%) + vitamin C (0.2%)	a	DMBA	7.5 mg ig	SD female rats	∅	—	Ip (1986)
Corn oil (5%) + vitamin C (0.5%)	a	DMBA	7.5 mg ig	SD female rats	∅	—	Ip (1986)
Corn oil (5%) + vitamin C (1%)	a	DMBA	7.5 mg ig	SD female rats	∅	—	Ip (1986)
Linoleic acid (2%) + α-tocopherol (0.2%)	b + d + a	DMBA	10 mg ig	SD female rats	∅	—	McCay et al. (1981)
Linoleic acid (2%) + α-tocopherol (0.2%)	b + a	DMBA	10 mg ig	SD female rats	∅	—	King and McCay (1983)
DL-α-tocopherol-acetate deficiency (7.5 ppm)	b + d + a	DMBA	5 mg ig	SD female rats	←	∅	Ip (1982)
Vitamin A–palmitate (100000 IU/1000 kcal) + α-tocopherol (3300 IU/1000 kcal) + 12% fat[c]	a	NMU	25 mg/kg iv	SD female rats	↑ / →	—	Aksoy et al. (1985)
Vitamin A–palmitate (50000 IU/1000 kcal) + α-tocopherol (225 IU/1000 kcal) + 25% fat[c]	a	NMU	25 mg/kg iv	SD female rats	∅	∅	Beth et al. (1987b)
Vitamin A–palmitate (100000 IU/1000 kcal) + α-tocopherol (3300 IU/1000 kcal) + 45% fat[c]	a	NMU	25 mg/kg iv	SD female rats	∅	—	Aksoy et al. (1985)
Vitamin A–palmitate (50000 IU/1000 kcal) + α-tocopherol (225 IU/1000 kcal) + 45% fat[c]	a	NMU	25 mg/kg iv	SD female rats	∅	∅	Beth et al. (1987b)

[a] Conventional with high linoleic acid.
[b] Mutant with high linolic acid.
[c] Energy %.

Table 9.13. The Effect of Protein and Different Combinations on Mammary Gland Carcinogenesis

Diet	Feeding schedule	Carcinogen	Dose/duration	Species, strain/sex	Tumor incidence	No. of tumors/ tumor-bearing animal	Reference
Protein (16%)	b + d + a	DMBA	20 mg/kg ig	SD female rats	∅	∅	Clinton et al. (1984a)
Protein (32%)	b + d + a	DMBA	20 mg/kg ig	SD female rats	∅	∅	Clinton et al. (1984a)
Protein (33%)	b + d + a	NMU	2 × 50 mg/kg iv	SD female rats	∅ →	↑	Hawrylewicz et al. (1986)
Protein (16 en%) + corn oil (24en%)	b + d + a	DMBA	20 mg/kg ig	SD female rats	∅	∅	Clinton et al. (1984a)
Protein (16 en%) + corn oil (48en%)	b + d + a	DMBA	20 mg/kg ig	SD female rats	∅ ↓	∅	Clinton et al. (1984a)
Protein (32en%) + corn oil (24 en%)	b + d + a	DMBA	20 mg/kg ig	SD female rats	∅	∅	Clinton et al. (1984a)
Protein (32%) + corn oil (48 en%)	b + d + a	DMBA	20 mg/kg ig	SD female rats	∅ ↓	∅	Clinton et al. (1984a)
Casein (14%) + L-arginine (5%)	b + d + a	DMBA	7.5 mg ig	SD female rats	∅	∅	Burns and Milner (1984)
Casein (14%) + L-arginine (5%)	b + d + a	NMU	40 mg/kg iv	SD female rats	∅	∅	Burns and Milner (1984)
Casein (3%) + beef tallow (30%)	b + d + a	DMBA	10 mg ig	SD female rats	∅	—	Rogers and Wetsel (1981)
Casein (3%) + beef tallow (30%)	b + d + a	DMBA	20 mg ig	SD female rats	∅	—	Rogers and Wetsel (1981)
Casein (3%) + beef tallow (30%)	b + d + a	AAF	0.02%/2 weeks	SD female rats	∅	—	Rogers and Wetsel (1981)
Casein (3%) + beef tallow (30%)	b + d + a	AAF	0.0125%/11 weeks	SD female rats	∅	—	Rogers and Wetsel (1981)
Casein (22%) + beef tallow (30%)	b + d + a	DMBA	10 mg ig	SD female rats	∅	—	Rogers and Wetsel (1981)
Casein (22%) + beef tallow (30%)	b + d + a	DMBA	20 mg ig	SD female rats	∅	—	Rogers and Wetsel (1981)

Diet	Treatment	Carcinogen	Dose	Strain	Effect		Reference
Casein (22%) + beef tallow (30%)	b + d + a	AAF	0.02%/2 weeks	SD female rats	∅ →	—	Rogers and Wetsel (1981)
Casein (22%) + beef tallow (30%)	b + d + a	AAF	0.0125%/11 weeks	SD female rats	∅ →	—	Rogers and Wetsel (1981)
Casein (16 en%) + corn oil (24 en%)	b + a	DMBA	20 mg/kg ig	SD female rats	∅	∅	Clinton et al. (1986)
Casein (8 en%) + corn oil (24 en%) and casein (16 en%) + corn oil (24 en%)	b and a	DMBA	20 mg/kg ig	SD female rats	∅	∅	Clinton et al. (1986)
Casein (8 en%) + corn oil (48 4n%) and casein (16 en%) + corn oil (24 en%)	b and a	DMBA	20 mg/kg ig	SD female rats	∅ ↓	∅	Clinton et al. (1986)
Casein (16 en%) + corn oil (12 4n%) and casein (16 en%) + corn oil (24 en%)	b and a	DMBA	20 mg/kg ig	SD female rats	∅	∅	Clinton et al. (1986)
Casein (16 en%) + corn oil (48 4n%) and casein (16 en%) + corn oil (24 en%)	b and a	DMBA	20 mg/kg ig	SD female rats	∅ ↓	∅	Clinton et al. (1986)
Casein (32 en%) + corn oil (12 4n%) and casein (16 en%) + corn oil (24 en%)	b and a	DMBA	20 mg/kg ig	SD female rats	∅	∅	Clinton et al. (1986)
Casein (32 en%) + corn oil (24 en%) and casein (16 en%) + corn oil (24 en%)	b and a	DMBA	20 mg/kg ig	SD female rats	∅	∅	Clinton et al. (1986)
Casein (32 en%) + corn oil (48 4n%) and casein (16 en%) + corn oil (24 en%)	b and a	DMBA	20 mg/kg ig	SD female rats	↑ ↓	∅	Clinton et al. (1986)

Table 9.14. The Effect of Dextrose in Combination with Corn Oil on Mammary Gland Carcinogenesis

Diet	Feeding schedule	Carcinogen	Dose/duration	Species, strain/sex	Tumor incidence	No. of tumors/ tumor-bearing animal	Reference
Dextrose (19.6 g)[a] + corn oil (25 g)[a]	b + d + a	NMU	50 mg/kg iv	Fischer, Long Evans, and SD female rats	∅	∅	Chan and Dao (1981)
Dextrose (19.6 g)[a] + corn oil (25 g)[a]	b or a	NMU	50 mg/kg iv at day 90	Fisher female rats	∅	∅	Dao and Chan (1983)
Dextrose 64.5 (g)[a] + corn oil 5 (g)[a]	b + d + a	NMU	50 mg/kg iv or 40 mg/kg 30 mg/kg 20 mg/kg 10 mg/kg	Fischer female rats	→→→→∅ ∅	→→→→∅ ∅	Dao and Chan (1983)
Dextrose (64.5 g)[a] + corn oil (5 g)[a]	b + d + a	NMU	50 mg/kg iv	Fischer, Long Evans, and SD female rats	∅	∅	Dao and Chan (1983)
Dextrose (64.5 g)[a] + corn oil (5 g)[a]	b + d + a	NMU	50 mg/kg iv at day 35, 50, 90 or 130 of age	Fischer female rats	→	∅	Chan and Dao (1983)
Dextrose (64.5 g)[a] + corn oil (5 g)[a]	b + d + a	NMU	50 mg/kg iv at day 50, 90, 133	Fischer female rats	→	—	Dao and Chan (1983)
Dextrose (73 g) + corn oil free	a	DMBA	5 mg ig	SD female rats	∅	→	Davidson and Carroll (1982)

[a]g/100 g of diet.

Table 9.15. *The Effect of Calories on Mammary Gland Carcinogenesis*

Diet	Feeding schedule	Carcinogen	Dose/duration	Species, strain/sex	Tumor incidence	No. of tumors/tumor-bearing animal	Reference
The Effect of Caloric Restriction on Mammary Gland Carcinogenesis							
Caloric restriction by 20%	a	—	—	SPF Wistar female rats	→	—	Tucker (1979)
Caloric restriction by 25% + corn oil (20%)	b + d + a	DMBA	5 mg ig	SD female rats	→	→	Kritchevsky et al. (1986)
Caloric restriction by 25% (39 kcal/rat/day) + corn oil (26.6%)	b + d + a	DMBA	5 mg ig	SD female rats	→	→	Kritchevsky et al. (1986)
Caloric restriction by 30% (35 kcal/rat/day)	a	NMU	25 mg/kg iv	SD female rats	↓ →	→	Beth et al. (1987a)
Caloric restriction by 38%	a	—	—	C3H female mice	→	—	Sarkar et al. (1982)
Caloric restriction by 38%	a	—	—	C3H/Umc female mice	→	—	Fernandes et al. (1976)
Caloric restriction by 40% (39 kcal/rat/day) + corn oil (13.1%)	b + d + a	DMBA	5 mg ig	SD female rats	→	→	Kritchevsky et al. (1986)
Caloric restriction by 40% + corn oil (13.1%)	a	DMBA	5 mg ig	SD female rats	→	→	Klurfeld et al. (1987)
Caloric restriction by 50%	b + a	DMBA	5 mg iv	SD female rats	→	→	Sylvester et al. (1982)

(continued)

Table 9.15. (Continued)

Diet	Feeding schedule	Carcinogen	Dose/duration	Species, strain/sex	Tumor incidence	No. of tumors/ tumor-bearing animal	Reference
Caloric restriction by 50%	a[b]	DMBA	5 mg ig	SD female rats	↓	—	Leung et al. (1983)
Caloric restriction by 50%	a	DMBA	5 mg/rat ig	SD female rats	↓	→	Kritchevsky et al. (1984)
Caloric restriction by 50%	a	DMBA	5 mg iv	SD female rats	∅	∅	Sylvester et al. (1982)
Caloric restriction (34 kcal/day/rat) + corn oil (30%)	a	DMBA	65 mg ig	F344 female rats	↓	—	Boissonneault et al. (1986)
Caloric restriction	b + d + a	DMBA	5 mg iv	SD female rats	↓ →	—	Sylvester et al. (1981)
Caloric restriction	b + a	DMBA	20 mg/kg ig	SD female rats	→	—	Clinton et al. (1986)
The Effect of a High Caloric Intake on Mammary Gland Carcinogenesis							
High calories (57.1 kcal/day/rat)	a	DMBA	5 mg ig	SD female rats	↑ ↓	↑*	Thompson et al. (1988)
High calories	b + d + a	DMBA	20 mg ig	SD female rats	↑	∅	Clinton et al. (1984b)
High calories + low fat (5%)	b + a	DMBA	5 mg ig	SD female rats	∅	∅	Kritchevsky et al. (1984)
High calories + high fat (20%)	a	NMU	25 mg/kg iv	SD female rats	↑ ↓	—	Thompson et al. (1985)

[a] The entire experimental period.
[b] When tumor of > 1 cm was manifest.

Table 9.16. The Effect of Seaweeds and Brussel Sprouts on Mammary Gland Carcinogenesis

Diet	Feeding schedule	Carcinogen	Dose/duration	Species, strain/sex	Tumor incidence	No. of tumors/ tumor-bearing animal	Reference
Seaweeds (2%): *Laminaria angustata, angustata* var. *longissima, japonica* var. *ochotensis, religiosa, pinnatifida, porphyra tenera*	b + d + a	DMBA	20 mg/kg ig	SD female rats	∅ ∅ ∅→↑ ∅→↑	— — — — — —	Yamamoto *et al.* (1987)
Brussel sprouts (20%)	d	DMBA	60 mg/kg po	SD female rats	→	—	Stoewsand *et al.* (1988)

Table 9.17. The Effect of Coffee on Mammary Gland Carcinogenesis

Diet	Feeding schedule	Carcinogen	Dose/duration	Species, strain/sex	Tumor incidence	No. of tumors/ tumor-bearing animal	Reference
Coffee (moderate strength)	a	DMBA	5 mg/rat ig	SD female rats	∅	∅*	Welsch et al. (1988b)
Coffee (moderate strength)	a	DMBA	5 mg/rat ig	SD female rats	∅	∅*	Welsch and DeHoog (1988)
Coffee (moderate strength)	b + d + a	DMBA	20 mg/kg iv	SD female rats	∅	→*	Welsch et al. (1988b)
Coffee (full strength)	a	DMBA	5 mg/rat ig	SD female rats	∅	∅*	Welsch et al. (1988b)
Coffee (full strength)	b + d + aᵃ	DMBA	20 mg/kg iv	SD female rats	∅	→*	Welsch et al. (1988b)
Coffee (decaffeinated, moderate strength)	a	DMBA	5 mg/rat ig	SD female rats	∅	∅*	Welsch et al. (1988b)
Coffee (decaffeinated, moderate strength)	a	DMBA	5 mg/rat ig	SD female rats	∅	∅*	Welsch and DeHoog (1988)
Coffee (caffeinated, moderate strength)	b + d + aᵃ	DMBA	20 mg/kg iv	SD female rats	∅	∅*	Welsch and DeHoog (1988)
Coffee (decaffeinated, moderate strength) + caffeine (430 mg/liter dw)	b + d + aᵃ	DMBA	20 mg/kg iv	SD female rats	∅	→*	Welsch and DeHoog (1988)
Coffee (decaffeinated, full strength + caffeine (860 mg/liter dw)	b + d + aᵃ	DMBA	20 mg/kg iv	SD female rats	∅	→*	Welsch et al. (1988b)
Coffee (caffeinated, moderate strength)	a	DMBA	5 mg/rat ig	SD female rats	∅	∅*	Welsch and DeHoog (1988)
Coffee (decaffeinated, moderate strength) + caffeine (430 mg/liter dw)	a	DMBA	5 mg/rat ig	SD female rats	∅	∅*	Welsch and DeHoog (1988)

Coffee (decaffeinated, full strength)	a	DMBA	5 mg/rat ig	SD female rats	∅	∅*	Welsch et al. (1988b)
Coffee (decaffeinated, moderate strength)	b + d + a[a]	DMBA	20 mg/kg iv	SD female rats	∅	∅*	Welsch and Dehoog (1988)
Coffee (decaffeinated, moderate strength)	b + d + a[a]	DMBA	20 mg/kg iv	SD female rats	∅	∅*	Welsch et al. (1988b)
Coffee (decaffeinated, full strength)	b + d + a[a]	DMBA	20 mg/kg iv	SD female rats	∅	∅*	Welsch et al. (1988b)
Caffeine (100 mg/liter dw)	a	DMBA	5 mg/rat ig	SD female rats	∅	∅*	Welsch et al. (1988b)
Caffeine (200 mg/liter dw)	a	DMBA	5 mg/rat ig	SD female rats	∅	∅*	Welsch et al. (1988b)
Caffeine (400 mg/liter dw)	a	DMBA	5 mg/rat ig	SD female rats	∅	∅*	Welsch et al. (1988b)
Caffeine (430 mg/liter dw)	a	DMBA	5 mg/rat ig	SD female rats	∅	∅*	Welsch et al. (1988b)
Caffeine (430 mg/liter dw)	a	DMBA	5 mg/rat ig	SD female rats	∅	∅*	Welsch and DeHoog (1988)
Caffeine (600 mg/liter dw)	a	DMBA	5 mg/rat ig	SD female rats	∅	↓*	Welsch et al. (1988b)
Caffeine (700 mg/liter dw)	a	DMBA	5 mg/rat ig	SD female rats	∅	∅*	Welsch et al. (1988b)
Caffeine (800 mg/liter dw)	a	DMBA	5 mg/rat ig	SD female rats	∅	∅*	Welsch et al. (1988b)
Caffeine*	b + d + a	DMBA	20 mg ig	SD female rats	∅→↑	↑	Minton et al. (1983)
Caffeine (100 mg/liter dw)	b + d + a	DMBA	20 mg/kg iv	SD female rats	∅	↓*	Welsch et al. (1988b)
Caffeine (200 mg/liter dw)	b + d + a[a]	DMBA	20 mg/kg iv	SD female rats	∅	↑*	Welsch et al. (1988b)
Caffeine (300 mg/liter dw)	b + d + a[a]	DMBA	20 mg/kg iv	SD female rats	∅	↓*	Welsch et al. (1988b)
Caffeine (430 mg/liter dw)	b + d + a	DMBA	20 mg/kg iv	SD female rats	∅	∅	Welsch and DeHoog (1988)

(continued)

Table 9.17. (*Continued*)

Diet	Feeding schedule	Carcinogen	Dose/duration	Species, strain/sex	Tumor incidence	No. of tumors/ tumor-bearing animal	Reference
Caffeine (430 mg/liter dw)	b + d + a[a]	DMBA	20 mg/kg iv	SD female rats	Ø	→*	Welsch and DeHoog (1988)
Caffeine (860 mg/liter dw)	b + d + a[a]	DMBA	20 mg/kg iv	SD female rats	Ø	→*	Welsch et al. (1988b)
Caffeine (430 mg/liter dw) + corn oil (5%)	a	DMBA	5 mg/rat ig	SD female rats	Ø	Ø*	Welsch and DeHoog (1988)
Caffeine (430 mg/liter dw) + corn oil (20%)	a	DMBA	5 mg/rat ig	SD female rats	Ø	Ø*	Welsch and DeHoog (1988)
Caffeine (430 mg/liter dw) + corn oil (5%)	b + d + a[a]	DMBA	20 mg/kg iv	SD female rats	Ø	→*	Welsch and DeHoog (1988)
Caffeine (430 mg/liter dw) + corn oil (20%)	b + d + a	DMBA	20 mg/kg iv	SD female rats	Ø	→*	Welsch and DeHoog (1988)
Caffeine[b] + fat (20%)[c] (vegetable fat unsaturated)	b + d + a	DMBA	20 mg/rat ig	SD female rats	←↓	←	Minton et al. (1983)
Caffeine (250 mg/liter dw)	d	—	—	C3H female mice	Ø	←*	Welsch et al. (1988a)
Caffeine (500 mg/liter dw)	d	—	—	C3H female mice	Ø	←*	Welsch et al. (1988a)
Caffeine (250 mg/liter dw)	a	DMBA	1 mg/wk ig for 6 wks	BD2F1 female mice	Ø	←*	Welsch et al. (1988a)
Caffeine (500 mg/liter dw)	a	DMBA	1 mg/wk ig for 6 wks	BD2F1 female mice	Ø	←*	Welsch et al. (1988a)

[a]Only 3 days after.
[b]The amount of caffeine that each rat received per day was equivalent to 500 mg of caffeine in a 50-ig woman.
[c]Vegetable fat, unsaturated.
[d]From week 8 until the end of the experiment.

Table 10.1. The Effect of Oils on Pancreas Carcinogenesis

Diet	Feeding schedule	Carcinogen	Dose/duration	Species, strain/sex	Tumor incidence	No. of tumors/ tumor-bearing animal	Reference
Corn oil (2%)	d + a	Azaserine	6 × 10 mg/kg/wk ip then 10 × 10 mg/kg/4 wks ip	Wistar/Lewis male rats	∅	∅	Roebuck *et al.* (1981b)
Corn oil (20%)	b	Azaserine	6 × 10 mg/kg/wk ip	Wistar/Lewis male rats	∅	∅	Roebuck *et al.* (1981a)
Corn oil (20%)	d + a	Azaserine	6 × 10 mg/kg/wk ip then 10 × 10 mg/kg/4 wks ip	Wistar/Lewis male rats	↑	↑	Roebuck *et al.* (1981b)
Corn oil (20%)	a	Azaserine	6 × 10 mg/kg/wk ip	Wistar/Lewis male rats	↑	↑	Roebuck *et al.* (1981a)
Corn oil (20%)	a	Azaserine	30 mg/kg ip	Wistar male rats	∅	—	Roebuck *et al.* (1987)
Corn oil (23%)	a	BOP	4 × 5 mg/kg/wk sc	Syrian golden male and female hamsters	↑	∅	Birt *et al.* (1988)
Corn oil (21 en%)	b	BOP	10 mg/kg sc	Syrian golden male and female hamsters	∅	∅	Birt *et al.* (1981b)
Corn oil (21 en%, with 25 kcal/day/rat)	a	BOP	10 mg/kg sc	Syrian golden male and female hamsters	∅	∅	Birt *et al.* (1981b)
Corn oil (41 en%)	b	BOP	10 mg/kg sc	Syrian golden male and female hamsters	∅	∅	Birt *et al.* (1981b)

(continued)

Table 10.1. (Continued)

Diet	Feeding schedule	Carcinogen	Dose/duration	Species, strain/sex	Tumor incidence	No. of tumors/ tumor-bearing animal	Reference
Corn oil (42 en%)	b	BOP	10 mg/kg sc	Syrian golden male and female hamsters	∅	∅	Birt et al. (1983a)
Corn oil (41 en%), with 32 kcal/day/rat)	a	BOP	10 mg/kg sc	Syrian golden male and female hamsters	∅	↑	Birt et al. (1981b)
Corn oil (42 en%)	a	BOP	10 mg/kg sc	Syrian golden male and female hamsters	∅	∅	Birt et al. (1983a)
Linoleic acid (C18:2) (17.7 en% from corn oil and sunflower oil)	a	—	—	Brown Norway female rats	∅	∅	Kort et al. (1985)
Safflower oil (20%)	a	Azaserine	6 × 10 mg/kg/wk ip	Wistar/Lewis male rats	↑	∅	Roebuck et al. (1981b)
Coconut oil (18%)	b	Azaserine	6 × 10 mg/kg/wk ip	Wistar/Lewis male rats	∅	∅	Roebuck et al. (1981b)
Coconut oil (18%)	d + a	Azaserine	6 × 10 mg/kg/wk ip then 10 × 10 mg/kg/4 wks ip	Wistar/Lewis male rats	∅	∅	Roebuck et al. (1981b)
Coconut oil (18%)	a	Azaserine	6 × 10 mg/kg/wk ip	Wistar/Lewis male rats	∅	∅	Roebuck et al. (1981b)

[a] The entire experimental period.

Table 10.2. *The Effect of Vitamin A and Synthetic Retinoids on Pancreas Carcinogenesis*

Diet	Feeding schedule	Carcinogen	Dose/duration	Species, strain/sex	Tumor incidence	No. of tumors/ tumor-bearing animal	Reference
Retinyl acetate (250 ppm)	a	Azaserin	8 × 10 mg/kg ip 5-day intervals	W/LEW male rats	∅	—	Longnecker et al. (1981)
13-*Cis*-retinoic acid (0.1 mM/kg)	a	BOP	40 mg/kg sc	Syrian golden male and female hamsters	∅	∅	Birt et al. (1981a)
13-*Cis*-retinoic acid (0.05 mM/kg)	a	BOP	40 mg/kg sc	Syrian golden male and female hamsters	∅	∅	Birt et al. (1981a)
13-*Cis*-retinoic acid (0.2 mM/kg)	a	BOP	40 mg/kg sc	Syrian golden male and female hamsters	∅	∅	Birt et al. (1981a)
13-*Cis*-retinoic acid (0.4 mM/kg)	a	BOP	10 mg/kg sc	Syrian golden male and female hamsters	∅	∅	Birt et al. (1983b)
13-*Cis*-retinoic acid (0.4 mM/kg)	a	BOP	40 mg/kg sc	Syrian golden female hamsters	←	←	Birt et al. (1983b)
13-*Cis*-retinoic acid (0.4 mM/kg)	a	BOP	40 mg/kg sc	Syrian golden male hamsters	∅	←	Birt et al. (1983b)
13-*Cis*-retinoic acid (0.8 mM/kg)	a	BOP	10 mg/kg sc	Syrian golden male and female hamsters	∅	∅	Birt et al. (1983b)
13-*Cis*-retinoic acid (0.8 mM/kg)	a	BOP	40 mg/kg sc	Syrian golden female hamsters	←	←	Birt et al. (1983b)
13-*Cis*-retinoic acid (0.8 mM/kg)	a	BOP	40 mg/kg sc	Syrian golden male hamsters	∅	←	Birt et al. (1983b)

(continued)

Table 10.2. *(Continued)*

Diet	Feeding schedule	Carcinogen	Dose/duration	Species, strain/sex	Tumor incidence	No. of tumors/ tumor-bearing animal	Reference
N-ethylretinamide (0.05 mM/kg)	a	BOP	40 mg/kg sc	Syrian golden male and female hamsters	Ø	Ø	Birt et al. (1981a)
N-ethylretinamide (0.1 mM/kg)	a	BOP	40 mg/kg sc	Syrian golden male and female hamsters	Ø	Ø	Birt et al. (1981a)
N-ethylretinamide (0.2 mM/kg)	a	BOP	40 mg/kg sc	Syrian golden male and female hamsters	Ø	Ø	Birt et al. (1981a)
N-ethylretinamide (0.5 mM/kg)	a	BOP	10 mg/kg sc	Syrian golden male and female hamsters	Ø	Ø	Birt et al. (1983b)
N-ethylretinamide (0.5 mM/kg)	a	BOP	40 mg/kg sc	Syrian golden female hamsters	Ø	↑	Birt et al. (1983b)
N-ethylretinamide (0.5 mM/kg)	a	BOP	40 mg/kg sc	Syrian golden male hamsters	↑	↑	Birt et al. (1983b)
N-ethylretinamide (1 mM/kg)	a	BOP	10 mg/kg sc	Syrian golden male and female hamsters	Ø	Ø	Birt et al. (1983b)
N-ethylretinamide (1 mM/kg)	a	BOP	40 mg/kg sc	Syrian golden female hamsters	Ø	↑	Birt et al. (1983b)
N-ethylretinamide (1 mmol/kg)	a	BOP	40 mg/kg sc	Syrian golden male hamsters	↑	↑	Birt et al. (1983b)
N-phenylretinamide (0.5 mM/kg)	a	BOP	10 mg/kg sc	Syrian golden male and female hamsters	Ø	Ø	Birt et al. (1983b)
N-phenylretinamide (0.5 mM/kg)	a	BOP	40 mg/kg sc	Syrian golden female hamsters	Ø	Ø	Birt et al. (1983b)
N-phenylretinamide (0.5 mM/kg)	a	BOP	40 mg/kg sc	Syrian golden male hamsters	Ø	↑	Birt et al. (1983b)
N-phenylretinamide (1 mM/kg)	a	BOP	10 mg/kg sc	Syrian golden male and female hamsters	Ø	Ø	Birt et al. (1983b)
N-phenylretinamide (1 mM/kg)	a	BOP	40 mg/kg sc	Syrian golden female hamsters	Ø	Ø	Birt et al. (1983b)

Compound (dose)		Carcinogen	Dose	Animal			Reference
N-phenylretinamide (1 mM/kg)	a	BOP	40 mg/kg sc	Syrian golden male hamsters	∅	↑	Birt et al. (1983b)
N-(2-hydroxyethyl)-retinamide (0.5 mmole/kg)	a	BOP	10 mg/kg sc	Syrian golden male and female hamsters	∅	∅	Birt et al. (1983b)
N-(2-hydroxyethyl)-retinamide (0.5 mmole/kg)	a	BOP	40 mg/kg sc	Syrian golden female hamsters	∅	∅	Birt et al. (1983b)
N-(2-hydroxyethyl)-retinamide (0.5 mmole/kg)	a	BOP	40 mg/kg sc	Syrian golden male hamsters	↑	↑	Birt et al. (1983b)
N-(2-hydroxyethyl)-retinamide (1 mmole/kg)	a	BOP	40 mg/kg sc	Syrian golden female hamsters	∅	∅	Birt et al. (1983b)
N-(2-hydroxyethyl)-retinamide (1 mmole/kg)	a	BOP	10 mg/kg sc	Syrian golden male and female hamsters	∅	∅	Birt et al. (1983b)
N-(2-hydroxyethyl)-retinamide (1 mmole/kg)	a	BOP	40 mg/kg sc	Syrian golden male hamsters	↑	↑	Birt et al. (1983b)
4-hydroxyphenyl-retinamide (0.05 mM/kg)	a	BOP	40 mg/kg sc	Syrian golden male and female hamsters	∅	∅	Birt et al. (1981a)
4-hydroxyphenyl-retinamide (0.1 mM/kg)	a	BOP	40 mg/kg sc	Syrian golden male and female hamsters	∅	∅	Birt et al. (1981a)
4-hydroxyphenyl-retinamide (0.2 mM/kg)	a	BOP	40 mg/kg sc	Syrian golden male and female hamsters	∅	∅	Birt et al. (1981a)
2-hydroxyethyl-retinamide (0.05 mM/kg)	a	BOP	40 mg/kg sc	Syrian golden male and female hamsters	∅	∅	Birt et al. (1981a)
2-hydroxyethyl-retinamide (0.1 mM/kg)	a	BOP	40 mg/kg sc	Syrian golden male and female hamsters	∅	∅	Birt et al. (1981a)
2-hydroxyethyl-retinamide (0.2 mM/kg)	a	BOP	40 mg/kg sc	Syrian golden male and female hamsters	∅	∅	Birt et al. (1981a)

Table 10.3. The Effect of Selenium on Pancreas Carcinogenesis

Diet	Feeding schedule	Carcinogen	Dose/duration	Species, strain/sex	Tumor incidence	No. of tumors/tumor-bearing animal	Reference
Sodium selenite (0.1 ppm)	b	BOP	20 mg/kg sc	Syrian golden male and female hamsters	∅	∅	Birt et al. (1986)
Sodium selenite (2.5 ppm)	b + d + a	BOP	20 mg/kg sc	Syrian golden male and female hamsters	∅	∅	Birt et al. (1988)
Sodium selenite (5 ppm)	b	BOP	20 mg/kg sc	Syrian golden male and female hamsters	∅	∅	Birt et al. (1986)
Sodium selenite (5 ppm)	b + d + a	BOP	4 × 5 mg/kg/wk sc	Syrian golden male and female hamsters	∅	∅	Birt et al. (1988)
Sodium selenite (0.1 ppm + 5 ppm)	b / a	BOP	20 mg/kg sc	Syrian golden male and female hamsters	∅	∅	Birt et al. (1986)
Sodium selenite (2.5 ppm) + corn oil (23%)	a	BOP	4 × 5 mg/kg/wk sc	Syrian golden male and female hamsters	∅	∅	Birt et al. (1988)
DL-Selenomethionine (2.5 ppm)	b + d + a	BOP	4 × 5 mg/kg/wk sc	Syrian golden male and female hamsters	∅	∅	Birt et al. (1988)

Table 10.4. The Effect of Protein on Pancreas Carcinogenesis

Diet	Feeding schedule	Carcinogen	Dose/duration	Species, strain/sex	Tumor incidence	No. of tumors/ tumor-bearing animal	Reference
Casein deficiency	b	BOP	10 mg/kg sc	Syrian golden male and female hamsters	∅	—	Pour *et al.* (1983)
Casein deficiency	b + d + a	BOP	10 mg/kg sc	Syrian golden male and female hamsters	∅	—	Pour *et al.* (1983)
Casein deficiency	a	BOP	10 mg/kg sc	Syrian golden male and female hamsters	∅	—	Pour *et al.* (1983)
Casein (9 g/385 kcal)	b	BOP	10 mg/kg sc	Syrian golden male hamsters	∅	∅	Pour and Birt (1983)
Casein (9 g/385 kcal)	b	BOP	10 mg/kg sc	Syrian golden female hamsters	∅	∅	Pour and Birt (1983)
Casein (9 g/385 kcal)	a	BOP	10 mg/kg sc	Syrian golden male hamsters	∅	∅	Pour and Birt (1983)
Casein (9 g/385 kcal)	a	BOP	10 mg/kg sc	Syrian golden female hamsters	→	∅	Pour and Birt (1983)
Casein (36 g/385 kcal)	b	BOP	10 mg/kg sc	Syrian golden male hamsters	∅	∅	Pour and Birt (1983)
Casein (36 g/385 kcal)	b	BOP	10 mg/kg sc	Syrian golden female hamsters	∅	∅	Pour and Birt (1983)

(continued)

Table 10.4. (Continued)

Diet	Feeding schedule	Carcinogen	Dose/duration	Species, strain/sex	Tumor incidence	No. of tumors/ tumor-bearing animal	Reference
Casein (36 g/385 kcal)	a	BOP	10 mg/kg sc	Syrian golden male hamsters	∅	∅	Pour and Birt (1983)
Casein (36 g/385 kcal)	a	BOP	10 mg/kg sc	Syrian golden female hamsters	↑	∅	Pour and Birt (1983)
Casein (11%, low protein)	b	Azaserine	6 × 10 mg/kg/wk ip	Wistar/Lewis male rats	∅	∅	Roebuck et al. (1981)
Casein (11%, low protein)	d + a	Azaserine	6 × 10 mg/kg/wk ip then 10 × 10 mg/kg/wks ip	Wistar/Lewis male rats	∅	∅	Roebuck et al. (1981)
Casein (11%, low protein)	a	Azaserine	6 × 10 mg/kg/wk ip	Wistar/Lewis male rats	∅	∅	Roebuck et al. (1981)
Casein (40 en%)	a	BOP	10 mg/kg sc ip	Syrian golden male and female hamsters	∅	∅	Birt et al. (1983a)
Casein (40 en%)	b	BOP	10 mg/kg sc	Syrian golden male and female hamsters	↑	∅	Birt et al. (1983a)
Casein (50 en%)	d + a	Azaserine	6 × 10 mg/kg/wk ip then: 10 × 10 mg/kg/4 wk ip	Wistar/Lewis male rats	→	∅	Roebuck et al. (1981b)

Table 10.5. The Effect of Protein in Combination with Fat on Pancreas Carcinogenesis

Diet	Feeding schedule	Carcinogen	Dose/duration	Species, strain/sex	Tumor incidence	No. of tumors/ tumor-bearing animal	Reference
Casein (40%) + corn oil (41%)	b	BOP	.10 mg/kc sc	Syrian golden male and female hamsters	↑	∅	Birt *et al.* (1983a)
Casein (40%) + corn oil (41%)	a	BOP	10 mg/kg sc	Syrian golden male and female hamsters	↑	↑	Birt *et al.* (1983a)
Raw soya flour (20%) + corn oil (20%)	a	Azaserine	30 mg/kg sc	Wistar male rats	∅	—	Roebuck *et al.* (1987)
Heated soya flour (20%) + corn oil (20%)	a	Azaserine	30 mg/kg sc	Wistar male rats	∅	—	Roebuck *et al.* (1987)

Table 10.6. The Effect of Soya Flour (Raw or Heated) on Pancreas Carcinogenesis

Diet	Feeding schedule	Carcinogen	Dose/duration	Species, strain/sex	Tumor incidence	No. of tumors/tumor-bearing animal	Reference
Raw soya flour	b[a] wk 31–60 / wk 61–90 / wk > 90 / wk 61–90 / wk > 90	Azaserine	5 mg/kg/wk ip for different times from wk 3–75	Wistar male rats	∅ ∅ ←∅ ←∅	—	McGuinness et al. (1981)
Raw soya flour	b + d + a	DHPN[c]	4 × 0.2 mg/wk ip then 20 × 0.1 mg/wk ip	Hooded male rats / Wistar male rats	∅	—	Levinson et al. (1979)
Raw soya flour (5%)	b + d + a	Azaserine	5 mg/kg/wk ip 85 weeks	Wistar male rats	↑	—	McGuinness and Wormsley (1986)
Raw soya flour (20%)	a	Azaserine	30 mg/kg ip	Wistar male rats	∅	—	Roebuck et al. (1987)
Raw soya flour (25%)	b + d + a	Azaserine	5 mg/kg/wk ip 85 weeks	Wistar male rats	↑	—	McGuinness and Wormsley (1986)
Raw soya flour (25%)	b + d + a[b]	Azaserine	5 mg/kg/wk ip 85 weeks	Wistar male rats	∅	—	McGuinness and Wormsley (1986)
Raw soya flour (42%)	b + d + a	Azaserine	110 mg/kg/wk ip 15 weeks	CFJ male mice	∅	—	Hasdai and Liener (1986)
Raw soya flour (50%)	b + d + a	Azaserine	5 mg/kg/wk ip 85 weeks	Wistar male rats	↑	—	McGuinness and Wormsley (1986)
Raw soya flour (50%)	b + d + a[b]	Azaserine	5 mg/kg/wk ip 85 weeks	Wistar male rats	∅	—	McGuinness and Wormsley (1986)
Raw soya flour (100%)	b + d + a	Azaserine	5 mg/kg/wk ip 85 weeks	Wistar male rats	↑	—	McGuinness and Wormsley (1986)
Raw soya flour (100%)	b + d + a[b]	Azaserine	5 mg/kg/wk ip 85 weeks	Wistar male rats	↑	—	McGuinness and Wormsley (1986)
Heated soya flour	b[a] wk 31–60 / wk 61–90 / wk > 90 / wk 61–90 / wk > 90	Azaserine	5 mg/kg/wk ip for different times from wk 3–75	Wistar male rats	∅ ∅ ←∅ ∅	—	McGuinness et al. (1981)
Heated soya flour (20%)	a	Azaserine	30 mg/kg ip	Hooded male rats / Wistar male rats	∅	—	Roebuck et al. (1987)
Heated soya flour (42%)	b + d + a	Azaserine	110 mg/kg/wk ip 15 weeks	CFJ male mice	∅	—	Hasdai and Liener (1986)

[a]Because of different effects, feeding schedule was differentiated.

Table 10.7. The Effect of Caloric Restriction on Pancreas Carcinogenesis

Diet	Feeding schedule	Carcinogen	Dose/duration	Species, strain/sex	Tumor incidence	No. of tumors/ tumor-bearing animal	Reference
Caloric restriction by 10%	b	Azaserine	6 × 10 mg/kg/wk ip	Wistar/Lewis male rats	→	→	Roebuck *et al.* (1981b)
Caloric restriction by 10%	a	Azaserine	6 × 10 mg/kg/wk ip	Wistar/Lewis male rats	∅	∅	Roebuck *et al.* (1981b)
Caloric restriction by 15%	d + a	Azaserine	6 × 10 mg/kg/wk ip then 10 × 10 mg/kg/4 wks ip	Wistar/Lewis male rats	→	→	Roebuck *et al.* (1981b)

6. References

Aksoy, M., Berger, M. R., and Schmähl, D., 1985, Effect of different diets on the ratio of plasma lipids/vitamin A and E in female Sprague–Dawley rats with MNU-induced mammary carcinomas, *Arch. Geschwulst-forsch.* **55**:443–450.

Albaner, T., 1987, Total calories, body weight and tumor incidence in mice, *Cancer Res.* **47**:1987–1992.

Ankerst, J., and Sjögren, H. O., 1982, Effect of selenium on the induction of breast fibroadenomas by adenovirus type 9 and 1,2-dimethylhydrazine-induced bowel carcinogenesis in rats, *Int. J. Cancer* **29**:707–710.

Arakawa, S., Okumura, M., Yamada, S., Ito, M., and Tejima, S., 1986, Enhancing effect of carrageenan on the induction of rat colonic tumors by 1,2-dimethylhydrazine and its relation to β-glucuronidase activities in feces and other tissues, *J. Nutr. Sci. Vitaminol.* **32**:481–485.

Aylsworth, C. F., Cullum, M. E., Zile, M. H., and Welsch, C. W., 1986, Influence of dietary retinyl acetate on normal rat mammary gland development and on the enhancement of 7,12-dimethylbenz[a]anthracene-induced rat mammary tumorigenesis by high levels of dietary fat, *J. Natl. Cancer Inst.* **76**(2):339–345.

Bansal, B. R., Rhoads, J. E., Jr., and Bansal, S. C., 1978, Effects of diet on colon carcinogenesis and the immune system in rats treated with 1,2-dimethylhydrazine, *Cancer Res.* **38**:3293–3303.

Barbolt, T. A., and Abraham, R., 1978, The effect of bran on dimethylhydrazine-induced colon carcinogenesis in the rat, *Proc. Soc. Exp. Biol. Med.* **157**:656–659.

Barbolt, T. A., and Abraham, R., 1980, Dose–response, sex difference, and the effect of bran in di-methylhydrazine-induced intestinal tumorigenesis in rats, *Toxicol. Appl. Pharmacol.* **55**:417–422.

Barch, D. H., Kuemmerle, S. C., Hollenberg, P. F., and Iannaccone, P. M., 1984, Esophageal microsomal metabolism of *N*-nitrosomethylbenzylamine in the zinc-deficient rat, *Cancer Res.* **44**:5629–5633.

Barnes, D. S., Clapp, N. K., Scott, D. A., Oberst, D. L., and Berry, S. G., 1983, Effects of wheat rice, corn and soybean bran on 1,2-dimethylhydrazine-induced large bowel tumorigenesis in F344 rats, *Nutr. Cancer* **5**(1):1–9.

Bauer, H. G., Asp, N-G., Öste, R., Dahlqvist, A., and Fredlund, P. E., 1979, Effect of dietary fiber on the induction of colorectal tumors and fecal β-glucuronidase activity in the rat, *Cancer Res.* **39**:3752–3756.

Bauer, H. G., Asp, N-G., Dahlqvist, A., Fredlund, P. E., Nyman, M., and Öste, R., 1981, Effect of two kinds of pectin and guar gum on 1,2-dimethylhydrazine initiation of colon tumors and on fecal β-glucuronidase activity in the rat, *Cancer Res.* **41**:2518–2523.

Becci, P. J., Thompson, H. J., Grubbs, C. J., Brown, C. C., and Moon, R. C., 1979, Effect of delay in administration of 13-*cis*-retinoic acid on the inhibition of urinary bladder carcinogenesis in the rat, *Cancer Res.* **39**:3141–3144.

Becci, P. J., Thompson, H. J., Strum, J. M., Brown, C. C., Sporn, M. B., and Moon, R. C., 1981, *N*-butyl-*N*-(4-hydroxybutyl) nitrosamine-induced urinary bladder cancer in C57BL/6 × DBA/2F₁ mice as a useful model for study of chemoprevention of cancer with retinoids, *Cancer Res.* **41**:927–932.

Beems, R. B., 1986, Dietary selenium and benzo[a]pyrene-induced respiratory tract tumours in hamsters, *Carcinogenesis* **7**(3):485–489.

Beems, R. B., and van Beck, L., 1984, Modifying effect of dietary fat on benzo[a]pyrene-induced respiratory tract tumours in hamsters, *Carcinogenesis* **5**(3):413–417.

Berry, E. M., Zimmerman, J., Peser, M., and Ligumsky, M., 1986, Dietary fat adiipose tisue composition and the development of carcinoma of the colon, *J. Natl. Cancer Inst.* **77**(1):93–97.

Beth, M., Berger, M. R., Aksoy, M., and Schmähl, D., 1987a, Comparison between the effects of dietary fat level and of calorie intake on methylnitrosourea-induced mammary carcinogenesis in female SD rats, *Int. J. Cancer* **39**:737–744.

Beth, M., Berger, M. R., Aksoy, M., and Schmähl, D., 1987b, Effects of vitamin A and E supplementation to diets containing two different fat levels on methylnitrosourea-induced mammary carcinogenesis in female SD-rats, *Br. J. Cancer* **56**:445–449.

Birt, D. F., Sayed, S., Davies, M. H., and Pour, P., 1981a, Sex differences in the effects of retinoids on carcinogenesis by *N*-nitrosobis(2-oxopropyl)amine in Syrian hamsters, *Cancer Lett.* **14**:13–21.

Birt, D. F., Salmasi, S., and Pour, P. M., 1981b, Enhancement of experimental pancreatic cancer in Syrian golden hamsters by dietary fat, *J. Natl. Cancer Inst.* **67**(6):1327–1332.

Birt, D. F., Lawson, T. A., Julius, A. D., Runice, C. E., and Salmasi, S., 1982, Inhibition by dietary selenium of colon cancer induced in the rat by bis(2-oxopropyl)nitrosamine, *Cancer Res.* **42**:4455–4459.

Birt, D. F., Stepan, K. R., and Pour, P. M., 1983a, Interaction of dietary fat and protein on pancreatic carcinogenesis in Syrian golden hamsters, *J. Natl. Cancer Inst.* **71**(2):355–360.

Birt, D. F., Davies, M. H., Pour, P. M., and Salmasi, S., 1983b, Lack of inhibition by retinoids of bis(2-oxopropyl)nitrosamine-induced carcinogenesis in Syrian hamsters, *Carcinogenesis* **4**(10):1215–1220.

Birt, D. F., Julius, A. D., Runice, C. E., and Salmasi, S., 1986, Effects of dietary selenium on bis(2-oxopropyl)nitrosamine-induced carcinogenesis in Syrian golden hamsters, *J. Natl. Cancer Inst.* **77**(6):1281–1286.

Birt, D. F., Julius, A. D., Hasegawa, R., St. John, M., and Cohen, S. M., 1987, Effect of L-tryptophan excess and vitamin B_6 deficiency on rat urinary bladder cancer promotion, *Cancer Res.* **47**:1244–1250.

Birt, D. F., Julius, A. D., Runice, C. E., White, L. T., Lawson, T., and Pour, P. M., 1988, Enhancement of BOP-induced pancreatic carcinogenesis in selenium-fed Syrian golden hamsters under specific dietary conditions, *Nutr. Cancer* **11**:21–33.

Black, H. S., Lenger, W., Phelps, A. W., and Thornby, J. I., 1984, Influence of dietary lipid upon ultraviolet light-carcinogenesis, *J. Environ. Pathol. Toxicol. Oncol.* **5**:271–282.

Boissonneault, G. A., Elson, C. E., and Pariza, M. W., 1986, Net energy effects of dietary fat on chemically induced mammary carcinogenesis in F344 rats, *J. Natl. Cancer Inst.* **76**(2):335–338.

Bollag, W., 1975, Prophylaxis of chemically induced epithelial tumors with an aromatic retinoic acid analog (RO 10-9359), *Eur. J. Cancer* **11**:721–724.

Boyd, J. N., Babish, J. G., and Stoewsand, G. S., 1982, Modification by beet and cabbage diets of aflatoxin B_1-induced rat plasma α-foetoprotein elevation, hepatic tumorigenesis, and mutagenicity of urine, *Food Chem. Toxicol.* **20**:47–52.

Braden, L. M., and Carroll, K. K., 1986, Dietary polyunsaturated fat in relation to mammary carcinogenesis in rats, *Lipids* **21**(4):285–288.

Broitman, S. A., Vitale, J. J., Jakuba, E. V., and Gottlieb, L. S., 1977, Polyunsaturated fat, cholesterol and large bowel tumorigenesis, *Cancer* **40**:2455–2463.

Brown, R. R., 1981, Effects of dietary fat on incidence of spontaneous and induced cancer in mice, *Cancer Res.* **41**: 3741–3742.

Bull, A. W., Soullier, B. K., Wilson, P. S., Hayden, M. T., and Nigro, N. D., 1979, Promotion of azoxymethane-induced intestinal cancer by high-fat diet in rats, *Cancer Res.* **39**:4956–4959.

Burns, R. A., and Milner, J. A., 1984, Effect of arginine on the carcinogenicity of 7,12-dimethylbenz-[a]anthracene and N-methyl-N-nitrosourea, *Carcinogenesis* **5**(12):1539–1542.

Byers, T., and Graham, S., 1984, The epidemiology of diet and cancer, *Adv. Cancer Res.* **41**:1–69.

Calvert, R. J., Klurfeld, D. M., Subramaniam, S., Vahouny, G. V., and Kritchevsky, D., 1987, Reduction of colonic carcinogenesis by wheat bran independent of fecal bile acid concentration, *J. Natl. Cancer Inst.* **79**(4):875–880.

Carr, B. I., 1985, Chemical carcinogens and inhibitors of carcinogensesis in the human diet, *Cancer* **55**:218–224.

Carroll, K. K., and Noble, R. L., 1987, Dietary fat in relation to hormonal induction of mammary and prostatic carcinoma in Nb rats, *Carcinogenesis* **8**(6):851–853.

Carter, C. A., Milholland, R. J., Shea, W., and Ip, M. M., 1983, Effect of the prostaglandin synthetase inhibitor indomethacin on 7,12-dimethylbenz(a)anthracene-induced mammary tumorigenesis in rats fed different levels of fat, *Cancer Res.* **43**:3559–3562.

Castleden, W. M., 1977, Prolonged survival and decrease in intestinal tumours in dimethylhydrazine-treated rats fed a chemically defined diet, *Br. J. Cancer* **35**:491–495.

Chan, P-C., and Dao, T. L., 1981, Enhancement of mammary carcinogenesis by a high-fat diet in Fischer, Long–Evans, and Sprague–Dawley rats, *Cancer Res.* **41**:164–167.

Chan, P-C., and Dao, T. L., 1983, Effects of dietary fat on age-dependent sensitivity to mammary carcinogenesis, *Cancer Lett.* **18**:245–249.

Chan, P-C., Head, J. F., Cohen, L. A., and Wynder, E. L., 1977, Influence of dietary fat on the induction of mammary tumors by N-nitrosomethylurea: associated hormone changes and differences between Sprague–Dawley and F344 rats, *J. Natl. Cancer Inst.* **59**(4):1279–1283.

Chan, P-C., Ferguson, K. A., and Dao, T. L., 1983, Effects of different dietary fats on mammary carcinogenesis, *Cancer Res.* **43**:1079–1083.

Charnley, G., and Tannenbaum, S. R., 1985, Flow cytometric analysis of the effect of sodium chloride on gastric cancer risk in the rat, *Cancer Res.* **45**:5608–5616.

Chen, W-F., Patchefsky, A. S., and Goldsmith, H. S., 1978, Colonic protection from dimethylhydrazine by a high fiber diet, *Surg. Gynecol. Obstet.* **147**:503–506.

Chester, J. F., Gaissert, H. A., Ross, J. S., Malt, R. A., and Weitzman, S. A., 1986, Augmentation of 1,2-dimethylhydrazine-induced colon cancer by experimental colitis in mice: role of dietary vitamin E, *J. Natl. Cancer Inst.* **76**(5):939–941.

Clapp, N. K., Henke, M. A., London, J. F., and Shock, T. L., 1984, Enhancement of 1,2-dimethylhydrazine-induced large bowel tumorigenesis in Balb/c mice by corn, soybean, and wheat brans, *Nutr. Cancer* **6**(2):77–85.

Clinton, S. K., Imrey, P. B., Alster, J. M., Simon, J., Truex, C. R., and Visek, W. J., 1984a, The combined effects of dietary protein and fat on 7,12-dimethylbenz(a)anthracene-induced breast cancer in rats, *J. Nutr.* **114**:1213–1223.

Clinton, S. K., Mulloy, A. L., and Visek, W. J., 1984b, Effects of dietary lipid saturation on prolactin secretion, carcinogen metabolism and mammary carcinogenesis in rats, *J. Nutr.* **114**:1630–1639.

Clinton, S. K., Alster, J. M., Imrey, P. B., Nandkumar, S., Truex, C. R., and Visek, W. J., 1986, Effects of dietary protein, fat and energy intake during an initiation phase study of 7,12-dimethylbenz[a]anthracene-induced breast cancer in rats, *J. Nutr.* **116**:2290–2302.

Cohen, L. A., and Chan, P-C., 1982, Dietary cholesterol and experimental mammary cancer development, *Nutr. Cancer* **4**(2):99–106.

Cohen, L. A., Thompson, D. O., Maeura, Y., Choi, K., Blank, M. E., and Rose, D. P., 1986, Dietary fat and mammary cancer. I. Promoting effects of different dietary fats on *N*-nitrosomethylurea-induced rat mammary tumorigenesis, *J. Natl. Cancer Inst.* **77**(1):33–41.

Cohen, S. M., Wittenberg, J. F., and Bryan, G. T., 1976, Effect of avitaminosis A and hypernitaminosis A on urinary bladder carcinogenicity of *N*-[4-(5-nitro-2-furyl)-2-thiazolyl]formamide, *Cancer Res.* **36**:2334–2339.

Cohen, S. M., Arai, M., Jacobs, J. B., and Friedell, G. H., 1979, Promoting effect of saccharin and DL-tryptophan in urinary bladder carcinogenesis, *Cancer Res.* **39**:1207–1217.

Conybeare, G., 1980, Effect of quality and quantity of diet on survival and tumour incidence in outbred swiss mice, *Food Cosmet. Toxicol.* **18**:65–75.

Cook, M. G., and McNamara, P., 1980, Effect of dietary vitamin E on dimethylhydrazine-induced colonic tumors in mice, *Cancer Res.* **40**:1329–1331.

Cruse, J. P., Clark, C. G., and Lewin, M. R., 1978, Failure of bran to protect against experimental colon cancer in rats, *Lancet* **2**:1278–1279.

Dao, T. L., and Chan, P-C., 1983, Effect of duration of high fat intake on enhancement of mammary carcinogenesis in rats, *J. Natl. Cancer Inst.* **71**(1):201–205.

Daoud, A. H., and Griffin, A. C., 1980, Effect of retinoic acid, butylated hydroxytoluene, selenium and sorbic acid on azo-dye hepatocarcinogenesis, *Cancer Lett.* **9**:299–304.

Davidson, M. B., and Carroll, K. K., 1982, Inhibitory effect of a fat-free diet on mammary carcinogenesis in rats, *Nutr. Cancer* **3**(4):207–215.

Dayton, S., Hashimoto, S., and Wollman, J., 1977, Effect of high-oleic and high-linoleic safflower oils on mammary tumors induced in rats by 7,12-dimethylbenz[a]anthracene, *J. Nutr.* **107**:1353–1360.

Diet, nutrition and cancer, executive summary of the report of the committee on diet, nutrition and cancer, 1983, *Cancer Res.* **43**:3018–3023.

Dogra, S. C., Khanduja, K. L., and Gupta, M. P., 1985, The effect of vitamin A deficiency on the initiation and postinitiation phases of benzo(a)pyrene-induced lung tumourigenesis in rats, *Br. J. Cancer* **52**:931–935.

Doll, R., and Peto, R., 1981, The causes of cancer: Quantitative estimates of avoidable risks of cancer in the United States today, *J. Natl. Cancer Inst.* **66**:1191–1308.

Dunham, M. B., Zuckerkandl, E., Reynolds, R., Willoughby, R., Marcuson, R., Barth, R., and Pauling, L., 1982, Effects of intake of L-ascorbic acid on the incidence of dermal neoplasms induced in mice by ultraviolet light, *J. Natl. Acad. Sci. USA* **79**:7532–7536.

El-Bayoumy, K., 1985, Effects of organoselenium compounds on induction of mouse forestomach tumors by benzo(a)pyrene, *Cancer Res.* **45**:3631–3635.

Elegbede, J. A., Maltzman, T. H., Verma, A. K., Tanner, M. A., Elson, C. E., and Gould, M. N., 1986, Mouse skin tumor promoting activity of orange peel oil and *d*-limonene: A re-evaluation, *Carcinogenesis* **7**(12):2047–2049.

Evarts, R. P., and Brown, C. A., 1977, Effect of L-tryptophan on diethylnitrosamine and 3'-methyl-4-*N*-dimethylaminoazobenzene hepatocarcinogenesis, *Food Cosmet. Toxicol.* **15**:431–435.

Fernandes, G., Yunis, E. J., and Good, R. A., 1976, Suppression of adenocarcinoma by the immunological consequences of calorie restriction, *Nature* **263**:504–507.

Fleiszer, D., MacFarlane, J., Murray, D., and Brown, R. A., 1978, Protective effect of dietary fibre against chemically induced bowel tumours in rats, *Lancet* **2**:552–553.

Fleiszer, D. M., Murray, D., Richards, G. K., and Brown, R. A., 1980, Effects of diet on chemically induced bowel cancer, *Can. J. Surg.* **23**(1):67–73.

Fong, L. Y. Y., Sivak, A., and Newberne, P. M., 1978, Zinc deficiency and methylbenzylnitrosamine-induced esophageal cancer in rats, *J. Natl. Cancer Inst.* **61**(1):145–150.

Fong, L. Y. Y., Lee, J. S. K., Chan, W. C., and Newberne, P. M., 1984, Zinc deficiency and the development of esophageal and forestomach tumors in Sprague–Dawley rats fed precursors of *N*-nitroso-*N*-benzylmethylamine, *J. Natl. Cancer Inst.* **72**(2):419–423.

Freeman, H. J., 1986, Effects of differing purified cellulose, pectin, and hemicellulose fiber diets on fecal enzymes in 1,2-dimethylhydrazine-induced rat colon carcinogenesis, *Cancer Res.* **46**:5529–5532.

Freeman, H. J., Spiller, G. A., and Kim, Y. S., 1980, A double-blind study on the effects of differing purified cellulose and pectin fiber diets on 1,2-dimethylhytdrazine-induced rat colonic neoplasia, *Cancer Res.* **40**:2661–2665.

Freeman, H. J., Sipller, G. A., and Kim, Y. S., 1984, Effect of high hemicellulose corn bran in 1,2-dimethylhydrazine-induced rat intestinal neoplasia, *Carcinogenesis* **5**(2):261–264.

Fukushima, S., Friedell, G. H., Jacobs, J. B., and Cohen, S. M., 1981, Effect of L-tryptophan and sodium saccharin on urinary tract carcinogenesis initiated by *N*-[4-(5-nitro-2-furyl)-2-thiazolyl]formamide, *Cancer Res.* **41**:3100–3103.

Fukushima, S., Hagiwara, A., Ogiso, T., Shibata, M., and Ito, N., 1983a, Promoting effects of various chemicals in rat urinary bladder carcinogenesis initiated by *N*-nitroso-*n*-butyl-4(4-hydroxybutyl)amine, *Food Chem. Toxicol.* **21**(1):59–68.

Fukushima, S., Imaida, K., Sakata, T., Okamura, T., Shibata, M. A., and Ito, N., 1983b, Promoting effects of sodium L-ascorbate on two-stage urinary bladder carcinogenesis in rats, *Cancer Res.* **43**:4454–4457.

Fukushima, S., Kurata, Y., Shibata, M. A., Ikawa, E., and Ito, N., 1984, Promotion by ascorbic acid, sodium erythorbate and ethoxyquin of neoplastic lesions in rats initiated with *N*-butyl-*N*-(4-hydroxybutyl)nitrosamine, *Cancer Lett.* **23**:29–37.

Fukushima, S., Shibata, M. A., Shirai, T., Tamano, S., and Ito, N., 1986, Roles of urinary sodium ion concentration and pH in promotion by ascorbic acid of urinary bladder carcinogenesis in rats, *Cancer Res.* **46**:1623–1626.

Gabrial, G. N., Schrager, T. F., and Newberne, P. M., 1982, Zinc deficiency, alcohol, and a retinoid: Association with esophageal cancer in rats, *J. Natl. Cancer Inst.* **68**(5):785–789.

Galloway, D. J., Owen, R. W., Jarrett, F., Boyle, P., Hill, M. J., and George, W. D., 1986, Experimental colorectal cancer: The relationship of diet and faecal bile acid concentration to tumour induction, *Br. J. Surg.* **73**:233–237.

Galloway, D. J., Jarrett, F., Boyle, P., Indran, M., Carr, K., Owen, R. W., and George, W. D., 1987, Morphological and cell kinetic effects of dietary manipulation during colorectal carcinogenesis, *Gut* **28**:754–763.

Garfinkel, L., 1986, Overweight and mortality, *Cancer* **58**:1826–1829.

Gensler, H. L., Watson, R. R., Moriguchi, S., and Bowden, G. T., 1987, Effects of dietary retinyl palmitate or 13-*cis*-retinoic acid on the promotion of tumors in mouse skin, *Cancer Res.* **47**:967–970.

Glauert, H. P., and Bennink, M. R., 1981, Enhancement of 1,2-dimethylhydrazine-induced colon carcinogenesis in mice by dietary agar, *Food Cosmet. Toxicol.* **19**:281–286.

Glauert, H. P., and Pitot, H. C., 1986, Influence of dietary fat on the promotion of diethylnitrosamine-induced hepatocarcinogenesis in female rats, *Proc. Soc. Exp. Biol. Med.* **181**:498–506.

Griffin, A. C., and Jacobs, M. M., 1977, Effects of selenium on azo dye hepatocarcinogenesis, *Cancer Lett.* **3**:177–181.

Grubbs, C. J., Moon, R. C., Sporn, M. B., and Newton, D. L., 1977, Inhibition of mammary cancer by retinyl methyl ether, *Cancer Res.* **37**:599–602.

Harada, T., Kitazawa, T., Maita, K., and Shirasu, Y., 1985, Effects of vitamin C on tumor induction by diethylnitrosamine in the respiratory tract of hamsters exposed to cigarette smoke, *Cancer Lett.* **25:**163–169.

Hasdai, A., and Liener, I. E., 1986, The failure of long-term feeding of raw soy flour, in the presence or absence of azaserine, to induce carcinogenic changes in the mouse pancreas, *Nutr. Cancer* **8:**85–91.

Hawrylewicz, E., Huang, H. H., and Liu, J. M., 1986, Dietary Protein, Enhancement of *N*-nitrosomethylurea-induced mammary carcinogenesis, and their effect on hormone regulation in rats, *Cancer Res.* **46:**4395–4399.

Heilbrun, L. K., 1986, Black tea consumption and cancer risk: A prospective study, *Br. J. Cancer* **54:**677–683.

Hicks, R. M., Chowaniec, J., Turton, J. A., Massey, E. D., and Harvey, A., 1982, The effect of dietary retinoids on experimentally induced carcinogenesis in the rat bladder, in: *Molecular Interrelations of Nutrition and Cancer* (M. S. Arnott, J. van Eys, and Y. M. Wang, eds.), Raven Press, New York, pp. 419–447.

Hopkins, G. J., and Carroll, K. K., 1979, Relationship between amount and type of dietary fat in promotion of mammary carcinogenesis induced by 7,12-dimethylbenz[a]anthracene, *J. Natl. Cancer Inst.* **62**(4):1009–1012.

Hopkins, G. J., West, C. E., and Hard, G. C., 1976, Effect of dietary fats on the incidence of 7,12-dimethylbenz(a)anthracene-induced tumors in rats, *Lipids* **11**(4):328–333.

Hopkins, G. J., Kennedy, T. G., and Carroll, K. K., 1981, Polyunsaturated fatty acids as promoters of mammary carcinogenesis induced in Sprague–Dawley rats by 7,12-dimethylbenz[a]anthracene, *J. Natl. Cancer Inst.* **66**(3):517–522.

Howarth, A. E., and Pihl, E., 1985, High-fat diet promotes and causes distal shift of experimental rat colonic cancer—Beer and alcohol do not, *Nutr. Cancer* **6**(4):229–235.

Imaida, K., Fukushima, S., Shirai, T., Masui, T., Ogiso, T., and Ito, N., 1984, Promoting activities of butylated hydroxyanisole, butylated hydroxytoluene and sodium L-ascorbate on forestomach and urinary bladder carcinogenesis initiated with methylnitrosourea in F344 male rats, *Jpn. J. Cancer Res.* **75:**769–775.

Ingram, D. M., and Castleden, W. M., 1981, Glucose Increases experimentally induced colorectal cancer: A preliminary report, *Nutr. Cancer* **2**(3):150–151.

Ip, C., 1980, Ability of dietary fat to overcome the resistance of mature female rats to 7,12-dimethylbenz(a)anthracene-induced mammary tumorigenesis, *Cancer Res.* **40:**2785–2789.

Ip, C., 1981, Prophylaxis of mammary neoplasia by selenium supplementation in the initiation and promotion phases of chemical carcinogenesis, *Cancer Res.* **41:**4386–4390.

Ip, C., 1982, Dietary vitamin E intake and mammary carcinogenesis in rats, *Carcinogenesis* **3**(12):1453–1456.

Ip, C., 1985, Attenuation of the anticarcinogenic action of selenium by vitamin E deficiency, *Cancer Lett.* **25:**325–331.

Ip, C., 1986, Interaction of vitamin C and selenium supplementation in the modification of mammary carcinogenesis in rats, *J. Natl. Cancer Inst.* **77**(1):299–303.

Ip, C., and Ip, M. M., 1980, Inhibition of mammary tumorigenesis by a reduction of fat intake after carcinogen treatment in young versus adult rats, *Cancer Lett.* **11**(1):35–42.

Ip, C., and Ip, M. M., 1981, Serum estrogens and estrogen responsiveness in 7,12-dimethylbenz[a]anthracene-induced mammary tumors as influenced by dietary fat, *J. Natl. Cancer Inst.* **66**(2):291–295.

Ip, C., and Sinha, D., 1981a, Anticarcinogenic effect of selenium in rats treated with dimethylbenz[a]anthracene and fed different levels and types of fat, *Carcinogenesis* **2**(2):435–438.

Ip, C., and Sinha, D. K., 1981b, Enhancement of mammary tumorgenesis by dietary selenium deficiency in rats with a high polyunsaturated fat intake, *Cancer Res.* **41:**31–34.

Ip, C., and White, G., 1986, BCG-modulated mammary carcinogenesis is dependent on the schedule of immunization but is not affected by dietary fat, *Cancer Lett.* **31:**87–96.

Jacobs, L. R., 1983, Enhancement of rat colon carcinogenesis by wheat bran consumption during the stage of 1,2-dimethylhydrazine administration, *Cancer Res.* **343:**4057–4061.

Jacobs, L. R., and Lupton, J. R., 1986, Relationship between colonic luminal pH, cell proliferation, and colon carcinogenesis in 1,2-dimethylhydrazine treated rats fed high fiber diets, *Cancer Res.* **46:**1727–1734.

Jacobs, M. M., 1983, Selenium inhibition of 1,2-dimethylhydrazine-induced colon carcinogenesis, *Cancer Res.* **43:**1646–1649.

Jacobs, M. M., Jansson, B., and Griffin, A. C., 1977, Inhibitory effects of selenium on 1,2-dimethylhydrazine and methylazoxymethanol acetate induction of colon tumors, *Cancer Lett.* **2:**133–138.

Jacobs, M. M., Forst, C. F., and Beams, F. A., 1981, Biochemical and clinical effects of selenium on dimethylhydrazine-induced colon cancer in rats, *Cancer Res.* **41:**4458–4465.

Jones, F. E., Komorowski, R. A., and Condon, R. E., 1984, The effects of ascorbic acid and butylated hydroxyanisole in the chemoprevention of 1,2-dimethylhydrazine-induced large bowel neoplasms, *J. Surg. Oncol.* **25:**54–60.

Jurkowski, J. J., and Cave, W. T., Jr., 1985, Dietary effects of menhaden oil on the growth and membrane lipid composition of rat mammary tumors, *J. Natl. Cancer Inst.* **74**(5):1145–1149.

Kalamegham, R., and Carroll, K. K., 1984, Reversal of the promotional effect of high-fat diet on mammary tumorigenesis by subsequent lowering of dietary fat, *Nutr. Cancer* **6**(1):22–31.

Kawasaki, H., Morishige, F., Tanaka, H., and Kimoto, E., 1982, Influence of oral supplementation of ascorbate upon the induction of *N*-methyl-*N'*-nitro-*N*-nitrosoguanidine, *Cancer Lett.* **16:**57–63.

King, M. M., Bailey, D. M., Gibson, D. D., Pitha, J. V., and McCay, P. B., 1979, Incidence of growth of mammary tumors induced by 7,12-dimethylbenz[a]anthracene as related to the dietary content of fat and antioxidant, *J. Natl. Cancer Inst.* **63**(3):657–663.

King, M. M., and McCay, P. B., 1983, Modulation of tumor incidence and possible mechanisms of inhibition of mammary carcinogenesis by dietary antioxidants, *Cancer Res.* **43:**2485s–2490s.

Klurfeld, D. M., Weber, M. M., and Kritchevsky, D., 1987, Inhibition of chemically induced mammary and colon tumor promotion by caloric restriction in rats fed increased dietary fat, *Cancer Res.* **47:**2759–2762.

Kollmorgen, G. M., King, M. M., Roszel, J. F., Daggs, B. J., and Longley, R. E., 1981, The influence of dietary fat and non-specific immunotherapy on carcinogen-induced rat mammary adenocarcinoma, *Vet. Pathol.* **18:**82–91.

Konishi, N., Kitahori, Y., Shimoyama, T., Takahashi, M., and Hiasa, Y., 1986, Effects of sodium chloride and alcohol on experimental esophageal carcinogenesis induced by *N*-nitrosopiperidine in rats, *Jpn. J. Cancer Res.* **77:**446–451.

Kort, W. J., Zondervan, P. E., Hulsman, L. O. M., Weijma, I. M., Hülsmann, W. C., and Westbroek, D. L., 1985, Spontaneous tumor incidence in female brown norway rats after lifelong diets high and low in linoleic acid, *J. Natl. Cancer Inst.* **74**(2):529–536.

Kritchevsky, D., Weber, M. M., and Klurfeld, D. M., 1984, Dietary fat versus caloric content in initiation and promotion of 7,12-dimethylbenz(a)anthracene-induced mammary tumorigenesis in rats, *Cancer Res.* **44:**3174–3177.

Kritchevsky, D., Weber, M. M., Buck, C. L., and Klurfeld, D. M., 1986, Calories, fat and cancer, *Lipids* **21**(4):272–274.

Laurier, C., Tatematsu, M., Rao, P. M., Rajalakshmi, S., and Sarma, D. S. R., 1984, Promotion by orotic acid of liver carcinogenesis in rats initiated by 1,2-dimethylhydrazine, *Cancer Res.* **44:**2186–2191.

LeBoeuf, R. A., Laishes, B. A., and Hoekstra, W. G., 1985, Effects of dietary selenium concentration on the development of enzyme-altered liver foci and hepatocellular carcinoma induced by diethylnitrosamine or *N*-acetylaminofluorene in rats, *Cancer Res.* **45:**5489–5495.

Lee, D. J., Sinnhuber, R. O., Wales, J. H., and Putnam, G. B., 1978, Effect of dietary protein on the response of rainbow trout (*Salmo gairdneri*) to aflatoxin B₁ 1978, *J. Natl. Cancer Inst.* **60**(2):317–320.

Lee, S. Y., and Rogers, A. E., 1983 Dimethylbenzanthracene mammary tumorigenesis in Sprague–Dawley rats fed diets differing in content of beef tallow or rapeseed oil, *Nutr. Res.* **3:**361–371.

Leung, F. C., Aylsworth, C. F., and Meites, J., 1983, counteraction of underfeeding-induced inhibition of mammary tumor growth in rats by prolactin and estrogen administration, *Proc. Soc. Exp. Biol. Med.* **173:**159–163.

Levinson, D. A., Morgan, R. G. H., Brimacombe, J. S., Hopwood, D., Coghill, G., and Wormsley, K. G., 1979, Carcinogenic effects of di(2-hydroxypropyl)nitrosamine (DHPN) in male Wistar rats: Promotion of pancreatic cancer by a raw soya flour diet, *Scand. J. Gastroenterol.* **14:**217–224.

Longnecker, D. S., Roebuck, B. D., Lilja, H. S., Yager, J. D., and Siegmund, B., 1981, Pancreatic carcinoma in azaserine-treated rats: Induction, classification and dietary modulation of incidence, *Cancer* **47:**1562–1572.

Luo, X. M., Wei, H. J., and Yang, S. P., 1983, Inhibitory effect of molybdenum on esophageal and forestomach carcinogenesis in rats, *J. Natl. Cancer Inst.* **71**(1):75–80.

Marshall, M. V., Arnott, M. S., Jacobs, M. M., and Griffin, A. C., 1979, Selenium effects on the carcinogenicity and metabolism of 2-acetylaminofluorene, *Cancer Lett.* **7**:331–338.

McCay, P. B., King, M. M., and Pitha, J. V., 1981, Evidence that the effectiveness of antioxidants as inhibitors of 7,12-dimethylbenz(a)anthracene-induced mammary tumors is a function of dietary fat composition, *Cancer Res.* **41**:3745–3748.

McCormick, D. L., and Moon, R. C., 1982, Influence of delayed administration of retinyl acetate on mammary carcinogenesis, *Cancer Res.* **42**:2639–2643.

McCormick, D. L., Burns, F. J., and Albert, R. E., 1980, Inhibition of rat mammary carcinogenesis by short dietary exposure to retinyl acetate, *Cancer Res.* **40**:1140–1143.

McCormick, D. L., Burns, F. J., and Albert, R. E., 1981, Inhibition of benzo[a]pyrene-induced mammary carcinogenesis by retinyl acetate, *J. Natl. Cancer Inst.* **66**(3):559–564.

McCormick, D. L., Becci, P. J., and Moon, R. C., 1982a, Inhibition of mammary and urinary bladder carcinogenesis by a retinoid and a maleic anhydride–divinyl ether copolymer (MVE-2), *Carcinogenesis* **3**(12):1473–1476.

McCormick, D. L., Mehta, R. G., Thompson, C. A., Dinger, N., Caldwell, I. A., and Moon, R. C., 1982b, Enhanced inhibition of mammary carcinogenesis by combined treatment with *N*-(4-hydroxyphenyl)retinamide and ovariectomy, *Cancer Res.* **42**:508–512.

McCormick, D. L., Sowell, Z. L., Thompson, C. A., and Moon, R. C., 1983, Inhibition by retinoid and ovariectomy of additional primary malignancies in rats following surgical removal of the first mammary cancer, *Cancer* **51**:594–599.

McGuinness, E. E., and Wormsley, K. G., 1986, Effects of feeding partial and intermittent raw soya flour diets on the rat pancreas, *Cancer Lett.* **32**:73–81.

McGuinness, E. E., Morgan, R. G. H., Levison, D. A., Hopwood, D., and Wormsley, K. G., 1981, Interaction of azaserine and raw soya flour on the rat pancreas, *Scand. J. Gastroenterol.* **16**:49–56.

Minton, J. P., Abou-issa, H., Foecking, M. K., and Sriram, M. G., 1983, Caffeine and unsaturated fat diet significantly promotes DMBA-induced breast cancer in rats, *Cancer* **51**:1249–1253.

Mirvish, S. S., Cardesa, A., Wallcave, L., and Shubik, P., 1975, Induction of mouse lung adenomas by amines or ureas plus nitrite and by *N*-nitroso compounds: Effect of ascorbate, gallic acid, thiocyanate, and caffeine, *J. Natl. Cancer Inst.* **55**(3):633–636.

Mirvish, S., Pelfrene, A. F., Garcia, H., and Shubik, P., 1976, Effect of sodium ascorbate on tumor induction in rats treated with morpholine and sodium nitrite, and with nitrosomorpholine, *Cancer Lett.* **2**:101–108.

Miyakawa, M., and Yoshida, O., 1980, Protective effects of DL-tryptophan on benzidine-induced hepatic tumor in mice, *Jpn. J. Cancer Res.* **71**:265–268.

Miyata, Y., Tsuda, H., Matayoshi-Miyasato, K., Fukushima, S., Murasaki, G., Ogiso, T., and Ito, N., 1978, Effect of vitamin A acetate on urinary bladder carcinogenesis induced by *N*-butyl-*N*-(4-hydroxybutyl)-nitrosamine in rats, *Jpn. J. Cancer Res.* **69**:845–848.

Mizutani, T., and Mitsuoka, T., 1982, Effect of konjac mannan on spontaneous liver tumorigenesis and fecal flora in C3H/He male mice, *Cancer Lett.* **17**:27–32.

Mizutani, T., and Mitsuoka, T., 1983, Effect of konjac mannan on 1,2-dimethylhydrazine-induced intestinal carcinogenesis in Fischer 344 rats, *Cancer Lett.* **19**:1–6.

Moon, R. C., Grubbs, C. J., Sporn, M. B., and Goodman, D. G., 1977, Retinyl acetate inhibits mammary carcinogenesis induced by *N*-methyl-*N*-nitrosourea, *Nature* **267**:620–621.

Moon, R. C., McCormick, D. L., Becci, P. J., Shealy, Y. F., Frickel, F., Paust, J., and Sporn, M. B., 1982, Influence of 15 retinoic acid amides on urinary bladder carcinogenesis in the mouse, *Carcinogenesis* **3**(12):1469–1472.

Mori, S., Kurata, Y., Takeuchi, Y., Toyama, M., Makino, S., and Fukushima, S., 1987, Influences of strain and diet on the promoting effects of sodium L-ascorbate in two-stage urinary bladder carcinogenesis in rats, *Cancer Res.* **47**:3492–3495.

Murasaki, G., Miyata, Y., Babaya, K., Arai, M., Fukushima, S., and Ito, N., 1980, Inhibitory effect of an aromatic retinoic acid analog on urinary bladder carcinogenesis in rats treated with *N*-butyl-*N*-(4-hydroxybutyl)nitrosamine, *Jpn. J. Cancer Res.* **71**:333–340.

Muto, Y., and Moriwaki, H., 1984, Antitumor activity of vitamin A and its derviatives, *J. Natl. Cancer Inst.* **73**(6):1389–1393.

Narisawa, T., Reddy, B. S., Wong, C. Q., and Weisburger, J. H., 1976, Effect of vitamin A deficiency on rat colon carcinogenesis by *N*-methyl-*N'*-nitro-*N*-nitrosoguanidine, *Cancer Res.* **36**:1379–1383.

Nauss, K. M., Locniskar, M., and Newberne, P. M., 1983, Effect of alterations in the quality and quantity of dietary fat on 1,2-dimethylhydrazine-induced colon tumorigenesis in rats, *Cancer Res.* **43**:4083–4090.

Nauss, K. M., Locniskar, M., Sondergaard, D., and Newberne, P. M., 1984, Lack of effect of dietary fat on *N*-nitrosomethyl urea (MNU)-induced colon tumorigenesis in rats, *Carcinogenesis* **5**(2):255–260.

Nauss, K. M., Bueche, D., Soule, N., Fu, P., Yew, K., and Newberne, P. M., 1986, Effect of dietary selenium levels on methylbenzylnitrosamine-induce esophageal cancer in rats, *Cancer Lett.* **33**:107–116.

Nauss, K. M., Bueche, D., and Newberne, P. M., 1987, Effect of vitamin A Nutriture on experimental esophageal carcinogenesis, *J. Natl. Cancer Inst.* **79**(1):145–147.

Nettesheim, P., and Williams, M. L., 1976, The influence of vitamin A on the susceptibility of the rat lung to 3-methylcholanthrene, *Int. J. Cancer* **17**:351–357.

Nettesheim, P., Cone, M. V., and Snyder, C., 1976, The influence of retinyl acetate on the postinitiation phase of preneoplastic lung nodules in rats, *Cancer Res.* **36**:996–1002.

Nettesheim, P., Snyder, C., and Kim, J. C. S., 1979, Vitamin A and the susceptibility of respiratory tract tissues to carcinogenic insult, *Environ. Health Perspect.* **29**:89–93.

Newberne, P. M., and Suphakarn, V., 1977, Preventive role of vitamin A in colon carcinogenesis in rats, *Cancer* **40**:2553–2556.

Newberne, P. M., Weigert, J., and Kula, N., 1979, Effects of dietary fat on hepatic mixed-function oxidases and hepatocellular carcinoma induced by aflatoxin B$_1$ in rats, *Cancer Res.* **39**:3986–3991.

Newberne, P. M., Charnley, G., Adams, K., Cantor, M., Roth, D., and Suphakarn, V., 1986, Gastric and oesophageal carcinogenesis: Models for the identification of risk and protective factors, *Food Chem. Toxicol.* **24**(10/11):1111–1119.

Newberne, P. M., Charnley, G., Adams, K., Cantor, M., Suphakarn, V., Roth, D., and Schrager, T. F., 1987, Gastric carcinogenesis: A model for the identification of risk factors, *Cancer Lett.* **38**:149–163.

Nigro, N. D., Singh, D. V., Campbell, R. L., and Pak, M. S., 1975, Effect of dietary beef far on intestinal tumor formation by azoxymethane in rats, *J. Natl. Cancer Inst.* **54**(2):439–442.

Nigro, N. D., Bull, A. W., Klopfer, B. A., Pak, M. S., and Campbell, R. L., 1979, Effect of dietary fiber on azoxymethane-induced intestinal carcinogenesis in rats, *J. Natl. Cancer Inst.* **62**(4):1097–1102.

Nigro, N. D., Bull, A. W., Wilson, P. S., Soullier, B. K., and Alousi, M. A., 1982, Combined inhibitors of carcinogenesis: Effect on azoxymethane-induced intestinal cancer in rats, *J. Natl. Cancer Inst.* **69**(1):103–107.

Nishio, Y., Kakizoe, T., Ohtani, M., Sato, S., Sugimura, T., and Fukushima, S., 1986, L-Isoleucine and L-leucine: Tumor promoters of bladder cancer in rats, *Science* **231**:843–845.

Ohshima, M., Ward, J. M., and Wenk, M. L., 1985, Preventive and enhancing effects of retinoids on the development of naturally occurring tumors of skin, prostate gland, and endocrine pancreas in aged male ACI/segHapBR rats, *J. Natl. Cancer Inst.* **74**(2):517–523.

Overvad, K., Thorling, E. B., Bjerring, P., and Ebbesen, P., 1985, Selenium inhibits UV-light-induced skin carcinogenesis in hairless mice, *Cancer Lett.* **27**:163–170.

Oyaizu, N., Morii, S., Saito, K., Katsuda, Y., and Matsumoto, J., 1985, Mechanism of growth enhancement of 7,12-dimethylbenz[a]-anthracene-induced mammary tumors in rats given high polyunsaturated fat diet, *Jpn. J. Cancer Res.* **76**:676–683.

Pence, B. C., and Buddingh, F., 1985, Effect of dietary selenium deficiency on incidence and size of 1,2-dimethylhydrazine-induced colon tumors in rats, *J. Nutr.* **115**:1196–1202.

Philips, R. L., and Snowdon, D. A., 1985, Dietary relationships with fatal colorectal cancer among Seventh-Day Adventists, *J. Natl. Cancer Inst.* **74**:307–317.

Pollard, M., and Luckert, P. H., 1985, Tumorigenic effects of direct- and indirect-acting chemical carcinogens in rats on a restricted diet, *J. Natl. Cancer Inst.* **74**(6):1347–1349.

Pollard, M., Luckert, P. H., and Pan, G-Y., 1984, Inhibition of intestinal tumorigenesis in methylazoxymethanol-treated rats by dietary restriction, *Cancer Treat. Rep.* **68**(2):405–408.

Pour, P. M., and Birt, D. F., 1983, Modifying factors in pancreatic carcinogenesis in the hamster model IV. Effects of dietary protein, *J. Natl. Cancer Inst.* **71**(2):347–352.

Pour, P. M., and Birt, D. F., 1986, Effect of dietary protein on *N*-nitroso-bis(2-oxopropyl)amine-induced carcinogenesis and on spontaneious diseases in Syrian golden hamsters, *J. Natl. Cancer Inst.* **76**(1):67–72.

Pour, P. M., Birt, D. F., Salmasi, S. Z., and Götz, U., 1983, Modifying factors in pancreatic carcinogenesis in the hamster model. I. Effect of protein-free diet fed during the early stages of carcinogenesis, *J. Natl. Cancer Inst.* **70**(1):141–146.

Preussmann, R., 1985, Krebs and Ernährung, *Ernährungs-Umschau* **32**:28–35.

Quander, R. V., Leary, S. L., Strandberg, J. D., Yarbrough, B. A., and Squire, R. A., 1985, Long-term effect of 2-hydroxyethyl retinamide on urinary bladder carcinogenesis and tumor transplantation in Fischer 344 rats, *Cancer Res.* **45**:5235–5239.

Reddy, B. S., and Maeura, Y., 1984, Tumor promotion by dietary fat in azoxymethane-induced colon carcinogenesis in female F344 rats: Influence of amount and source of dietary fat, *J. Natl. Cancer Inst.* **72**(3):745–750.

Reddy, B. S., and Maruyama, H., 1986a, Effect of dietary fish oil on azoxymethane-induced colon carcinogenesis in male F344 rats, *Cancer Res.* **46**:3367–3370.

Reddy, B. S., and Maruyama, H., 1986b, Effect of different levels of dietary corn oil and lard during the initiation phase of colon carcinogenesis in F344 rats, *J. Natl. Cancer Inst.* **77**(3):815–822.

Reddy, B. S., and H. Mori, 1981, Effect of dietary wheat bran and dehydrated citrus fiber on 3,2FT-dimethyl-4-aminobiphenyl-induced intestinal carcinogenesis in F344 rats, *Carcinogenesis* **2**(1):21–25.

Reddy, B. S., and Ohmori, T., 1981, Effect of intestinal microflora and dietary fat on 3,2'-dimethyl-4-aminobiphenyl-induced colon carcinogenesis in F344 rats, *Cancer Res.* **41**:1363–1367.

Reddy, B. S., and Tanaka, T., 1986, Interactions of selenium deficiency, vitamin E, polyunsaturated fat, and saturated fat on axoymethane-induced colon carcinogenesis in male F344 rats, *J. Natl. Cancer Inst.* **76**(6):1157–1162.

Reddy, B. S., Narisawa, T., Vukusich, D., Weisburger, J. H., and Wynder, E. L., 1976a, Effect of quality and quantity of dietary fat and dimethylhydrazine in colon carcinogenesis in rats, *Proc. Soc. Exp. Biol. Med.* **151**:237–239.

Reddy, B. S., Narisawa, T., and Weisburger, J. H., 1976b, Effect of a diet with high levels of protein and fat on colon carcinogenesis in F344 rats treated with 1,2-dimethylhydrazine, *J. Natl. Cancer Inst.* **57**(3):567–569.

Reddy, B. S., Watanabe, K., and Weisburger, J. H., 1977, Effect of high-fat diet on colon carcinogens in F344 rats treated with 1,2-dimethylhydrazine, methylazoxymethanol acetate, or methylnitrosourea, *Cancer Res.* **37**:4156–4159.

Reddy, B. S., Cohen, L. A., McCoy, G. D., Hill, P., Weisburger, J. H., and Wynder, E. L., 1980, Nutrition and its relationship to cancer, *Adv. Cancer Res.* **31**:237–345.

Reddy, B. S., Mori, H., and Nicolais, M., 1981, Effect of dietary wheat bran and dehydrated citrus fiber on azoxymethane-induced intestinal carcinogenesis in F344 fats, *J. Natl. Cancer Inst.* **66**(3):553–557.

Reddy, B. S., Hirota, N., and Katayama, S., 1982, Effect of dietary sodium ascorbate on 1,2-dimethylhydrazine- or methylnitrosourea-induced colon carcinogenesis in rats, *Carcinogenesis* **3**(9):1097–1099.

Reddy, B. S., Maeura, Y., and Wayman, M., 1983, Effect of dietary corn bran and autohydrolyzed lignin on 3,2'-dimethyl-4-aminobiphenyl-induced intestinal carcinogenesis in male F344 rats, *J. Natl. Cancer Inst.* **71**(2):419–423.

Reddy, B. S., Tanaka, T., and El-Bayoumy, K., 1985, Inhibitory effect of dietary *p*-methoxybenzeneselenol on azoxymethane-induced colon and kidney carcinogenesis in female F344 rats, *J. Natl. Cancer Inst.* **74**(6):1325–1328.

Reddy, B. S., Wang, C-X., and Maruyama, H., 1987, Effect of restricted caloric intake on azoxymethane-induced colon tumor incidence in male F344 rats, *Cancer Res.* **47**:1226–1228.

Reddy, B. S., Sugie, S., Maruyama, H., and Marra, P., 1988, Effect of dietary excess of inorganic selenium during initiation and postinitiation phases of colon carcinogenesis in F344 rats, *Cancer Res.* **48**:1777–1780.

Rensburg, van S. J., du Bruyn, D. B., and van Schalkwyk, D. J., 1980, Promotion of methylbenzylnitrosamine-induced esophageal cancer in rats by subclinical zinc deficiency, *Nutr. Rep. Int.* **22**(6):891–899.

Rensburg, van S. J., Hall, J. M., and du Bruyn, D. B., 1985, Effects of various dietary staples on esophageal carcinogenesis induced in rats by subcutaneously administered *N*-nitrosomethylbenzylamine, *J. Natl. Cancer Inst.* **75**(3):561–566.

Rensburg, van S. J., Hall, J. M., and Gathercole, P. S., 1986, Inhibition of esophageal carcinogenesis in corn-fed rats by riboflavin, nicotinic acid, selenium, molybdenum, zinc, and magnesium, *Nutr. Cancer* **8**:163–170.

Roebuck, B. D., Yager, J. D., Jr., Longnecker, D. S., and Wilpone, S. A., 1981a, Promotion by unsaturated fat of azaserine-induced pancreatic carcinogenesis in the rat, *Cancer Res.* **41**:3961–3966.

Roebuck, B. D., Yager, J. D., Jr., and Longnecker, D. S., 1981b, Dietary modulation of azaserine-induced pancreatic carcinogenesis in the rat, *Cancer Res.* **41**:888–893.

Roebuck, B. D., Kaplita, P. V., Edwards, B. R., and Praissman, M., 1987, Effects of dietary fat and soybean protein on azaserine-induced pancreatic carcinogenesis and plasma cholecystokinin in the rat, *Cancer Res.* **47**:1333–1338.

Rogers, A. E., and Wetsel, W. C., 1981, Mammary carcinogenesis in rats fed different amounts and types of fat, *Cancer Res.* **41**:3735–3737.

Rogers, A. E., Connor, B., Boulanger, C., and Lee, S., 1986, Mammary tumorigenesis in rats fed diets high in lard, *Lipids* **21**(4):275–280.

Rose, D. G., Boyar, A. G., and Wynder, E. L., 1986, International comparisons of mortality rates for cancer of the breast, ovary, prostate and colon and per capita food consumption, *Cancer* **58**:2363–2371.

Sakaguchi, M., Hiramatsu, Y., Takada, H., Yamamura, M., Kioki, K., Saito, K., and Yamamoto, M., 1984, Effect of dietary unsaturated and saturated fats on azoxymethane induced colon carcinogenesis in rats, *Cancer Res.* **44**:1472–1477.

Sakita, M., Imai, H., Kasuga, M., Kageyama, N., Imaki, S., Tamai, M., Fujita, Y., and Majima, S., 1983, Effect of a protein-bound polysaccharide preparation, PS-K, on dimethylhydrazine induction of intestinal tumors in rats, *Jpn. J. Cancer Res.* **74**:351–359.

Sarkar, N. H., Fernandes, G., Telang, N. T., Kourides, I. A., and Good, R. A., 1982, Low-calorie diet prevents the development of mammary tumors in C3H mice and reduces circulating prolactin level, murine mammary tumor virus expression, and proliferation of mammary alveolar cells, *Proc. Natl. Acad. Sci. USA* **79**:7758–7762.

Sato, A., Nakajima, T., Koyama, Y., Shirai, T., and Ito, N., 1984, Dietary carbohydrate level as a modifying factor of 3'-methyl-4-dimethylaminoazobenzene liver carcinogenesis in rats, *Jpn. J. Cancer Res.* **75**:665–671.

Schmähl, D., and Habs, M., 1978, Experiments on the influence of an aromatic retinoid on the chemical carcinogenesis in rats by butyl-butanol-nitrosamine and 1,2-dimethylhydrazine, *Arzneim. Forsch./Drug. Res.* **28**:49–51.

Schmähl, D., and Habs, M., 1981, Experiments on the influence of an aromatic retinoid on the chemical carcinogenesis induced by *N*-nitroso-methyl benzylamine in rats, *Arzneim.-Forsch./Drug Res.* **31**:677–679.

Schmähl, D., Danisman, A., Habs, M., and Diehl, B., 1976, Experimental investigations on the influence upon the chemical carcinogenesis, *Z. Krebsforsch.* **86**:89–94.

Schmähl, D., Habs, M., Wolter, S., and Kuenstler, K., 1979, Experimental investigation on the influence upon chemical carcinogenesis: 4th communication, *J. Cancer Res. Clin. Oncol.* **93**:57–66.

Schmähl, D., Habs, M., and Habs, H., 1983, Influence of a non-synthetic diet with a high fat content on the local occurrence of colonic carcinomas induced by *N*-nitroso-acetoxymethylmethylamine (AMMN) in Sprague–Dawley rats, *Hepato-gastroenterology* **30**:30–32.

Schrauzer, G. N., White, D. A., and Schneider, C. J., 1978, Selenium and cancer: Effects of selenium and of the diet on the genesis of spontaneous mammary tumors in virgin inbred female C_3H/St, *Bioinorg. Chem.* **8**:387–396.

Scotto, J. M., Stralin, H. G., Lageron, A., and Lemonnier, F. J., 1975, Influence of carbon tetrachloride or riboflavin on liver carcinogenesis with a single dose of aflatoxin B1, *Br. J. Exp. Pathol.* **56**:133–138.

Selenskas, S. L., Ip, M. M., and Ip, C., 1984, Similarity between trans fat and saturated fat in the modification of rat mammary carcinogenesis, *Cancer Res.* **44**:1321–1326.

Shibata, M. A., Nakanishi, K., Shibata, M., Masui, T., Miyata, Y., and Ito, N., 1986, Promoting effect of sodium chloride in 2-stage urinary bladder carcinogenesis in rats initiated by *N*-butyl-*N*-(4-hydroxybutyl)-nitrosamine, *Urol. Res.* **14**:201–206.

Shimizu, H., Mack, T. M., Ross, R. K., and Henderson, B. E., 1987, Cancer of the gastrointestinal tract among Japanese and white immigrants in Los Angeles county, *J. Natl. Cancer Inst.* **78**:223–228.

Shirai, T., Imaida, K., Fukushima, S., Hasegawa, R., Tatematsu, M., and Ito, N., 1982, Effects of NaCl, Tween 60 and a low dose of *N*-ethyl-*N'*-nitro-*N*-nitrosoguanidine on gastric carcinogenesis of rat given a single dose of *N*-methyl-*N'*-nitro-*N*-nitrosoguanidine, *Carcinogenesis* **3**(12):1419–1422.

Shirai, T., Fukushima, S., Ohshima, M., Masuda, A., and Ito, N., 1984, Effects of butylated hydroxyanisole, butylated hydroxytoluene, and NaCl on gastric carcinogenesis initiated with *N*-methyl-*N'*-nitro-*N*-nitro-soguanidine in F344 rats, *J. Natl. Cancer Inst.* **72**(5):1189–1198.

Shirai, T., Ikawa, E., Hirose, M., Thamavit, W., and Ito, N., 1985, Modification by five antioxidants of 1,2-dimethylhydrazine-initiated colon carcinogenesis in F344 rats, *Carcinogenesis* **6**(4):637–639.

Silverman, J., Shellabarger, C. J., Holtzman, S., Stone, J. P., and Weisburger, J. H., 1980, Effect of dietary fat on X-ray-induced mammary cancer in Sprague–Dawley rats, *J. Natl. Cancer Inst.* **64**(3):631–634.

Silverman, J., Katayama, S., Zelenakas, K., Lauber, J., Musser, T. K., Reddy, M., Levenstein, M. J., and Weisburger, J. H., 1981, Effect of retinoids on the induction of colon cancer in F344 rats by *N*-methyl-*N*-nitrosourea or by 1,2-dimethylhydrazine, *Carcinogenesis* **2**(11):1167–1172.

Smith, D. M., Rogers, A. E., Herndon, B. J., and Newberne, P. M., 1975a, Vitamin A (retinyl acetate) and benzo(a)pyrene-induced respiratory tract carcinogenesis in hamsters fed a commercial diet, *Cancer Res.* **35**:11–16.

Smith, D. M., Rogers, A. E., and Newberne, P. M., 1975b, Vitamin A and benzo(a)pyrene carcinogenesis in the respiratory tract of hamsters fed a semisynthetic diet, *Cancer Res.* **35**:1485–1488.

Soloway, M. S., Cohen, S. M., Dekernion, J. B., and Persky, L., 1975, Failure of ascorbic acid to inhibit fat-induced bladder cancer, *J. Urol.* **113**:483–486.

Soullier, B. K., Wilson, P. S., and Nigro, N. D., 1981, Effect of selenium on azoxymethane-induced intestinal cancer in rats fed high fat diet, *Cancer Lett.* **12**:343–348.

Sporn, M. B., Squire, R. A., Brown, C. C., Smith, J. M., Wenk, M. L., and Springer, 1977, 13-*Cis*-retinoic acid: Inhibition of bladder carcinogenesis in the rat, *Science* **195**:487–489.

Squire, R. A., Sporn, M. B., Brown, C. C., Smith, J. M., Wenk, M. L., and Springer, S., 1977, Histo-pathological evaluation of the inhibition of rat bladder carcinogenesis by 13-*cis*-retinoic acid, *Cancer Res.* **37**:2930–2936.

Stemmermann, G. N., Nomura, A. M., and Heilbrun, L. K., 1984, Dietary fat and the risk of colorectal cancer, *Cancer Res.* **44**:4633–4637.

Stenbäck, F., Mu, B., and Williams, G., 1987, Retinyl acetate effects on the life span and the incidence of cryptogenic neoplasms in C3H mice, *Nutr. Cancer* **10**(3):119–128.

Stinson, S. F., Reznik, G., and Donahoe, R., 1981, Effect of three retinoids on tracheal carcinogenesis with *N*-methyl-*N*-nitrosourea in hamsters, *J. Natl. Cancer Inst.* **66**(5):947–951.

Stoewsand, G. S., Anderson, J. L., and Munson, L., 1988, Protective effect of dietary brussels sprouts against mammary carcinogenesis in Sprague–Dawley rats, *Cancer Lett.* **39**:199–207.

Sumiyoshi, H., 1985, Effects of vitamin E deficiency on 1,2-dimethylhydrazine-induced intestinal carcinogenesis in rats, *Hiroshima J. Med. Sci.* **34**(3):363–369.

Sylvester, M. R., Ip, M. M., and Ip, C., 1985, Comparative effects of animal and vegetable fats fed before and during carcinogen administration on mammary tumorigenesis, puberty and hormone levels in rats, *Proc. Annu. Meet. Am. Assoc. Cancer Res.* **26**:126.

Sylvester, P. W., Aylsworth, C. F., and Meites, J., 1981, Relationship of hormones to inhibition of mammary tumor development by underfeeding during the "critical period" after carcinogene administration, *Cancer Res.* **41**:1384–1388.

Sylvester, P. W., Aylsworth, C. F., Vaun Vugt, D. A., and Meites, J., 1982, Influence of underfeeding during the "critical period" or thereafter on carcinogen-induced mammary tumors in rats, *Cancer Res.* **42**:4943–4947.

Sylvester, P. W., Ip, C., and Ip, M. M., 1986a, Effects of high dietary fat on the growth and development of ovarian-independent carcinogen-induced mammary tumors in rats, *Cancer Res.* **46**:763–769.

Sylvester, P. W., Russell, M., Ip, M. M., and Ip, C., 1986b, Comparative effects of different animal and vegetable fats fed before and during carcinogen administration on mammary tumorigenesis, sexual maturation, and endocrine function in rats, *Cancer Res.* **46**:757–762.

Szepsenwol, J., 1978, Gastro-intestinal tumors in mice of three strains maintained on fat-enriched diets, *Oncology* **35**:143–152.

Takahashi, M., and Hasegawa, R., 1986, Enhancing effects of dietary salt on both initiation and promotion stages of rat gastric carcinogenesis, in: *Diet, Nutrition and Cancer* (Y. Hayashi, M. Nagao, T. Sugimura, S. Takayama, L. Tomahs, L. W. Wahenberg, G. A. Wogan, eds.), VNU Science Press, Tokyo, pp. 169–182.

Takahashi, M., Kokubo, T., Furukawa, F., Kurokawa, Y., Tatematsu, M., and Hayashi, Y., 1983, Effect of high salt diet on rat gastric carcinogenesis induced by *N*-methyl-*N'*-nitro-*N*-nitrosoguanidine, *Jpn. J. Cancer Res.* **74**:28–34.

Takahashi, M., Kokubo, T., Furukawa, F., Kurokawa, Y., and Hayashi, Y., 1984, Effects of sodium chloride, saccharin, phenobarbital and aspirin on gastric carcinogenesis in rats after initiation with *N*-methyl-*N'*-nitro-*N*-nitrosoguanidine, *Jpn. J. Cancer Res.* **75**:494–501.

Takahashi, M., Furukawa, F., Toyoda, K., Sato, H., Hasegawa, R., and Hayashi, Y., 1986, Effects of four antioxidants on *N*-methyl-*N'*-nitro-*N*-nitrosoguanidine initiated gastric tumor development in rats, *Cancer Lett.* **30**:161–168.

Tanaka, T., Reddy, B. S., and El-Bayoumy, K., 1985, Inhibition by dietary organoselenium, *p*-methoxybenzenselenol, of hepatocarcinogenesis induced by azoxymethane in rats, *Jpn. J. Cancer Res.* **76**:462–467.

Tatematsu, M., Takahashi, M., Fukushima, S., Hananouchi, M., and Shirai, T., 1975, Effects in rats of sodium chloride on experimental gastric cancers induced by *N*-methyl-*N'*-nitro-*N*-nitrosoguanidine or 4-nitroquinoline-1-oxide, *J. Natl. Cancer Inst.* **55**(1):101–107.

Tatsuta, M., Iishi, H., Yamamura, H., and Taniguichi, H., 1988, Effect of a defined diet in liquid form on gastric carcinogenesis induced by *N*-methyl-*N'*-nitro-*N*-nitrosoguanidine in Wistar rats, *Arch. Geschwulstforsch.* **58**:29–34.

Temcharoen, P., Anukarahanonta, T., and Bhamarapravati, N., 1978, Influence of dietary protein and vitamin B_{12} on the toxicity and carcinogenicity of aflatoxins in rat liver, *Cancer Res.* **38**:2185–2190.

Temple, N. J., and El-Khatib, S. M., 1987, Effect of high fat and nutrient depleted diets on colon tumor formation in mice, *Cancer Lett.* **37**:109–114.

Thompson, H. J., and Becci, P. J., 1979, Effect of graded dietary levels of selenium on tracheal carcinomas induced by 1-methyl-1-nitrosourea, *Cancer Lett.* **7**:215–219.

Thompson, H. J., Becci, P. J., Brown, C. C., and Moon, R. C., 1979, Effect of the duration of retinyl acetate feeding on inhibition of 1-methyl-1-nitrosourea-induced mammary carcinogenesis in the rat, *Cancer Res.* **39**:3977–3980.

Thompson, H. J., Becci, P. J., Moon, R. C., Sporn, M. B., Newton, D. L., Brown, C. C., Nürrenbach, A., and Paust, J., 1980, Inhibition of 1-methyl-1-nitrosourea-induced mammary carcinogenesis in the rat by the retinoid axerophthene, *Arzneim.-Forsch./Drug Res.* **30**(7):1127–1129.

Thompson, H. J., Meeker, L. D., and Becci, P. J., 1981a, Effect of combined selenium and retinyl acetate treatment on mammary carcinogenesis, *Cancer Res.* **41**:1413–1416.

Thompson, H. J., Becci, P. J., Grubbs, C. J., Shealy, Y. F., Stanek, E. J., Brown, C. C., Sporn, M. B., and Moon, R. C., 1981b, Inhibition of urinary bladder cancer by *N*—(ethyl)-all-*trans*-retinamide and *trans*-retinamide and *N*—(2-hydroxyethyl)-all-*trans*-retinamide in rats and mice, *Cancer Res.* **41**:l933–936.

Thompson, H. J., Meeker, L. D., Becci, P. J., and Kokoska, S., 1982a, Effect of short-term feeding of sodium selenite on 7,12-dimethylbenz[a]anthracene-induced mammary carcinogenesis in the rat, *Cancer Res.* **42**:4954–4958.

Thompson, H. J., Meeker, L. D., Tagliaferro, A. R., and Becci, P. J., 1982b, Effect of retinyl acetate on the occurrence of ovarian hormone responsive and nonresponsive mammary cancers in the rat, *Cancer Res.* **42**:903–905.

Thompson, H. J., Meeker, L. D., and Kokoska, S., 1984, Effect of an inorganic and organic form of dietary selenium on the promotional stage of mammary carcinogenesis in the rat, *Cancer Res.* **44**:2803–2806.

Thompson, H. J., Meeker, L. D., Tagliaferro, A. R., and Roberts, J. S., 1985, Effect of energy intake on the promotion of mammary carcinogenesis by dietary fat, *Nutr. Cancer* **7**:37–41.

Thompson, H. J., Ronan, A. M., Ritacco, K. A., Tagliaferro, A. R., and Meeker, L. D., 1988, Effect of exercise on the induction of mammary carcinogenesis, *Cancer Res.* **48**:2720–2723.

Topping, D. C., and Visek, W. J., 1976, Nitrogen intake and tumorigenesis in rats injected with 1,2-dimethylhydrazine, *J. Nutr.* **106**(11):1583–1590.

Toth, B., 1984, Effect of metamucil on tumour formation by 1,2-dimethylhydrazine dihydrochloride in mice, *Food Chem. Toxicol.* **22**(7):573–578.

Toth, B., and Patil, K., 1983, Enhancing effect of vitamin E on murine intestinal tumorigenesis by 1,2-dimethylhydrazine dihydrochloride, *J. Natl. Cancer Inst.* **70**(6):1107–1111.

Trudel, J. L., Senterman, M. K., and Brown, R. A., 1983, The fat/fiber antagonism in experimental colon carcinogenesis, *Surgery* **94**(4):691–696.

Tucker, M. J., 1979, The effect of long-term food restriction on tumours in rodents, *Int. J. Cancer* **23**:803–807.

Vitale, J. J., Broitman, S. A., and Vavrousek-Jakuba, E., 1977, The effect of iron deficiency and the quality and quantity of fat on chemically induced cancer, *Adv. Exp. Med. Biol.* **91**:229–242.

Wagner, G., Habs, M., and Schmähl, D., 1983, Inhibition of the promotion phase in two-step carcinogenesis in forestomach epithelium of mice by the aromatic retinoid etretinate, *Arzneim.-Forsch./Drug Res.* **33**:851–852.

Wakabayashi, K., Inagaki, T., Fujimoto, Y., and Fukuda, Y., 1978, Induction by degraded carrageenan of colorectal tumors in rats, *Cancer Lett.* **4**:171–176.

Ward, J. M., Sporn, M. B., Wenk, M. L., Smith, J. M., Feeser, D., and Dean, R. J., 1978, Dose response to intrarectal administration of *N*-methyl-*N*-nitrosourea and histopathologic evaluation of the effect of two retinoids on colon lesions induced in rats, *J. Natl. Cancer Inst.* **60**(6):1489–1493.

Warzok, R., Thust, R., Mendel, J., Herbst, C., and Eismann, C., 1981, The influence of sodium selenite on tumor induction by methylnitrosourea (MNU) in rats, *Arch. Geschwulstforsch.* **51**(6):503–508.

Watanabe, K., Reddy, B. S., Wong, C. Q., and Weisburger, J. H., 1978, Effect of dietary undegraded carrageenan on colon carcinogenesis in F344 rats treated with azoxymethane or methylnitrosourea, *Cancer Res.* **38**:4427–4430.

Watanabe, K., Reddy, B. S., Weisburger, J. H., and Kritchevsky, D., 1979, Effect of dietary alfalfa, pectin, and wheat bran on azoxymethane or methylnitrosourea-induced colon carcinogenesis in F344 rats, *J. Natl. Cancer Inst.* **63**(1):141–145.

Waxler, S. H., Brecher, G., and Beal, S. L., 1979, The effect of fat-enriched diet on the incidence of spontaneous mammary tumors in obese mice, *Proc. Soc. Exp. Biol. Med.* **162**:365–368.

Wells, P., Aftergood, L., and Alfin-Slater, R. B., 1975, Effect of varying levels of dietary protein on tumor development and lipid metabolism in rats exposed to aflatoxin, *J. Am. Oil Chem. Soc.* **53**:559–562.

Welsch, C. W., and DeHoog, J. V., 1983, Retinoid feeding, hormone inhibition, and/or immune stimulation and the genesis of carcinogen-induced rat mammary carcinomas, *Cancer Res.* **43**:585–591.

Welsch, C. W., and DeHoog, J. V., 1988, Influence of caffeine consumption on 7,12-dimethyl-benz(a)anthracene-induced mammary gland tumorigenesis in female rats fed a chemically defined diet containing standard and high levels of unsaturated fat, *Cancer Res.* **48**:2074–2077.

Welsch, C. W., Brown, C. K., Goodrich-Smith, M., Chiusano, J., and Moon, R. C., 1980, Synergistic effect of chronic prolactin suppression and retinoid treatment in the prophylaxis of *N*-methyl-*N*-nitrosourea-induced mammary tumorigenesis in female Sprague–Dawley rats, *Cancer Res.* **40**:3095–3098.

Welsch, C. W., DeHoog, J. V., and Moon, R. C., 1984, Lack of an effect of dietary retinoids in chemical carcinogenesis of the mouse mammary gland: Inverse relationship between mammary tumor cell anaplasia and retinoid efficacy, *Carcinogenesis* **5**:1301–1304.

Welsch, C. W., DeHoog, J. V., and O'Connor, D. H., 1988a, Influence of caffeine consumption on carcinomatous and normal mammary gland development in mice, *Cancer Res.* **48**:2078–2082.

Welsch, C. W., DeHoog, J. V., and O'Connor, D. H., 1988b, Influence of caffeine and/or coffee consumption on the initiation and promotion phases of 7,12-dimethylbenz(a)anthracene-induced rat mammary gland tumorigenesis. *Cancer Res.* **48**:2068–2073.

Wenk, M. L., Ward, J. M., Reznik, G., and Dean, J., 1981, Effects of three retinoids on colon adenocarcinomas, sarcomas and hyperplastic polyps induced by intrarectal *N*-methyl-*N*-nitrosourea administration in male F344 rats, *Carcinogenesis* **2**(10):1161–1166.

Wetzel, W. C., Rogers, A. E., and Newberne, P. M., 1981, Dietary fat and DMBA mammary carcinogenesis in rats, *Cancer Detection Prevention* **4**:535–543.

Whanger, P. D., Schmitz, J. A., and Exon, J. H., 1982, Influence of diet on the effects of selenium in the genesis of mammary tumors, *Nutr. Cancer* **3**(4):240–248.

Willett, W. C., Stampfer, M. J., Colditz, G. A., Rosner, B. A., Hennekens, C. H., and Speizer, F. E., 1984, Dietary fat and the risk of breast cancer, *N. Engl. J. Med.* **316**:22–28.

Wilpart, M., and Roberfroid, M., 1987, Intestinal carcinogenesis and dietary fibers: The influence of cellulose or fybogel chronically given after exposure to DMH, *Nutr. Cancer* **10**:39–51.

Wilson, R. B., Hutcheson, D. P., and Wideman, L., 1977, Dimethylhydrazine-induced colon tumors in rats fed diets containing beef fat or corn oil with and without wheat bran, *Am. J. Clin. Nutr.* **30**:176–181.

Yamamoto, I., Maruyama, H., and Moriguchi, M., 1987, The effect of dietary seaweeds on 7,12-dimethyl-benz[a]anthracene-induced mammary tumorigenesis in rats, *Cancer Lett.* **35**:109–118.

Yamamoto, R. S., 1980, Effect of vitamin B_{12}-deficiency in colon carcinogenesis, *Proc. Soc. Exp. Biol. Med.* **163**:350–353.

Yanagi, S., Tsuda, H., Sakamoto, M., Fuse, E., and Ito, N., 1984, Effects of margarine on hepatocarcinogenesis by *N,N'*-2,7-fluorenylenebisacetamide in mice, *Oncology* **41**:101–105.

Yarita, T., Nettesheim, P., and Mitchell, T. J., 1980, Failure of two retinoids to inhibit tracheal carcinogenesis in hamsters, *Carcinogenesis* **1**:255–262.

Zaridse, D. G., 1983, Environmental etiology of large bowel cancer, *J. Natl. Cancer Inst.* **70**:389–400.

Index